Community-Oriented Primary Care

Community-Oriented Primary Care

From Principle to Practice

Edited by Paul A. Nutting, M.D.

University of New Mexico Press ▼ Albuquerque

Library of Congress Cataloging-in-Publication
Data

Community-oriented primary care : from principle
   to practice / edited by Paul A. Nutting.
      p.   cm.
   Reprint. Originally published: [Rockville,
Md.?] : U.S. Dept. of Health and Human
Services, Public Health Service, Health Resources
and Services Administration, Office of Primary
Care Studies, 1987.
   Includes bibliographical references.
   ISBN 0-8263-1230-6 : $19.95
   1. Community health services.
   2. Community health services—United States.
   I. Nutting, Paul A.
   [DNLM: 1. Community Health Services—
United States.   2. Delivery of Health Care—
United States.   3. Primary Health Care—
United States.   WA 546 AA-C6853 1987a]
RA425.C773   1990
362.1'0425—dc20
DNLM/DLC
for Library of Congress   90-12627
                                                   CIP

First published in 1987 by the Government
Printing Office for the Office of Primary Care
Studies, Health Resources and Services
Administration, U.S. Public Health Service,
Department of Health and Human Services.

University of New Mexico Press edition published
1990.

Acknowledgments

This book could not have been produced except for the efforts of a number of people. I am grateful to the authors for their commitment to primary care and for laboring under the burden of an unreasonable publication schedule. Their enthusiasm for this project has made the task of editor an experience of pure delight. I am indebted to James Calvert, Kaia Gallagher, and Douglas Kamerow for their editorial assistance and wise counsel and to Ron Carlson for his support of the total effort. The preparation of the manuscript proceeded smoothly, despite the very tight schedule, due to the skill and diligence of James Walker and Peter L. Petrakis. A special note of gratitude is due Sue Nagel, Doris Martin, and Jacqueline Painter, without whose effort neither the conference that allowed the authors to compare notes, nor the book would have been possible.

Paul A. Nutting, M.D.
    Editor

Table of Contents

List of Contributors

Editor
Paul A. Nutting, M.D.
Director, Research Program
Indian Health Service

Mark Andrews, M.D.
Center Director
Mountain View Medical Center
P.O. Box 82
Hays, NC 28635

Marc E. Babitz, M.D.
Regional Clinical Coordinator
Public Health Service, Region VIII
1961 Stout Street
Denver, CO 80294

Leatrice H. Berman, M A
Chicago Department of Health
Richard J. Daly Center
50 W. Washington Street, Room 219
Chicago, IL 60602

Mary B. Breckenridge, Ph.D.
Department of Family Medicine
University of Medicine and
    Dentistry of New Jersey
Robert Wood Johnson Medical School
One Robert Wood Johnson Place CN-19
New Brunswick, NJ 08903-0019

Raynald Bujold, M.D.
M.P.H. Degree Candidate
University of California, Berkeley
School of Public Health
Berkeley, CA 95720

James F. Calvert, M.D.
Assistant Professor
Department of Family and Community
    Medicine
Georgetown University
School of Medicine
Washington, DC 20007

Lynn P. Carmichael, M.D.
Professor and Chairperson
Department of Family Medicine
University of Miami
P.O. 016700
Miami Beach, FL 33101

Terry Conway, M.D.
Cook County Hospital
1900 W. Polk
Chicago, IL 60612

Larry Culpepper, M.D.
Family Health Center
Brown University
89 Pond Street
Pawtucket, RI 02860

Carol A. Delany, M.S.S.
Division of Primary Care Services
Bureau of Health Care Delivery
    and Assistance
5600 Fishers Lane, Room 7A-55
Rockville, MD 20857

Carolee A. DeVito, Ph.D., M.P.H.
Vice Chairperson
Department of Family Medicine
University of Miami
P.O. Box 016700
Miami Beach, FL 33101

Daniel B. Doyle, M.D.
New River Family Health Center
P.O. Box 337
Scarbro, WV 25917

Mona Ellerbrock, M.P.H.
M.P.H. Degree Candidate
University of California, Berkeley
School of Public Health
Berkeley, CA 94720

Eugene S. Farley, M.D., M.P.H.
Chairman
Department of Family Medicine
University of Wisconsin
777 S. Mills Street
Madison, WI 53715

William L. Freeman, M.D., M.P.H.
Director, Diabetes Program
Portland Area Indian Health Service
2592 Kwina Road
Bellingham, WA 98226

Kathleen E. Furey Martin, Ph.D.
Director, Division of Health Facilities
   Planning/ORM/OM
Parklawn Building, Room 17A-10
5600 Fishers Lane
Rockville, MD 20857

Sim S. Galazka, M.D.
Department of Family Medicine
Case Western Reserve University
2119 Abington Road
Cleveland, OH 44106

Kaia M. Gallagher, Ph.D.
Rural Health Office
Department of Family and Community
   Medicine
University of Arizona
3131 E. 2nd Street
Tucson, AZ 85716

Laura Gardner, M.D.
Preventive Medicine Resident
U.C. Berkeley School of Public Health
Berkeley, CA 94720

David R. Garr, M.D.
Department of Family Medicine
Medical University of South Carolina
171 Ashley Avenue
Charleston, SC 29425

H. Jack Geiger, M.D.
City College of New York
School of Biomedical Education
138th Street at Convent Avenue J-920
New York, NY 10031

Marthe Gold, M.D.
Department of Family Medicine
University of Rochester
885 S. Avenue
Rochester, NY 14620

Jeffrey B. Gould, M.D , M.P.H.
Assoc. Professor of Maternal and
   Child Health
University of California, Berkeley
School of Public Health
Berkeley, CA 94720

Jim Hartye, M.D.
Family Physician
Clingman Medical Center
P.O. Box 100
Ronda, NC 28670

David L. Hawk, M.D., M.P.H.
Thomas M. Hart Family Practice
   Center at the York Hospital
1001 South George Street
York, PA 17405

Norman Hearst, M.D., M.P.H.
Division of Family and Community
   Medicine
University of California, San Francisco
400 Parnassus, AC9
San Francisco, CA 94143

Carol Horowitz, M.P.H.
Public Health Analyst
Bureau of Health Care Delivery
  and Assistance
5600 Fishers Lane, Room 7A-55
Rockville, MD 20857

Sylvia Hutchison, B.S.N., M.P.H.
Behavioral Science Program
University of California, Berkeley
School of Public Health
Berkeley, CA 94720

Joseph Jacobs, M.D., M.B.A.
Medical Director, New Program
  Development
AETNA Life Insurance Company
151 Farmington Avenue, MC 17
Hartford, CT 06156

Douglas B. Kamerow, M.D., M.P.H.
Director, Clinical Preventive
  Services Staff
Office of Disease Prevention and
  Health Promotion
Room 2132 Switzer Building
330 C Street, S.W.
Washington, DC 20201

Arthur Kaufman, M.D.
Director, Division of Family Medicine
University of New Mexico School of
  Medicine
2400 Tucker, N.E.
Albuquerque, NM 87131

William L. Kissick, M.D., Ph.D.
George Seckel Pepper Professor of
  Public Health and Preventive
  Medicine
Department of Research Medicine
NEB-2L/Room 224
Philadelphia, PA 19104-6020

Robert S. Kohl
Executive Director
Near North Health Service Corporation
1276 N. Clybourn
Chicago, IL 60610

Richard Kozoll, M.D., M.P.H.
Director of Health Services
State of New Mexico
725 St. Michael Drive
P.O. Box 968
Santa Fe, NM 87504-0968

Lewis Kraus, M.P.H.
M.P.H. Degree Candidate
University of California, Berkeley
School of Public Health
Berkeley, CA 94720

Marshall Kreuter, Ph.D.
Director, Division of Health Education
Center for Health Promotion
  and Education
Centers for Disease Control
Atlanta, GA 30333

Joyce C. Lashof, M.D.
Dean and Professor of Public Health
School of Public Health
University of California, Berkeley
19 Earl Warren Hall
Berkeley, CA 94720

Robert C. Like, M.D., M.S.
Department of Family Medicine
University of Medicine and Dentistry
  of New Jersey
Robert Wood Johnson Medical School
One Robert Wood Johnson Place CN-19
New Brunswick, NJ 08903-0019

Joanne E. Lukomnik, M.D.
Associate Professor of Community
  Health and Social Medicine
City University of New York
  Medical School
136th Street and Convent Avenue
New York, NY 10031

William R. Maas, D.D.S., M.P.H.
Project Officer
Agency for Health Care Policy &
  Research
Parklawn Building, Room 18-A30
5600 Fishers Lane
Rockville, MD 20857

Donald L. Madison, M.D.
Professor of Social Medicine
University of North Carolina
  at Chapel Hill
Chapel Hill, NC 27514

Robert J. Massad, M.D.
Chairman, Department of Family
  Medicine
Montefiore Medical Center
3412 Bainbridge Avenue
Bronx, NY 10467-2490

Thomas M. Mettee, M.D.
Department of Family Medicine
Case Western Reserve University
2119 Abington Road
Cleveland, OH 44106

Angela D. Mickalide, Ph.D.
Staff Liaison
U.S. Preventive Services Coordinating
  Committee
Office of Disease Prevention and
  Health Promotion
Switzer Building, Room 2132
330 C Street, S.W.
Washington, DC 20201

Fitzhugh Mullan, M.D.
Director, Center for Medical
  Effectiveness Research
Agency for Health Care Policy
  and Research
5600 Fishers Lane, Room 18-46
Rockville, MD 20857

Charles F. Nelson
Patch Coordinator
Division of Health Education
Center for Health Promotion &
  Education
Centers for Disease Control
Atlanta, GA 30333

Jeffrey Newman, M.D.
Medical Epidemiologist
Division of Diabetes Translation
Mail Stop E08
Centers for Disease Control
Atlanta, GA 30333

Paul A. Nutting, M.D.
Director, Research Program
Indian Health Service
7900 South J. Stock Road
Tucson, AZ 85746

Emilie H. S. Osborn, M.D., M.P.H.
Division of Family and Community
  Medicine
University of California, San Francisco
400 Parnassus, AC9
San Francisco, CA 94143

Frank M. Reed, M.D.
AMC Cancer Research Center
Comprehensive Cancer Assessment
  and Prevention (C-CAP)
1600 Pierce Street
Denver, CO 80214

Robert L. Rhyne, M.D.
Assistant Professor, Dept. of Family,
  Community and Emergency Medicine
University of New Mexico School of
  Medicine
2400 Tucker, N.E.
Albuquerque, NM 87131

Karen T. Rivo, R.N., M.S.P.H.
Providence Hospital
1150 Varnum Street, N.E.
Washington, DC 20017

Marc L. Rivo, M.D., M.P.H.
Deputy Administrator for Preventive
  Health Services Administration
Department of Human Services
1660 L. Street, N.W.
Washington, DC 20036

Craig Robinson
New River Family Health Center
P.O. Box 337
Scarbro, WV 25917

David N. Rose, M.D.
Internal Medicine Associates
1200 Fifth Avenue
New York, NY 10029

Walter W. Rosser, M.D.
Chairman
Department of Family Medicine
McMaster University
1200 Main Street
Hamilton, Ontario, Canada

Charles E. Schlager, M.D.
Thomas M. Hart Family Practice
  Center at the York Hospital
1001 South George Street
York, PA 17405

Milton H. Seifert, Jr., M.D.
Family Physician
675 Water Street
Excelsior, MN 55331

J. Christopher Shank, M.D.
Director, Family Practice Residency
  of Fairview General Hospital
Hassler Center for Family Medicine
18200 Lorain Avenue
Cleveland, OH 44111

Cecil Sheps, M.D., M.P.H.
Taylor Grandy Distinguished Professor
  of Social Medicine
Campus Box 7490, Chase Hall
The University of North Carolina
  at Chapel Hill
Chapel Hill, NC 27599-7490

Patricia Shonubi, M.S., R.N.
Assistant Professor of Clinical Nursing
Columbia University, School of Nursing
Community Care Division
617 West 168th Street
New York, NY 10032

Betty Skipper, Ph.D.
Department of Family, Community and
  Emergency Medicine
University of New Mexico
School of Medicine
2400 Tucker, N.E.
Albuquerque, NM 87131

Brian Stewart, P.A., M.P.H.
Office of Primary Care Epidemiology
Department of Health and Environment
725 St. Michael Drive
P.O. Box 968
Santa Fe, NM 87504

Ronald R. Stoddard
Public Health Advisor
Division of Health Education
Center for Health Promotion &
  Education
Centers for Disease Control
Atlanta, GA 30333

A. H. Strelnick, M.D.
Residency Program in Social Medicine
Montefiore Hospital and Medical
  Center
3412 Bainbridge Avenue
Bronx, NY 10467

Henry Taylor, M.D.
Pendleton Community Care, Inc.
Box 100
Franklin, WV 26807

Alan Trachtenberg, M.D., M.P.H.
Adjunct Assistant Professor
  of Epidemiology
Institute of Health Policy Studies
University of California
  at San Francisco
San Francisco, CA 94143

Ronald E. Voorhees, M.D., M.P.H.
Medical Epidemiologist
New Mexico Health and Environment
  Department
Harold Runnels Building
1190 St. Francis Drive
Santa Fe, NM 87503

Gregory R. Wagner, M.D.
Department of Family and Community
  Health
Marshall University School of Medicine
1801 Sixth Avenue
Huntington, WV 25701

Nancy B. Watkins
Public Health Specialist
Division of Health Education
Center for Health Promotion &
  Education
Centers for Disease Control
Atlanta, GA 30333

Donald L. Weaver, M.D.
Director of Divison of National
  Health Service Corp.
Bureau of Health Care Delivery
  and Assistance
5600 Fishers Lane, Room 7A-39
Rockville, MD 20857

Maurice Wood, M.D.
Professor and Director of Research
Department of Family Practice
Medical College of Virginia
MCV Station, Box 251
Richmond, VA 23298

William Zubkoff, Ph.D., M.P.H.
Executive Director
South Shore Hospital and Medical
  Center
Miami, FL

Stephen Zyzanski, Ph.D.
Department of Family Medicine
School of Medicine
Case Western Reserve University
2119 Abington Road
Cleveland, OH 44106

Robert B. Walker, M.D.
Department of Family & Community
  Health
Marshall University School of Medicine
1801 Sixth Avenue
Huntington, WV 25701

Preface

Since the late 1940s, the health care system of this country has hitched its wagon to the subspecialty star, and as a result, medical science has enjoyed tremendous expansion of its technical capability. Progress, however, has exacted its price in terms of explosive growth in the costs of health care and increasing isolation of both the physician and the patient from the primary care relationship that has been the foundation of medical practice for centuries. As the health care system struggles to rediscover and restore primary care to the base of the health care pyramid, primary care practitioners also seek to discover new and appropriate ways in which the partnership between patient and physician can be strengthened and used to improve health.

Community-oriented primary care (COPC) may offer just such an opportunity. The principles of COPC expand the primary care model to include a defined population and a process by which the health problems of that population are systematically identified and addressed. As a marriage of the principles of epidemiology and the practice of primary care, COPC challenges practitioners to broaden their scope of concern beyond the care of the individual patient.

One of the problems facing practitioners who wish to incorporate the principles of COPC into their practice is the lack of tools and techniques needed to define and characterize the community, identify its priority health problems, and monitor the impact of changes made in the organization and delivery of primary care services. Clearly methods exist in the parent disciplines of epidemiology, demography, and evaluation research, but have not been adapted for use by busy clinicians in the hectic primary care setting. To be useful, COPC tools must be "quick and dirty" enough to be feasible for routine use, yet rigorous enough to offer practitioners a credible basis for confidently modifying the primary care program.

While the state of the art of COPC is in its infancy, our general experience with primary care in the United States is growing rapidly. A sizeable body of experience in identifying and addressing health problems of defined populations has accumulated over the last two decades. This book attempts to harvest the fruit of that experience. To assemble this volume, we assembled a group of primary care practitioners, educators, and researchers from varied backgrounds and with different perspectives on COPC. Their commonality, however, is a commitment to primary care and a deep-seated belief that primary care can be improved by focusing on the health care of a defined population.

The book is written for practitioners with a commitment to primary care, and who are interested in expanding their primary care activities beyond the confines of the examining room. It is not our intention to argue that COPC is the only legitimate form of primary care, or even that it is better than the traditional primary care model. Nor do we expect that practitioners will embrace the COPC model in its entirety. It is our intention to describe a population-based approach to primary care—one that has applicability in all primary care settings of the United States—and to offer a variety of simple tools and techniques that will allow practitioners to move toward the principles of COPC in simple stages, tailoring their strategies and pace to their own practice.

This is not a textbook. Our knowledge base is still too thin to produce a definitive text. But it does represent a start, a collection of approaches to COPC that may provide a staging area for those who wish to enter this largely uncharted territory. In the following chapters, tools and techniques will be found that will not be applicable in all settings, although it is hoped that all readers will find a few that are of use to them.

Community-Oriented Primary Care: From Principle to Practice

Introduction

Paul A. Nutting, M.D.

PURPOSE AND OVERVIEW OF THE BOOK

Community-oriented primary care (COPC) is a modification of the traditional model of primary care in which a primary care practice or program systematically identifies and addresses the health problems of a defined population. The practice of COPC combines primary care skills and the principles of epidemiology. While not the prevailing form of primary care in this country, the challenges of COPC have nonetheless attracted a great deal of interest and attention among primary care practitioners, educators, and researchers.

One of the serious obstacles to the more widespread practice of COPC is the lack of tools and techniques for the clinician. While the general methods exist in the parent disciplines of epidemiology, demography, biostatistics, health services and evaluation research, and in several of the behavioral sciences, they have not been well adapted for use in the primary care setting. Substantial progress has been made, however, over the last several years as practitioners, researchers, and educators have begun the task of adapting methods for COPC. This book describes for

the interested practitioner a series of strategies and techniques for implementing COPC, in the differing health care settings that typify primary care in the United States. Most of the chapters focus on those techniques that will be of interest to the practitioner in the early stages of development of a COPC practice. Tools and methods are described as well for those who have taken the initial steps and are seeking additional challenges. Due to the diversity of practice settings and the wide variety of tools needed, any reader may find that some techniques described will not be useful in his or her practice. An effort has been made in the introduction to each Part to provide some clue to the reader as to the content and applicability of each chapter. At the end of each Part, a Coda,[1] written by a notable leader in either primary care, community medicine, or public health, adds an additional perspective to the general subject.

The book consists of nine Parts, and the first examines COPC from several

---

[1] In music a coda is a relatively independent passage placed at the end of a diverse set of passages, introduced to bring the composition to a satisfactory close.

perspectives, offering general insights into the nature of COPC. The next four Parts deal with the functional activities of COPC: defining and characterizing the community (Part II), identifying the community's important health problems (Part III), developing emphasis programs (Part IV), and monitoring the impact of program modifications (Part V). Part VI addresses the important topic of patient and community involvement, describing its application and value in different settings, and offering suggestions for incorporating the patient and community participants into the COPC process.

Part VII discusses practice management techniques that promote COPC. Of particular importance are the techniques for initiating and sustaining changes within the practice that support a particular emphasis program. With the increased emphasis on data that attends COPC, several chapters focus on techniques for data acquisition and management. Part VIII covers getting started with COPC and provides a great deal of important advice and guidance in developing allies, finding resources, and generally achieving a critical mass for COPC. Part IX details information sources that will be of use to the COPC practitioner, with individual chapters describing the structure and content of several national data sets, information resources for health promotion and disease prevention, and an annotated bibliography of the COPC literature. Finally, the Conclusion addresses the challenges to COPC and suggests a general strategy for moving toward a COPC practice.

COMMUNITY-ORIENTED PRIMARY CARE IN THE U.S. CONTEXT

The notion of community-oriented primary care has only recently become part of the vocabulary of primary care. The general concepts, however, have been expressed by primary care advocates in the United States for some time. The writings of Kerr White (1-4), Cecil Sheps (5-8), Jack Geiger (9-12), Robert Haggerty (13-16), Kurt Deuschle (17-18), and others have stressed the need to harness and direct the technical capability of our health care system toward addressing the health and health care needs of defined populations. Each has argued for a central strategy that marries epidemiology and primary medical care.

The term COPC, itself, was first popularized by Sidney Kark, writing first on his work in South Africa and more recently with Joseph Abramson in Israel (19-22). They characterize COPC as "a strategy whereby elements of primary health care and of community medicine are systematically developed and brought together in a coordinated practice" (23). They define the fundamental features of COPC as: the use of epidemiology and clinical skills; a defined population for which the program has assumed responsibility; defined programs to address the community's health problems; community involvement; and accessibility to the program's services. Discussing COPC from a U.S. perspective, Donald Madison characterizes a community-responsive practice as "one which assumes a larger than ordinary share of responsibility for safeguarding the health of a community, and which follows through on this responsibility by taking action beyond the traditional mode of treating the complaints and problems of patients as they approach the practice one-by-one" (24). Writing on the future of COPC in the United States, Fitzhugh Mullan characterizes COPC as "the reunion of the traditions of public health and personal clinical health services" (25).

The principles of COPC have provided the philosophical foundation of publicly funded health programs for many years. In response to policy and environmental forces in the health care arena, two applications of COPC have evolved in the

United States over a number of years. The community health center program grew out of the original Neighborhood Health Center experiment of the Office of Economic Opportunity (OEO) and provides primary care services to medically needy populations. Community health centers are located in underserved areas and strive to address the health problems of the local community. Community involvement in the health center is an integral philosophical underpinning of the program. On another front, the Public Health Service (through the Indian Health Service) assumed the responsibility for the health care of American Indians and Alaskan natives in 1955. In its 30-year history, the Indian Health Service has developed a comprehensive program of integrated primary care and community health services, operating within and tailored to the health needs of particular Indian communities.

More recently, elements of COPC have emerged in the private sector as well. Prepaid group practices have flourished over the last decade following the patterns established by the Kaiser-Permanente organization in the 1940s. With a contractual obligation to a fixed enrollment, the HMOs have an economic incentive to respond to the perceived health needs of their enrolled communities. More generally, the specialty of family practice has begun, over the last decade, to shift the focus of clinical attention from care of the individual to care of the family. As an important step toward systematically addressing intervention strategies within the larger context of the community, family medicine offers the best hope for incorporating the central principles of COPC into the mainstream of primary care.

Each of these applications of COPC represents a legitimate variation on the general model of community-oriented primary care, although each stresses different aspects of the model and uses quite different methods to address the particular health needs of their target communities. A recent study from the Institute of Medicine (IOM) described the implementation of COPC principles in differing U.S. primary care settings. The study concluded that while not a prevalent form of primary care practice, the COPC approach offers great promise as a form of primary care that is responsive to the health care needs of defined populations, ranging from geopolitical communities to the enrolled populations of prepaid health plans (26). Seven case studies demonstrated the feasibility, if not always the practicality, of COPC in vastly different health care environments. The case studies illustrated the spectrum of COPC expression in settings typical of today's U.S. health care system (27).

THE COMPONENTS OF COPC

To be applicable to a wide audience of primary care clinicians, the basic elements of COPC must be adaptable to the unique environments of clinicians practicing in different communities, under different organizational structures, and financed through different fiscal arrangements. Such a model has been proposed to accommodate differing expressions of COPC while providing enough structure to support research, education, and practice (28). The basic COPC model consists of three essential components—a primary care program or practice, a defined population, and a process by which the major health problems of the community are addressed. While all three components are expected to vary widely, each must be represented in some form.

Primary Care Practice or Program

The practice of primary care assumes a variety of faces in this country. Practices or programs with a single specialty (family medicine, general internal medicine, pediatrics) often differ widely from those with a mixed-specialty orientation. Practices also differ in their organizational structures and methods of financing.

The COPC model can accommodate any mixture of structural characteristics. Of critical importance is that the practice meet the basic characteristics of primary care, namely that it offer an array of personal health services that are accessible and acceptable to the patient, comprehensive in scope, coordinated and continuous over time, and for which the practitioner is accountable for the quality and potential effects of services. The primary care component of the model speaks to the services a practice provides, but not to the composition or organization of the practitioners, nor the manner by which the costs are reimbursed (directly or indirectly by the patient, patient groups, or third parties).

The Community

The community represents the target population of the practice—those individuals for whose health care the practice has assumed responsibility. In some settings, the COPC practice will address "true" communities, those sharing common social, cultural, economic, and political systems. Alternatively, the community may consist of less clearly defined, and perhaps less organized, groups such as individuals enrolled in a health plan, occupational or workplace populations, or school populations. Where the community is difficult to define, the COPC practice may address its active patient population or a practice community, the latter consisting of all members of households of active patients.

Involving the community is an important feature of COPC, but the manner and extent to which the community participants collaborate in the COPC process will vary widely across different settings. The range of possibilities for patient and community participation will differ widely

between a small fee-for-service practice in a rural area, a large urban HMO, and a publicly funded community health center. However, the range of variation can be described in terms of the organization and mechanisms of input, the level of involvement, and the focus of attention. The latter feature is critical to COPC. Just as practitioners have a tendency to focus their attention on their active patients (the numerator of the practice), patients and community participants may also develop a "numerator bias." For example, consumer boards often focus on administrative issues surrounding the daily operation of the health facility. When the focus of attention is broadened to the "denominator" population, community involvement can add a distinctly new and vitally important dimension to the identification of community health problems. As described later, group consensus techniques can enhance the involvement of consumers and practitioners in setting priorities among competing health needs and in allocating constrained resources among competing health programs. The critical role for the patient and community participants is to develop a "denominator bias" and to represent the interests of the entire target population while participating in the functions of the COPC process.

The COPC Process

The third component of the model is the process by which the major health problems of the community are identified and systematically addressed. This process can be described as a set of activities that fall into four functional categories.

Defining and Characterizing the Community. The first step, defining and characterizing the target population, forms the basis for the subsequent practice activities. While the tradition of primary care has stressed the importance of understanding the community from which individual patients present for care, the COPC model extends this notion to the denominator group, recommending that the health status of the population be recorded and analyzed with the same rigor that the practitioner uses when approaching the individual patient. The practitioner needs to know precisely who are the individuals who comprise the denominator population, where they live, and how their behavior influences their health, where and when they seek care for ailments, and how they perceive and finance their care. Ideally, the practitioner should be able to list all the individuals in the denominator population as a basis for identifying and focusing on high risk individuals.

Identifying the Community Health Problems. The second step entails the activities necessary to identify the major health problems of the community, characterize their determinants and correlates, and set priorities among them. At the most basic level, important health problems can be identified from practice impressions and the perceptions of community members. Use of group process techniques can add a level of rigor to this function. Additional information can often be obtained at reasonable expense through secondary data sources (vital statistics, epidemiologic studies). While practice impressions and secondary data may suggest the presence of a health problem, new data often are needed to define the extent and severity of the problem and to examine its correlates and determinants. Finally, identifying the major health problems of the community must be followed by efforts to set priorities among them.

Developing Emphasis Programs. After identifying a priority health problem, the third COPC step modifies the health care program to address the problem more effectively. In some cases an appropriate emphasis program can be developed entirely within the primary care practice. For many problems, however, an emphasis program requires cooperation among the primary care practice and other health-related programs and agencies within the community. Often the intended recipients of the emphasis program are not active users of the health care system and efforts to target high-risk individuals and mount aggressive outreach activities may be necessary to achieve the desired effect.

Monitoring Impact of Program Modifications. To determine the extent to which the health problem has been resolved, the effectiveness of the emphasis program should be monitored and evaluated. Results of the monitoring activity lead naturally to further modifications of the emphasis program. This final step in the COPC process rarely receives adequate attention although most practitioners agree with its importance. Although it is tempting to move to the next health problem, some level of effort should be devoted to assessing the impact of program modifications. In addition to identifying refinements that may increase the impact of emphasis programs, monitoring practice activities permits elimination of those activities with little or no benefit, thus freeing up energies and resources for program activities with potentially higher impact.

PROBLEMS AND OBSTACLES

The development of a COPC practice or program is not without problems (29,30). While the exact nature of the problems may vary with the practice setting, they nonetheless tend to fall into seven general categories.

First, for many practices the community may be extremely complex and difficult to define, particularly in urban areas where the community can be subdivided into neighborhoods, each with a unique ethnic and social structure. Many communities, especially suburban communities, are served by a multitude of practices and health programs, making it difficult for practitioners to distinguish their own community from those of other practices. Indeed, many families and individuals do not look to a single practice or program for all of their health care services, instead using multiple practitioners.

Second, most practitioners will find that they have a limited set of resources at their disposal that can be directed to the COPC activities. It is uncommon to find a primary care practice that has an abundance of financial reserves, staff commitment, or time and energy to be devoted to activities beyond direct patient care.

Third, many potential COPC practitioners are alone among their immediate colleagues in their interest and commitment to expanding the focus of their primary care practice. While COPC does not require the full commitment of all professional staff members (26), it does require support for the individual(s) who are carrying the responsibility for analyzing and reviewing data, meeting with other community programs, and planning emphasis programs. Attempting this in a practice in which one's colleagues are totally unsympathetic could be very difficult.

Fourth, most practices have only a basic data system, in most cases limited to the hard copy of the medical record. While many practices are moving rapidly into data automation, most computer systems in primary care are devoted to billing and other practice management tasks. Even those programs with well developed patient care information systems often find that data are limited to their active patients and do not serve well in identifying and characterizing the health problems of the larger target population.

Fifth and perhaps most frustrating to the practitioner, is the lack of skill, knowledge, and experience in the principles, strategies, and methods of COPC. This lack is reminiscent of the predicament of the medical graduates of two decades ago.

Upon entering a primary care practice, young physicians found that they lacked many of the skills necessary to provide care for those common problems that were prevalent in their patient population, but rare in the teaching curriculum of the tertiary care centers where they trained. The current dilemma is an extension of the old problem: while training programs in primary care are now providing much improved training in the care of primary care problems, they are deficient in training practitioners to address and deal with health problems within their target population or community. Much has been accomplished through academic departments of community medicine, but regrettable gaps remain in the training for primary care, community medicine, and public health.

Sixth, there is a relative lack of quantitative tools and techniques that are feasible for COPC activities in most primary care settings. While methods have been well developed in the parent disciplines of demography, epidemiology, anthropology, health services and evaluation research, and biostatistics, they have not been distilled and fitted to the unique needs of the busy primary care setting. To be useful and to support the practice of COPC, tools and techniques must strike a careful balance between the ease and simplicity with which they can be used and the rigor required to confidently alter the health care program. There is of course a clinical analogy. Often working diagnoses are made with an information base that could be challenged if submitted for publication in a leading medical journal. Nonetheless, they are quite adequate in the primary care setting where care is continuous and vigilant enough to detect early changes in health status.

Finally, the most vexing problem facing COPC, and indeed facing all of primary care, is that the current mechanisms of reimbursement do not support, much less encourage, the additional activities of COPC. Many new practice forms are developing in an attempt to gain an edge in the increasingly competitive medical care marketplace; unfortunately, none provide clear incentives for the additional activities of COPC. Even HMOs do not find a clear incentive to act prospectively to improve the health of a population that is free to disenroll before the impact of an emphasis program may be realized.

AN INCREMENTAL APPROACH TO COPC

While the impediments to implementing a COPC practice are formidable, it is quite possible to integrate the COPC principles into the practice of primary care in an incremental fashion. A general model of COPC has been offered (26,28) in which each of the steps is described according to stages of development, where the highest stage represents the ideal and the intermediate stages describe a developing COPC practice or program. This particular model is useful for research and education, but the needs of the practitioner in the early stages of developing a COPC practice are better served by a scheme that encourages a simple stepwise transition to a COPC program.

To many practitioners the decision to develop a COPC practice is seen as one requiring momentous and largely irreversible changes in the practice or program. Since the COPC literature in the last several years has described relatively well developed forms of COPC, many perceive a gulf between most current practices and the COPC practice model, which has, in turn, discouraged many potential COPC practitioners from taking the first steps.

In reality, the transition to a COPC practice involves the addition of only two elements to a primary care practice—a definition of the target population and the development of activities that systematically address the health problems of that population. Both of the additional elements can be approached incrementally and at a pace appropriate to the individual setting.

Starting with a Definable Community

Many practitioners may find it difficult to address the health problems of their total community. The community may be complex and disorganized, consisting of many ethnic subgroups and political factions. In addition, the community may be served by a number of other primary care programs, making it difficult for the practitioner to distinguish his or her population from that of other practices, and calling into question the appropriateness of the practitioner assuming responsibility for the patients of another practice or program. In such cases, the COPC process might be started by targeting a community consisting of the active patients of the practice or a "practice community," consisting of the active patients and all members of their households. Similarly, other target populations may be addressed, such as populations defined by location (e.g., school or workplace), by health problem (e.g., hypertension, homeless), age group (e.g., elderly, infancy), or risk group (e.g., teenage pregnancy). COPC is an iterative process and the practice starting with a "bite-size" subset of the community can expand its scope later.

Starting with Simple Tools

Similarly, the process of addressing the community's health problems can be seen as a set of alternative strategies that can vary widely, ranging from the simple to the often more rigorous activities of the mature COPC practice. The activities of each of the four functions can be approached at differing levels of rigor with differing costs and requirements for practitioner time and energy. At the most basic level, practitioners can rely on subjective information gleaned from the practice impressions of their professional colleagues and the wealth of information that can be mined from the opinions and experience of individuals from the community. Subjective information of this sort can be obtained with little expense; the rigor of this information can be further enhanced through the use of group process techniques (31), which aid in eliciting, analyzing, and interpreting subjective data. Integration of subjective data from the health professional and consumer can offer a richness of information not often possible with quantitative data. Moreover, through collaboration, professionals and consumers can cooperatively approach the difficult task of setting priorities among competing health problems.

The use of secondary (or existing) data offers another inexpensive alternative for initiating the COPC functions. Most communities have a wealth of data available, ranging from census data to vital statistics. The appropriateness of secondary data will, of course, vary across settings and will largely be a function of the "fit" between the target population of the practice and the population for which the data were collected.

The practitioner hoping to move a step toward the mature COPC model can move independently on either dimension. A two dimensional matrix, shown in Table 1, can assist in locating the current mode of practice and identifying opportunities for any given practice to move one step closer to the mature model. For example, the matrix of Table 1 may describe the appropriate steps for a small fee-for-service private practice. On one dimension the increasing rigor of the processes of COPC can be described in terms of stages of development. At Stage I, the practice may be characterizing the community and identifying health problems using the subjective impressions of the practitioners and/or patients. At Stage II, secondary data may be used for the same functional activities, while at Stage III, new data are collected and analyzed to describe the community and its health problems.

Table 1. Levels of the target community

	Active patients	Practice community	Total community
Stage I: use of subjective information			Teen-age pregnancy
Stage II: use of secondary data		Hypertension	
Stage III: use of newly collected and analyzed data	Urinary tract infections		

Similarly, on the other dimension, a COPC practice can define its denominator population at three levels. The first is the population of active patients, defined as all individuals who have contacted the practice within the previous two years. The next level is the practice community, which includes all members of the household to which active patients belong. Finally, there is the larger population whose health needs can be addressed, encompassing, for example, school populations, the enrolled members of a health plan, participants in a work-place health program, and/or a geographic community.

Viewed in this context, any practitioner may locate his or her current pattern of practice and identify small and feasible steps toward a more rigorous practice of COPC. Many practices may be operating simultaneously in more than one cell of the matrix, when examined by service category. For example, a practice that has a strong quality assurance activity may be engaged in activities at Stage III in examining the quality of care for urinary tract infections among their active patients. Simultaneously, the practitioners may be concerned about members of the practice community with undiagnosed or untreated hypertension, based on prevalence figures extrapolated from secondary data (Stage II). Finally, the practice may be collaborating with other community programs to address the problem of unwanted teenage pregnancy based on subjective information within the larger community (Stage I). If the practice is involved in an HMO or has a contract with a major employer in the community for occupational health services, other denominator populations may be addressed at differing stages of refinement of the COPC process.

The level of development of the COPC activities and the denominator population addressed may differ among the four COPC functions as well. For example, in any COPC effort the activities that iden-

tify the major health problems of the community and the activities that monitor the impact of the intervention may be undertaken at different stages of development. Similarly, the practice that is addressing more than one problem may be doing so at differing levels, and those levels may change over time.

While the matrix scheme implies higher value associated with higher stages of development and higher levels of the community and more specific definitions of the target population, the appropriateness of COPC activities on either dimension will be specific to local requirements. In some settings, the philosophy of the practitioners or the needs of the area may argue for defining the denominator population as a social, cultural, or geographic community, while other practices or programs may find it more appropriate to address a practice community. On the other dimension, Stage III may represent a high level of development for a given function, but attaining the ideal in a practical world may not always be worth the marginal cost. For example, some programs may be able to extract more information about their community from the diligent use of secondary data than from the use of a sophisticated, but undoubtedly more expensive, data system.

WHY COMMUNITY-ORIENTED PRIMARY CARE?

Since the mid-1940s, the medical profession has ridden the crest of unprecedented growth in knowledge and technology. This has produced many miracles of modern medicine, but it has also led to an unfortunate overemphasis on the technology of health care, that by the mid-1960s had nearly eliminated the practice of primary care. Fortunately, the pendulum has begun to reverse its swing. With the emergence of the specialty of family medicine and the increased emphasis on general internal medicine and pediatrics, primary care is again gaining prominence and public support, and once again is being recognized as the foundation of the U.S. health care system.

As primary care has gained prominence, it has been accompanied by a renewed interest in COPC. No longer considered to be limited to publicly funded health programs for underserved populations, the principles of COPC are beginning to appear in private practices and for-profit health programs as well.

What is the appeal of COPC to such a wide audience of primary care practitioners? First, COPC offers a context for the practitioner to expand beyond the focus of the examining room, and to systematically consider the larger community from which active patients emerge for care.

Second, COPC provides a strategy for defining and addressing a target population and an opportunity to market primary care services that are appropriate to the health needs of that population. Although most clinicians are hesitant to join the competitive marketplace with overt marketing practices, COPC provides an acceptable strategy for defining a target population and reaching out to offer services that are truly needed.

Third, in an educational setting, COPC offers the structure for defining and exploring the health problems of a population that leads to an appreciation of the breadth of common problems that present to a primary care practice. Attempting to engender in clinicians-in-training an appreciation of population rates (e.g., incidence and prevalence) in the absence of a community to serve as a living laboratory is often discouraging.

In sum, COPC offers a set of strategies and techniques that can assist the clinician in assuming a leadership role by dealing with the priority health problems of his community. Moreover, the fundamental principles of COPC catalyze a colle-

gial relationship with the community and its leaders and provide a means for collective discussions of the myriad health and health care issues relevant to the community.

COPC provides a mechanism for tracking the extent and severity of health problems in the community. The clinician engaged in a COPC practice should be more sensitive to early changes in the profile of community health problems and thereby able to mobilize community health resources for an early response.

Perhaps most importantly, engaging in a COPC practice can lead to a deeper sense of satisfaction with the practice of primary care. In a health care arena that values and rewards high technology over primary care, COPC offers an opportunity to act fully on the important principles that have guided the practice of medicine for centuries.

FROM PRINCIPLE TO PRACTICE

This book offers practitioners a number of helpful strategies for integrating the principles of COPC into their primary care practices or programs. It is important to remember that the entire COPC model does not have to be implemented in a single step; rather it can be approached incrementally. Tools and techniques for doing so serve as the foci for many of the subsequent chapters.

An early, and perhaps the most critical, decision to be made is that of defining the target community. As discussed above, addressing large and complex communities may seem overwhelming in the early stages, and it is wise to start with a population that is definable and readily accessible to the practice. Starting with the active patients of the practice, the practice community, or predefined groups within the population may ease the transition to a COPC practice, as described in the early chapters of Part II.

The beginning practitioner should start

with simple activities for identifying and addressing the community's health problems. Techniques for using subjective data, systematically gathered from the impressions of consumers and health professionals, and methods for using secondary data, gathered from national and local data sources, are described in Parts II and III. These data can be gathered relatively inexpensively, and offer the practitioner an opportunity to examine the characteristics of the community and its health problems. Most importantly, these data provide a point of departure for discussions of the community's health with fellow practitioners and community members.

The early involvement of the community, itself, can often provide the impetus necessary to move toward a COPC form of practice. In addition to the valuable knowledge and insight that can come only from lay members of the community, the community participants have access to resources that may be unavailable to the practice, for example, resources for community surveys. Methods for involving and working with patients and community participants in a variety of practice settings are described in Part VI.

At the outset it is important to achieve a critical mass of people, time, energy, and resources. The startup costs of COPC will be less burdensome if spread among those practices, agencies, and institutions with a shared concern for the health of the community. Consequently, a critical first challenge for the potential COPC practice is to develop contact with the other health programs that also serve the community. At the most basic level, two or more practices may find an advantage in collaborating in the COPC activities that describe and address community health problems, while maintaining independence in their primary care clinical activities. Similarly, a substantial amount of support can be realized through collaboration with institutions within the community that share an interest or an incentive for addressing the health problems of defined communities. Of particular importance are the local health department and increasingly the community hospital which may be economically motivated to collaborate in a COPC effort. These and other strategies for attaining a critical mass for making the transition to a COPC practice are described in Part VIII.

REFERENCES

1. White, K.L. Health care arrangement in the United States: AD 1972. *Milbank Memorial Fund Quarterly* 1972; 50:17.

2. White, K.L. Primary care research and the new epidemiology. *Journal of Family Practice* 1976; 3:579.

3. White, K.L. Contemporary epidemiology. *International Journal of Epidemiology* 1974; 3:295.

4. White, K.L. Epidemiologic intelligence requirements for planning personal health services. *Acta Socio-Medica Scandinavica* 1972; 2:143.

5. Sheps, C.G. Education for what? A decalogue for change. *Journal of the American Medical Association* 1977; 238:232.

6. Sheps, C.G. Primary care—The problem and the prospect. *Annals of the New York Academy of Science* 1978; 310:265.

7. Sheps, C.G. The modern crisis in health services—Professional concerns and the public interest. *Israel Journal of Medical Science* 1981; 17:71.

8. Sheps, C.G., and Bachar, M. Rural areas and personal health services: current strategies. *American Journal of Public Health* 1981; 71:71.

9. Geiger, H.J. The neighborhood health center. *Archives of Environmental Health* 1967; 14:912.

10. Geiger, H.J. Community control—or community conflict? In: *Neighborhood Health Centers*, R.M. Holister, B.M. Kramer, and S.S. Bellin, (eds.). Lexington, MA: D.C. Heath and Co., 1974.

11. Geiger, H.J. A health center in Mississippi. A case study in social medicine. In: *Medicine in a Changing Society*, Lorey, L., Saltman, S.E., and Epstein, M.F. (eds.). Saint Louis: C.V. Mosby Co., 1972.

12. Geiger, H.J. The meaning of community oriented primary care in an American context. In: *Community Oriented Primary Care—New Directions for Health Services*, Connor, E.C. and Mullan, F. (eds.). Washington, DC: National Academy Press, 1983.

13. Haggerty, R.J. Community pediatrics. *New England Journal of Medicine* 1968; 278:15.

14. Haggerty, R.J. Effectiveness of medical care. *New England Journal of Medicine* 1973; 289:7.

15. Haggerty, R.J. Changing lifestyles to improve health. *Preventive Medicine* 1977; 6:276.

16. Haggerty, R.J.; Roghmann, K.J.; and Pless, I.B. *Child Health and the Community*. New York: John Wiley and Sons, 1975.

17. Deuschle, K.W. Community-oriented primary care: Lessons learned in three decades. *Journal of Community Health* 1982; 8:13.

18. Deuschle, K.W., and Bosch, S.J. The community medicine-primary care connection. *Israel Journal of Medical Science* 1981; 17:2.

19. Kark, S.L. *Community-Oriented Primary Health Care*. New York: Appleton-Century-Crofts, 1981.

20. Kark, S.L., and Abramson, J.H. Community-focused health care.

21. Kark, S.L. From medicine in the community to community medicine. *Journal of the American Medical Association* 1974b; 228:1585.

22. Abramson, J.H.; Epstein, L.M.; Kark, S.L. et al. The contribution of a health survey to a family practice. *Scandinavian Journal of Social Medicine* 1973; 1:33.

23. Abramson, J.H., and Kark, S.L. Community oriented primary care: Meaning and scope. In: *Community Oriented Primary Care—New Directions for Health Services*, Connor, E.C. and Mullan, F. (eds.). Washington, DC: National Academy Press, 1983.

24. Madison, D.L., and Shenkin, B.N. *Leadership for Community-Responsive Practice—Preparing Physicians to Serve the Underserved*. Chapel Hill, NC: The Rural Practice Project, 1978.

25. Mullan, F. Community-oriented primary care: An agenda for the '80s. *New England Journal of Medicine* 1982; 307:1076.

26. Institute of Medicine. *Community-Oriented Primary Care: A Practical Assessment, Vol. I, The Committee Report*. Washington, DC: National Academy Press, 1984.

27. Institute of Medicine. *Community-Oriented Primary Care: A Practical Assessment, Vol. II, The Case Studies*. Washington, DC: National Academy Press, 1984.

28. Nutting, P.A. Community-oriented primary care: An integrated model for practice, research, and education. *American Journal of Preventive Medicine*. 1986; 2:140.

29. Madison, D.L. The case for community-oriented primary care. *Journal of the American Medical Association* 1983; 49:1279.

Israel Journal of Medical Science 1981; 17:65.

30. Rogers, D.E. Community-oriented primary care. *Journal of the American Medical Association* 1982; 248:1622.

31. Fink, A.; Kosecoff, J.; Chassin, M.; and Brook, R.H. Consensus methods: Characteristics and guidelines for use. *American Journal of Public Health* 1984; 74:979.

Part I.
Perspectives on COPC

CHAPTER 1

William N. Pickles, M.D.: A Country Doctor with a Naturalist's Interest in Illness

Thomas M. Mettee, M.D.

When a physician comes to a district previously unknown to him, he should consider both its situation and its aspect to the winds. The effect of any town upon the health of its population varies according as it faces north or south, east or west. This is of greatest importance. Similarly, the nature of the *water* supply must be considered. Is it mushy and soft, hard as it is when it flows from high and rocky ground or salty with a hardness which is permanent? Then think of the *soil*; whether it be bare and waterless or thickly covered with vegetation and well-watered; whether in a hollow and stifling, or exposed and cold. Lastly, consider the life of the *inhabitants* themselves; are they heavy drinkers and eaters and consequently unable to stand fatigue or, being fond of work and exercise, eat wisely but drink sparingly?

Airs, Waters, Places
Hippocrates

This translation of *Air, Waters, Places* from the Hippocratic Corpus was first translated into English in 1849 by the English surgeon, Francis Adams, whose hobby was the translation of the works of Hippocrates from Latin. Will Pickles, an English country doctor who eventually came to be called "The Grand Old Man of General Practice," was strongly influenced by the ideas expressed in the Hippocratic Corpus. In his book, *Epidemiology In Country Practice*, published in 1939 when he was 50 years old, Pickles records his 7 years of meticulous observations, from 1931 to 1938, on the natural history of infectious diseases and describes the methods he used to make his observations.

Will Pickles showed the relationship between chicken pox and shingles, the incubation period of epidemic catarrhal jaundice or infectious (Type A) hepatitis, and the infectious etiology of epidemic myalgia, also known as Devils Grip, Bornholm Disease, or pleurodynia. His book is considered a classic in the field of epidemiology, "written with deceptive simplicity of real art." A professor of epidemiology at the London School of Hygiene and Tropical Medicine called the book "The most outstanding happening in epidemiology in the last 25 years." The book also has much to offer when contemplating the meaning of community-oriented primary care.

Will Pickles, the second of six sons, was born in 1889 in a delivery that was supervised by his general practitioner father, who delivered 2,700 babies during his years in practice. All six sons entered medical training, and five of them entered medical practice. In 1913, at the age of 24, Will joined a partnership in Aysgarth, a village of 438 people in the district of Wensleydale. The district, a country valley in Yorkshire running 10 miles along the River Ure, had eight villages, 4,267 people, and two physicians. One of the physicians was Will. The other was his partner, a physician as curious as Will was about the transmission of infectious diseases.

Among Will Pickles' several appointments outside his practice was that of Medical Officer of Health to the Aysgarth Rural District. To perform his duties he traveled by foot, horseback, bicycle, or motorcycle. Since his motorcyle had only one gear it had to be pushed up steep hills. Eventually Pickles acquired a Model T Ford. Sometimes when the wind was strong, Will would take a train to the end of the practice and bicycle home with the wind behind him, visiting his patients on the way. He dispensed medicines from local post offices and practiced without a phone for 18 years.

In 1931, at the age of 42 and after 18 years in practice, Will began systematically recording the *name*, *date*, *village*, and *diagnosis* of all infectious diseases he encountered, with an insatiable curiosity that is said to have bordered on "nosiness." He epitomized John Ryle's description of the naturalist as someone who has never lost the native curiosity of childhood.

Will believed that "valuable knowledge can be accumulated by a team of doctors in conjunction with each other and keeping accurate records over a long term of years." He was assisted in his efforts by the Ministry of Health, but also by his wife Gerty and his daughter Patience, both of whom helped him chart his meticulous observations. Pickles commented later, "in the absence of family help I believe it would be possible for anyone who is similarly interested to obtain the services of some neat (and discreet) child to relieve most of the drudgery" in recording numerous observations.

Pickles reviewed the history of epidemics in Wensleydale and studied mortality by reviewing parish records for clusters of deaths. He also studied local geography. "No book on the epidemiology of a country district," said Pickles, "would be complete without some reference to the water supplies . . . water supplies cannot be understood unless the geology of the district is described." His book includes a cross-sectional diagram of the rock strata in Wensleydale, which he obtained from a geologist. He also included photographs

TABLE 1. The Will Pickles "COPC Team"

Team member	Function
Family—wife & daughter	Recording data
Partner	Collective curiosity
"Those kindly cooperative patients"	Subjects
James Mackenzie (gen. practitioner)	Charismatic leadership
Ministry of Health	Records, maps
Epidemiologist	Guidance
Geologist	Charts, water supply
Photographer	Lay of the land
School mistresses	Amateur epidemiologists
Headmaster	"Quarantine officer"
Clergy	Mortality records

3

of the district obtained from a local photographer. A plan of the district detailing rivers, towns, schools, and churches was also included to help the reader understand the community.

He recruited key members of the community to help in his work (Table 1). A number of school mistresses were transformed by Will into enthusiastic epidemiologists using, among other things, the attendance registers for monitoring illness rates. The headmaster of the local grammar school, a man who was enthusiastic about epidemiology and also had the power to quarantine, was his ally in preventing the spread of diseases.

Will Pickles was a tall, handsome, broad-shouldered man who was at ease with almost everyone. He was an early riser and a nonstop worker who allowed himself only 15 minutes for lunch. He was enthusiastic, modest, warm, and friendly. His courtesy, cheerfulness, gentleness, generosity, culture, and impish sense of humor endeared him to patients and friends alike. All of these characteristics were combined with a youthful zest know to what was going on around him. These characteristics, combined with the mental toughness, patience, and industry of a Yorkshireman, made up the personality of William Pickles.

His knowledge of his subject matter was extensive. He described standing on the summit of one of the noble hills of Wensleydale watching the "Eight" train creep up the valley, with its pauses at three stations. As the setting sun lit up the foreground he could make out each of the villages one by one with their thin clouds of smoke. In all of those villages,

> . . . there was hardly a soul — man, woman, or child — of whom he did not know the Christian name . . . [W]ithout conscious effort the country doctor knows about all his patients . . . [We] know a great deal about each other in country districts . . . [T]he village doctor with his numerous friends and acquaintances, well over 3,000 in many practices, has probably a greater knowledge than any other single inhabitant. He knows the markets they frequent, the schools which their children attend, and the memorable trips to the seaside or the pantomime.

Will Pickles was especially grateful to the "kindly, cooperative patients who were of invaluable assistance to him in completing his study of infectious diseases."

A number of aspects of Will Pickles' experience are relevant to the modern physician who wishes to practice community-oriented primary care. He lived with and worked with a *geographically defined community* or denominator population. His intimate knowledge of them and the district provided his primary data source. He carefully studied *community history and community records*. He walked, rode, cycled, and drove all over his community seeking to understand its geologic and geographic *physical characteristics*. He used maps, photographs, charts, and other *ancillary data* to understand the relationship between the physical and human environment; he honored the advice of the Hippocratic Corpus. He identified *community problems*. He enlisted the support of *community institutions* — the Ministry of Health, post offices, churches, schools — to carry out his studies and treatment programs.

Pickles was inspired by charismatic physicians such as James Mackenzie, who wrote "emphatically on the advantages of general practice as a medium for research, contending that it was the family doctor who alone saw disease in its true perspective as he had the advantage of observing early symptoms and following an illness from beginning to end."

Pickles served as the first President of the Research Committee of the Royal College of General Practitioners. In 1969, the year family practice became a specialty in the United States, the journal *Lancet* called Pickles, then 80 years old, "The Grand Old Man of General Practice."

In summary, Will Pickles, over time, gathered a community history, performed a community physical exam, and carried out a number of ancillary laboratory tests that led to several specific community diagnoses. With the cooperation of his community he was able to intervene in their behalf. Hence, Will Pickles' accomplishments were really those of a primary care physician leading a "community care team" that included his family, his partners, his patients, charismatic leadership, the Ministry of Health, epidemiologists, a geologist, a photographer, school mistresses, a headmaster, and the clergy (Table 1). This team, carefully coordinated and orchestrated by Pickles, led to the enjoyment of a hobby, the advancement of knowledge in infectious diseases, and improved health in Wensleydale. In short, Will Pickles was a pioneer in the practice of community-oriented primary care.

It is unlikely that Will Pickles would describe himself as the leader of a COPC Team. Yet his personality, curiosity, and practice melded together all the elements of clinical care, epidemiology, and behavioral science that compose our definition of COPC today.

REFERENCES

1. Pemberton, John, *Will Pickles of Wensleydale. The Life of a Country Doctor.* London: Geoffrey Bles, 1970.

2. Pickles, W. N., *Epidemiology in Country Practice.* London: The Devonshire Press Ltd. Reissued 1972.

CHAPTER 2

COPC as a
Marketing Strategy

David R. Garr, M.D.

During the past decade in the United States, health care has been increasingly viewed as a business. The term "marketing" has arisen to describe the efforts of health care providers to inform the public about the services they offer. This paper reviews the evolution of health care marketing in this country, examines the four distinct elements of an effective marketing strategy, and demonstrates how community-oriented primary care (COPC) fulfills each of these four strategies. Some of the potential problems that may be encountered in using COPC as a marketing strategy are also discussed.

EVOLUTION IN
HEALTH CARE MARKETING

Marketing is an attempt to anticipate and influence the behavior of groups of people. Applied to health care, it means that a practice identifies the needs of its patients and matches its services to those needs. The concept of marketing in health care has gained prominence only in the past 15 years (1). There are several reasons for little marketing effort prior to that time. First, ethical standards within the medical profession restricted physicians from advertising their services. Physicians began to market their services only after the Federal Trade Commission in 1975, and Supreme Court in 1977, found that these standards were unfair restraints of trade. Second, during parts of this century, particularly in the 1960s and 1970s, the number of physicians has been insufficient to provide optimal health care. This deficiency lessened as a result of increased medical school enrollment, and as a result, physicians are now competing for patients. This need to compete has stimulated interest in marketing. Third, the acceptance and development of competition in the medical community has generated a need for physicians to market their services. In order to keep up with their colleagues, physicians who had been opposed to marketing have now initiated marketing programs within their own practices and within their own communities.

Initially, marketing was primarily done by large, for-profit health care corporations. These organizations had the expertise and the financial resources needed to support extensive marketing efforts. Now the situation has changed, and marketing has increased. Today, all types and sizes of health care practices are vigorously marketing their services. Fee-for-service, as well as pre-paid programs, preferred provider organizations, and nonphysician health providers are all implementing marketing programs.

THE FOUR ELEMENTS OF A GENERAL MARKETING STRATEGY

In recent years, several textbooks (2-4) and hundreds of articles have been published on the subject of marketing. This short chapter cannot address this topic comprehensively. Rather, the author will explain how the general principles of marketing can be satisfied by a practice that emphasizes COPC.

Four elements are essential for effective marketing: market analysis, positioning, favorable service, and promotion.

Market Analysis

An effective market analysis identifies the services being provided within the community. Once the inventory of existing services is completed, the practice can then identify the unmet community needs and offer these services.

A COPC practice assesses the types and quality of services it presently provides as well as those provided by other health professionals in the community. The practice uses community and epidemiological input to guide its provision of health care services.

Example: A community of 15,000 people had three groups of physicians. One group was particularly interested in obstetrics. The four family physicians in this group recognized that an increasing number of women were obtaining their obstetrical care from doctors in the urban area 40 miles away. These physicians analyzed data from the state's Office of Vital Statistics, met with representatives from the childbirth education group and other interested lay people, and conducted a survey of women from the community who had given birth during the preceding sev-

eral years. The information they gathered led to the creation of a task force which identified ways to better meet the needs of obstetrical patients. The result of this COPC project was to reverse the trend of women going elsewhere for obstetrical care, and to increase the number of patients cared for by local physicians.

Positioning

Positioning refers to the process of finding a place in a health care marketplace where certain services best fit. The followup step is to design and modify services in order to maximize the public's interest in what is being offered.

A COPC practice develops programs and services that meet the community's needs. The central principle of any COPC project is that it indeed addresses the needs of the people. A COPC practice also specifies the target population within the community for whom new programs and services are being developed.

Example: A group of five family physicians were practicing in a community of 20,000 people. There were 12 additional doctors in town distributed among four other groups. All five family physicians in the one group were interested in geriatrics and recognized a need in the community for better health and social services for the elderly. These physicians met with senior citizens and local leaders and learned that these people shared this perception of unmet needs. These initial conversations led to the creation of a Senior Citizens Task Force, and two of the physicians were asked to serve on the task force. Over a period of several months, the group accomplished several things: surveyed community residents over age 65 to identify their needs; completed an inventory of existing services for the elderly; visited other communities that had active health and social programs for the elderly. This COPC project, initiated by the physician group but placed in the hands of local residents, resulted in extensive improvements in health care and social services for the elderly. The five-physician practice acquired a reputation for being informed about and interested in the needs of the elderly. They noted a substantial increase in the number of people aged 65 and over in their practice.

Favorable Service

To be competitive, a COPC practice must consider and deal realistically with financial, cultural, and geographic barriers. Some barriers may have to persist if the practice is to survive.

A COPC practice designs its services to maximize accessibility and to limit barriers. These factors account for the success of practices which implement COPC programs.

Example: A five-physician practice in the intermountain west was located on the eastern edge of a county that extended 100 miles further west. There were 1,500 residents in the western portion of the county who had to travel 100 miles in either direction for the nearest health care. The five physicians met with representatives from the community and indicated their willingness to help establish a small health care facility. During a period of several months, and with the assistance of the state health needs assessment, a planning committee was formed. The committee then used the results of the survey and other sources (i.e., census data, information from the state health department) to set up a local clinic staffed by a physician's assistant. The five physicians provided backup to the physician's assistant by means of on-site visits, telephone consultations, and acceptance of referrals from the physi-

cian's assistant. The project improved the access of health care for the people in the small community and created valuable positive publicity and more patients for the physician's practice.

Promotion

Promotion refers to the use of advertising and effective public relations in marketing one's services. Advertising is only one component of an effective program. Most people consider only the advertising component of the marketing strategy.

The publicity generated by the COPC projects in a community increases the visibility of the practice. In addition, positive COPC experiences by patients and other community members direct attention to the practice, its programs, and its philosophy.

Example: A group of six physicians provided care to a large number of patients, including many with diabetes. The physicians distributed a questionnaire to these diabetic patients, and the survey results revealed that the patients desired more diabetes education. The physicians worked with representatives from the American Diabetes Association and organized a series of seminars. They publicized the sessions and made them available to all interested diabetics in the community. The result was the creation of a support group of parents of young diabetics and a range of new services for adult diabetics. The group of physicians who organized the initial program received favorable publicity for their work and enhanced their reputation in the community. The physicians identified diabetes as a COPC project which they supported for several years.

POTENTIAL PROBLEMS IN USING COPC AS A MARKETING STRATEGY

Introducing COPC as a focus within a practice is not without risk. Several issues may arise. Some are listed below, and others may develop, depending on the particular circumstances of the locale:

1. The practice may overcommit its financial and personnel resources by undertaking overly ambitious COPC projects. The result may jeopardize the future of the practice or the physicians within that practice.
2. The practice conducting the COPC project may make promises, either real or implied, that it cannot fulfill.
3. The specific project may not be accessible to people who would like to take advantage of it. The practice and/or the practitioners may thus be criticized.
4. The COPC project may prove to be divisive in the community.
5. The practice may be stereotyped as only having an interest/expertise in the area selected for the COPC project. As a result, other services available from the practice may not be well known or accepted.
6. The COPC project may be viewed with suspicion. For example, some community residents may perceive that the motivation for carrying out the COPC project is only as a marketing strategy and not as a demonstration of interest in the community and the community's needs.

CONCLUSION

The chapter examines the four distinct elements of a general marketing strategy and shows how a COPC project addresses all four elements. Conducting a COPC project is not without risks; there are some potential problems. It is clear that marketing is an integral part of health care in the United States and will likely increase in coming years. COPC enables a practice to meet its community's needs and to market itself simultaneously. As COPC becomes more widely applied, COPC practices will become more visible in their communities and will develop a competitive advantage.

REFERENCES

1. Fried, R.A., and Stine, C.C. Developing a marketing plan for a residency practice. *Family Medicine* 1985; 17:251.
2. Sweeney, D.R.; Beck, L.C.; and Anders, G.T. Marketing — what does it mean to physicians? *Pennsylvania Medicine* December 1984, 78.
3. Young, M.G. Physician advertising — legal and ethical considerations. *Texas Medicine* 1983; 79:79.
4. Dever, G.E.A. *Epidemiology in Health Services Management.* Rockville, MD: Aspen Systems Corp., 1982.
5. Cooper, P.D., and Robinson, L.M. *Health Care Marketing Management.* Rockville, MD: Aspen Systems Corp., 1982.
6. Brown, S.W., and Morley, A.P. *Marketing Strategies for Physicians.* New Jersey: Medical Economics Books, 1986.

CHAPTER 3

Reflections on Financing COPC

William L. Kissick, M.D., Dr. P.H.

Community-oriented primary care can be conceptualized as an effort to synthesize two traditionally disparate dimensions of medical care — private practice and public health. This generalization, while ignoring the precise definition and requisite ingredients of COPC, does capture the essence of a combination of the essential reactive mode of most patient care with the anticipatory strategies of organized community health programs. The prevailing fee-for-service payments associated with solo practice and the salaried, tax-supported employment of the public health physician dramatize the disparity between the principle components of COPC.

Community-oriented primary care has been defined as:

The provision of primary care services to a defined community coupled with systematic efforts to identify and address the major health problems of that community through effective modification in *both the primary care services and other appropriate community health programs* (1). (Emphasis added.)

The authors further specify the three essential components as follows: acces-

sible, comprehensive, coordinated, continuous, and accountable primary care; responsibility for a defined community; interactive process to (a) define community, (b) identify problems, (c) modify health programs to address priorities, and (d) monitor effectiveness.

Virtually all of the early COPC programs launched in the United States have been centrally budgeted, as in the public health model, using the salary system to compensate physicians and other health professionals. The current ferment in the Nation's health care enterprise suggests that pluralistic financing strategies must be sought to facilitate and reinforce the goals of COPC. This chapter discusses some of the implications of different strategies and reviews one approach in search of pluralism and cost-effectiveness in primary care financing.

PRIMARY CARE FINANCING

Primary care physicians or family physicians, traditionally thought of as general practitioners, like their peers in the medical specialties, have been compensated predominantly by fees for their services. The salaried arrangements have been exceptions.

When the Office of Economic Opportunity launched Neighborhood Health Centers in 1964 as one of the historical forerunners of COPC, salaried arrangements for physicians were adopted. This approach was easier to administer and monitor through grant funding.

The main challenge for any human service enterprise, as in the remainder of the economy, is value for money. Stated in the current vernacular, are the services cost-effective? Derivative questions focus on incentives for productivity, quality, and consumer satisfaction. How can the physician be best rewarded for productivity and quality of care?

Although fee-for-service is the dominant financial arrangement in the United States between physician and patient, capitation and salary arrangements are increasingly used. An analysis of the pros and cons of each mechanism in the pure form reveal advantages and disadvantages to the provider, the consumer, and the institution or community.

Incentives for overuse or underuse of medical care are obvious concerns. Fee-for-service stimulates the physician to provide services, whether necessary or unnecessary. Capitation can provoke the physician to underutilization. Compensation, by salary has been criticized as sustaining a physician who is underproductive and unresponsive to patient need or demand. Can the advantages of fees, capitation, and salary be maximized at the same time the disadvantages are minimized?

EVOLUTION OF FEDERAL ROLE IN PRIMARY CARE

The Migrant Health Act of 1962 launched Federal involvement in primary care policy. This act, and its subsequent amendments, provided Federal grants to support clinics offering services to domestic migratory farm workers and their families.

The Office of Economic Opportunity (OEO) created in 1963 soon recognized the importance of adequate health care to the overall issue of poverty. The Neighborhood Health Centers were funded under demonstration authority. The 1966 amendments to the Act led to the replication of the Neighborhood Health Center Model as developed by Drs. Jack Geiger and Count Gibson, Jr. By the end of 1968 the OEO had funded 52 such centers. Section 202 of the 1965 Appalachian Regional Act authorized Federal funds ". . . for the construction, equipment, and operation of multicounty demonstration health facilities." These grants were to cover 100 percent of operational costs for the first 2 years and up to 50 percent for the subsequent 3 years. Section 314(e) of the Partnership for Health enacted in 1966 authorized Project Grants for Health Services Development.

The early 1970s brought several changes for the Neighborhood Health Centers. Administrative control was changed from OEO to DHEW. A renewed interest in financial self-sufficiency developed. Section 330 replaced this authority in 1975.

Direct Federal intervention to bring health professionals into underserved areas began with implementation of the Emergency Health Personnel Act of 1970. The 1972 Amendments added the National Health Service Corps Scholarship Training Program to provide scholarship money to medical students who would agree to represent the Corps in underserved areas. The Health Underserved Rural Areas (HURA) Program, created under Section 1110 of the Social Security Act in 1974, was established to "attract physician assistants and nurse practitioners to rural scarcity areas."

The Rural Health Initiative (RHI) and Urban Health Initiative (UHI) began as an administrative effort of the Bureau of Community Health Service (BCHS) designed to coordinate the activities of the existent Federal programs including the Community Health Centers, the National Health Service Corps, the Health Underserved Areas, the Migrant Health Program, and the Appalachian Health Program. Finally, the Health Services and Centers Amendments of 1978 continued authorization of the RHI and UHI and most of the programs. In sum, a decade and a half of ferment in primary care in the Federal Government saw many initiatives and a search for coherence, or what many would call community-oriented primary care.

SHIFTING SUBSIDIES

The late 1970s brought questions concerning the continuation of subsidies for community health clinics. The Claude Worthington Benedum Foundation, long committed to supporting projects to increase access to primary care in West Virginia, became concerned about the long-range financial viability of community health clinics. They approached the School of Medicine and the Leonard Davis Institute of Health Economics of the University of Pennsylvania to study the alternatives.

The project undertook financial and organizational analysis of primary health care clinics in West Virginia and the formulation of strategies to promote clinic cost-effectiveness. The initial analysis identified three major issues: financial viability, provider productivity, and adequacy of reimbursement. All are critically interdependent. Each is the result of a variety of factors, including population density, the structure of government subsidy, health care reimbursement, and the availability of health personnel.

A major national study of primary care published at that time compared the characteristics of sponsored and self-sufficient clinics (2). While self-sufficient clinics confined themselves to basic medical care in service areas greater than 2,500 popula-

tion and provided 7,500 encounters per year at a minimum, the sponsored clinic attempted comprehensive services for a limited service area and reported less than 4,200 encounters per year. The self-sufficient clinic conducted an active hospital practice, employed minimum support staff, and enjoyed relatively higher reimbursement against lower operating costs. In contrast the sponsored clinics had a limited hospital practice and utilized more support staff, contributing to higher operating costs compounded by lower reimbursement.

The clinic administrators in the project verified these findings and were unanimous in the conviction that sponsored clinics lacked incentives for efficiency and productivity. Self-sufficiency, on the other hand, would require limiting the scope of ambulatory services with an eye toward fee-for-service reimbursement, restricting service, and engaging in an active hospital practice. It was concluded that primary care clinic financing in West Virginia required an intermediate alternative.

A middle-ground strategy was sought that would combine the productivity and efficiency incentives of self-sufficient clinics with sufficient support to assure access to health care. The design of the financing strategy would ensure that health services were available in underserved areas by providing a subsidy; encourage health promotion, preventive services, and comprehensive care; stimulate productivity and reward organizational efficiency; and have the potential to create long-term financial viability.

Conceptual Background

In 1974 Dr. Sidney Lee of the Faculty of Medicine of McGill University advanced the concept of "The Three-Layered Cake — A Plan for Physician Compensation" (3) based on the planning and operation of primary care systems for the Province of

Quebec under Canadian national health insurance. Specifically he proposed a payment scheme to meet the interests of the medical profession, society, and the paying agent. The objectives and characteristics of each layer were as follows:

Basic compensation (Salary) (50-60% of earnings) ". . .payable to all physicians engaged in full-time medical activity within a given geographic area."

Personal Incentives (Weighted Capitation) (30-40% of earnings) ". . . to reflect personal accomplishments and responsibilities" such as educational attainment, participation in continuing education, years of experience, and geographic location.

Systems Incentive (Bonus Fees) (10-20% of earnings) to ". . . encourage reduced infant mortality rates, increased preventive services, or decreased rates of hospitalization."

The British National Health Service has de facto implemented its own version of a "three-layered cake" for general practitioners in its version of community-oriented primary care.[1] General practitioners in the National Health Service are responsible for panels of registered patients numbering 2,300 on average. Patients usually reside in a neighborhood or defined service area. The Department of Health and Social Security pays each GP a practice allowance, essentially a salary subsidy, to cover overhead and other expenses. Most GPs practice out of "surgeries" or solo offices situated in their own homes, although increasingly they are situated in health centers. The major financial relationship between the NHS and the GP is a capitation fee per panel member per year. This accounts for 60 percent of the GP's income. Finally, the government pays fees for priority services; e.g., immunization, family planning, cervical screening, and home visits to the elderly.

SIR Model

The Primary Care Study Group in West Virginia developed a similar approach. The Subsidy-Incentive-Reimbursement (SIR) model was designed to address the middle-ground strategy by incorporating the three basic mechanisms for compensating physicians; i.e., salary (Subsidy), capitation (Incentive for enrollment), and fee-for-service (Reimbursement) to provide positive incentives for efficiency and productivity (4).

A 50 percent salary subsidy was proposed for physicians, physician extenders, and dentists. This guarantees a contribution toward compensating these health professionals. Since many underserved areas cannot support, demographically or economically, primary care professionals, salary support constitutes a minimum subsidy to bring access to health care to these areas. The National Health Service Corps, by contrast, provided a 100 percent salary subsidy. A smaller subsidy shifts some risk to the clinic encouraging attention to productivity.

The second strategy is the enrollment incentive. The registration and screening of patients, health promotion, and preventive services generate a per capita annual fee called an enrollment incentive. The capitation mechanism assures that these services will be available to users of the clinic while allowing the clinic to tailor its program to its local needs.

The third strategy, fee reimbursement, is the most common method of financing services rendered, particularly for diagnosis, treatment, and followup. The fee would be paid by the patient, Medicare, Medicaid, other third-party, or out-of-pocket. Since fees are linked to services rendered, revenue will vary directly with

---

[1] Personal communication from Sir George Godber, former Chief Medical Officer, British National Health Service, August 23, 1985.

13

the activity of the clinic measured as encounters.

Finally, a provision was developed to reward a clinic for increases in productivity. A clinic would receive a bonus based on the surplus generated. Subsequently a simulation of the SIR model was conducted. Each administrator sought to increase enrollments and encounters in his clinic. Staffing costs, fixed costs, and variable costs were recorded.

A simulation using the SIR model was conducted, even though actual financial arrangements with the Federal Government remained unchanged. Each administrator worked for a bonus to be awarded as a proportional allocation of a pool established with grant funds from the Benedum Foundation. All five clinics earned a bonus as calculated by the SIR model.

FROM PUBLIC TO PRIVATE SECTOR FUNDING

The three financing schemes that seek to blend fee-for-service, capitation, and salary compensation for physicians were all designed for funding by the public sector — the Province of Quebec, the British National Health Service, and the State of West Virginia utilizing the Primary Care Block Grant. What are the prospects for synthesizing private practice and public health financial strategies in COPC? In the primary care component of COPC the patient can assume financial responsibility by paying the physician a fee for service. The physician could serve simultaneously as a public health physician and receive a salary from the community for the broader health responsibilities. This approach has been attempted in some settings over time.

The three essential components of COPC are:

Accessible, comprehensive, coordinated, continuous, and accountable primary care;

Responsibility for a defined community; and

Interactive process to define community, identify problems, modify health programs to address priorities, and monitor effectiveness.

These components suggest the need for pluralism in financial arrangements. Fees alone cannot address the public goods addressed to community needs. Salary or capitation have a broader scope but a different mix of incentives and disincentives.

Given the developments in health affairs in the United States *circa* 1986, one suspects that the future of COPC rests on the financial incentives to be found in an increasingly pluralistic and private sector orientation. Yet much of our existing health care financing can frustrate efforts to combine a comprehensive approach for the individual with a focus on the community context. Preferred Provider Organizations, and Hospital/Joint Ventures could hardly be better designed to undermine COPC. Competing financial strategies must be developed. A pluralistic model would seem to be most compatible with the special requirements of COPC.

The Robert Wood Johnson Foundation announced in January 1986 the Primary Care Health Center Management Program (5). The intent, stated as follows:

. . . initiative aimed at strengthening the management capabilities of not-for-profit care health centers located in communities lacking adequate medical resources. The purpose of this program is to help *selected centers sustain* and *improve* their *overall financial* and *managerial operations*, as well as ensure their future viability. (emphasis added)

suggests an excellent opportunity to attempt viable strategies for financing the synthesis of primary care and community health. Observations of numerous health center initiatives over the past couple of decades suggest to the author that some mix of salary, capitation, and fee-for-service will best approach cost-effectiveness in COPC.

REFERENCES

1. Nutting, P.A.; Wood, M.; and Conner, E.M. Community-oriented primary care in the United States: A status report. *Journal of the American Medical Association* 1985; 253:March 22/29.

2. Wallack, S.S., and Kretz, S.E. Self-sufficiency in rural medical practice: Obstacles and solutions. Health Policy Consortium and Florence Heller School, Brandeis University, 1979. Working Paper.

3. Lee, S.S., and Butler, L.M. The three-layered cake—A plan for physician compensation. *New England Journal of Medicine* 1974; 291: August.

4. *The SIR Model Procedure Manual.* Primary Care Financing Project, Department of Research Medicine, University of Pennsylvania, School of Medicine and West Virginia Primary Care Study Group, 1980.

5. *Primary Care Health Center Management Program* (brochure). The Robert Wood Johnson Foundation, January 1986.

CHAPTER 4

The Use of Community-Oriented Primary Care Techniques in Health Maintenance Organizations

James F. Calvert, M.D.

By definition, COPC must include comprehensive, high-quality ambulatory care, and it is well documented that health maintenance organizations (HMOs) do provide primary care of excellent quality (1-5). On the other hand, good primary care need not necessarily use COPC techniques (6), although as we shall see, HMOs have used numerous COPC techniques to develop their ambulatory-based health care delivery systems. Many HMOs routinely canvass their enrolled members for perceptions of the quality and accessibility of services and the need and/or demand for additional services, then use this information to modify their health care programs. Clearly this exemplifies the principles of COPC, as described in some detail for the Kaiser-Permanente Medical Program of Oregon in the recent report from the Institute of Medicine (18).

Some HMOs have gone beyond their enrolled population to address issues facing the community as a whole. If we consider the case of an HMO like the Group Health Cooperative of Puget Sound, for example, which includes 20 percent of the Seattle area population in its membership, we will see that the extensive health services research which this organization carries out among its members amounts to a statistically meaningful look at the entire community, and that many of the preventive and outreach programs developed by the cooperative have benefited the entire Seattle community, and indeed the national community.

Historically, the HMO movement had a slow start, but in recent years it has had tremendous growth and there are now 15 million Americans enrolled in 323 HMOs (7). While the earliest prepaid group practices in the United States were started in the Seattle area in the nineteenth century to serve a trade union population, the first truly modern HMO, Group Health of Washington, D.C., was founded in 1936 by community members who felt their health needs were not being met by the fee-for-service sector. Thus community participation and the goal to meet defined health needs of the community were with the HMO movement from its origins. Both consumer governance and competitive pressures on prepaid group practices have led them to a style of practice that in some instances meets many criteria for community-oriented primary care.

It follows, then, that HMOs have

administrative and economic incentives to deliver care that meets the criteria for accessibility, comprehensiveness, continuity, and accountability that have traditionally defined high-quality primary care (8), as well as including extensive community control in their governance system. The motivation to do this comes from a combination of market forces, in the sense that good ambulatory care is seen as a method of lowering costs, and philosophical ones as well, in that from their founding these prepaid group practice plans were designed to meet the perceived unmet health care needs of their patients through an ambulatory-based, patient-controlled practice.

COMMUNITY CONTROL OF PREPAID GROUP PRACTICES

Many nonprofit HMOs have extensive consumer involvement in governance and decisionmaking at all levels. Group Health Cooperative of Puget Sound, for example, is administered primarily by a board of trustees, all of whom are consumers of the plan and are elected in a mail ballot system by all members of the cooperative. The board of trustees has full administrative authority in the cooperative, which serves as an important element of community involvement in a COPC practice. Additionally, however, the board at GHC/Puget Sound has shown a firm commitment to researching the health needs of the population it serves and modifying its program to meet them.

The board does much of its research through the cooperative's Center for Health Studies, which among other activities, conducts extensive mail surveys of the enrolled members. These surveys cover the level of satisfaction of members with services, but also seek their opinions on matters of policy. The results of the surveys are conveyed to the board which may often use them to set policy.

For instance, the board has recently started a project to develop membership awareness of bioethical problems such as abortion and major organ transplantation and to develop consensus policies on these issues. This program is modeled on a similar program started in Oregon by the State Public Health Department (9). The program involves both extensive consumer education on these issues and also involves polling every enrolled member so their opinion on these issues is known. While the board is not bound by the vote of the membership on such controversial issues, there is no doubt that the opinion of the membership is widely sought.

In another example, the board, in response to an increasing geriatric practice, has recently added a "Senior Initiative" section to the cooperative's overall philosophical document, its "Strategic Plan." The Senior Initiative provides information services and coordination of programs such as home health care with clinic and hospital care, and is also examining the possibility of extending care for elderly members after they lose work-related eligibility for HMO care.

Yet another example of community involvement by the board is its Foundation for Group Health, which sponsors biological research. The foundation has sponsored programs for educating teenage mothers, studying bone marrow transplant for cancer treatment, and primary treatment of diabetic retinopathy, among others. Many of these programs benefit non-enrolled as well as enrolled members.

The board has consistently promoted preventive approaches to care, with a theme of "Partners in Prevention," emphasizing the role of the patient. In addition, numerous industrial health plans have been started by the cooperative at plants whose members are part of the GHC plan.

As noted above, the board has taken an increasingly policy-oriented role in recent years, and has set up three regional councils which are involved more in the day-to-day administrative aspects of health care delivery. In addition, on the clinic level, each health center has a similar board composed of members elected from its service population. These boards deal with grievances about care delivery, clinic hours, special clinics, etc. at the local level. This network of grass roots administrative controls, closely linked to a central policymaking board, represents a mature form of community-oriented primary care, and also is an effective way to separate out the purely administrative issues from the broader health issues of COPC community involvement (10).[1]

HEALTH EDUCATION AND OTHER PREVENTIVE ACTIVITIES IN HMOS

Several HMOs have developed health education programs based on needs surveys of their constituencies; this can be seen as a modification of the program in response to statistically defined needs of the community. For example, the George Washington University HMO, in Washington, D.C., surveyed its members to find out what new services they felt were needed to enhance the plan, and found a strong, unanticipated interest in education about various health problems. In particular, members expressed a desire for education about anxiety and stress, physical fitness, methods to lose weight, and CPR training. Classes were established, generally conducted by HMO staff during evening hours. The program is still in effect and attendance remains high. Additional surveys showed that members wanted written material on subjects such as the interpretation of blood tests and various women's health problems; staff members developed handouts in some cases and reference lists for patients desiring more detailed information (11).

This type of activity has occurred in numerous HMOs, and in fact a whole literature has grown up describing it (12,

13). Most plans have emphasized education about the value of preventive health services such as blood pressure control, women's health issues, immunizations, and prevention of sexually transmitted diseases, along with health promotion activities such as smoking cessation and prudent alcohol use, as well as accident prevention and industrial safety among trade union members. Consistent with the thesis that economic motives underlie many community-based HMO activities, the literature has emphasized the cost effectiveness and marketing value of these activities (12,13). Whatever the motivation for performing these activities, however, they probably fit working definitions of COPC.

ROLE OF RESEARCH IN COPC ACTIVITIES OF HMOS

Health services research in the American population is greatly hampered by the difficulty in defining the population studied. This has been called the denominator problem (14). Since most HMOs have a computerized data base defining the demographic characteristics of the enrolled population, and since most enrollees obtain essentially all their health care in the HMO, these researchers have a much better handle on the denominator problem than their colleagues working in the fee-for-service sector.

Health services research among the enrollees of HMOs has often focused on problems that were considered costly to the HMOs. Programs have been instituted based on these findings to reduce morbidity due to these conditions and, it is hoped, their subsequent costs. Good examples include research on alcoholism

---

[1] The facts about Group Health Cooperative of Puget Sound were confirmed by discussion with its public relations officer, Wiley Brooks.

in Rhode Island Group Health Association (15) and Kaiser-Permanente (16). The Rhode Island study led to an increased emphasis on alcohol treatment benefits in the plan, based on study conclusions that this would reduce inpatient costs, which were found to be higher among alcoholics than sober members of the practice.

The Kaiser alcoholism study provides an example of the kind of epidemiologic research that can be done in the closed population of an HMO practice. The Kaiser study was able to select four groups of 2,000 persons, each with different drinking patterns. Because of the closed practice of an HMO, there was relative certainty of defining all health care costs and pathologic consequences of drinking in the group studied. The study provided the most complete and detailed look at the pathologic effects of alcohol consumption on a typical American population that we have had to date. It confirmed, for example, previous studies showing that modest alcohol consumption leads to a reduced mortality relative to no consumption, but that progressively higher consumption leads to progressively increasing ill effects. This extremely important study was conducted entirely with Kaiser money, with a basic motivation, presumably, to save money for Kaiser. However, the importance of the findings to our overall understanding of the health consequences of alcoholism was profound (16).

Additional examples along these lines would include the Group Health of Minnesota plan to reduce premature deliveries (17). This project uses the group health data base to identify prenatal patients with known high-risk characteristics and institute a prevention program that has been demonstrated in other centers to reduce prematurity, emphasizing preventive techniques and educating providers and patients on the signs of early labor to facilitate very early institution of tocolytic therapy.

Other examples of the use of community-oriented health services research in prepaid group practices are cited in the Institute of Medicine report, that included the Kaiser/Oregon HMO among its COPC models. Described there are programs in preventive services for children, health care for the elderly, and sudden infant death syndrome (18). In the SIDS intervention, all babies in the prepaid group practice who were at high risk for SIDS (low birthweight, known apneic spells, etc.) were identified and monitored at home; parents were educated about SIDS and instructed in CPR, and in methods (such as warming the environment) thought to reduce the risk of SIDS. Since initiation of this protocol, the incidence of SIDS deaths in the Kaiser population has dropped to 30 percent of the previous level, while that of the rest of the Oregon population has not changed. This project is a remarkable example of the combination of applied health services research (to identify the problem), biomedical research (to identify potential solutions), and clinical skills (to carry out the program) in a COPC environment.

The Group Health Cooperative of Puget Sound has a Center for Health Studies, that conducts top quality health services research within the context of the enrolled population. The Center has received a $1.8 million grant to do smoking cessation research among the cooperative's members, and has been involved in numerous cancer prevention studies as well. The Center is currently engaged in about 60 internally directed research projects, the results of which are conveyed to the Board of Directors. The Board has the authority to translate the results into policy at the delivery level. The Center then carries on studies to monitor the effects of policy changes. This would meet COPC criteria for identifying, addressing, and monitoring health problems of the populations served (6).

SUMMARY AND CONCLUSIONS

Recent studies have confirmed that HMOs can deliver care comparable to that of the fee-for-service sector at reduced costs. It appears that HMOs achieve their reduced costs almost entirely by decreased hospital utilization and reliance on ambulatory services in their place (19). In an increasingly competitive and cost-conscious health care delivery environment, there is little doubt that these studies have done much to stimulate the entry of the for-profit medical care sector into the HMO market. It is these corporate sponsored HMOs that have primarily been responsible for the movement's recent growth (20,21).

Clearly, the examples cited above demonstrate that COPC techniques can be and have been used by HMOs, and there is little doubt that especially among the nonprofit (consumer directed) HMOs many COPC projects have an altruistic incentive, as well as an economic one. However, as Federal support for HMOs has gradually disappeared, competitive pressures on them are increasing. This has made them less willing to take on high risk groups (22) such as those from impoverished backgrounds who might most benefit from their preventive services (23). There is increasing evidence, in fact, that disadvantaged populations may not get the same quality of health benefits from HMOs that middle-class patients do, perhaps because of their inability to deal with the system, which can be more complex than a private office (24,25).

In fact, the innovative community-oriented health care described here has evolved in nonprofit HMOs that were founded as consumer cooperatives. Due to competitive pressures, it is becoming increasingly difficult for these HMOs to maintain their nonprofit status. The problem is that when HMOs were perceived as quirky, alternative health care delivery systems they were relatively free from competitive pressure. Now that the Rand study (19) has shown them to be cost-effective, the corporate world has moved strongly into the HMO market, and HMO stocks have done very well in the for-profit sector (20). In addition, many fee-for-service providers are bonding together to form their own prepaid practice plans (these are sometimes called IPAs, Individual Practice Associations). These developments taken together mean an increasingly competitive market for the nonprofit HMO cooperatives, and as increasing numbers of for-profit corporations enter the marketplace, it becomes increasingly difficult for nonprofit groups to compete for capital (20,26).

In response to this pressure, four of the most prestigious nonprofit HMOs—Group Health Cooperative of Puget Sound, Group Health of St. Paul, Harvard Community Health Plan, and the Health Insurance Plan of Greater New York—are considering forming a for-profit company to develop new HMO "markets" (20). It is to be hoped that competitive pressures will continue to stimulate HMOs to provide preventive health services for their clients. In addition, it remains to be seen whether activities sponsored by HMOs such as Kaiser/Permanente and GHC of Puget Sound, which do benefit many community members not enrolled in the HMO, will continue as the financial screws are tightened more and more, and whether these major nonprofit HMOs will retain their community control when they have a corporate board of directors, as well as a consumer board, to answer to.

REFERENCES

1. Deuschle, J. M.; Alvarez, B.; Logsden, D. N. et al. Physician performance in a prepaid group practice. *Medical Care* 1982; 20:127.

2. Cunningham, F., and Williamson, J. W. How does the quality of care in

HMOs compare to that in other settings? An analytic literature review. *Group Health Journal* 1980:1.

3. Donabedian, A. The quality of care in a health maintenance organization: A personal view. *Inquiry* 1983; 20:218.

4. Wright, C. H. Obstetric care in health maintenance organization and a private fee-for-service practice: A comparative analysis. *American Journal of Obstetrics and Gynecology* 1984; 149:848.

5. Yelin, E. H.; Henke, C. J.; Kramer, J. S. et al. A comparison of the treatment of rheumatoid arthritis in health maintenance organizations and fee for service practices. *New England Journal of Medicine* 1985; 312:962.

6. Nutting, P. A., and Connor, E. M. (eds.). *Community Oriented Primary Care: A Practical Assessment*, Volume I: The Committee Report. Washington D.C.: National Academy Press, 1984.

7. Mayer, T. R., and Mayer, G. G. HMOs: Origins and development. *New England Journal of Medicine* 1985; 312:590.

8. Silver, H. K., and McAtee, P. R. The essentials of primary health care. *Journal of Family Practice* 1977;4:151.

9. Crawshaw, R.; Garland, M. J.; Hine, B. et al. Oregon Health Decisions: An experiment with informed community consent. *Journal of the American Medical Association* 1985;22:3213.

10. MacColl, W. A. *Group Practice and Prepayment of Medical Care*. Washington, D.C.: Public Affairs Press, 1966.

11. Donaldson, M. A.; Nicklason, J. A.; and Ott, J. E. Needs-based health promotion program serves as HMO marketing tool. *Public Health Reports* 1985; 100:270.

12. Deeds, S. G., and Mullen, P. D.

(eds.). Health education in HMOs: Part one. *Health Education Quarterly* 1981; 8:279.

13. Howard, D. M. Health education needs assessment in an HMO: A case study. *Health Education Quarterly* 1982; 9:23.

14. Cherkin, D. C.; Phillips, W. R.; and Berg, A. O. A method for estimating the population at risk in primary care practices by applying correction factors to the active patient census. *Journal of Family Practice* 1984; 19:355.

15. Putnam, S. L. Alcoholism, morbidity, and care seeking: The inpatient and ambulatory service utilization and associated illness experience of alcoholics and matched controls in a health maintenance organization. *Medical Care* 1982; 20:97.

16. Klatsky, A. L.; Friedman, G. D.; and Siegelaub, A. B. Alcohol and mortality: A ten year Kaiser-Permanente experience. *Annals of Internal Medicine* 1981; 95:139.

17. Mark, P. A., and Eggen, D. Group health program to reduce the incidence of preterm deliveries. *Minnesota Medicine* Sept 1984; 509.

18. Nutting, P. A., and Connor, E. M. (eds.). *Community Oriented Primary Care: A Practical Assessment*, Volume II: The Case Studies. Washington, D.C.: National Academy Press, 1984.

19. Manning, W. G.; Liebowitz, A.; Goldberg, G. A. et al. A controlled trial of the effect of a prepaid group practice on use of services. *New England Journal of Medicine* 1984; 310:1505.

20. Iglehart, J. K. HMOs (for-profit and not-for-profit) on the move. *New England Journal of Medicine* 1984; 310:1203.

21. Saward, E. W., and Fleming, S. Health maintenance organizations. *Scientific American* 1980; 243:47.

22. Birnbaum, R. W. Community rating and underlying HMO reimbursement issues. *Topics in Health Care Financing* 1981; 51.

23. Wise, P. H.; Kotelchuk, M.; Wilson, M. L. et al. Racial and socioeconomic disparities in childhood mortality in Boston. *New England Journal of Medicine* 1985; 313:360.

24. Mechanic, D.; Weiss, N.; and Cleary, P. D. The growth of HMOs: Issues of enrollment and disenrollment. *Medical Care* 1983; 21:338.

25. Mullooly, J. P., and Freeborn, D. K. The effect of length of membership upon the utilization of ambulatory care services: A comparison of disadvantaged and general populations in a prepaid group practice. *Medical Care* 1979; 17:922.

26. Capital requirements and capital financing in a hospital based group practice prepayment plan. *Topics in Health Care Financing* Winter 1981:1.

CHAPTER 5

COPC:
Doing Something Is Better
Than Doing Nothing

Marc E. Babitz, M.D.

I am a recent convert to the formal concept of community-oriented primary care. As a practicing primary care physician who is community oriented, I had a variety of experiences that upon retrospective analysis could have easily formed the basis for a COPC system. That experience, which I believe is similar to the practice experience of most primary care physicians, is what I wish to share with the reader. Nearly all primary care physicians have the capability and resources to convert elements of their primary care practices into true COPC. Currently, the physicians who are interested and active in promoting and practicing COPC seem to be but a small subset of the total pool of primary care physicians who potentially are interested in doing more for their patients than can be accomplished within the confines of an examination room. I hope readers will identify with elements of my experiences and discern ways by which they may begin to incorporate COPC into their practices.

To most primary care physicians the philosophy and practice of COPC, to at least some degree, is perceived as an effective, qualitative, and quantitative means of providing primary care. I have found that the biggest barrier discouraging physicians from getting started is that they feel overwhelmed by the "requirements" of COPC, and feel themselves to be without financial, personnel, and statistical resources. My message is simply that the only "required" resource for COPC is your own interest in doing something beyond seeing patients in your office every day!

Once health care professionals have identified that personal resource, they have taken the first step into a public health (COPC) approach to health care; they have accepted the principle that some health problems are better approached in a broader, medical-social context. The experience of some early successes in one's initial COPC endeavors simplifies the advancement to the more rigorous concepts of COPC detailed in subsequent chapters of this book.

Let me now share my own experiences in taking those first steps. I must confess that I was not familiar with the theory, concept, or application of COPC, by that name, until early in 1984. I am a board certified family physician who began my practice experience with 9 years of National Health Service Corps (NHSC) field service after residency training. My practice was in a semi-rural community in Sonoma County, California. I was assigned to a community-owned and -operated, non-profit health center. Although this area is one of the famous wine-growing regions of northern California, the western half of this county is poor and relatively isolated. As a well-trained, somewhat idealistic, and motivated new physician I encouraged our health center to engage in the appropriate health promotion/disease prevention activities I learned about as a resident physician. These activities included sponsoring free blood pressure screening clinics, providing a variety of educational patient handouts on several common health problems, "stop smoking" classes, and weight loss programs. I, and the other professional staff, also made ourselves available to community groups as speakers who would discuss any health topic requested. In reflecting on these activities, I consider them reasonable attempts to practice good primary care, but since these activities were not targeted to serve a specific population or a defined problem in that community, and were not monitored for effectiveness, they do not serve as examples of a fully developed COPC practice. Something else happened in my practice that began my conversion to the principles and practice of COPC, although I did not realize it at the time.

By definition, our NHSC site was serving two rural Health Manpower Shortage Areas (HMSAs), which covered nearly 400 square miles and included nearly 20,000 people. The population was relatively young and included many women of childbearing age. The population was poor, most receiving some form of welfare support, and eligible for Medi-Cal (Medicaid for California residents). There was little or no public transportation available for most of the residents of these two HMSAs, and the nearest hospital was 20 miles from our clinic. As I looked at my patient population, it was apparent that compared to other family physicians in my area I was carrying a heavy obstetrical (OB) patient load, averaging 4 - 5 deliveries a month. In addition, I had been asked to provide physician staffing for a county public health clinic that was providing prenatal care one-half day each week to a group of pregnant women who had chosen not to seek their care in the private sector. The reasons were multiple for women to choose to use this county public health clinic, but there were two major themes: first, many who were poor and were not eligible for Medi-Cal could not afford other sources of care; and second, many of these women practiced "alternative" lifestyles and were planning home deliveries with lay midwives and felt ostracized from the regular OB community.

Since I provided prenatal care for my own patients and the public health clinic patients, I was very concerned with finding ways to improve the outcomes of these pregnancies, especially for the high-risk women; major risk factors in this population included poverty, poor nutrition, lack of regular prenatal care, lack of prenatal education (childbirth classes, parenting classes, nutrition information, etc.), and planned home deliveries in the face of obvious complications. My partner, a fellow family physician, was faced with an equally heavy OB load, and we felt that we needed to do something beyond our examination rooms to improve the care for this population.

As I look back on my OB patient population, it is now clear to me that I could have easily "defined" my community with some simple assistance from outside public agencies. Our geographic service area was well defined, and population statistics could have easily been obtained. These would have included the number of women of childbearing age. By using data for the county fertility rate, or by using zip code information about births in the county, I could have determined the total potential OB population that our prenatal care programs might try to reach. I realize now that all of this statistical data was readily available.

We essentially defined our target population as all the pregnant women in our service area, although, at the time, we didn't formally declare this as our "community." We defined the problem based on our personal experience and that of the local hospital; namely that many adverse or potentially adverse outcomes could be prevented in this group.

The county public health department clearly felt the same way, which is why they established the prenatal clinic in our area. We did not have a statistical base upon which to compare our target group with another control which could show that we had a special problem (although I suspect that data was also discernible from the birth records, which list pregnancy complications). However, in obstetrics it can be painfully clear when a problem is unpredictable as opposed to one which is preventable or predictable. Our goal, of course, was to eliminate the predictable and preventable problems to the greatest degree possible.

Our resources assessment was also done mostly on a subconscious level. For personnel we had the support of our health center staff, the public health clinic staff, and fortunately many of the lay midwives. Had it been necessary, I am sure we could have also received help from some of our patients and from members of our Board of Directors. Financial resources were not an initial item of concern, but as we began to propose specific projects my health center board of directors was willing to provide small amounts of money, and the use of our facility, when needed. As mentioned before, we didn't even consider the need or desirability for statistical resources

since we were not aware that we were getting started in the practice of COPC.

Over the next couple of months we set up several projects designed to address specific aspects of the problem. To combat poor nutrition we set up formal referral systems for our patients to the Women, Infants, and Children (WIC) staff; we developed numerous patient education handouts on nutrition that were appropriate for women of low income and those living alternate lifestyles (e.g., vegetarians); we arranged for our patients to be given prescription prenatal vitamins at cost or for free (at center expense) since even Medi-Cal would not cover this item; and we involved the women in the monitoring of their own nutritional status (e.g., charting weight gain, and noting hematocrit results). We offered free prenatal classes, and while we taught natural childbirth, we discussed nutrition, risk factors in pregnancy and delivery, conduct of labor, family planning, and parenting. The free classes also served to bring our counter-culture patients into our health center where they could meet and speak with our providers without having to enter into a formal patient-doctor relationship. We worked with the local lay midwives to improve rapport, which would facilitate earlier referral of problems. We developed a formal risk assessment system, which they accepted as criteria for deciding when their patients needed physician and/or hospital care. We worked with patient groups to overcome superstitions and prejudices held by each side regarding the health care beliefs of the other. Finally, we worked with the local hospital and consultant staff to allow more family-centered, natural, childbirth experiences to occur whenever possible. All these activities were continually evaluated informally and modified, as needed, to reach the maximum number of patients in our area.

Had we considered it, it would have

been relatively simple to define better which risk factors were most predominant in our population through chart review and/or questionnaires. We then could have formalized our assessment of the specific health problems in our OB population on which we should focus. Had we included this COPC element, we would have established criteria by which we could have evaluated our success (or failure) to affect outcome.

As I have implied, we did not formally evaluate our health program for improving obstetrical outcomes. From a purely subjective viewpoint, those involved in this program felt that it achieved significant results. This viewpoint was based on the apparent decrease in patients arriving at the hospital with problems, and without prenatal care or records; the apparent increase in the number of home-birth patients who voluntarily came to the hospital for care when recommended; and a general feeling, shared by our consultants, that we were seeing healthier babies and healthier mothers with fewer complications. In this area also, it would have been relatively easy for us to have reviewed hospital birth records from patients in our population to determine statistically whether changes in outcome were occurring following the implementation of our improved pregnancy program.

I don't really know at what point we became a COPC practice as we took that first big step beyond the confines of a typical primary health care delivery system. We were rewarded by a feeling of success and achievement, and that feeling is what sustained our desire to do more. Given the perspective of my current position with the NHSC, which is primarily administrative, my present knowledge of COPC, and my past clinical experiences as a family physician in the Public Health Service, I want to summarize my experience with this message about COPC.

COPC is a public health tool. It is a

tool that can help us care for our patients. All health care professionals are hopefully seeking ways to improve the health status of their patients, the practice in which they are located, and the community in which they serve. If these professionals are better able to care for their patients and their community, they are more likely to derive professional and personal satisfaction in their efforts as health care providers.

The typical primary care provider in underserved settings, such as those in the NHSC, will face a seemingly limitless need for health care services, in an environment of limited resources and restricted options. The health care professional working in well-served communities also faces limited resources and other barriers to the implementation of a COPC practice. In addition, the primary care skills of the average health professional are often inadequate tools to effect the desired changes in the health status of the patients and their community. Those providers seeking to make a greater impact on their practice and on the health of their community, beyond that achievable by providing good primary care, may wish to learn and practice the simple public health technique known as community-oriented primary care (COPC).

The incorporation of COPC into one's primary care practice can be as simple or as rigorous as one has the time, resources, and inclination. To me COPC is the systematic process of: definition of the population in which a change in health status is desired; identification of the specific health problem(s) to be addressed; implementation of a plan to effect the desired change; evaluation of the plan's effectiveness; and modification of the plan as needed.

There are additional aspects that can easily be added to this process, and there are clearly differences in the degree to which one explores and addresses each step. However, any interested primary care provider has the ability to understand and use the essentials of COPC, and appreciate the measurable benefits of improved community health status.

This book has been designed to offer a broad view of COPC, to demonstrate several unique methods of approach, and of problem-solving, for each step in the process. In this way interested health professionals can begin to identify which technique or situation is most likely to be applicable in their own practice settings.

It is my hope that this book will encourage others to join the growing number of primary health professionals who practice their caring by direct intervention combined with COPC.

CHAPTER 6

COPC and the Challenge
of Public Health

Fitzhugh Mullan, M.D.

The short history of community-oriented primary care in the United States
has taken place almost entirely within the
confines of the primary care movement.
The National Health Service Corps and
the Community Health Center Program
have provided a natural environment for
COPC concepts to germinate and take
root. The North American Primary Care
Research Group (NAPCRG) and the
Society of Teachers of Family Medicine
(STFM) have supplied academic interest
and legitimacy to the concept. The clinicians who have grasped the COPC idea
and are using it to modify and improve
their practices are, almost without exception, practitioners of primary care.

The reasons for the trend are obvious.
COPC, after all, addresses the practice of
primary care and while its principles could
well be applied to many elements of clinical practice, family physicians, general
internists, and general pediatricians are
its most natural audience. If the primary
care community remains the only participant in the COPC movement, however,
a major opportunity to disseminate the
benefits of the discipline will be lost. A
major ally with important historical roots
as well as responsibility for a great deal of

the Nation's health is the public health
community. COPC, in fact, draws heavily
on skills for which public health has long
been the custodian — epidemiology and
biostatistics. Enlisting the enthusiasm,
abilities, and support of practitioners of
public health and public health institutions in the development of COPC will
be an enormously important undertaking
over the next few years.

The history of public health in the
United States dates back to the last century when a number of larger cities established health departments to oversee sanitary reforms and monitor vital statistics.
Through the latter part of the 19th century and the early years of this century,
all states and many counties followed suit
in delegating public health authority to
an established body. At the outset, health
departments tended to have only a regulatory function, but over time more and
more of them took on responsibility for
certain health service functions — maternal and child health, the treatment of
venereal diseases, the care of populations
institutionalized for mental illness or retardation. The service delivery aspects of
State and local health departments were
driven in large part by Federal funding

that became increasingly abundant as the century progressed. Yet the relationship between regulation and health service delivery within State and local health authorities was never a clear one and, as a result, some local health departments have a tradition of active and creative service delivery while others do not.

Primary care as a concept emerged in the 1960s and 1970s as the result of a national consensus that medical care, particularly general medical care, was in short supply. Everyone was at risk in what many termed "the health care crisis," but rural people, the poor, and the institutionalized populations suffered the most pronounced lack of medical services. The Federal Government responded with a variety of legislative actions that reconstructed the landscape of health care. Foremost among these were programs designed to supply physicians to serve poor and isolated people — the Office of Economic Opportunity's Neighborhood Health Centers, the Maternal and Infant Care and the Children and Youth Programs, the Migrant Health Program, grants to stimulate the development of family medicine, and the National Health Service Corps and its scholarship program. These programs and the providers practicing in them, or because of them, provided a greatly expanded clinical capability in dealing with the needs of the underserved. It is these people and programs that have constituted the primary participants in the COPC movement.

The principal constituency of both the public health programs and the primary care programs are poor, isolated, and institutionalized people who cannot afford or cannot gain access to private medical care. The synonymity of interest between the public health and the primary care programs ought to drive them together into a single, dynamic force for improving the health care for those Americans who have least. Yet, with a few notable exceptions,

this has not happened. The reasons are multiple, including, I believe, the separate history and traditions that have spawned the two movements.

The primary care programs have a Federal base while the public health activities are the domain of State and local governments. The one salutes the notions of preventive medicine, categorical programming, and population-based care while the other aims for curative care with a comprehensive and personal approach. There are arguments to be made for both approaches, but they pale in comparison to the potential for better health services that could be achieved by the coordination of skills, resources, and energies from the two systems.

Because it has a foot firmly planted in both camps, COPC has the promise to bring about collaboration between practitioners of primary care and public health for the benefit of the system as a whole. Practical examples of this approach include State, local, and municipal health agencies taking the lead in assembling representatives of primary care clinics to discuss COPC programming and coordinated activities. Target projects could include the development of consortia, collaborative data base development, conjoint health promotion/disease prevention programs, and COPC methodology troubleshooting.

State and local public health leaders have proven effective in working with primary care leaders to lobby legislative bodies for support. State laboratories; family planning resources; immunizations; Women, Infants, and Children's (WIC) contracts; and Emergency Medical Services (EMS) programs are all areas where increased collaboration will result in improved and more cost effective services for clients of the public programs. In every case, a population-based approach using numerate, epidemiological assessments as the basis for the conjoint activity will bring the two camps together and provide a format understood by both. The winners will be the clients of the public programs.

In our enthusiasm to make COPC a more prominent part of the American medical landscape, the oft-neglected valley between primary care and public health needs to be mapped, seeded, and watered. Both movements will benefit from the process, and, most important, so will their constituencies.

Part II.
Defining and Characterizing the Community

Introduction

The COPC process begins with defining and characterizing the community for which the practice has accepted responsibility. The resulting knowledge of the total community forms the foundation upon which the subsequent functions of COPC are based. The practice of medicine in any primary care setting has traditionally stressed the importance of understanding the community from which patients present for care. COPC extends this notion to systematically examining the community, recording, and analyzing the results with the same rigor that the practitioner uses when understanding a particular patient. Many primary care practitioners through years of practice and observation will have developed a basic knowledge of the community, based on subjective analysis of information gained from patients and the fact of his/her living and often raising a family in the community. In the absence of a systematic approach to collecting and analyzing the data on the community, however, primary care practitioners may erroneously generalize patterns of health and health behavior from their most familiar patients (the numerator) to the target community (the denominator). In COPC, the practitioner needs to know more precisely who and where are the individuals and households who comprise his community, how they live and behave in ways that influence their health, where and when they seek care for ailments, and how they perceive and finance their care. Ideally, the practitioner would be able to actually list all the individuals in the community as a basis for subsequent identifying and focusing on high risk individuals and groups.

Among the important characteristics of the activities of this function is the rigor and precision of the methods used to gather information on the community. Methods which yield a wide scope of detailed and relevant data are clearly of value, as are techniques that yield the less quantitative information on the social and cultural values of the community or its many important subsets.

USE OF SUBJECTIVE INFORMATION

For the practitioner beginning to incorporate some of the COPC principles into his/her practice, an expansion of the subjective information base may be most appropriate. This can be started by thinking of the community in a systematic manner and documenting observations and impressions, similar to the manner in which a new patient is approached. This process can be enriched by involving members of the community either formally or informally. While most practitioners can subjectively describe their active patient population, fewer can describe the socioeconomic, cultural, and health-related behavioral patterns within a larger community. In turning attention to the larger community, one should be cautioned against relying too heavily on extrapolation from the active patients to the community. Most physicians can recall an experience from medical school of being told of the importance of some obscure disease, because from the specialty perspective it appeared to be common.

USE OF SECONDARY DATA

In many instances a great deal of information on the community can be gained through the use of secondary data. Large area statistics may be particularly useful in the early development of an information base on the community. Several drawbacks, however, should be kept in mind. Large area data often do not describe exactly the target community for which the practice has accepted responsibility, often do not lend themselves to more in-depth analysis of issues of particular interest, and do not permit an enumeration of all individuals within the community. Clearly secondary data are most useful when drawn from an area that corresponds closely to the definition of the community.

USE OF PRIMARY DATA

In some settings the practitioner may wish or need to engage in primary data collection, either as the foundation of a community data base or as a supplement to subjective information and a base of secondary data. In some cases a reasonable community data base may be developed from a practice data system that has been in operation for some time and includes active users of health services. In single-practice communities such a data base may eventually include the majority of a larger community. The major drawback of a data base constructed in this fashion is the inconsistency and lack of currency of data elements for those individuals who have sought care infrequently. Increasingly health maintenance organizations (HMOs) are developing data bases on their enrolled populations, and a comprehensive data system developed by the Indian Health Service are examples of the feasibility, in some settings, of a data base that contains information for each individual and permits a careful analysis of the demography and socioeconomic status of the target population or community.

The chapters of this section cover a broad range of topics relevant to defining and characterizing the target community in a wide variety of practice settings. Obviously the manner in which the information base is assembled, its reliance on subjective or objective data, each drawn from either primary or secondary data sources will be a function of the type of community or population to be addressed and the availability of information or data on that community. In turn there is a great

deal of variation in the way in which the COPC practice can define its target community. In Chapter 7, Strelnick confronts several difficult conceptual and definitional issues in the use of the terms "community" and "population" and describes the relationships that exist between them.

The next three chapters describe steps in an incremental approach to addressing a target population. In Chapter 8, Hawk and Calvert offer suggestions for starting with the active patients of one's practice. Nutting describes, in Chapter 9, an approach with particular relevance to family practice that defines as the target community all members of the households of active patients of the practice. Finally, Reed discusses the manner in which a practice can address the health problems of pre-defined populations, and gives an example of addressing the school-age population (Chapter 10).

In Chapter 11, Mettee describes the concept of community diagnosis as a process that integrates the basic and applied sciences of clinical care, epidemiology, and behavioral science. He outlines a general approach to gathering and analyzing a variety of subjective and objective information, using both primary and secondary data sources. In order to develop an accurate and comprehensive understanding of the characteristics of the community, he stresses the importance of developing a team approach consisting of health professionals, patients, and citizens of the community.

The next series of chapters describes methods for using practice data and secondary data to develop estimates of the practice denominator and to define and characterize the target population. Chapter 12, by Rhyne, Kozoll, and Stewart, describes the use of census data for deriving a count of the practice denominator and describing the demographic characteristics of that population. The authors describe the anatomy of the census and

33

make recommendations for when and how to use census data. Next in Chapter 13, Hearst reviews the several techniques and the results of attempting to estimate the total patient population of a practice or program. Although the results of these methods have been somewhat discouraging, the problem of estimating a denominator in order to convert practice-based observations into meaningful rates continues to deserve emphasis.

In companion chapters Zyzanski and Galazka describe methods for defining the community from which one's active patients come for care (Chapter 14), and techniques for comparing the demographic characteristics of the active patients to those of the larger community (Chapter 15). In their approach the practice denominator is defined as the population of the geographic area in which the active patients of the practice reside. In Chapter 16, Breckenridge and Like offer some "pencil and paper" techniques of demography that will assist in organizing and displaying secondary data.

The next two chapters describe approaches that may be useful in different settings, but are particularly applicable to community health centers. Chapter 17, by Trachtenberg, Gardner, Gould, and Hutchison, describes a process for developing an interactive community data base, by combining primary and secondary data. They offer suggestions on data sources as well as hardware and software requirements for developing a similar system in other settings. Kohl and Conway, in Chapter 18, describe the use of the Need-Demand Assessment (NDA), required for federally funded community health centers, as an important tool for the practice of COPC. Modifications in the NDA are suggested to make it more compatible with the principles of COPC and the changing environment of the community health centers.

The next two chapters address approaches to collecting primary data on the community. In Chapter 19, Berman reviews the most widely applied techniques for conducting community surveys and discusses the advantages and disadvantages of these approaches. Ellerbrock, Kraus, Osborn, and Bujold describe, in Chapter 20, an approach to defining a transient population, a vexing problem of growing proportions in most urban areas.

Finally in the Coda, Maurice Wood reflects on the contribution that more widespread adoption of COPC principles could have on the system of primary care in this country. He notes that many of the principles of COPC are (or at least should be) a fundamental part of primary care physicians' views of their role in society.

CHAPTER 7

The Community-Defining
Process in COPC

A. H. Strelnick, M.D.

Gone are the days of the horse-and-buggy doctor whose rich knowledge of his community was unconsciously acquired over a lifetime of growing up, living and practicing in a stable hometown or neighborhood. Mobility and change now profoundly affect most Americans, their families, and communities, including physicians. Like their contemporaries, physicians often commute to their practices, in locations far from the roots of their childhood and youth. For optimal primary care practice physicians need alternative, systematic approaches for learning about their communities in which they practice and for developing their relationship with those communities. Community-oriented primary care (COPC) is the model for one such approach, the essence of which is the conscious broadening of the relationship between medical practitioners and their communities.

As with other relationships, the community-practitioner relationship develops and grows incrementally, a montage composed over time of chance encounters and formal meetings, carefully designed studies and crash programs, rigorous statistical research and casual observations, false starts and profound successes. Defining "community" is a part of this process and is an essential, and often imposing, component of the COPC model (1,2). Defining the community or communities that a medical practice serves is particularly challenging in urban settings where geography is not destiny, patients have a choice of providers, and civic and functional boundaries rarely correspond. The process of defining community in urban primary care can be likened to putting together a thousand-piece jigsaw puzzle of a Jackson Pollack action painting without having the corner and border pieces with their straight edges. It would take a month of rainy Sunday afternoons for even the most patient, fastidious, and diligent art lovers to complete the puzzle (i.e., define "community") if they set their task as fitting all one thousand pieces together in their proper places. Most of us would quit or never even start. However, if the task were to compose a "Jackson Pollack" mosaic from the same puzzle pieces, fitting together only the obvious pieces while capturing the general composition, color, and movement of the painting, most of us could succeed during the commercials of the Superbowl. Since the office of our local or State health department and the

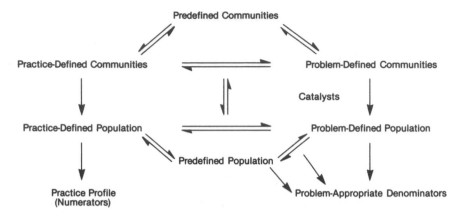

Figure 1. The Community-Population Denominator Definition Process.

Census Bureau can supply each of us with our own thousand-piece puzzles, the questions become how complete and clear a "picture" of our community is needed for COPC and what pieces are missing that we have to generate ourselves?

Joining clinical medicine with epidemiology in COPC poses the potential of confusing logical types (3). The COPC literature has implied that COPC is identical with "population-based" or "denominator-based" medicine. A "community" (derived from the Latin *comunite* meaning "commons" or "fellowship") is not only people and places but bricks and mortar, power structures, historical traditions, social values and customs, and a myriad of unquantifiable and often undefinable but essential features. Different disciplines have attempted to define "community" including anthropology, sociology, urban studies, and political science. A population (from the Latin *populus* meaning "people") is a class or a group of people that is both more clearly definable and quantifiable than a community (in the abstract if not always in real life practice) — all the inhabitants of a given country or area considered together, the whole collection of units from which a sample may be drawn.

A denominator (derived from the Latin root *denominare* meaning "to name") is by definition a number that is used to divide another, a part of a ratio. Each term functions at a different level of discourse derived from a different field (i.e., common speech, demography or epidemiology, and mathematics, respectively). Each term has a hierarchical relationship to the others in COPC with each a subset of its predecessor. "Community" represents the most comprehensive term and the most difficult to define. Rigorous methods for its assessment have been developed in anthropology, sociology, and urban studies. Rigorous quantitative methods from demography and epidemiology can be applied to "populations" and from mathematics and biostatistics to "denominators." But as Kozoll points out (5), in COPC a "population" may serve as either a numerator or denominator. In general, comprehensiveness and methodological rigor will be inversely related.

THE COMMUNITY-PRACTICE DIALECTIC

Defining a "community" — and therefore a population and denominator — is an ongoing, dialectical process between a practice and its human environment (Figure 1).

36

Predefined Communities

Urban communities may be defined independent of the practice by public agencies in civic units (e.g., school districts, health areas, boroughs), by geographic and geologic serendipity (e.g., steep hills, highways, bodies of water), by social or economic function (e.g., the garment district, South Bronx, North Shore, or Gold Coast), or by historical neighborhood traditions (e.g., Chinatown, Little Italy, Georgetown).

Practice-Defined Communities

A practice may define its community in a number of different ways that emphasize geographic proximity (e.g., Kark's "Initial Defined Area" (6), contiguous census tract clusters, etc.), receiving responsibility (e.g., catchment area), programmatic or practice resource commitment (e.g., target areas or markets), or historical patient utilization (e.g., patient origin, market penetration). Practices that limit their services to or serve specific subgroups (e.g., women, gays, the poor, Native Americans, students) may define their communities along ethnic, racial, gender, or sexual-preference boundaries. In a fee-for-service, freedom-of-choice medical system the relationship between a practice's patients and its community is always somewhat arbitrary. In a prepaid, capitated panel system, such as a health maintenance organization, that relationship is clearer, although enrollees do not necessarily constitute a community. A clear mission or purpose will help a practice define a community. As noted above, a community is more than a sum of its population.

Problem-Defined Communities

Communities are also defined by common experiences, problems, or exposures, a definition process close to the hearts and purses of funding and granting agencies. Communities may be organized around these problems, their "common ground,"
such as environmental exposure (e.g., Love Canal, Lead Belt, "the South Bronx is burning"), sexually transmitted diseases (the gay or singles community), and other infectious diseases (e.g., refugee, homeless communities).

Problem-Defined Populations

When problems are defined as being identifiable characteristics of people rather than social, geographic, or cultural phenomena that transcend their aggregate as individuals, then a population is the appropriate level of focus. The presence or absence of the relevant problem (or characteristic) or being at risk for it defined the population. We readily understand what is meant by the population of hypertensives in a workplace, the population at high risk for AIDS, or the homeless. Research designs define populations and then draw representative samples that permit extrapolation of the findings in the sample to the whole. Grants are frequently targeted for at-risk populations such as those to prevent teenage pregnancy or to reduce low birth weight babies (7).

Practice-Defined Populations

A practice may define a population from its active patients, those who have enrolled in it through an insurance contract (like an HMO or IPA), or those who share households with these groups. Because of the patient's initiative in joining the practice population (skewed selection), it cannot be said to be fully representative of larger or broader groups. Subgroups within a practice (e.g., chronic "no-shows") may also be defined. Descriptions of these populations constitute a "practice-profile" and serve as numerators for community-based denominators.

Predefined Populations

Populations of interest to COPC may be defined outside the practice of medicine: employees of a factory, members of a union, registered voters of a municipality.

Occasionally, "community" is applied to a population where a set of values are being promoted (e.g., the "hospital or IBM community") or "population" is applied to a community to avoid judging or stereotyping (e.g., the "black" or "gay" population). Such shifts in logical types in common usage makes clarity between "community" and "population" more difficult. As can be readily seen in Figure 1, these categories are interactive. A given practice may use one or more of these defined groups as denominators or target populations and serve many communities.

CATALYSTS FOR DEFINITION

A variety of catalysts promote initial and further definition of community and practice. *Community boards* bring an outside, nonmedical perspective to community problems, needs, priorities, and values and provide formal channels for practice-community dialogue. *Categorical grants* target defined problems and/or populations but often require a broader needs assessment and evaluation process. A grant may lead to the definition of a target or catchment area that best meets the funding criteria rather than "true" community. *Clinical experience* exposes the tip of the community iceberg but not what is below the surface; it can alert a practice to areas for special investigation. Motivated *individuals with special interests*, whether provider, staff, or patient, can stimulate further investigation and/or activity into a problem or a neighborhood. This may also occur through *the media*. Targeted *research* — both academic and market-oriented — assists in the definition of practice mission and community responsiveness. A formal *needs assessment* may be employed for program development or service packaging. Resources and measurement units for *vital statistics* may determine the data available for comparison and, thus, define the denominator. Because of need for catalysts and their serendipity, the process of building toward COPC may be both opportunistic and rational (8).

URBAN BOUNDARY SETTING

Units of measurement (e.g., census tracts, health areas for vital statistics), and limitations of resources and data will greatly affect the arbitrariness of boundary setting. Coterminous boundaries may not be possible for all projects but contribute to the composition of a broader montage and mosaic picture of the community.

Projects and all the other parts of the compositional process may be evaluated by their *contribution* to the picture of the community as a whole, their *process* in engaging with members of the community in dialogue, their *function* to improve the quality, responsiveness, and mix of health services in the practice, or their *progress* in improving health status of the community beyond the practice's own population.

CONCLUSION

COPC in an urban setting, to return to the art metaphor, is an unending process of mosaic and montage building where the mathematical rigors of color field analysis and super-realism may be combined with the value-laden messages of pop and primitive art with arbitrary and shifting frames to capture a meaningful portrait of a community. To paraphrase Maurice Woods, it is better to be approximate and active than precise, perplexed, and paralyzed.

REFERENCES

1. Abramson, J. H., and Kark, S. L. Community oriented primary care: Meaning and scope. In: Connor, E., Mullan, F. (eds.). *Community Oriented Primary Care: New Directions for Health Service Delivery*. Washington, DC: National Academy Press, 1983, p. 21.

2. Nutting, P. A., and Connor, E. M. (eds.). *Community Oriented Primary*

Care: A Practical Assessment, Vol. I. Washington, DC: National Academy Press, 1984.

3. Whitehead, A. N., and Russell, B. *Principia Mathematica*. Cambridge: Cambridge University Press, 1913.

4. Last, E. D. A *Dictionary of Epidemiology*. New York: Oxford University Press, 1983.

5. Kozoll, R. Community oriented primary care: Problem characterization schema — sequentially smaller measurable populations. In: *Community-Oriented Primary Care — From Principle to Practice*. Washington, DC: National Academy Press, 1986.

6. Kark, S. L. *Epidemiology and Community Medicine*. New York: Appleton, 1974.

7. Nutting, P. A., and Connor, E. M. (eds). Montefiore Family Health Center. In: *Community Oriented Primary Care: A Practical Assessment*, Vol. II. Washington, DC: National Academy Press, 1984, p. 115.

8. Strelnick, A. H., and Shonubi, P. A. Integrating community-oriented primary care into training and practice: A view from the Bronx. *Family Medicine*, in press.

CHAPTER 8

The Active Patients in a Clinical Practice: The First Step Toward a Definable Community

David L. Hawk, M.D., M.P.H.
James F. Calvert, M.D.

Busy practitioners considering the use of COPC techniques in their practices may be overwhelmed with the prospects of defining and characterizing their community. Difficulty with the first step may discourage any effort to initiate the program at all. One solution is to begin the COPC process by addressing (as the "community") the active patients in the practice. This initial focus will allow time to gain experience with the process and to engender enthusiasm among fellow practitioners, while concentrating on the traditional scope of responsibility of the practice. Some practitioners may appropriately see the application of the COPC principles to the active population as an extension of their quality assurance program.

After gaining experience with the process, some practitioners may wish to expand their COPC efforts at a later date to include a larger definition of the community. At that point, it will be important to remember, however, that the health problems in the practice population may not be representative of those of the larger community. With this in mind the practitioner can develop proficiency in identifying and addressing health problems in the narrowly defined community of his prac-

tice, and once this proficiency is achieved, apply his expertise to a more broadly defined population, if appropriate, at a later date.

The basic principles of practice analysis, such as describing the composition of the practice, are discussed in this chapter. These are in essence the principles of COPC, applied to a practice population, but in application are somewhat easier to implement. This should leave more energy and time for subsequent activities of developing and monitoring an emphasis program, which may be more rewarding.

GENERAL CONSIDERATIONS

Data collection and organization can be time consuming, tedious, and expensive. Careful planning should go into the decision to allocate resources to develop a practice data base. The difficulty of the task will vary depending on the amount of data kept and the complexity of the analysis desired; such decisions should not be made lightly. The purpose for which the data will be collected should be determined even before the data gathering begins. Otherwise, even the most simple description of an active practice can become a burdensome task. Careful selection of a few key factors can have a greater impact than large amounts of data unanalyzed and of little interest.

It is often best to assign the actual responsibility for collecting data to a nonphysician within the office, such as a billing clerk or receptionist. Some physicians, however, may prefer to be personally involved in data collection because of specific research interests.

DEFINITION OF ACTIVE PATIENTS

The problem of defining a practice population may at first glance seem to be a trivial one. However, it is one of the most complex problems in primary care research. Usually this problem is called the denominator problem. In this sense the numerator would be a subgroup of the practice, such as all obstetric patients within the practice. The practical problems, which many consider insurmountable, in arriving at the practice denominator accurately include the fact that many members of a practice may only very rarely, or even not at all, come in to see the doctor, even though they might identify the practice as their source of care if asked. In addition, in the American system, many of us have several doctors who we have sorted out in various ways and we may in fact be part of several practices. This problem is discussed at length by Norman Hearst in another chapter of this section.

For our purposes, however, we will limit our definition of practice population to what might be considered the active practice population. This definition in itself will inevitably be a controversial one, since there is no uniformly accepted standard, although many practitioners define an active patient as a patient who has had an office visit within the previous 2 years. It should be kept in mind, however, that this is a compromise, and patients who have not been seen in 2 years (or in any chosen time interval) may still consider

themselves as members of the practice.

Many practices use a simple marking or coding system on the outside of the patient's chart which allows rapid identification of inactive patients. For instance, the first time a patient visits in a given year, the color tape for that year is placed on the back of the chart. Thus, if in 1986 the last tape noted on a chart is from 1983 this means that a patient has been inactive for 2 years. Many practices purge inactive charts once a year using this system.

Once inactive charts are removed from the active files, a count of the active charts can then be made. The count of the active charts or patients can be said to represent the number of active patients in the practice.

AGE-SEX REGISTRY

After the active patient count, the age-sex registry is frequently the next information gathered to describe a practice. This registry lists individual patients along with their age and gender data. The data may be stored on index cards kept in a file box for each category. Marginal perforations on the cards can be used to further stratify them within categories. In some cases, it can be helpful to place such lists in a computerized data base. If the practice uses a computerized billing system, often this system can be used to generate an age-sex register with minimal effort; however, care needs to be taken to insure that the lists generated by the billing computers correspond accurately to the preset definition of active patients, with all active patients included and inactive patients purged. Identification of a study sample of patients of a particular age and/or sex allows easy retrieval for further analysis (e.g., immunization review for boys and girls under 2 years of age).

This data set reveals a lot about the practice. Age groupings can be established, and numbers of males and females in each age cell can be determined, as shown for

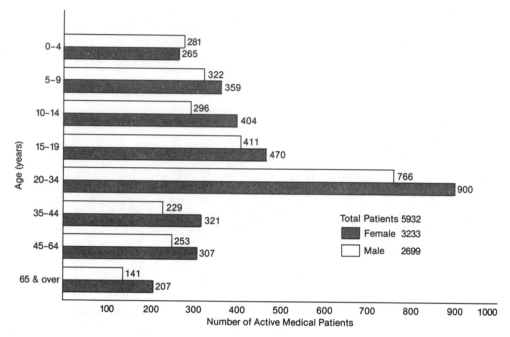

Figure 1. Age–Sex Profile, York Health Corporation, 1985.

a typical practice in Figure 1. The expansion rate of the practice over time can be determined and future personnel or space needs predicted. The clinician can use the list to plan preventive services specific to particular age and gender groups (Pap smears for adult women, home stool occult blood tests for adults 50 years of age and older, or influenza immunizations for the elderly). Finally, the age-sex distribution of the practice can be compared with that of the larger community to suggest underserved groups (e.g., middle-aged males) or groups for which emphasis services may be marketed (e.g., infants, the elderly, etc.)

RACIAL OR ETHNIC DISTRIBUTION

Knowledge of the ethnic makeup of a practice may also enable the clinician to select and plan certain services for the active patients. This data is more difficult to collect than the age-sex registry, since it may be necessary to specifically question

patients on this point. Such data will probably not have been collected for billing purposes, and it may be necessary to obtain it sequentially as patients are seen in the practice. Once the information is collected, however it is done, it can be organized in a manner analogous to the age-sex registry, as shown in Figure 2.

Genetic counseling programs, interpreter needs, determining shifts in racial composition of the practice, and awareness of ethnic attitudes toward health care are a few examples of the advantages of having this information available. Certain medical problems are strongly associated with given ethnic groups; for instance the prevalence of hypertension is increased among black males. Efforts to detect hypertension or followup on known cases might be increased if a large number of black males were noted in a practice. Such efforts would not necessarily need to be limited to the ethnic group identified as being at risk, though in some cases they might be; the point is that a choice of preventive programs to institute might be based on an awareness of the ethnic composition of a practice.

Other enumerated data about the active patients may also be of interest to the clinician, and numerous factors could be selected depending on the diversity of the practice. Religion, education level, occupation, income level, geographic location, and household or family size are examples of data often collected. In a new practice in which COPC is planned, such information can be obtained from each patient as they first contact and register. In established practices patients can be interviewed as they come in for visits or they could be contacted by a mail survey. Alternatively, statistical or demographic techniques could be used to give estimates of some parameters. For instance, in larger cities the census data can provide information about incomes and ethnic composition broken down by census tract, and such information correlated with patient address data.

DIAGNOSIS OR MORBIDITY DATA

The frequency distribution of the various patient problems or diagnoses shared by

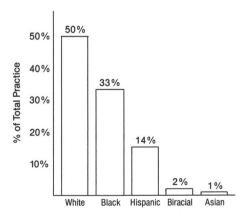

Figure 2. Racial Distribution, York Health Corporation, 1985.

patients can be very helpful to the clinician; this type of information can further define a practice which has previously been stratified by demographic characteristics as noted above. A log of problems managed during each encounter can be maintained by a manual or automated system. In many cases such a log can be created by billing personnel based on the physician's billing diagnosis, or, the practitioners can augment the log themselves as each patient is seen. The data for a period of time is then summarized, as shown in Table 1.

A list of frequently encountered problems may indicate the need for new programs or personnel, or may suggest continuing education topics or audit topics. Logs of patients with common, chronic illnesses such as hypertension, diabetes, or of patients requiring special types of care like prenatal patients can be kept. Protocols can be developed for management of these patients and those who have not received the quality of care desired can be contacted and asked to come in for needed care.

SUMMARY

Practitioners interested in initiating a COPC approach within their practice setting may find it useful to first define the "community" as the active patients of the practice. This provides a workable target population with which to gain familiarity with the activities of COPC. Analysis of the practice population will identify areas for improving the mix and array of services offered, and often raise questions that suggest more detailed epidemiologic questions. The practitioner may wish then to have a look at the larger denominator population, or to coordinate COPC efforts with other providers in the community. The procedures to be followed in expanding this initial definition of community are discussed in subsequent chapters of this section.

TABLE 1. Rank Order of Diagnosis By Frequency
York Health Corporation January through December 1985
Total Diagnoses 13,700

Rank	ICHPPC	Description	Number (% Total)	Cumulative %
1.	V70	Medical Exams	2362 (17.2%)	17.2%
2.	V03	Prophylactic Immunizations	835 (6.1%)	23.3%
3.	460	Upper Respiratory Infection	742 (5.4%)	28.7%
4.	278	Obesity	323 (2.4%)	31.0%
5.	466	Bronchitis	322 (2.3%)	33.3%
6.	401	Hypertension	312 (2.3%)	35.6%
7.	098	Gonorrhea	235 (1.7%)	37.3%
8.	692	Contact & Other Dermatitis NEC	216 (1.6%)	38.9%
9.	3920	Otitis Media	214 (1.6%)	40.5%
10.	V654	Advice & Health Instruction	207 (1.5%)	42.0%
11.	3000	Anxiety Disorder	190 (1.4%)	43.3%
12.	520	Teeth & Support Structure Disease	178 (1.3%)	44.6%
13.	6161	Vaginitis NOS, Vulvitis	171 (1.2%)	45.9%
14.	3051	Tobacco Abuse	170 (1.2%)	47.1%
15.	V01	Contact/Carrier, Inf/Parasit Dis	159 (1.2%)	48.3%
16.	7890	Abdominal Pain	149 (1.1%)	49.4%
17.	V255	Oral Contraceptives	147 (1.1%)	50.4%

CHAPTER 9

Defining a Practice Community: An Approach to COPC for Family Medicine

Paul A. Nutting, M.D.

In many practice settings it can be very difficult to address the health problems of the entire community. In urban areas, the community is often complex, transient, and composed of multiple social and ethnic neighborhoods. Often suburban communities share none of the usual attributes of a community, other than geographic proximity, and continue to seek health care from sources determined in part by location of employment, schools, and shopping patterns. Moreover, most practitioners would be very hesitant to actively assume responsibility for a population that may include patients of another practice.

The COPC process can be applied very appropriately, however, to a "practice community" that consists of the household members of active patients of the practice. An excellent example of addressing a practice community was described in the Institute of Medicine report on COPC (1). The Crow Hill practice defined its community as all members of each household in which any member was an active patient (i.e., they had made contact with the practice within the past 24 months). Based on these criteria, the practice assumed responsibility for a practice community of 2,183 families or 7,280 individuals, many of whom were not active users of the practice. A data system captured a minimal data set on all members of the practice community, collected when a new patient registers with the practice. Use of this data base allowed the practice to define precisely their "practice community," to identify health problems, and to pinpoint high-risk individuals.

The practice community represents a denominator population for which most family physicians feel a professional responsibility, and for which reaching out to offer needed health services is entirely appropriate. A major problem in addressing this population, however, is the lack of an appropriate data base. The data needed to manage a practice community, however, may be more available than is readily apparent. Many practitioners could develop a modest data base on all members of the practice community at the time of patient registration, collecting such items as age, sex, occupation, major health problems, height, weight, and smoking and exercise habits. These data could then be analyzed to pinpoint specific individuals potentially in need of a variety of screening, educational, and therapeutic services.

A growing body of evidence suggests that much of the burden of chronic disease can be reduced by early detection and prevented altogether by changes in personal behaviors. Family medicine is ideally postured to incorporate a variety of health promotion and disease prevention services into its practice. However, family physicians are also well aware that the ailing patient is receptive to a limited body of new information related to his presenting problem but not overly receptive to health education on a separate topic. Consequently, health promotion services are usually deferred to followup visits or reserved for periodic physical examinations. By expanding the scope of these health promotion and disease prevention efforts to all members of the patient's household, the effectiveness of these activities can be enhanced by soliciting family support for changes in the patient's behavior and by encompassing potential risk behaviors of other family members.

The cause of health promotion and disease prevention in the primary care setting can be enhanced by the practice that assumes responsibility for a denominator population. With the modest data base described above, the practitioner can identify specific individuals at risk or with adverse risk profiles for preventable illness. With simple analysis of the data base and a modest outreach effort, important and needed services can be offered to the at-risk individuals in the practice community. For example, listing all individuals over the age of 65 years or individuals with cardiovascular or chronic pulmonary disease can identify a subset of the denominator population potentially at increased risk for complications of influenza. For this subset, the physician could compose a letter outlining the epidemiologic patterns of influenza and the relative protec-

tion afforded by annual immunization. The letter could further indicate that the immunization is available from the practice or could be requested from the patient's usual source of physician care. This modest data base could further be used to identify subsets of the denominator population who would benefit from specific services related to cancer screening (e.g., Papanicolaou smear, mammography, rectal examination, flexible sigmoidoscopy), needed immunizations (e.g., DPT and polio series in children), or health promoting behaviors (e.g., smoking cessation, weight reduction, appropriate exercise patterns). While some physicians would be hesitant to give the impression of "advertising" their services, this problem could be offset by an appropriate expression of concern for the health of all members of the family. Families who indicate a desire not to be approached in this way could easily be "flagged" in the data base and not included in subsequent efforts.

The advent of microprocessor applications to office practice will offer new opportunities to automate a number of the activities required to address health problems of the target population. By linking current data base management and word processing software, the physician can compose health education material and target it on relevant at-risk individuals in the practice community, avoiding much of the labor-intensive cost associated with preparing personalized correspondence and addressing envelopes.

DISCUSSION

The activities inherent in identifying and addressing the health services requirements of a denominator population will be associated with certain marginal costs—those incurred above and beyond the baseline costs of operating the practice. At the same time, however, the process will lead to a marginal improvement in the health status of the denominator population, and an increment in the revenue generated by a fee-for-service practice. The magnitude of these costs, benefits, and revenues are largely unknown, but in a chapter of Part VII, Reed offers a simple approach to estimating the cost of registering and collecting a modest data set on the practice community. In its recent study, the Institute of Medicine study found very little data to suggest the marginal cost and benefit associated with these activities, and virtually no data to describe the change of revenue resulting from the marketing value of the process itself (2). Whether the costs of the activities themselves will be offset by an increase in service demand and revenue generated remains an unanswered, but testable, hypothesis.

REFERENCES

1. Institute of Medicine. *Community-Oriented Primary Care: A Practical Assessment, Vol. II, The Case Studies.* Washington, DC: National Academy Press, 1984.

2. Institute of Medicine. *Community-Oriented Primary Care: A Practical Assessment, Vol. I, The Committee Report.* Washington, DC: National Academy Press, 1984.

CHAPTER 10

The School-Age Community: Addressing a Predefined Population

Frank M. Reed, M.D.

Several of the previous chapters have described particular populations that are easily accessible to the practitioner attempting to initiate a COPC process within their practice. One important approach that can be used by practices in any setting, whether financed under public or private funding sources, involves addressing the health problems of a predefined population. Such populations may take a variety of forms, but one that is easily accessible in any setting is the school population. Depending on the practitioner's interest and the local educational structures and priorities, one might get involved with nursery or preschool programs, elementary schools, or middle and high schools. In any event, most schools have the data necessary to enumerate the school population, and in many cases basic health-related data useful in the early COPC process. Through collaboration with other health-oriented individuals such as public health nurses and school nurses, the school population becomes a logical target community.

Initially, it may be particularly important to develop goals that are mutual priorities. Collaboration and cooperation will be strengthened if the COPC activity also helps the school attain a health-oriented goal. Legally required immunizations for elementary school children, and mandated athletic examinations for secondary school children, offer the potential for COPC activities where collaboration between school and medical practice may help enhance health in the community and assist the local school in complying with local or State statutes. Examples are discussed later in this chapter.

It is also important that the presentation of COPC activities be professional and perceived as appropriate. If the practice is perceived as merely attempting to gain patients, the community will often shun the effort. Furthermore, if there are higher health priorities in the community, COPC activities may be perceived as misguided and inappropriate. For example, if a community considered the establishment of a rescue squad/ambulance service a number one priority, a COPC activity aimed at school-age children could be deemed a premature, low-priority endeavor. On the other hand, it is likely that if the school sees COPC activities in its own best interest, other community agencies can be brought into play with relative ease.

IMMUNIZATIONS

Most States require basic immunizations for all students attending public school, and in many areas schools maintain records on the immunization status of their students. By working with the school a list of students with current immunization status can be obtained. By auditing health records in the practice, comparisons between children registered in the practice and those who are not, and an overall immunization rate for enrolled school-age children can be developed. Subsequent campaigns to encourage immunization either at the public health office or at the practice site can be undertaken, supported through mailings and announcements in local newspapers.

A more sophisticated method involves mailing postcards or making telephone calls to homes of children who are not in compliance, and scheduling followup at a subsequent date. This also provides an opportunity to disseminate information about immunizations, particularly on those topics that have recently become increasingly controversial. Thus general health education may be conducted through such an immunization audit program.

The main deterrent to this type of operation involves the allocation of resources for auditing what is often a large number of records. Computer technology, both in the schools and the medical office, offers the potential for more rapid screening of records, and it is anticipated that before long many schools will have computerized lists of immunization status as well as computerized mailing labels.

ATHLETIC SCREENING

Another area for COPC in the school-age group involves athletic screening. Most States require annual physical evaluations prior to participation in high school sports. By cooperating with the schools, the COPC practice can provide comprehensive sports screening, and this can involve many segments of the professional community, including the medical practice, paramedics and EMTs, and physical therapists, as well as other volunteers from the community. A screening form for such a program is shown in Figure 1. The COPC practice may ask the school to identify the target population (competitive athletes) and then set aside 2 days, perhaps a weekend, for a mass physical screening session, with the various health care segments of the community providing the physicals. Often the school will pay for local advertising in the newspapers, and sometimes newspapers provide free advertising for such events. This approach has the advantage of providing a standardized examination, and if conducted properly it can often predict individuals at risk, decreasing the incidence of serious injury by focusing especially on orthopedic weaknesses. Such a screening examination is illustrated in Figure 1.

If these physicals are performed either at the school or at the medical facility outside regular hours, they can be offered at greatly reduced cost to the community and without regard to whether an athlete is a patient in the practice. The development of suitable record forms in the practice allows information from the examination to be included in the athlete's chart, if the student is an active patient, or the information can be sent to the practice where the athlete normally receives care. With increasing emphasis on sports-oriented medicine, athletic screening can become an increasingly popular, yet relatively simple, activity for COPC.

CONCLUSION

Addressing the school-age community provides an opportunity for the potential COPC practitioner to collaborate with an important community institution and address the health problems of an important subset of the community. For the

Name _____ Grade _____ Date _____

School _____ Date of Birth _____ Age _____ Sex _____

Address _____ Phone Number _____

Sports You Participate In _____

Positions You Play _____

Parents' Names _____

BP _____   P _____   Urine _____   Height _____   Weight _____

Station 1: Previous Medical History (check if problem)

Concussion ____   Glasses/Contacts (hard/soft) ____   Allergies ____
Dental Injuries ____   Asthma ____   Seizures (epilepsy) ____
Diabetes ____   Arrhythmia ____   Hernia ____
Back/Neck Injuries ____   Muscle Injuries ____   Sprains ____
Menstrual Problems ____   Fractures ____   Rheumatic Fever ____
Previous Surgeries and Dates _____
Loss of a Paired Organ _____
Medications _____
Comments:

Station 2: Flexibility (check if problem)

Hamstrings ____   Number on Sit and Reach ____
Piriformis ____   Quads ____   Calf ____
Comments:

Station 3: Percent Body Fat

Sex/Age Dependent = _____ %

Station 4: Range of Motion (check if problem)

Wrist ____   Elbow ____   Hand ____   Shoulder ____
Grip Strength: right ____   left ____
Comments:

Foot ____   Ankle ____   Knee ____   Hip ____
Comments:

Station 5: Quad/Hamstring Strength

	mod. resist. Q/H (4)	max. resist. Q/H (6)
Right		
Left		

Right H/Q ratio ____ %
Left H/Q ratio ____ %
Comments:

Station 6: Vision

Distance Vision: without glasses L ____   R ____
                         with glasses L ____   R ____

Station 7: Heart/Lung (check if problem)

Arrhythmia ____   Murmur ____   Lungs ____
Abdomen ____   Hernia ____
Blood Pressure ____   Resting Pulse ____
Urinalysis ____
Comments:

Station 8: Risks/Recommendations

Figure 1. Reporting Form for Athletic Screening Examination.

practitioner hesitant to define a target population beyond that of the active patients,
the school-age population offers an ideal
starting point. In most communities the
health of this population is an undisputed
priority, and often the school officials welcome the help of a local physician. There
are opportunities to address important
health problems at all grade levels from
preschool through high school. Through
the use of lists developed by the educational system, the COPC practice can
often attain relatively easy access to those
students in need of the particular service.
In addition to providing increased health
care access to school-age children, these
activities facilitate collaborative relationships among agencies providing various
segments of health care throughout the
community and provide a model for evaluating the outcome of COPC activities.

CHAPTER 11

Community Diagnosis:
A Tool for COPC

Thomas M. Mettee, M.D.

Community diagnosis is one of the major components of an operational model of COPC. It specifically represents one of the functional elements whose purpose is to define and characterize the community. This paper presents concepts of community diagnosis and describes a method for community diagnosis that can be used by the office-based primary care physician.

The definition of COPC as presented by the Community Oriented Primary Care Planning Committee of the Institute of Medicine in their report of June 1981 (1) is particularly useful in developing this model. COPC is defined in this report as "an approach to health care delivery that undertakes responsibility for the health of a defined population which is practiced by combining epidemiologic study and social intervention with the clinical care of individual patients, so that the primary care practice itself becomes a community medicine program. Both the individual patient and the community or population are the foci of diagnosis, treatment and ongoing surveillance."

This definition clearly states that in addition to the biomedical knowledge required to carry out clinical care one must incorporate epidemiologic and behavioral science in order to achieve a complete understanding of the community for diagnosis, community cooperation, intervention, and evaluation. The Venn diagram in Figure 1 illustrates these important relationships.

In developing a diagnostic approach using this model it is important to keep in mind that clinical care derives from the basic sciences of biology, chemistry, and physics with their specific application to clinical biological sciences such as genetics, anatomy, microbiology, biochemistry, nutrition, physiology, biophysics, and pathology. *Epidemiology* is rooted in the basic science of mathematics and is clinically applied as one of the community health sciences along with biostatistics, human ecology, and public health practice. The basic *behavioral sciences* include anthropology, psychology, sociology, political science, and economics and have their clinical applications in such fields as demography; human geography; education; applied anthropology, psychology, sociology, and economics; law; and public administration. The basic and clinical fields of knowledge that blend in this model of care are so broad that a

"THE COMMUNITY RESPONSIVE PRACTICE"

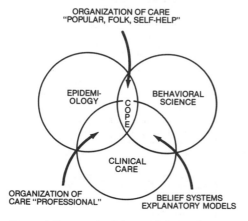

Figure 1. Community-Oriented Primary Care.

single individual could not achieve competence in their integration. Thus a community-oriented primary care *team* is a prerequisite to accomplishing such an indepth understanding.

An example of the application of medical anthroplogy to this model is shown in Figure 1. Arthur Kleinman (2) has made popular the concept of sectors in the health care system, including the professional, popular, and folk sectors. In addition, he has encouraged the use of patients' belief systems and explanatory models in understanding the cultural richness of the phenomenon of illness and recovery. Another example of the application of behavioral science to COPC is represented in Figures 2 and 3.

Abraham Maslow presented his concept of individual self actualization through a hierarchy of needs built upon the physical requirements of nutrition and shelter, which allow for social requirements of inter- and intrapersonal relationships that lead to the integrative and even spiritual level of independence and growth. By borrowing this concept and applying it to the community as if it were the patient, one can construct a "community hierarchy of needs," which is built upon physical factors and protections that lead to social interactions and eventually economic growth and prosperity.

These examples of applied behavioral science serve only to emphasize the importance of considering disciplines beyond the biomedical when developing an understanding of the community for diagnosis.

The etymology of the term *community diagnosis* is helpful in understanding the process. Diagnosis is an action noun that literally means to distinguish, discern, know thoroughly, or perceive asunder. Community derives from the Latin *communis* or fellowship and means a body of people organized around a commonality

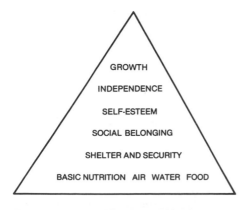

Figure 2. Maslow's Hierarchy of Needs.

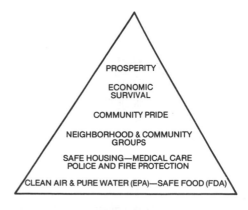

Figure 3. A Community Hierarchy of Needs.

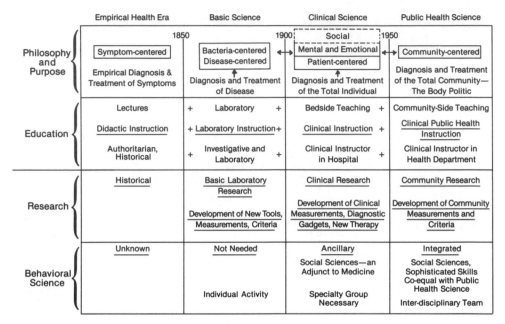

	Empirical Health Era	Basic Science	Clinical Science	Public Health Science
	1850	**1900**	Social **1950**	
Philosophy and Purpose	Symptom-centered	Bacteria-centered Disease-centered ◄─►	Mental and Emotional ◄─► Patient-centered	Community-centered
	Empirical Diagnosis & Treatment of Symptoms	Diagnosis and Treatment of Disease	Diagnosis and Treatment of the Total Individual	Diagnosis and Treatment of the Total Community— The Body Politic
Education	Lectures	+ Laboratory +	Bedside Teaching +	Community-Side Teaching
	Didactic Instruction	+ Laboratory Instruction +	Clinical Instruction +	Clinical Public Health Instruction
	Authoritarian, Historical	+ Investigative and Laboratory +	Clinical Instructor in Hospital +	Clinical Instructor in Health Department
Research	Historical	Basic Laboratory Research	Clinical Research	Community Research
		Development of New Tools, Measurements, Criteria	Development of Clinical Measurements, Diagnostic Gadgets, New Therapy	Development of Community Measurements and Criteria
Behavioral Science	Unknown	Not Needed	Ancillary	Integrated
			Social Sciences—an Adjunct to Medicine	Social Sciences, Sophisticated Skills Co-equal with Public Health Science
		Individual Activity	Specialty Group Necessary	Inter-disciplinary Team

Figure 4. Evolutionary Development of Medical and Health Science.

TABLE 1. Knowledge of the Social Sciences to Diagnose Community Ills

I. Community Economy
II. Social Structure of the Community
III. Cultural Patterns of the Different Groups of the Community
IV. Impact of Cultural, Nutritional, Recreational, Religious, Moral, and Ethnical Patterns Upon Health Practices
V. Community Organization
   a. Power Structure of the Community
   b. Political Structure
   c. Health Laws and Regulations
VI. Community Attitudes that Determine Acceptance or Rejection of Change and Development
VII. Education and Educational Methods
VIII. Mores and Morals that Affect the Growth and Development of Community Consciousness and Community Action

TABLE 2. Knowledge of Epidemiology to Diagnose Community Ills

I. Community Measurements — Demographic Characteristics

II. Biostatistical Techniques of Collection and Analysis of the Data

III. Geographical Base that Determines Isolation, Transportation, and Resources

IV. Sanitary Science: Air, Water, Food

V. Community Mental Health

VI. Techniques to Assess the Early Symptoms of Community Illness (Physical or Mental)

VII. Mass Nutrition

VIII. Mass Disease or Epidemic Phenomena

such as a geographic, political, municipal, social, religious, or even health care entity. Hence, community diagnosis simply means to know thoroughly a body of people who serve as a defined population with something in common. The process involves collecting information, assessing resources and needs, and identifying problems at the community level. It means assessing the community as if it were the patient.

HISTORICAL BASIS OF COMMUNITY DIAGNOSIS

The concept of viewing the community as patient is not new and can be traced in the literature to the mid-1950's with the work of Edward McGavran, Dean of the School of Public Health at the University of North Carolina in Chapel Hill (3). He makes the case that public health is, in fact, the scientific diagnosis and treatment of the community as a patient. He points out the concept is difficult to grasp since it represents a developmental shift from the era of clinical science to the era of public health science. Figure 4, a matrix graph from his 1956 paper, demonstrates the evolutionary development of medical and health science and shows very nicely the need to integrate the behavioral sciences and to use an interdisciplinary team of public health scientists. In addition he identifies eight areas of knowledge of social sciences and eight areas of knowledge of epidemiology that are prerequisites to diagnosing community ills. These areas of knowledge are included in Tables 1 and 2. Thirty years later McGavran's concepts and ideas are grist for the COPC mill.

A PROBLEM-ORIENTED APPROACH

If one is a physician and chooses to view the community as patient, then the clinical methods of individual diagnosis can be applied to community diagnosis. The description of the foregoing concepts

SUBJECTIVE	Qualitative Data (History) Profile of Symptoms Explanation of Problem(s) Perception of Resources
OBJECTIVE	Direct Observations (Signs) Indirect Observations (Quantitative Data)
ASSESSMENT	"The Diagnostic Process"
PROGNOSIS	Knowledge of the Natural History of the Problem
PLAN	Education Intervention Further Data Collection

Figure 5. Outline—The Problem Oriented Clinical Method.

emphasizing basic and clinical sciences and the importance of their integration points out the complexity of the task of community diagnosis and the need for a team approach with multiple inputs. This approach is no different than that used for the complex individual case whose primary physician has received the input of many consultants in order to chart a safe and appropriate course of treatment.

Most physicians are now trained in the problem-oriented clinical method. A brief outline is presented in Figure 5. The only difference in this outline from that originally proposed by Weed is the insertion of *prognosis* between *assessment* and *plan*. Although prognosis is rarely confronted openly, we carry a number of assumptions about the natural history of a disease process if intervention is not undertaken. We no doubt share similar assumptions about a "disease process" in the community even though we may have less knowledge of its natural history. Fundamentally one compares an observed outcome with an expected outcome and attempts to measure the difference. That is the fundamental principle upon which a chi square test is based and thus represents an application of epidemiology to individual and community medicine. Figure 6 presents the SOAP process in a matrix format which compares the individual to the community level of application.

	INDIVIDUAL	COMMUNITY
SUBJECTIVE		
OBJECTIVE		
ASSESSMENT		
PROGNOSIS		
PLAN		

Figure 6. An Individual-Community Problem Oriented Matrix.

If one considers the classifications of *subjective data* that are collected in an individual patient history, the analogy with the community is direct. Both written and oral histories of the community are easily obtained if one has access to senior citizens who have spent most of their lives in the community. The local library and historical society are also excellent resources. Present day community issues (symptoms) are easily identified in media headlines. They are also available through discussion with key informants such as civic leaders or executive officers who serve in the economic and social resources of the community. The office-based physician's patients are a steady resource of information about neighborhoods, schools, churches, pharmacies, and police and fire protection. By putting this information together with data from other sources — churches, pharmacies, police — the physician becomes an ethnographer. Thus the methods of medical anthropology can broaden our conventional approach to the medical history. Therefore, the citizens' explanations of the community problems and their perceptions of community resources to meet those problems are suggested as part of the history or subjective data.

Objective data include both the physical examination and laboratory tests. Direct observations of the natural and man-made resources, barriers, and hazards in the community are best made by using the five senses and touring the community's streets, houses, workplaces, parks, schools, restaurants, stores, and service institutions.

Indirect observations or laboratory tests essentially constitute secondary data. If one has the opportunity to screen a large number of community members, primary data can be collected. Photographs and maps of all sorts as well as data from the United States Census, the local health department, and hospitals are easily obtained and are extremely useful. Figure 7 presents an integrated individual-community problem-oriented matrix that details the application of individual diagnosis to community diagnosis.

USE OF MAPS

Maps of various kinds are extremely useful in understanding the community. A highway or street map is essential for locating addresses. A large wall-size map is especially useful if it is on display for patients to point out the location of their homes or places of business. Zip code maps (phone book, blue pages) are useful for displaying health care utilization data from hospitals or clinics since the locator is an address rather than census tract. Political wards, state legislative districts, and congressional districts represent maps with constantly changing boundaries. Transportation maps showing the routes of the mass transit system provide insight into accessibility of the practice site. The U.S. Geological Society provides topographical maps that carefully identify all landmarks. Even a geologist's chart of the rock formations provides information about underwater aquifers, surface water runoff, earthquake faults, and old river beds. Such data were especially useful in locating the

"A CLASSIFICATION OF INFORMATION"

	INDIVIDUAL	COMMUNITY
SUBJECTIVE QUALITATIVE DATA	"the medical history"	written & oral history of community
PROFILE OF SYMPTOMS	patient symptoms	community symptoms
EXPLANATION OF PROBLEM(S)	patient's explana-tion(s) of illness	community member's explana-tion(s) of problem(s)
PERCEPTION OF RESOURCES	patient's perception of personal resources	community member's percep-tion of community resources
OBJECTIVE DIRECT OBSERVATIONS	physical findings (signs)	observations of. . . —natural & manmade resources barriers & hazards —institutional resources
INDIRECT OBSERVATIONS (QUANTITATIVE DATA)	results of laboratory tests and ancillary investigations	findings from. . . —photographs & maps —data sets
ASSESSMENT "THE DIAGNOSTIC PROCESS"	individual problem & resource list	community problem & resource list
	INTEGRATED ASSESSMENT	
PROGNOSIS KNOWLEDGE OF THE NATURAL HISTORY	—of individuals in health & disease "individual life cycle"	—of communities & cultures in adaptive & maladaptive states "community life cycle"
PLAN —EDUCATION —INTERVENTION —FURTHER DATA COLLECTION	patient education and advice —medications —individual counseling	community education and advice —working with community based providers —programs and jobs

Figure 7. An Individual-Community Problem Oriented Matrix.

source of toxic contamination of drinking water in the Love Canal area. An ethnic map locating clusters of nationality or racial groups may be available from a local university anthropology or urban planning department. Census maps (4) are perhaps the most useful because so much data can be superimposed and displayed. The best example of this is the Urban Atlas published by the United States Bureau of the Census Manpower Administration. It represents the application of computerized geographic files assisted by a laser beam line-following digitizer and displays 12 maps of selected socioeconomic characteristics for 65 standard metropolitan statistical areas (SMSAs). The color shading is nothing short of exquisite! The Users Guide (4) to the 1980 Census of Population and Housing details several map sizes ranging from United States and State SMSA outline maps, to urbanized area, metropolitan, place, county, county subdivision, and census tract outline maps.[1]

A TEAM APPROACH

The collection of community data, especially as broad as has been suggested, may seem overwhelming. However, if the primary care physicians consider themselves as members of a team the problem becomes more manageable. Medical students who participate in an office practice educational activity can be encouraged to carry out brief community projects. Examples of such projects at the Cleveland Metropolitan General Hospital Family Practice Center include: the acquisition and mounting of a three- by five-foot lot line map of our target area; a survey of primary care physicians in the target area; the evaluation of Puerto Rican folk medicine beliefs within the Hispanic community; the identification of all pharmacies within the target area and their hours of operation; the geographic distribution of industrial workplaces in the target areas; the development of nutritional assessment for homebound patients; a patient satisfaction questionnaire; a brief survey of airborne lead monitoring in the target area; an evaluation of the Public Health Department; an assessment of teenage pregnancy; an analysis of sexuality education in the public schools; an assessment of barriers to health care as perceived by eastern European elderly immigrants in one neighborhood of the target area. All of these student projects helped us develop a greater appreciation of the population and improved our ability to serve.

Patients are also helpful in the collection of data. We have asked patients to attend educational conferences specifically to inform us about community history or a specific community problem. Patients together with key informants in the community often provide lively dialogue regarding the cause or treatment of a specific community problem. They are usually very interested in our perceptions, data displays, maps, and diagnosis of the community and gain a new appreciation for community-oriented physicians.

SUMMARY

This chapter has reviewed the concept of Community Diagnosis emphasizing the complex integration of basic and clinical sciences as they apply to clinical care, epidemiology and behavioral science and viewing the community as patient in the SOAP diagnostic process. The use of maps to display diagnostic data is encouraged. A team approach involving students, patients, citizens of the community, and educational institutions is essential for a comprehensive diagnosis.

---

[1] These maps are available through Customer Services (Maps), Data User Services Division, Bureau of the Census, Washington, D.C. 20233 (301) 763-4100.

REFERENCES

1. Institute of Medicine. Report on a meeting of the Community Oriented Primary Care Planning Committee. Washington, DC: National Academy of Sciences, June 1981.

2. Kleinman, A. Concepts and a model for the comparison of medical systems as cultural systems. *Social Science and Medicine* 1978; 12:85.

3. McGavran, E. G. Scientific diagnosis and treatment of the community as a patient. *Journal of the American Medical Association* 1956; 162:723.

4. *User's Guide, Part A Text, 1980 Census of Population and Housing.* Washington, DC: United States Department of Commerce, Bureau of the Census, March 1982, p. 60.

CHAPTER 12

Defining the Practice
Population with Census Data

Robert L. Rhyne, M.D.
Richard Kozoll, M.D., M.P.H.
Brian Stewart, P.A., M.P.H.

Anytime one wishes to express data as a rate, a ratio, or a proportion, defining a denominator is of utmost importance. In the practice of COPC identifying the denominator is the first and most basic step of the entire process. That denominator will then be used throughout the remaining steps and will determine how accurately the problem can be identified and characterized. The methods one must use to determine the denominator are currently being developed, and no single method has been shown to be most effective for accurately defining practice for community denominators.

The methods being developed depend largely on what kind of setting is being considered. The primary care providers in a community can identify their practice service population or the community from which they draw their patients as the denominator population, depending upon whether the health problem under consideration is practice or community based. In rural and geographically well defined areas, the decennial U.S. Census is probably the most complete data source that can be used to calculate denominators. In urban areas and areas where geographic definition of the target population is not

possible, statistical methods and extrapolation techniques using practice data will probably be the most effective means of identifying denominators, but these methods are still being developed and are not at the level of sophistication where practitioners can use them easily.

This chapter is not intended to be an exhaustive review of these methods. It will, however, concentrate on how to use geographic census data and is intended to be an introduction and orientation to the use of the U.S. Census.

CHOOSING AN APPROACH

We will first consider the pros and cons of using census data. Even though the census is collected only every 10 years, it is the best population-based demographic data source and can usually be accessed easily through a local clearinghouse for census data. (Another chapter will discuss the availability and use of these external data sources.) As mentioned earlier, and again here for completeness, the census data are probably best used when the population being defined is rural or can be geographically defined. The success of this approach depends on two things. First, providers must be able to specifically define their practice service areas using the geographic maps associated with the most recent census. And second, the area that defines the denominator population must also be definable using the geographic subdivisions used by the census to collect data. If a denominator population is more easily defined by one of the variables collected by the Census Bureau, i.e., ethnicity or educational level, census data are probably still the best source to use.

The factors that make the census difficult to use are important to keep in mind when using these data. Smaller areas are more difficult to define, and the practitioner must be careful when defining the denominator in these areas. Comparatively larger areas have more data tables generated for them than the smaller areas, and the tables for larger areas are more readily available. Also, more detailed data are collected for larger areas. It is important to remember, when dealing with smaller areas, that certain data may be suppressed in order to protect confidentiality of those living in these areas. Suppression means that certain data are omitted from the reports that are generated from the census because by reporting these data, individuals could potentially be identified. When compiling census denominator data, it is important that the provider ask the agent through which the census is being accessed whether or not data are being suppressed at the particular level that the provider is attempting to define.

Another potential problem when dealing with smaller and less populated areas is sampling error. While some data are collected by the census using 100 percent counts of the population, other data are generated from samples of the population. When dealing with sample data, not 100 percent counts, smaller populations are subject to more statistical sampling error than larger populations. While the extent of this potential error has not been de-

fined, it is important to realize that it could potentially affect the accuracy of the denominator estimate.

Intercensal comparisons are difficult because many of the boundaries used to collect and tabulate census data change between the 10-year counts. This is discussed in greater detail in the following section. When denominators are being defined for years between census counts, the previous census data are not always applicable to the year for which the denominator is being defined. It is difficult to make population projections for years between census counts, and demographic expertise is usually needed to help with these projections.

When theorizing about how geographic denominators can be estimated, the question often arises about how accurate census zip code data are. It seems reasonable that smaller populations could be enumerated geographically by where they receive their mail. The problem is, however, that the census bureau did not report zip code data on their 100 percent counts, and these data are available only on a limited basis. In 1970, zip code data were collected only on limited data sets for metropolitan areas. In 1980, the census bureau planned to produce zip code files as a part of their regular tabulation program, but was forced to cancel those plans due to budgetary constraints. As a result, the zip code data were prepared only as a special tabulation of a sample estimate file, not for the 100 percent tabulations. In future census tabulations, these zip code files may prove to be more useful than in the 1970 or 1980 tabulations.

Another potential problem with using zip code areas is that they do not necessarily coincide with the geographic census areas. Since the 1980 zip code data are estimated using sampling techniques, it is important to cross-check these estimates by comparing them to the 100 percent census counts for the same variables. Further study of these differences is needed. While in subsequent census counts zip code data may be a good way of identifying denominator populations, one must be aware of the limitations involved when using 1980 census zip code data.

When choosing a method to define one's community or practice denominator, extrapolation techniques using practice or multi-practice data must be considered. These techniques are usually based on chart reviews and assume that the practice can identify the active patients who define its current practice population. One method that has been reported (Cherkin et al., JFP, 1984; 19:355) adjusts practice age and sex strata obtained by chart review using standardized data based on the National Health Interview Survey (HIS). The HIS defines health-seeking behavior by age and sex groups that can then be used to estimate the population from which the practice draws its patients. This method assumes that the practice and community populations are similar to that of the national HIS population and that the health-seeking behavior of the primary care practice community is also similar to those of the HIS.

Survey data from multiple practices in a community can be used, but may be difficult to obtain. The records may not be accessible from practice to practice, and the active patient population in these communities may overlap between practices, causing the estimation of the total population to be artificially inflated. This points to the difficulty encountered when trying to define denominator populations in communities with more than one provider. In these middle-sized towns and cities, if the providers cannot geographically define their practice population, the census may not be the best method to use, and one of these extrapolation techniques may be more accurate.

Data sources used to define denominator populations may differ depending on the community and the method used. In one-practice communities, the practice records may more accurately reflect the demographics of the community than the census estimates. In these communities, where most people are registered in the practice, a chart review to define the demographic composition of the community may be more accurate than the potentially undercounted census estimates. We encountered an example of differences in data sources when we attempted to define a denominator for an American Indian population. In this example, the estimates from the 1980 U.S. Census differed from those using the Bureau of Indian Affairs data and the tribal census data by as much as 100 percent. We are currently investigating these differences.

In conclusion, the most accurate method seems to be to use the census when geographically well-defined communities can be identified. It is important to recognize that all methods used to define denominators have yet to be validated and are currently under study. Until these studies are published, it seems most reasonable to use the census if at all possible, because it is the best demographic definition of our population that is available.

ANATOMY OF THE CENSUS

This section briefly outlines the specific geographic units that are used to collect and report U.S. Census data. The reader can use it as a guide when considering which specific units to use in calculating a denominator population. It summarizes a section in Chapter 4 of the *1980 Census Users Guide*, published by the U.S. Department of Commerce, Bureau of the Census. For a more complete description and discussion of the 1980 Census, the reader can refer directly to this *Users Guide*, which can be accessed through most offices where census data are available. It will quickly be seen that this is a complicated subject and that the specific units are not mutually exclusive and many overlap.

Political and governmental areas represent one major category under which data are organized and areas defined. These include States and the District of Columbia, congressional districts, counties, minor civil divisions, incorporated places, American Indian reservations, and election precincts. All these subdivisions have legally prescribed boundaries, powers, and functions.

Statistical and administrative areas represent the other major organizational structure under which data are defined and collected. These areas are not defined by governmental or political boundaries, but are used solely for the organization of data collection and reporting by the census. There are four major census regions (West, South, Northeast, North Central), each containing up to three "divisions" that

are defined by groups of States that are usually contiguous within that division (Figure 1).

Standard metropolitan statistical areas (SMSAs) represent the urban areas in this country and consist of cities of 50,000 or more, plus the counties where the cities are located. In 1970 there were 247 SMSAs across the country, and in 1980 there were 363.

Urbanized areas define urban areas more specifically than SMSAs because they consist of cities and closely relating surrounding territories (suburbs). They are usually determined by the population density in an area and differ from SMSAs in that they do not include rural counties of urban centers (Figure 2). In fact, they usually divide urban from rural areas.

Census county divisions (CCDs) are statistical areas that subdivide counties in States that do not use minor civil divi-

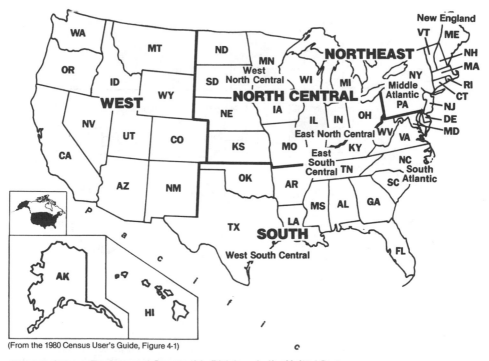

(From the 1980 Census User's Guide, Figure 4-1)

Figure 1. Census Regions and Geographic Divisions in the United States.

Metropolitan

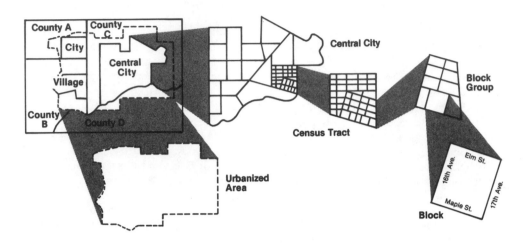

Nonmetropolitan

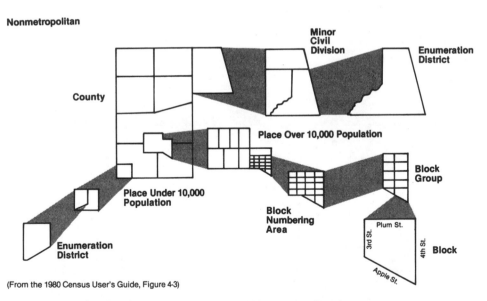

(From the 1980 Census User's Guide, Figure 4-3)

Figure 2. Geographic Hierarchy in Metropolitan and Nonmetropolitan Areas.

sions (MCDs) for statistical data collection. Both CCDs and MCDs are subdivisions of counties and MCDs are usually political or administrative subdivisions of counties, whereas CCDs are purely statis-

tical subdivisions. In 1980, CCDs were defined in 20 States; the remaining States used MCDs (Figure 3).

Census designated places are concentrations of populations that do not legally

These figures illustrate the principal hierarchical or "nesting" relationships among census geographic areas. Note that the hierarchies overlap, e.g., counties are subdivided into MCD's or CCD's (part A), into urban and rural components (part C), and, inside SMSA's, also into census tracts (part B).

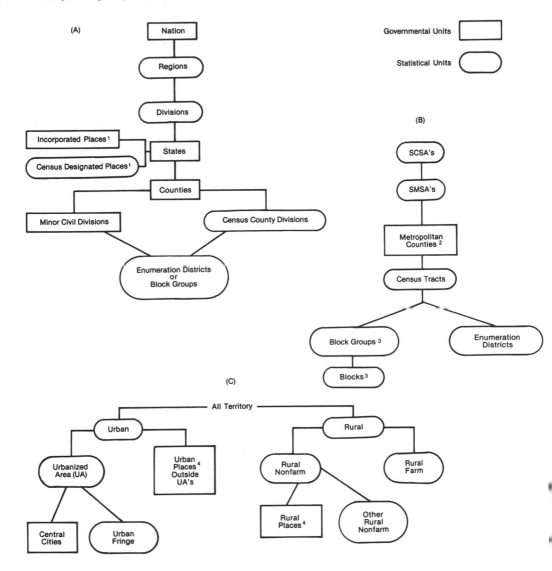

1 Places are not shown in the county, MCD, and CCD hierarchy since places may cross the boundaries of these areas. ED and BG summaries do, however, respect place boundaries.
2 In New England, metropolitan towns (MCD's) and cities replace counties as the components of SMSA's.
3 In SMSA's, blocks and block groups generally cover only the urbanized area and places of 10,000 or more.
4 Includes both incorporated places (governmental units) and census designated places (statistical units).
(From the 1980 Census User's Guide, Figure 4-4.)

Figure 3. Principal Hierarchical Relationships Among Geographic Units.

define corporate limits. In 1970 they were called "unincorporated places." These areas are based on a population density of 1,000 per square mile or greater. In 1970 there were 2,000 census designated places; in 1980 there were 3,000.

Census tracts are statistical areas that consist of approximately 4,000 population. Counties that are defined by SMSAs are subdivided into census tracts. In addition, 252 counties outside SMSAs and five entire States (Delaware, Hawaii, New Jersey, Rhode Island, and Connecticut) are defined by census tracts. These boundaries do not change from census to census and thus provide a consistent geographic boundary from census to census. When the population increases in a census tract, it may be subdivided to make additional census tracts, but the original boundaries are not violated. In 1970 there were 34,600 census tracts; in 1980, there were 43,300. Figure 2 is a pictorial representation of a census tract, and Figure 3 shows how census tracts are related to SMSAs.

Neighborhoods are areas that were defined for the first time in 1980. They consist of sub-areas that are foci of citizen participation. Because they were new in 1980, only those areas that requested to participate are included under this category. This may hold promise for COPC in the future, if these areas are defined throughout the Nation.

Enumeration districts (EDs) were the principal statistical data collection and tabulation units used by the census in 1980. They are the administrative units under which census field operations are organized and average about 600 people each. Because they are census administrative units and are set by local governments, their boundaries usually change between census counts. EDs are used mainly in nonmetropolitan areas (Figure 2).

Block groups are groups of city blocks consisting of about 1,100 population and are the equivalent to EDs in cities, or areas where block statistics are prepared. Because block groups and EDs represent principal data collection units in metropolitan and nonmetropolitan areas respectively, together they cover the entire area of the Nation.

Block numbered areas (BNAs) are groupings of city blocks each assigned a specific number that represents that collection of blocks. BNA's are used in areas where census tracts are not defined (Figure 2).

Blocks are the smallest type of area and consist of approximately 70 population. They are usually rectangular areas that are defined and bounded by four streets. They are defined in all incorporated municipalities with 10,000 or more population.

The geographic units discussed above are used for tabulating and reporting statistical data. The relationship between these geographic units can be seen in Figures 1-3. It is important to note again that these statistical and governmental units overlap and that theoretically 100 percent of the Nation's population can be represented by a combination of these different types of areas.

USE OF CENSUS DATA IN FOUR COPC PRACTICES IN NEW MEXICO

Examples may serve to illustrate how different geographic census units can be used in four different practice settings in the state of New Mexico. At each site the health providers were able to specifically outline the community from which their patient population was drawn; however, for each site, a different geographic census unit was used to most appropriately define the denominator. La Clinica del Pueblo is in a geographically isolated area where there are two towns in close proximity, each served by a different provider. To define the practice's community denominator, enumeration districts were used to compile data. From Table 1, it is evident that this site is rural and over 80 percent Hispanic. The "Other" category under the race variable represents the large number of Hispanic people that do not consider themselves "white."

In compiling the Carrizozo denominator, census county divisions (CCDs) were used (Table 2) because there were no population centers within those CCDs that were not served by that primary care practice. The Gallup denominator, on the other hand, had to be calculated from Block Numbered Areas (Table 3) because the practice is located in a mid-sized town where there are a number of providers. Fortunately, the providers doing the COPC project were able to map their ser-

vice populations geographically within the town. One can see that this mid-sized town is not classified as either rural or urban, but still conforms to the geographic units described above.

Table 4 describes the denominator for an Indian Health Service practice that serves three separate American Indian tribes. Women own the real property in these societies and are thus considered by Western society as the heads of the households or "Female Householders."

PROCESS FOR DEFINING DENOMINATORS USING CENSUS DATA

The steps outlined below can be used as a general guide when one has determined that the census method is the best one to

TABLE 1. Demographic Characterization of La Clinica del Pueblo Service Area (1980 Census)

CHARACTERISTIC	Geographic Census Units (Enumeration Districts)				TOTAL
	678	679	681	682	
POPULATION					
Rural	732	684	107	433	1,956
Urban	0	0	0	0	0
SEX					
Male	352	337	55	229	973
Female	380	347	52	204	983
RACE					
White	510	247	49	149	955
American Indian	1	11	0	0	12
Other	221	426	58	284	989
SPANISH ORIGIN	621	518	77	401	1,617
Mexican	259	102			
Other Spanish	362	416			
Not Spanish	111	166	30	32	339
Percent Hispanic	84.8	75.7	72.0	92.6	82.7
FAMILIES					
Number	178	185	30	93	486
Persons/Family	4.11	3.70	3.57	4.66	4.02

TABLE 2. Demographic Characterization of Carrizozo Health Center Service Area (1980 Census)

CHARACTERISTIC	Geographic Census Units (Census County Divisions)		TOTAL
	010 (Carrizozo)	015 (Corona)	
POPULATION			
Rural	1476	550	2026
Urban	0	0	0
SEX			
Male	743	274	1017
Female	733	276	1009
RACE			
White	1167	453	1620
American Indian	11	1	12
Other	298	96	394
SPANISH ORIGIN	723	151	874
Mexican	359	101	460
Other Spanish	364	50	414
Not Spanish	753	399	1152
Percent Hispanic	49	27.5	43.1
FAMILIES			
Number	386	162	548
Persons/Family	3.37	3.12	
HOUSEHOLDS			
Number	543	199	742
Persons/Household	2.72	2.76	2.73

use to define the COPC denominator population.

Identify and choose a user agency. To gain access to the census and develop expertise in its use, it is advisable to identify a local agency that is responsible for disseminating census data. By working closely with this agency, one can usually obtain assistance in approaching the census. Once the agency has been identified, it is advisable to obtain and read as much of the user's guide as is necessary to complete your project.

Examine and choose geographic units. If one's practice area or community is geographically well defined, census maps can be used to outline those areas. Once out-

lined it usually becomes obvious which geographic census units must be used to define the entire denominator population.

Examine and choose variables of interest. After choosing the geographic units and before going directly to the data, it is advisable to identify which specific variables one is most interested in and can best describe the denominator.

Aggregate data into the largest practical geographic unit. The largest geographic units that define the denominator geographic area are the most practical to use because the data are more complete and detailed for these larger units. One must be sure to avoid the smaller areas if possible, where data may be suppressed for reasons of confidentiality.

Estimate/project population figures to the present date. If one feels the denominator population has changed dramatically since the previous census count, it is important to project population figures to the date of interest. Demographers usually do this by using regression analysis and factoring in fertility, mortality, and migration rates in and out of the area. Methods are currently being developed that will make it easier for the individual provider to estimate these projections.

Narrow the population to fit a specific problem denominator. Once the practice or community denominator is defined by age

and sex, one can then narrow the population to fit the specific problem that the COPC project is targeting. For example, if the project concerns teen pregnancy as the community problem, then the denominator population would be narrowed to include all teens in the area.

CONCLUSIONS AND RECOMMENDATIONS

If providers can describe their service areas or communities in terms of well-defined geographic census units, the census is probably the best method to define COPC denominators. It is the most complete collection of demographic data available, but

TABLE 3. Demographic Characterization of Gallup Family Health Clinic Service Area (1980 Census)

| CHARACTERISTIC | Geographic Census Units | | | TOTAL |
| | Block Numbered Areas (Block Groups) | | | |
	9903 (1,2,3,7)	9904 (1,2,3,6)	9905 (1,2,3,4)	
POPULATION				
Rural	0	0	0	0
Urban	0	0	0	0
Total	2781	2229	2840	7850
SEX				
Male	1318	1126	1398	3842
Female	1463	1103	1442	4008
RACE				
White	1182	744	1676	3602
American Indian	637	303	566	1506
Black	50	53	74	177
Other	921	1129	525	2575
SPANISH ORIGIN				
Mexican	1092	1035	771	2898
Other Spanish	689	424	358	1470
Not Spanish	1000	771	1711	2482
Percent Hispanic	6.40	65.4	39.8	55.6
FAMILIES				
Number	664	516	673	1853
Persons/Family	3.74	3.67	3.80	3.75

TABLE 4. Demographic Characterization of Acoma-Canoncito-Laguna Service Area (1980 Census)

CHARACTERISTIC	ACOMA PUEBLO	CANONCITO RESERVATION	LAGUNA PUEBLO	TOTAL
SEX				
Male	1063	477	1699	3239
Female	1205	492	1865	3562
Total	2268	969	3564	6801
AGE				
under 5	275	124	486	885
5-17	691	345	962	1995
18-64	1104	473	1828	3405
over 65	198	27	288	513
Median	21.3	18.6	23.0	
SOCIETY				
Married Couples	264	137	589	990
Female Householders	95	45	174	314
Persons/Household	4.95	3.85	3.77	

there are drawbacks if the geographic areas are small. This implies that rural areas are most suited to using census data to define denominators. Areas with multiple providers, such as middle-size towns or urban areas, may have to rely on adjustment or statistical methods until new methods are developed. These methods depend on practice data, and it is difficult to correlate multiple practices to calculate denominators. None of these methods has been validated by rigorous population-based survey studies, so at this time, denominator estimation of primary care practice communities is still being developed.

While specific steps can be recommended to providers that will allow them to calculate denominators from census data, individual providers may not have the time, energy, or funds to develop the expertise needed to perform this task. It largely depends on identifying a cooperative user agency through which these data can be identified. We recommend that those who are interested in performing COPC projects find external sources of technical assistance to help them with the important task of identifying appropriate denominators.

CHAPTER 13

The Denominator Problem in Community-Oriented Primary Care

Norman Hearst, M.D., M.P.H.

A key element of community-oriented primary care (COPC) is the application of epidemiologic methods to identify community health problems and to monitor the effectiveness of interventions designed to address these problems. As outlined in the Institute of Medicine model of COPC (1), the first step in this process is to define the community of interest. Identifying the community for a COPC practice may involve geographic, social, ethnic, and political considerations. This chapter, however, concentrates on the epidemiologic aspect of this process: the primary care denominator problem.

The basis of epidemiology is rates: mortality rates, disease rates, utilization rates, etc. A rate, by definition, is derived from a numerator and a denominator, such as infant deaths per 1,000 live births, or known diabetics per 100 female patients age 40-60. Without denominators, it is impossible to calculate rates, and epidemiology is reduced to a simple tally of events.

Suppose, for example, that a clinician in a community clinic has the clinical impression that diabetes is unusually common among his patient population. To test this hypothesis, he organizes a chart review (or perhaps uses his clinic's computer system) and discovers that his clinic has had 600 visits from 250 individuals with diabetes over the past 6 months. Is this high or is it low? While this numerator might be useful in program planning (e.g., deciding whether it would be worthwhile to have a special diabetes clinic), it cannot, by itself, answer the clinician's question.

One denominator the clinician might use is the total number of patient encounters during the same period. Thus, if the clinic had 10,000 patient encounters, he can calculate that 6 percent of all visits were for diabetes. This figure could be compared with other clinics or with national data from the National Ambulatory Care Survey. Such a comparison might be of value, especially if it reveals dramatic differences from what might be expected. However, such a comparison will be affected by many factors other than the prevalence of diabetes in the community. For example, a clinic in a community with a normal prevalence of diabetes might have a higher than expected proportion of patient visits attributed to diabetes for any of the following reasons:

  1. Clinicians in the clinic might see their diabetic patients at more fre-

quent intervals than the national average.

2. Patients might have fewer clinic visits for other diseases (e.g., in an uninsured population that cannot afford visits for less serious problems).

3. Clinicians in the clinic might have diagnostic or coding criteria that cause them to attribute more visits to diabetes. For example, they may be in the habit of coding visits for multiple problems (such as diabetes and hypertension) under diabetes.

4. Clinic patients might have a different age distribution than the national average. For example, a family planning clinic would be expected to have far fewer visits for diabetes than a clinic for the elderly. This problem can be avoided by making age-adjusted or age-specific comparisons.

What the clinician would really like to know is the prevalence of diabetes in the community that his clinic serves. If the clinic defines its community in geographic terms, the denominator can usually be obtained from the census. The problem here, however, becomes the numerator. Unless the clinic is really the only source of medical care for this population, such as in an isolated rural area, it is impossible to obtain accurate numerators from clinic data (i.e., some diabetics will receive treatment elsewhere). A survey or some other community-wide data source would be necessary. Our findings from a survey in a small town in California's Central Valley with a community clinic as its only medical care provider were that only 13 percent of the community identified this clinic as their main source of medical care. The rest traveled 30 miles or more to receive their medical care in larger neighboring cities. The situation is even

more complicated in urban areas where multiple sources of medical care may be available and where people using a community clinic (or any other single provider) probably differ in important ways from the rest of the community.

What, then, is the appropriate denominator for our clinician to use? He knows that 250 individuals have been seen for diabetes in 6 months, which is probably a good estimate of the number of known diabetics being served by his clinic. The appropriate denominator to go with this numerator would be the total number of all patients being served by the clinic. This is often referred to as the *practice population*.

In some settings, the size of a clinic's practice population may be accurately known. In England, for example, each general practitioner has a roster of individuals for whose care he is responsible. A similar situation exists in some health maintenance organizations in the United States. But for most practices in this country, it is impossible to determine an exact practice population. Instead, various methods can be used to estimate it.

The most time-honored method is the patient registry, in which a practice maintains a roster of its individual patients. Such registries are notoriously difficult to maintain, but clinics that have computerized billing systems can often retrieve the same information from their computer, if data has been stored by individual (rather than, for example, by billing unit). Such a clinic might construct a list of its *attending patients* (those seen within the last year). This might serve as a denominator of sorts; the problem is that many patients who are a part of the practice population (i.e., who consider the clinic their source of medical care, and who would use the clinic if they had diabetes) may pass a year or more without seeking medical attention. In England, where the number of nonattending patients is known, the percentage of registered patients with no visits in one year varies among practices from 23 percent to 69 percent (2). Using *visiting patients* instead (those seen within the past 2 years) will include a higher percentage of the patients in the practice population, but will also include more people who have died, moved away, or changed their source of medical care.

Patient registries (or computer systems) are thus unable to give an exact denominator because they cannot count the number of nonattending patients. To address this problem, statistical methods have been developed over the past decade to use information about patients who do attend to make projections about the number of nonattenders. These methods share the assumption that within a given practice, the number of visits (or, in some cases, the number of new illnesses) of individuals follows a predictable mathematical distribution. Thus the number of patients with 1, 2, 3, etc. visits (or illnesses) defines the shape of a curve that can be extrapolated backwards to give an estimate of the number of patients with zero visits. Several mathematical models for doing this have been proposed; the two that have received the most attention are the negative binomial method (2) and the quadratic odds estimator method (3).

When tested on practices in England, where the number of patients with zero visits is known, the negative binomial method has had mixed success (2). Clearly it works better than simply guessing at the number of nonattenders in a practice; still, its projections are sometimes off by 30 percent or more. We have tested both methods on a registered population of 8,781 Kaiser patients in the San Francisco Bay Area. In the Kaiser population, which had an unusually low percentage of nonattenders (only 18 percent with no visits during the year), both methods tended to overestimate the number of

nonattenders, with the negative binomial method giving somewhat lower, and therefore more accurate, projections. The best results came from the negative binomial method, based upon the distribution for the number of new illnesses. Table 1 and Figures 1 and 2 summarize our results. When patients were separated by age and sex, denominator projections based on these smaller groups were often highly inaccurate.

TABLE 1: Result of Denominator Projection Methods in Kaiser Population (Total number of patients: 8781)

Estimates based on number of visits:	
Actual non-attenders	1600
Projected non-attenders	
Negative binomial method	1983
Quadratic odds estimator method	2059
Estimates based on number of new diagnoses:	
Actual number with no new diagnoses	2619
Projected number with no new diagnoses	
Negative binomial method	2861
Quadratic odds estimator method	3506

At present, these complex mathematical techniques require a moderate degree of programming skill and access to a mainframe computer. However, it is possible that software packages might eventually become available with which to add this capability to clinic microcomputers. Meanwhile, a simpler method, based on national figures for the percentage of people in different age and sex groups who have seen a doctor within the past two years, has been proposed (4). This alter-

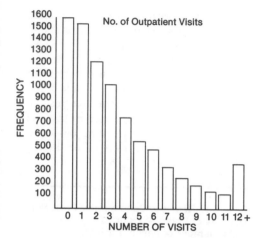

Figure 1. Distribution of Illness-Related Outpatient Visits in One Year Among 8,781 Patients of the Kaiser-Permanente Health Plan in the San Francisco Bay Area, 1979–1980.

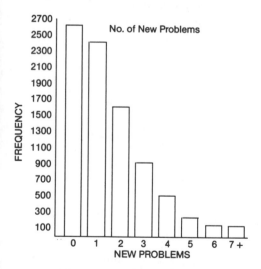

Figure 2. Distribution of Newly Made Diagnoses in One Year Among 8,781 Patients of the Kaiser-Permanente Health Plan in the San Francisco Bay Area, 1979–1980.

native method, while indeed simpler, has had disappointing results when tested on practices in England and Denmark (2).

In addition to the mathematical question of how well these models fit in regis-

tered populations, there remains a theoretical question of what their meaning is in a population that is free to seek medical care from numerous providers. Which nonattending patients should be counted in the practice population? Even if one could ask everyone in a community where they would go if they got sick tomorrow, some people might honestly not know. Others might go to their local community clinic if they got a cough, but would go to a chiropractor for a backache, or the emergency room for a lacerated finger. Thus a clinic's true denominator might be different for each disease. One further caveat is worth noting regarding the use of clinic data to estimate incidence or prevalence rates. Diabetes was used as an example because it is reasonable to assume that most known diabetics will have at least one visit for this problem in any 6-month period. Thus the 250 patients seen by the clinic is probably a good estimate of the number of known diabetics served by the clinic. This same assumption would not be reasonable in acute conditions for which patients might not always seek medical care, such as self-limiting infections, or in chronic conditions that do not always result in frequent clinic visits, such as arthritis. Clinic records can only give the frequency of *patient visits* for a given problem, which is not necessarily a true incidence or prevalence of the condition in the clinic's practice population. How close these numbers are likely to be will depend on the specific disease entity being examined.

We still haven't answered our clinician's question of what denominator he should use to calculate the prevalence of diabetes in his practice population. Unfortunately, there is no perfect answer, which is why the denominator problem remains a problem. Perhaps the best he can do for now is to use the clinic's roster of attending patients plus a fudge factor of about 30 percent to account for nonattenders (this might be adjusted based on the practice population's demographics and their barriers to receiving medical care). Or, if he has access to more expertise and has the time and energy to do so, he might consider using one of the projection methods to better estimate the number of nonattenders. In either case, it is essential to interpret resulting disease rates in the context of the age, sex, and ethnic distribution of the clinic's patient population.

Unless a better solution is found, the denominator problem will continue to limit the precision of the epidemiologic information that can be obtained from most practices in our present health care delivery system. Combined with the wide confidence intervals resulting from the small numbers of patients in most practices, this imprecision makes it difficult to document unusual health problems in a specific practice unless disease rates are substantially different from what might be expected. Indeed, it will often be impossible for individual COPC practices to identify their community's health problems using strict epidemiologic criteria applied to information gathered from their own practice; techniques such as synthetic estimation or nominal group process may be more realistic alternatives. An understanding of the denominator problem, while providing no easy solutions, can help a COPC practice to choose the best method for identifying the health problems of its community and to interpret and use available data more appropriately.

REFERENCES

1. Institute of Medicine, Division of Health Care Services. *Community-Oriented Primary Care: A Practical Assessment.* Washington, DC: National Academy Press, 1984.

2. Kilpatrick, S.J. Indirect estimation of non-attending patients using the negative binomial. In: *Primary Care Research*, Kilpatrick, S.J. and Boyle, R.M. (eds.). New York: Praeger Publishers, 1984, p. 41.

3. Smith, B.W.H., and Erickson, R.V. Solving the denominator problem in primary care epidemiology: six methods. Paper presented at the 1984 meeting of the North American Primary Care Research Group.

4. Cherkin, D.C.; Berg, A.O.; and Phillips, W.R. In search of a solution to the primary care denominator problem. *Journal of Family Practice* 1982; 14: 301.

CHAPTER 14

A Sampling Method
for Defining Community
in a Metropolitan Area

Stephen Zyzanski, Ph.D.
Sim S. Galazka, M.D.

The first step in the process of developing a community-oriented practice is to develop an operational definition of community served by the individual practice. Community can be understood from three different perspectives, as territory or space, as group membership, or as a set of social structures and organizations (1). While each perspective may be most appropriate for a given practice, a geographic definition often provides a clear picture of the population group to which the practice's services can be directed.

Several different criteria have been used to define a geographic community. One criterion that has been tried in metropolitan areas uses driving time or physical distance to the practice to define an area for targeting services (2). Other strategies are based on natural boundaries such as rivers, industrial areas, or wooded regions, while others arbitrarily define the community by applying specific street or community boundaries. Finally, the community can be defined as the geographic area bounding the locations of the residences of the patients who use the practice for their health care. This chapter will describe the latter approach and present a practical, accurate, and time-conservative method

for identifying the practice "community."

Four steps are required in this approach to defining the practice community:

1. A sample of the practice population is obtained.

2. Information from the sample, i.e., age, sex, address, is noted.

3. Addresses from the sample are plotted on a zip code map.

4. The distribution of the sample is compared with that of the general community.

DETERMINING SAMPLE SIZE

In order to draw a sample of patients from the practice, decisions must be made as to the number of patients to include in the sample, the criteria to be used in defining an active practice patient, as well as the method to be used to draw the sample. Any method used should be simple and time saving if it is to be practically applied in a busy practice.

The sample size is a prime determinant of the accuracy of the information obtained. Data gathered from an urban, Midwestern teaching practice will be used to help decide the number of patients' charts to include in the sample. Figure 1 illustrates the precision or efficiency of estimating the true mean age for a practice population of over 9,000 individuals. For each sample size, from 25 to 600, drawn from the practice, a 95 percent confidence interval was computed. This interval is a measure of the accuracy of the sample mean age when compared with the true practice mean age of 23 years.

As can be seen from Figure 1, as samples of larger size are drawn from this population, the confidence intervals become smaller and the precision or efficiency becomes greater. The general trend is for the confidence interval to decrease by half every time the sample size is quadrupled. For example, the confidence interval for N = 25 is from 15 to 31 years, an interval of 16 years. When the sample size is 100 (N = 100), the interval is 19-27 years, an interval of 8.0 years. When the sample size is increased to N = 400, the interval is again reduced by half from 21-25 years, an interval of 4.0 years. For the clinician trying to determine an appropriate sample size from which to define the practice community, Figure 1 illustrates two important points. First, to increase the precision to very high levels requires very large samples. Using the

quadruple rule to obtain a sample practice mean age with a confidence interval of 2 years would require that 1,600 charts be sampled. Second, the general shape of the curves connecting the upper and lower confidence interval points indicates that the level of precision tapers off markedly between sample sizes of 100 to 200 and that further improvement is at the cost of much larger increases in sample size.

To ensure that this approach holds for categorical variables such as sex, this same process was used to assess the percent of the patients who were female in the practice. The standard error of a proportion was used to estimate the precision and to compute confidence intervals for the same sample sizes as in Figure 1. The curves obtained for this categorical variable were comparable in shape to those for mean age. For samples between 100-200 the level of precision similarly tapers off. Thus, for either continuous characteristics such as age, or for categorical ones, such as sex, a sample size of N = 150-200 provides a level of accuracy that is adequate for many purposes. For purposes of defining the practice community, a sample size of 150-200 will provide accurate demographic information

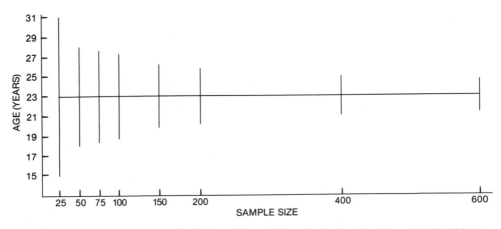

Figure 1. 95% Confidence Intervals for Selected Sample Sizes for the Practice Mean Age of 23 Years.

about the practice population for use in decisionmaking, without requiring the time and money necessary to work with larger sample sizes. Thus a sample of 150-200 charts can be drawn from any size practice and provide a relatively good level of precision.

DRAWING A SAMPLE

Once the sample size has been decided, the method for drawing the sample of practice charts must be determined. The method that ensures the greatest likelihood of a representative sample is a random selection. However, if the number of total practice charts is large, selecting a sample at random would require a numerical count of the charts as a part of the process. This time-consuming process may lead to total abandonment of the project in some cases, and to miscounting in others. An alternative to a purely random selection is to draw a systematic sample with a random start. To use this approach, an estimate of the total number of charts in the practice must be obtained. This can be done by computer if billing information is computerized. Alternatively, a rough estimate can be obtained by counting the charts on a single shelf and then multiplying by the number of shelves. An exact number is not essential. In fact, an underestimate will result in the drawing of a slightly larger sample, and the oversampling will ensure that the desired sample size will be achieved after charts that do not meet selection criteria are rejected.

Next, a sampling fraction is computed by dividing the estimated number of charts by the desired sample size. For an estimated chart number of 3,000 and a desired sample size of 150 charts, the sampling fraction is 3,000/150 or 20. Thus every 20th chart out of a total of 3,000 would need to be selected to have a sample of 150 upon completion. However, a certain number of charts will not meet the criteria defining an active patient. Some

charts may reflect patients who have died, moved, or not been in the office in years. Hence it is prudent to overestimate the desired sample size by 10 to 20 percent. A 10 percent increase in the sample size of the above example would require that 165 rather than 150 charts be initially chosen. Thus, 3,000/165 = 18, or every 18th rather than 20th chart is to be selected.

Next, a random number table is used to select a number at random between 1 and 18. For example if the random number selected from the table is 12, then the 12th chart and every 18th chart after that would be selected. Thus the selection would begin with the 12th chart on the first shelf followed by the 30th, then the 48th, 66th, 84th, etc., until the entire set of practice charts has been scanned. This process would produce at least 165 charts and perhaps a few more or a few less depending on whether the total practice chart estimate was high or low.

Once the first chart has been selected, it must be reviewed to determine whether it meets inclusion or exclusion criteria for the study. Excluded charts might include patients dropped or transferred from the practice, patients who have moved out of the area, and patients not seen in the office for a long time. For example "active patients" might be defined as patients who have been seen in the office within the last 2 years. In general the number and type of inclusion and exclusion criteria will vary depending upon the interests and intent of the individual practice.

EXTRACTING INFORMATION

Having defined the charts within the sample, the next step is to decide upon the information to be extracted from each chart. A minimum data base should include the following from each chart: address, zip code, age, sex, and date of the last visit. This data set allows each patient's residence to be located by zip code. This can be used to develop a geographic definition of the practice community. The address facilitates conversion of the patient's zip code to a census tract, enabling the use of the extensive descriptive data of the census to describe this community. In addition, an age/sex profile of the practice population is obtained. This is useful in designing services as well as for comparison with the surrounding community to determine how well the practice population represents the general community. The date of the last office visit can be used to examine whether active and inactive patients differ in important ways. Although this minimum set of variables provides a great deal of information, the practicing physician may wish to add other variables of interest. These may include items such as marital status, race, education, payment modality etc. The nature and size of the data base will vary depending on the interests of the practice and the availability of the information.

DEFINING THE PRACTICE COMMUNITY

The information obtained through the sampling process can be used to define and describe the practice population. The easiest way to proceed in developing a geographic definition of community for the practice is to list all of the separate zip codes for the patients in the sample and count the number of patients in each zip code. A scatter plot of this distribution can often present a useful visual display of this information. For the urban teaching practice used as an example, a sample of N = 149 charts were drawn which met the inclusion criteria of being valid and active patients. Figure 2 illustrates the distribution of the 29 zip codes listed in the sample. As shown, many zip codes are represented by only a few individuals. One strategy for defining the practice community is to select only those zip codes that represent at least 80 percent of the sample.

For the zip codes in Figure 2, the top 12 zip codes account for 85 percent of the sample selected, and the remainder of the zip codes are uniformly represented by a small number of patients. With a sample of 149, some errors in selecting zip codes could be expected, depending on how the sample was drawn and how representative it was of the true practice population. However, two different samples of 150 were drawn for this practice, one based on inclusion criteria of visits within the past 5 years and the other including only patients seen in the office within 2 years. Although the order differed in the two samples, the identical 12 zip codes were identified in both samples, accounting for 84 percent and 85 percent of the total sample respectively.

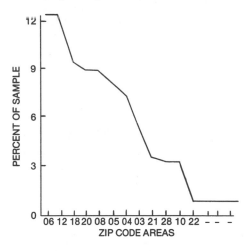

Figure 2. Distribution of Sample Patients by Zip Codes.

The next step in defining the geographic community for the practice is to display the zip code area as a map. The simplest method for developing this map is to trace the geographic area using the zip code map found in the local telephone directory. Tracing out the geographic area of the identified zip codes provides both visual and street boundaries for defining the practice community. The experience of the practice staff can be used to confirm the geographic area displayed. It should make sense. If it does not, then the sample size may have been too small or unrepresentative to include appropriate areas. A second sample of additional charts, following a similar procedure as related above, would likely resolve the inconsistency.

COMPARISONS WITH THE GENERAL POPULATION

The final step in defining the practice community is a comparative and descriptive one. This involved step is addressed in detail in the next chapter. However, two very important descriptions should be computed and contrasted at this point. First, for the zip code areas retained, the number of charts in each should be represented as a percentage of the total retained charts. This represents the "observed" percent of the defined community residing in each zip code. The next step is to locate

a census tract map of the area or a table indicating the number of census tracts in each zip code area. These are readily available at many public libraries. This information can be used to convert the zip code areas to census tracts. Then, census data can be used to describe the populations living in the census tracts in the practice community. When summed for each zip code and divided by the total population for the defined community, determined from the census data, an "expected" percent of the zip code areas can be calculated. This process is illustrated in Table 1 for the defined community. For example, 18 of the 126 charts comprising 85 percent of the sample were from zip code area 06. Thus, 18/126 or 14.3 percent of the sample practice charts were from zip code 06. Similarly, from the 1980 census figures, 41,860 out of a total of 517,643 persons living in the total area, live in zip code 06. The percent of the total, living in area 06 is then 41,860/ 517,643 or 8.1 percent.

TABLE 1: Practice vs Community Comparisons

ZIP CODE	#TRACTS	OBSERVED % OF PRACTICE	POPULATION	EXPECTED % OF PRACTICE	% OVER/ UNDER EXP
44106	15	14.5%	41,860	8.1%	+79%
44112	10	14.3%	40,020	7.7%	+85%
44118	12	11.1%	45,032	8.7%	+28%
44120	11	10.4%	54,519	10.5%	− 1%
44108	12	10.2%	46,608	9.0%	+14%
44105	23	9.4%	68,045	13.1%	−29%
44104	20	8.5%	42,428	8.2%	+ 3%
44103	21	6.4%	38,108	7.4%	−14%
44121	7	5.0%	42,594	8.2%	−40%
44128	9	4.2%	38,673	6.8%	−38%
44110	7	3.9%	29,756	5.8%	−32%
44122	7	2.1%	37,010	6.5%	−67%
TOTALS	155	100.0%	517,643	100.0%	

This example raises an additional point for individuals using this method of sampling to define and describe the practice population. In this example the selection of only those zip codes comprising 85 percent of the sample results in a decrease in the working sample size from the original sample size of N = 149 to a new sample size of N = 126. In order to maintain the actual working sample at about N = 150, a strong recommendation, the initial sample of charts should be increased appropriately. This reinforces the need to oversample in order to obtain the number of charts necessary to achieve a given confidence interval (Figure 1). If one assumes a 10 percent loss due to some patients not meeting study criteria, and a 15 percent loss due to infrequent zip code selections, then a 25 percent oversampling would be required to maintain a working sample at the pre-assigned level. Applied to the sample cited here, one would need to select N = 188 charts to be more certain that approximately 150 valid charts would be available for further analysis in describing the practice population and comparing it with the general community.

The most interesting comparison in Table 1 is a contrast of the percentage of the practice coming from each zip code area (the "observed" percent), with the percentage of the total area population living in each zip code area (the "expected" percent). If the practice population was representative of the community it serves, a logical relationship between the two percentages would be anticipated. The most logical relationship for a primary care practice would be to expect greater numbers of patients coming from zip code areas closer to the practice site and below expected numbers from areas which are farther from the practice site. Figure 3 is a visual representation of the data in the last column of Table 1 contrasting the "observed" and "expected" percentages for the twelve zip code areas.

Except for zip code area 12, the heaviest concentration of patients comes from the zip code area in which the family practice center resides. The immediately surrounding areas are drawing at expected levels and the more geographically distanced areas are drawing less. Zip code area 12 had the greatest number of patients over expected. This area contains a major traffic artery which serves as an access point to the practice site and the physicians and staff agreed with this and other findings. Comparison of the "observed" population with the "expected" population provides information which can highlight areas where the practice services have not penetrated and are useful in the planning process. In addition, the information in Figure 3 can be used to define a "core community" or neighborhood for this

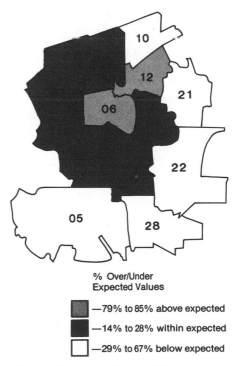

% Over/Under
Expected Values

[shaded] —79% to 85% above expected

[black] —14% to 28% within expected

[white] —29% to 67% below expected

Figure 3. Contrast of Observed Practice Population with Expected Community Population.

practice. Such an area would include zip code areas 03, 04, 06, 08, 12, 18, and 20.

Once a geographic community has been defined for a practice, one can, at a minimum, display by quartiles, the age and sex distribution of the practice. This can be contrasted with the age and sex distributions of the community. Major discrepancies can be used for future planning of practice services, e.g., to specific groups such as the elderly, or to new areas as in the development of services for an underserved area. This paper has focused on illustrating a simple cost-effective technique for defining the community served by an active practice in a metropolitan area. The following paper will illustrate the value of this geographically defined area in the process of describing this population as the next step in developing and planning a community-oriented primary care practice.

REFERENCES

1. Keith, R.J. *Old People New Lives*. Chicago: University of Chicago Press, 1977.

2. Lubin, J.W.; Reed, I.M.; Worstell, G.L. et al. How distance affects physician activity. *Modern Hospital* 1966; 107:80.

CHAPTER 15

How Representative
Is Your Practice Population
of the Community?

Sim S. Galazka, M.D.
Stephen Zyzanski, Ph.D.

The process of developing a community-oriented practice requires the clinician to discover descriptors of the community. Descriptors can be thought of as information that contributes toward the development of a meaningful and workable conceptualization and operationalization of the community (1). Examples of descriptors that can be useful in developing a community-oriented practice include impressions and perceptions of community members, impressions and perceptions of nonmembers or outsiders, as well as statistical indicator data derived from sources such as the United States Bureau of the Census and other public and private organizations.

Development of accurate descriptors of the community is a key to the accurate definition of community health, resources, and problems. Conversely, inaccurate input leads to inaccurate conclusions, and thus to actions in the name of community-oriented practice that may be inappropriate.

Information to describe a community may be derived from impressions and beliefs of members and nonmembers as well as from statistical data from various sources. This paper focuses specifically on the use of statistical indicator data as descriptors of community and on their use in comparing the practice population with the general community served by the practice. This type of comparison provides an index of how well the practice population represents the general community.

Describing the similarities and differences between these two population groups aids in the discovery of "hidden cohorts" within the general population not served by the practice and not immediately evident upon casual analysis. For example, an urban practice serving a predominantly black community found that its population was more heavily female than the general community. The black male population can be considered as a community group deserving further investigation as to health, illness, morbidity, mortality, and patterns of resort.

The methodology for determining how well the practice population represents the general community can be found within the basic precepts of epidemiology. Cohort analysis is the process of understanding morbidity and mortality in a group of persons who share a common experience within a defined time period (2). In analyzing a cohort, information can be displayed as a fraction, whose numerator is the number of cases and whose denominator is the total population at risk. This approach can be used in comparing the practice with the general community by comparing descriptors of the practice with similar descriptors of the general community. We will use three basic descriptors, age, sex, and location of residence to illustrate this technique.

METHODS OF COMPARISON

Defining Community

Developing a comparison between the practice population and the general community using statistical indicator data requires that a specific geographic area be designated as "community" for the practice. There are many methods to achieve this task, a number of which have been enumerated in previous chapters in this Section. The method described here to define the geographic practice community is especially appropriate for established practices. The strategy used to define the practice community was presented in the previous chapter and involves examining the actual practice composition and defining community from the locations of the residences of the patients. Once this step is complete, the process of describing the practice and community populations can begin.

Designating Descriptors

The next step requires the designation of a specific set of descriptors to be used in the comparison. A wealth of descriptors is available to describe the general community as defined in the previous step. Information from the United States Census Bureau provides a ready source of information about the general community and is available through public libraries or local planning agencies. Other sources of information that may prove useful include local health department vital statistics offices,

police and safety departments, and private foundations.

The sheer volume of available data can be overwhelming. Methods for limiting and refining this information have been developed (3). Usually, the variables used to develop a comparison between the practice population and the general community will be limited by the descriptors available for the practice population. The average practitioner interested in developing a community-oriented practice will either collect prospective data on the practice population that fits the designated descriptors, or will use descriptors currently collected and available in the practice. Prospective collection of a set of defined descriptors has the advantage of specificity and accuracy, but has the disadvantage of requiring a lengthy period of time (years). The use of data readily available in the practice is more time efficient but is limited to the information collected by the practice for other reasons, such as billing. Three variables available to most practices are age, sex, and location of residence of practice members. Other descriptors that can be used include income levels, race, ethnicity, occupation, and marital status.

Collecting the Data

The simple sampling technique discussed in the previous chapter can be used to measure the descriptors (variables) in the practice population. Display of this information along with data about the general population using mapping techniques rather than as tabular data facilitates a comparison between the practice and general populations. The following examples illustrate this process as applied to one urban community:

Age. Figure 1 illustrates a defined geographic community in which reside over 85 percent of the members of a sample of N = 149 active patients from an urban family practice center. The areas displayed

84

are zip code areas derived from a map in the phone book. The location of the practice is indicated by the black dot. The community defined by these 12 zip codes contained a population of 517,643 individuals in the 1980 census. The mean age for the population residing in this area is 31 years, compared with the mean age of

23 years for the patients of the family practice center. The difference of 8 years indicates that the practice population is heavily represented by young adults and children.

This age comparison can be further developed by contrasting the geographic distributions of the practice and community populations for extremes of age. To illustrate the comparison, data on two specific groups, the young and the old, are displayed. In Figure 2, the map on the right shows the distribution of the children in a sample of the practice (N = 149) age 5 years or less. This can be compared with the map on the left that shows the distribution of children in the general community derived from the 1980 census. The youth of the practice and the general community are displayed by plotting their respective distributions in quartiles. For the practice, the percent of the population 5 years old or under varies from 0 to 40 percent in any given area. For the general community, the percent of the population in this age group varies from 3.6 to

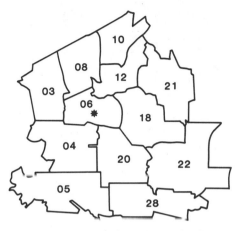

Figure 1. Community for an Urban Family Practice Center.

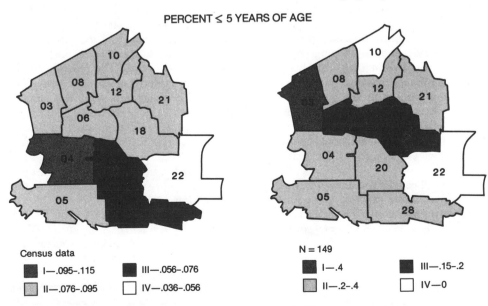

PERCENT ≤ 5 YEARS OF AGE

Census data

I—.095–.115   III—.056–.076

II—.076–.095   IV—.036–.056

N = 149

I—.4   III—.15–.2

II—.2–.4   IV—0

Figure 2. Comparison of Practice and Community Children 5 Years and Younger.

11.5 percent. The general distribution of the practice population seems to reflect the community distribution as a whole, with the exception of area 10, where the practice sample had no children. This represents a two quartile difference. Though this may reflect small sample variation, this information may indicate that children from this area are receiving care from sources other than the practice center. As mentioned earlier, data used for purposes of comparison may be limited by available practice data.

If indicators of socioeconomic status are not available for the practice population, useful comparisons can occasionally be made from community data alone. Figure 3 illustrates the distribution of individuals covered by Medicaid services in the general community. This map correlates well with the map showing the distribution of children 5 years or younger for the practice and the community. Note the smaller percent of Medicaid recipients in area 10 surrounded by areas with the highest percent. This information leads to the hypothesis that there may be a correlation between children and poverty within the practice community that should be further considered in developing services. Based on this information, this practice plays a significant role in care to children and young families in the general community. Attention to needs assessment, quality assurance, and program refinement for these individuals should continue to provide a major focus for practice activities.

Figure 4 provides a comparison of the distribution of the practice and community elderly populations. The practice population is especially underrepresented by patients in the older age groups when compared with the community population. For the majority of zip code areas illustrated in Figure 4, there were no elderly individuals represented in the practice sample. Zip code area 10 was the only area in

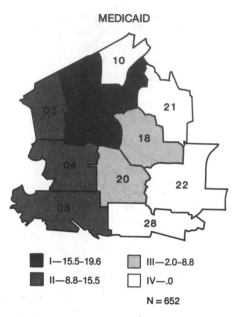

MEDICAID

■ I—15.5–19.6		▨ III—2.0–8.8	
■ II—8.8–15.5		□ IV—.0	

N = 652

Figure 3. Percent of Population Receiving Medicaid.

which the practice sample showed 15-20 percent of the individuals to be elderly. This figure also shows that the areas immediately surrounding the practice contain 12-17 percent elderly. These individuals are clearly not using this practice for their primary health care. The practice center is heavily underrepresented in the older population compared with the general community in close proximity. This information could lead the practice to further investigation of this phenomenon by additional survey of the aging population regarding health care service utilization, or could lead to outreach attempts to this population.

Sex. One would expect that for any community the female population would be approximately 50 percent. Census data for 1980 indicates that the percent female for census tracts in the practice community varies from 45 to 55 percent. This community is composed of approximately one-half males and one-half females dis-

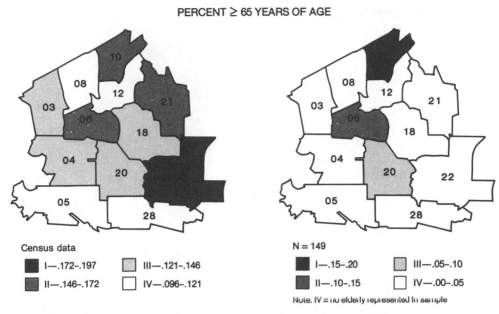

Figure 4. Comparison of Practice and Community Individuals 65 Years and Older.

tributed fairly homogeneously over the geographic area. Due to the evenness of the distribution throughout the community, visual display via mapping techniques does not add to the comparison and is not shown. For the family practice center the population is approximately 60 percent female and 40 percent male. Given the community demographics, this information would lead to the hypothesis that a "hidden cohort" of males may exist in the community toward which efforts could be potentially directed.

Residence Location. The location of the residences of the members of an urban practice can be used in comparison with the distribution of the population of the community at large as an index of the practice's penetration into this total population. If a sample is used in describing the practice population, the percent of the sample residing in each zip code area of the community at large can be calculated. This would then be the "observed"

population in each zip code area for the practice. This can then be contrasted with an "expected" population, calculated from the 1980 census data, that is the percent of the total population residing in each zip code area.

Figure 5 is a plot of observed versus expected percentages for the urban family practice center. For purposes of comparison, the percentage of the total area population living in each zip code area is calculated from census data clustered into the zip code areas comprising the general community. The most logical relationship to expect in a primary care practice would be that the practice population would include greater numbers of individuals residing close to the practice than farther away. Figure 5 indicates that this pattern is generally true for this particular practice. Zip code areas 6 and 12 had twice as many patients than expected, a statistically significant excess for these two areas. This area contains a major traffic corridor that eases access to the practice and is the most likely explanation for this difference. Areas 5, 10, 21, 22, 28 all had significantly fewer patients using the practice than would be expected by the population distribution. Based on this comparison, the practice may wish to redefine its target community to include only those zip code areas reflecting expected utilization rates, i.e., areas 3, 4, 6, 8, 12, 18, and 20 from Figure 5. This could be seen as a refinement in defining a practice's target community.

CONCLUSION

By defining community, designating descriptors, and collecting data describing the practice and general community, similarities and differences between these groups are noted and used an as index of how well the practice membership represents the community at large. This information can be used in targeting specific cohorts of individuals for specific services or for further information gathering by the community-oriented practice. In the examples above, data comparing differences in age between practice and community populations helps to designate the elderly as a potential group for practice outreach activities and reinforces this practice's need to refine and strengthen services to young families.

A practice is a dynamic entity, a group of living individuals with varying degrees of sickness and health. Multiple factors influence the help-seeking behavior of patients and their choice from multiple alternatives for meeting health care needs. Understanding the composition of the community and the practice is a step in the process of developing services that meet the needs of the community. In another sense, current times have increased the interest in marketing services and in health maintenance activities. Designing services that meet community needs can help in marketing. The first

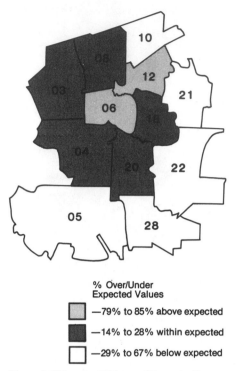

% Over/Under
Expected Values

☐ —79% to 85% above expected

■ —14% to 28% within expected

☐ —29% to 67% below expected

Figure 5. "Observed" Versus "Expected" Population Urban Family Practice Center.

step in this process is understanding the nature of the population toward which marketing efforts are directed.

In these examples statistical indicator data are used to compare the practice with the community at large. It is possible to make other comparisons, depending on the data collected and one's definition of community. The information obtained in this process can be used as a part of the planning process for the development of services that are oriented toward the needs of the given communities.

REFERENCES

1. Eckert, J.K., and Galazka, S.S. An anthropological approach to community diagnosis in family practice. *Family Medicine.* (in press).

2. Mausner, J.S, and Bahn, A.K. *Epidemiology: An Introductory Text.* Philadelphia: W.B. Saunders, 1974.

3. Zyzanski, S.J.; Mettee, T.M.; Metz, C. et al. Factor analysis as a tool in community diagnosis. *Fam Pract* 1984; 1:202-9.

4. Zyzanski, S.J. and Galazka, S.S. A sampling methodology for defining community in a metropolitan area. In *Community Oriented Primary Care: From Principle To Practice*, Nutting, P. (ed.).

CHAPTER 16

Practical Applications of Demography in Community-Oriented Primary Care

Mary B. Breckenridge, Ph.D.
Robert C. Like, M.D., M.S.

This chapter responds to the need for simple, informative techniques for working with COPC data. The goal of the chapter is to encourage the practitioner to take available, health-related data about a community of interest and put the data into graphic displays that elicit not a, "Hmm, well, yes . . . ", but rather, "Aha! Look at that!"

Specifically, we use some exploratory data analysis (EDA) techniques (1) that have been profitably applied in a number of fields and have recently proved valuable in demography in comparing two or more groups of people in regard to characteristics of interest (2).

Because the "demographic variables" most commonly used in comparing groups of people are age, sex, and race, it may be useful at the outset of our discussion to define demography in the much broader sense in which it is used in COPC. Demography is the study of the characteristics of populations—groups of people having some quality in common. In COPC that quality is being members of the same community by whatever definition of community you choose to use, and the concern is with a broad range of health-related characteristics. These may well begin with

age, sex, and race, and certainly include the morbidity and mortality information that are the focus of epidemiology. However, the population characteristics on which COPC planning is based also include such variables as family structure, access to transportation, health insurance coverage, living arrangement, ethnic identification, and source of medical care—all of which go beyond the traditional concerns of epidemiology but fall within the purview of medical demography.

Other chapters have discussed the various definitions of "community" and the sources of data that can be used to characterize a community. The data include information on the general population, and the information that you now record (or could record) about your own patients if you want to know whether they are representative of the communities in which they live, or whether they come from particular segments of those communities. This chapter asks you to make some choices about what you want to look at first. Then, using choices made by one practitioner (R.L.) as an example, the chapter illustrates some simple, pencil-and-paper techniques for looking at the selected characteristics of the selected community. Also, for those who have computerized the demographic information on their patient population, we propose computer-generated graphic displays of the same types, using readily available software for an office PC. Finally, for those interested in moving beyond pencil-and-paper techniques and office computers to a collaboration involving the use of a mainframe computer, we present some possibilities in computerized mapping of community and practice population characteristics.

DIALOGUE BETWEEN DEMOGRAPHER AND PRACTITIONER

Practitioner's question: I have a couple of hours on Wednesday afternoons, and I'm interested in looking at the community where I practice. What can a demographer offer me?

Demographer's response: I can offer you a practical set of demographic questions to ask and some simple graphic techniques that will enable you to describe the community at large and compare it with your practice community. Now let me ask you a question:

Demographer's Question: What definition of community do you want to use first? For example:

1. The town where the practice is located? Or the area bounded by specific streets?

2. The geographic area from which your patients come?

3. The geographic area from which you would like to draw patients? What towns does that include, or what are the geographic boundaries?

4. A geographic area defined by a population characteristic (e.g. "the Hispanic community") or a function (e.g. school district or parish)? What boundaries can you identify (or does the community itself identify)?

5. The "practice community"—all members of all households in which any one member is an active user of services—rather than a geographic area? (If you choose this definition, consider that you may also want to look at characteristics of the general population in the geographic areas in which these people live, that is, their human-environment context.)

Practitioner's Response: I'd like to start with the county where our two practice sites are located. About 70 percent of our enrolled patients come from Middlesex County, and many of the support services for our patients are administered on a county basis (e.g., the services of the Visiting Nurses Association) or by the 25 separate municipal units within the county. I do know that it's a very mixed county geographically, with several small cities, suburban areas, some small towns, and rural areas, and I'll later want to compare the distribution of the general population and the distribution of our patient population in relation to the type of area.

Demographer's Question 2: What characteristics of the people in the community (by whichever definition you have selected) do you want to know about first? For example:

1. Age? And are specific age groups of particular interest to you—Infants? School-age children? The elderly?

2. Sex?

3. How settled or transient the population is?

4. The racial or ethnic composition of the population?

5. Income distribution in the population? Or the number of persons (or families) below the poverty level in relation to the size of the total population?

6. Occupations?

7. The number of physicians in practice (by specialty) in relation to the size of the population?

Practitioner's Response: I'm interested first in the age composition of the population in Middlesex County, and particularly in the elderly population. We're considering some expanded services for the elderly (e.g., broader availability of home visits) and more coordination with community services for the elderly.

Demographer's Question 3: What form of the information about the age composition of Middlesex County would you like to examine first? You can look at data on a selected characteristic in a number of different forms, for example:

1. Actual numbers of people with a given characteristic (e.g., the number of persons aged 65 +, or the number of children born in a given year to women aged 15-19).

2. The percent of the total population that has a given characteristic (e.g., the percent of the total population that is 65 years or older).

3. The rate of occurrence of an event, that is, the number of deaths in a given year in a particular age group divided by the number of people in that age group, or the number of births in a given year to women aged 15-19 divided by the total number of women in that age group.

4. Change between two dates (e.g., decline or increase in population in a given geographic area or in a "practice community").

Practitioner's Response: I'd like to start with the simplest form of the information— the actual numbers of men and women in the different age groups. And then I'd like to compare the separate municipal units in regard to the percent of the population that is elderly.

WORKING WITH THE DATA

We are going to construct five types of visual displays: tables of numbers, histograms, box-and-whisker plots, stem-and-leaf displays, and cartographic displays. We will first work through the techniques at the pencil-and-paper level before considering the use of computers in generating the same types of displays.

For the simple pencil-and-paper techniques, you will need the following materials:

Graph paper—an 8 1/2" by 11" pad is convenient, with 10 squares to the inch and every 10th line heavy. (Paper with every 5th line medium heavy will make the plotting even easier.)

Pencil and a good eraser.

Clear ruler or straight edge (e.g. drafting triangle).

A simple map of the "community" with its components outlined will also be useful for reference. The map for the geographic area in the following examples was provided by the Middlesex County Planning Board. The area comprises 25 census Minor Civil Divisions (MCDs) which are designated in New Jersey as city, borough, or township. For simplicity, we will refer to them all as "municipalities."

Data Tables

The first step in developing graphic displays of data is to extract the numbers you want to use from their source and put them in your own data table. That way you have everything in hand that you want to graph but nothing extraneous, and there's no question later which data go with which graph. (It's well to note the data source on the table.) The census data used for our examples appear in Tables 1-4. (These data were available from the Middlesex County Planning Board. However, the practitioner's sources of census data will vary from State to

State. By calling the Data User Services Division of the Bureau of the Census, (301) 763-1580, you or your collaborator can learn who the primary participants in the State Data Center Program are in your State. The lead agency is usually within the State government. Primary participants are typically the State university and/or a major private university, and in many States the State library. Local planning boards and libraries are designated as local affiliates in many States.)

If you examine Tables 1-4, you will pick up some of the differences that interest you. However, the full array of differences and similarities is much harder to grasp in these tables than in the graphic displays we will construct from them in the following sections.

Age Histograms

Demographers often construct population pyramids, which show both age and sex structure in the same figure. (The number of males in each age group is indicated by bars to the left of a vertical line, and the number of females by bars to the right of the line.) However, in looking at small-area data for COPC, we have found age and sex differences easier to examine in separate groups—one, an age histogram for the total population, and the other, a graph showing the excess of female population over male population by age group (Figs. 1 and 2.)

TABLE 1. Population by Age Group for Three Selected Municipalities, Middlesex County, New Jersey, 1980.

Age Group	Number of Persons		
	New Brunswick	East Brunswick	Perth Amboy
0-4	2,321	2,134	2,804
5-9	2,165	3,041	2,885
10-14	2,418	4,143	2,887
15-19	6,345	3,778	3,269
20-24	8,901	2,677	3,465
25-29	3,864	2,486	3,004
30-34	2,536	3,034	2,911
35-39 } 40-44 }	2,843	6,080	3,745
45-49 } 50-54 }	2,666	5,053	3,957
55-59	1,854	2,080	2,309
60-64	1,800	1,290	2,385
65-69 } 70-74 }	2,178	1,320	3,178
75-79 } 80-84 }	1,179	476	1,741
85 +	372	119	411
Total	41,442	37,711	38,951

Data source: 1980 U.S. Census.

TABLE 2. Excess of Female Population Over Male Population by Age Group for Three Selected Municipalities, Middlesex County, New Jersey, 1980.

	Number of Persons					
Age Group	New Brunswick			East Brunswick		
	Female	Male	Female Excess	Female	Male	Female Excess
0-4	1129	1192	–63	1038	1096	–58
5-9	1113	1052	61	1520	1521	– 1
10-14	1175	1243	–68	1897	2246	–349
15-19	3675	2670	1005	1833	1945	–112
20-24	4848	4053	795	1291	1386	–95
25-29	1863	2001	–138	1231	1255	–24
30-34	1184	1352	–168	1744	1290	–454
35-39 } 40-44 {	1490	1353	137	3127	2953	174
45-49 } 50-54 {	1392	1274	118	2454	2599	–145
55-59	985	869	116	1021	1059	–38
60-64	939	861	78	652	638	14
65-69 } 70-74 {	1257	921	336	708	612	96
75-79 } 80-84 {	801	378	423	343	133	210
85 +	248	124	124	72	47	25
Total	22099	19343	2756	18931	18780	151

Age Group	Perth Amboy			Age Group	Perth Amboy		
	Female	Male	Female Excess		Female	Male	Female Excess
0-4	1300	1504	–204	55-59	1254	1055	199
5-9	1401	1484	– 83	60-64	1240	1145	95
10-14	1436	1451	– 15	65-69 } 70-74 {	1787	1391	396
15-19	1555	1714	–159				
20-24	1749	1716	33	75-79 } 80-84 {	1141	600	541
25-29	1569	1435	134				
30-34	1436	1475	– 39	85 +	341	97	217
35-39 } 40-44 {	1977	1768	209	Total	20314	18637	1667
45-49 } 50-54 {	2155	1802	353				

Data source: 1980 U.S. Census.

94

TABLE 3. Population Quartiles and Age at the Lower Quartile, Median, and Upper Quartile, for Six Selected Municipalities, Middlesex County, New Jersey, 1980.

	Municipality		
	New Brunswick	East Brunswick	Perth Amboy
Population (N)	41442	37711	38951
(1/4)N	10361	9428	9738
Age of (1/4)Nth person	18	15	16
(1/2)N (Median)	20721	18856	19476
Age of (1/2)Nth person (Median Age)	24	31	32
(3/4)N	31082	28283	29213
Age of (3/4)Nth person	43	46	58
	Highland Park	Metuchen	Monroe
Total Population (N)	13396	13762	15858
(1/4)N	3349	3441	3965
Age of (1/4)Nth person	20	18	17
(1/2)N (Median)	6698	6881	7929
Age of (1/2)Nth person (Median Age)	32	36	39
(3/4)N	10047	10322	11894
Age of (3/4)Nth person	52	55	62

Data source: 1980 U.S. Census.

A histogram of the age composition of the total population is usually shown for 5-year age groups. (However, if you want to focus on the school-age population, the census reports population by single year of age for many of the ages under 22.) A histogram permits you to see at a glance whether some age groups have much larger or smaller numbers of people than other age groups. For example, histograms show very prominent differences in the age structure of three Middlesex County municipalities (New Brunswick, East Brunswick, and Perth Amboy) with very close to the same 1980 total population, about 40,000.

To construct an age histogram:

Step 1. For all the municipalities to be compared, collect in a data table the total number of people in each 5-year age group (or 10-year age group when a smaller age group is not given). For our example, the data for New Brunswick, East Brunswick, and Perth Amboy are shown in Table 1. Note that the readily available printed census data for MCDs report population for ages 35-44, 45-54, 65-74, and 75-84 only by 10-year age groups. With some additional effort you can obtain data for the 5-year age groups in these ranges if this is important to you.

Step 2. For each municipality, construct the successive bars by age group as in Figure 1, (which used one square per 100 persons on the horizontal line of the grid, not shown in the figure, and three squares in height for each 5-year

TABLE 4. Total Population, Population Aged 65+, and Percent Aged 65+ for the 25 Municipalities of Middlesex County, New Jersey, 1980.

	Total Population	Age 65+	% Age 65+
Carteret	20598	2100	10.2
Cranbury	1927	287	14.9
Dunellen	6593	777	11.8
East Brunswick	37711	1917	5.1
Edison	70193	5716	8.1
Helmetta	955	97	10.2
Highland Park	13396	1701	12.7
Jamesburg	4114	391	9.5
Metuchen	13762	1596	11.6
Middlesex	13480	1190	8.8
Milltown	7136	826	11.6
Monroe	15858	3455	21.8
New Brunswick	41442	3740	9.0
North Brunswick	22220	1914	8.6
Old Bridge	51515	3440	6.7
Perth Amboy	38951	5341	13.7
Piscataway	42223	1919	4.5
Plainsboro	5605	163	2.9
Sayreville	29969	2609	8.7
South Amboy	8322	1134	13.6
South Brunswick	17127	1069	6.2
South Plainfield	20521	1399	6.8
South River	14361	1871	13.0
Spotswood	7840	495	6.3
Woodbridge	90074	7585	8.4

Data source: 1980 U.S. Census.

age group). Where the number of persons is given only for a 10-year age group, that number is divided evenly between the component 5-year age groups as an approximation; that is, the bar is drawn half as wide and twice as high.

In Figure 1, we see that the age histogram for New Brunswick is dominated by the young adult age groups, reflecting the student population of a major university located in this city. Note also the relative paucity of people in the prime working ages, 35-55. In contrast, East Brunswick has a prominent component in the prime working ages, 35-55, a more prominent elementary and high school age component than New Brunswick, and relatively few elderly. Perth Amboy has more pre-school children (ages 0-4) than either New Brunswick or East Brunswick, and a larger elderly component than either. We can identify male-female differences in the age composition of the population of these municipalities by constructing a display closely related to these histograms.

To display male-female differences in population age composition:

Step 1. For each municipality, subtract the number of males from the number

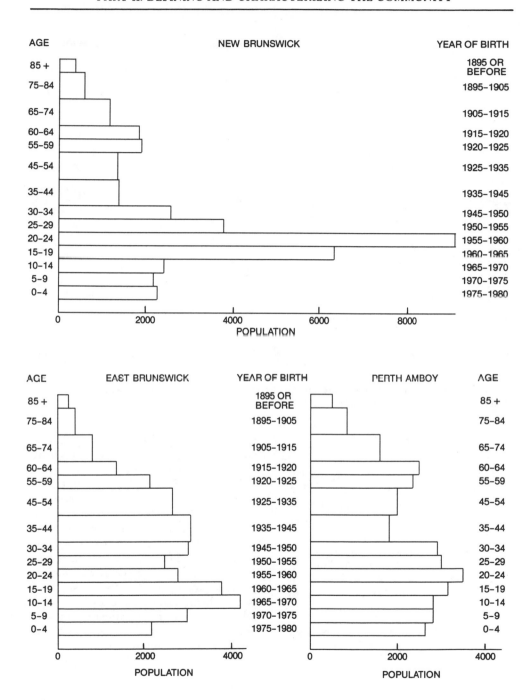

Figure 1. Population by Age Group for Three Selected Municipalities, Middlesex County, New Jersey, 1980.

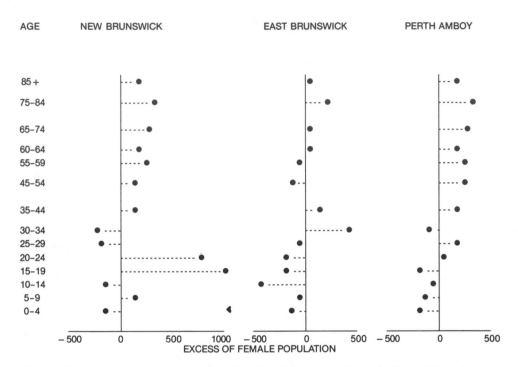

Figure 2. Excess of Female Population Over Male Population by Age Group for Three Selected Municipalities, Middlesex County, New Jersey, 1980.

of females in each age group (Table 2).

Step 2. For each municipality, display these differences about a vertical line at zero: if an age group has an excess of females, show a circle at the corresponding distance along the "plus" scale on the right. If there is an excess of males, show a circle on the "minus" scale on the left (Fig. 2). Link each circle by a dashed horizontal line to the vertical line at zero.

In Figure 2, we see New Brunswick's large excess of females in age groups 15-19 and 20-24, East Brunswick's excesses of females in age group 30-34 (young working age) and of males in age group 10-14. We can note also the near balance of males and females at ages 35 and above in East Brunswick, whereas New Brunswick

and especially Perth Amboy have a noticeably greater number of women than men at all ages 35 and above.

Additional data available from the census can further differentiate these populations by health-related characteristics. For example, in your consideration of strategies for expanded health care services for the elderly in different municipalities, you will probably want to compare the municipalities graphically on the number of persons below poverty level by age, marital status of the elderly population by sex, and the number of the elderly living in single-person households. Data on yearly Medicare enrollment by 5-year age groups by zip code permit you to look at changes in the number of elderly since the 1980 census, although by areas that may not be congruent with the geographic census areas.

We will now look at some other techniques for comparing the age composition of Middlesex County municipalities.

Box-and-Whisker Plots

Discussions of population characteristics often mention "median age." This tells you that half of the population is younger than that age and half is older. Box-and-whisker plots (reference 1, p. 39) offer a simple, convenient way of displaying more information about the age composition of municipal units or communities without constructing the entire age histogram. Five numbers needed are obtained by dividing the total population into quartiles—four groups, each containing one quarter of the population, from the youngest quarter to the oldest quarter—and noting the lowest age, the highest age, and the ages at the three boundaries between quartiles. The box-and-whisker plots (Fig. 3) show not only the median age but also the upper limit of the age range for the youngest quarter of the population, the lower limit

of the age range for the oldest quarter of the population, and how evenly the ages of the center half of the population are spread around the median age. (See also reference 3 for discussion of a closely related graphic display, the boxplot, that is useful in making comparisons for one or more batches of individual data values.) The example in Figure 3 uses the same three municipalities examined in the age histograms of Figure 1 and also three smaller municipalities with similar population sizes around 15,000.

To construct a box-and-whisker plot:

Step 1. List the population numbers in tabular form (as in Table 1 for the construction of age histograms).

Step 2. Divide each municipality's population into quartiles. For example, East Brunswick, with a total population of 37,711, would have 9,428 persons in each quartile (see Table 3).

Step 3. Identify the age of the person at the 1/4, 1/2, and 3/4 points by add-

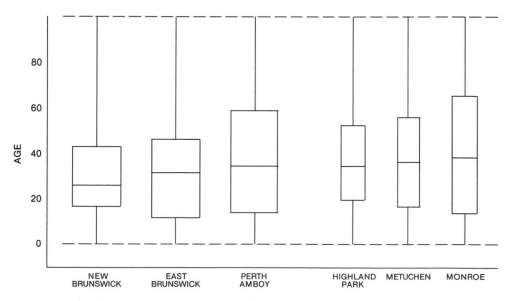

Figure 3. Box-and-Whisker Plots of the Age Distribution of the Population for Six Selected Municipalities, Middlesex County, New Jersey, 1980.

ing the population in successive age groups. For East Brunswick, this means identifying (or approximating by interpolation) the age of the person who is 9,428th, 18,856th, and 28,283rd from the youngest (see Table 3).

Step 4. Transfer this information to graph paper, with a box covering the age range for the middle half of the population, and the median age shown by a horizontal line inside the box. A solid line extending from the lower end of the box to zero covers the age range for the youngest quarter of the population; a solid line extending from the upper end of the box to age 85 or over covers the age range for the oldest quarter of the population (Fig. 3). The horizontal dashed lines indicate these extreme ages. The boxes can either be drawn all the same width or with the width roughly proportional to the size of the total population. The latter choice is shown in Figure 3, where three of the municipalities have approximately 2.5 times the population of the other three.

In Figure 3 we see that three municipalities (East Brunswick, Perth Amboy, and Highland Park) have almost identical median ages for their populations, but quite different age ranges for the oldest quarter of the population. We had already seen in the age histograms the extent to which Perth Amboy exceeded East Brunswick in elderly residents, and we find now that Highland Park lies between the two in this regard. We see too that Monroe has a quarter of its population older than age 62, reflecting the development of several retirement communities in this township, which was largely rural until recently. East Brunswick and Perth Amboy have the lowest ages (15 and 16) at the interquartile boundary for the youngest quarter of the population, indicating that they have somewhat higher proportions of children than the other four communities. The

significance of age composition differences for COPC planning is discussed in other chapters.

Stem-and-Leaf Display

A stem-and-leaf display permits us to examine a batch of numbers not only for symmetry and dispersion (as box-and-whisker plots do) but also for patterns, concentrations and gaps in the values, and outliers (1, 4). The display retains information about the individual data entries while revealing concentrations around particular values and values that are very different from the rest (see Figs. 4 and 5). We include two examples here to show quite different data distributions that you may encounter. In a later section, we use these examples to illustrate the mapping of COPC data.

To construct a stem-and-leaf display (using percent of total population aged 65+ as an example):

Step 1: List the total population and the number of residents aged 65 and older for each of the 26 municipalities (Table 4, columns 1 and 2).

Step 2: For each municipality, divide the number of persons aged 65 + by the total population to obtain the percent of the population aged 65 + (Table 4, column 3).

Step 3. Find the smallest percent aged 65 + and the largest percent (2.9 and 21.8) to use as the lower and upper limits of the stem-and-leaf display.

Step 4. Decide where you are going to split the values to form the stems. This is a key step. In the "percent aged 65 + " example, the leading digits of the data values become the stem; the first decimal digit of each value becomes a leaf:

Data value	Split	Stem and Leaf
21.8	21.8	21 and 8

(In a later example, with data values ranging from 14.5 to 240.1 percent, we drop the decimal digit and split each value between the tens digit and the ones digit to form the stem and leaf.) When complete the display then has one leaf for each original data value.

Step 5. Set up a skeleton of stems, and form the stem-and-leaf display (see Fig. 4). The first display you construct will have the leaves in the order in which they come from the data values; that is, the stems roughly sort the percentages from low to high, but the leaves on a line may not be in ascending order. It is often useful to tidy up the display by putting the leaves in ascending order of the data values for each piece of stem as in Figures 4 and 5.

The stem-and-leaf display for the percent of the total population aged 65 + (Fig. 4) reveals a relatively symmetric distribution around the median value of 9.0 but a wide range of 2.9-21.8 percent aged 65 + in these 25 municipalities. Monroe, at 21.8 percent, is a prominent outlier. We

become aware that the overall county value of 8.8 percent aged 65 + conceals important differences between municipalities within the county. We will consider this point further when we map the municipality information in a later section.

In our second example of a stem-and-leaf display we examine a contextual variable for elderly residents — the percent change in the total population between 1970 and 1980 in the 25 municipalities (Fig. 5). We find a wide range, from 14.5 percent loss to 240.1 percent gain in population (Fig. 5A). With the decimal digit dropped and the percentages ranked in ascending order, the stem-and-leaf display (Fig. 5B) reveals a distribution in which 14 of 25 municipalities lost population, while a small number of municipalities had very prominent gains. Again, we become aware that the overall county value of 2.1 percent gain cannot reveal important differences within the county. We will consider these differences further in the section on cartographic displays.

```
Stem (unit = 1%) | Leaf (unit = .1%)

              2  | 9                          Plainsboro
              3  |
              4  | 5                          Piscataway
              5  | 1                          East Brunswick
              6  | 2  3  7  8
              7  |
              8  | 1  4  6  7  8
              9  | 0  5
             10  | 2  2
             11  | 6  6  8
             12  | 7
             13  | 0  6  7
             14  | 9                          Cranbury
             15  |
             16  |
             17  |
             18  |
             19  |
             20  |
             21  | 8                          Monroe
```

Figure 4. Stem-and-Leaf Display for Percent of Total Population Aged 65 + , 25 Municipalities of Middlesex County, New Jersey, 1980.

101

A. Data for stem-and-leaf display

Municipality	% change
Carteret	− 11.0
Cranbury	− 14.5
Dunellen	− 6.8
East Brunswick	10.4
Edison	4.6
Helmetta	0.0
Highland Park	− 6.9
Jamesburg	− 10.3
Metuchen	− 14.2
Middlesex	− 10.4
Milltown	10.3
Monroe	73.5
New Brunswick	− 1.1
North Brunswick	33.1
Old Bridge	5.7
Perth Amboy	0.4
Piscataway	15.9
Plainsboro	240.1
Sayreville	− 7.8
South Amboy	− 10.9
South Brunswick	21.8
South Plainfield	− 2.9
South River	− 6.9
Spotswood	− 0.6
Woodbridge	− 9.0

B. Formation of stem-and-leaf display by splitting after the tens digit

Stem (unit = 10%)	Leaf (unit = 1%)
− 1	4 4 1 0 0 0
− 0	9 7 6 6 6 2 1 0
+ 0	0 0 4 5
+ 1	0 0 5
+ 2	1
+ 3	3
+ 4	
+ 5	
+ 6	
+ 7	3
+ 8	
+ 9	
+ 23	
+ 24	0

Figure 5. Stem-and-Leaf Display for Percent Change in Total Population in the 25 Municipalities of Middlesex County, New Jersey, 1970–1980.

These same pencil-and-paper displays—age histogram, box-and-whisker plots, stem-and-leaf displays—can be constructed for your patient population if you have a means of extracting the demographic information from your patient records. Then, for example, the patient age distribution can be compared graphically with the age distribution of the population in the geographic areas from which the patients come.

Practitioners who have computerized the demographic information on their patient population can use an office desktop computer to obtain graphic displays like the pencil-and-paper ones. This will involve using one of the available software packages, such as Minitab, PSTAT, or STATGRAPHICS, that include exploratory data analysis techniques, with boxplots and stem-and-leaf displays among their graphics capabilities.

Cartographic Displays

Mapping geographic variations in health-related characteristics of interest in COPC can be done by hand on a simple outline map similar to the computer-generated maps shown in Figures 6 and 7. Practitioners who choose to move beyond pencil-and-paper techniques and office computers can seek collaboration in a variety of places—academic, State health department, industry—to tap mainframe computer capabilities very useful in COPC planning. We take the example of academic collaboration to illustrate two of these computer capabilities: the generation of maps that show the distribution of a given variable by municipality or by census tract; and the matching of patient addresses with census tracts and tract characteristics in order to map the distribution of patients and permit examination of the community context of the patient population.

In mapping, the computer program plots the coordinates of the municipal boundaries or census tract boundaries and shades each municipality or tract on the basis of designated value-intervals for the variable under consideration. Usually four or five categories are the most that can be easily distinguished in viewing a map. Stem-and-leaf displays can help you to choose the groups of areas to be shaded in the same way.

One example, Figure 6, maps the data that we examined in the stem-and-leaf display of Figure 4—the percent of the total population that is aged 65 +. Based on the median and interquartile range, four intervals for the mapping were constructed for the main body of the data with a range of 2.9 to 14.9 percent. The single outlier, the 21.8 percent for Monroe, was given a separate designation.

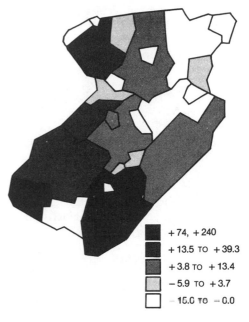

+ 74, + 240
+ 13.5 TO + 39.3
+ 3.8 TO + 13.4
− 5.9 TO + 3.7
− 15.0 TO − 0.0

Figure 7. Percent Change in Total Population by Minor Civil Division, Middlesex County, New Jersey, 1970–1980.

A second example, Figure 7, maps the data that we examined in the stem-and-leaf display of Figure 5: the percent change in total population between 1970 and 1980. Here, to determine the interval cuts for mapping, we consider that the median value is for a municipality with a slight loss of population, and that the median ± one-fourth the interquartile range represents areas of relative stability in population size (−2.9% to +0.4% change). By using a multiple of the interquartile range as a "unit of measure," we also identify an interval which includes the municipalities with greater population loss (−6.8% to −14.5% change), an interval including population gains of similar degree (+4.6% to +10.4% change), an interval of more prominent gains (+15.9% to +33.1% change), and two outliers (gains of 73.5% and 240.1%). The procedures used to select the interval cuts for these

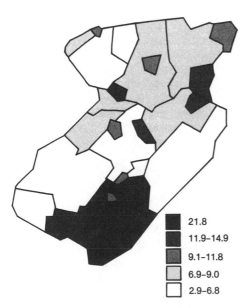

21.8
11.9–14.9
9.1–11.8
6.9–9.0
2.9–6.8

Figure 6. Percent of Total Population Aged 65 + by Minor Civil Division, Middlesex County, New Jersey, 1980.

maps are shown in Tables 5 and 6. You will note that we do not propose a set formula, as in the commonly used procedures of dividing the values into 4 or 5 groups containing an equal number of values, or dividing the range of the values into 4 or 5 equal segments. Instead, we use information about the spread of the data and the presence of outliers to make intelligent and systematic choices while capitalizing on natural separations and groupings.

When we compare Figures 6 and 7, we observe the following: 10 of the 12 municipalities with percentages of elderly above the median of 9.0 percent are longer established communities that exhibited either marked decline or little change in popula-

tion over the decade. Only one municipality, Monroe, with a high percent of elderly in 1980 (21.8 percent) was also an area of prominent growth (74.5 percent); however, the growth was due to the building of several retirement communities in a sparsely settled, largely rural area. The implications of total population change for the planning of COPC will be quite different for this one municipality than for the others with above-the-median percentages of elderly residents.

In the section "Stem-and-leaf displays," we noted how poorly the overall county values for the variables would have served us because of the geographic diversity within the county. Even values for municipalities may not give us the localization

---

TABLE 5. Preparation for Mapping of Percent of Total Population Aged 65+ by Municipality, Middlesex County, New Jersey, 1980.

A. Determination of interval cuts for mapping

Statistic	Rank	Value
Median $(n+1)/2$, where $n = 25$ municipalities	13	9.0
Quartiles (rank of median) + 1)/2		
Lower quartile	7	6.8
Upper quartile	19	11.8
Interquartile range (difference in value between upper and lower quartiles, representing range for center half of data)		5.0
Outlier cutoffs (using the interquartile range, IQR, as the "unit of measurement")		
Lower quartile -1.5(IQR)		-0.7
Upper quartile $+1.5$(IQR)		19.3
Outside values		21.8

B. Intervals for map based on median and IQR

Interval	Range	Rank	Values in interval
Lower quartile and below	0-6.8	1-7	2.9-6.8
Median to lower quartile	6.8-9.0	8-13	8.1-9.0
Median to upper quartile	9.0-11.8	14-19	9.5-11.8
Upper quartile to outlier cutoff	11.8-19.3	20-24	12.7-14.9
Outside values	> 19.3	25	21.8

TABLE 6. Preparation for Mapping of Percent Change in Total Population by Municipality, Middlesex County, New Jersey, 1970-1980.

A. Determination of interval cuts for mapping

Statistic	Rank	Value
Median $(n+1)/2$, where $n = 25$ municipalities	13	−1.1
Quartiles ((rank of median) + 1)/2		
Lower quartile	7	−9.0
Upper quartile	19	+ 10.3
Interquartile range (difference in value between upper and lower quartiles, representing range for center half of data)		+ 19.3
Outlier cutoffs (using the interquartile range, IQR, as the "unit of measurement")		
Lower quartile −1.5(IQR)		−38.0
Upper quartile + 1.5(IQR)		+ 39.3
Outside values		+ 74, + 240

B. Intervals for map based on median and IQR and centered on median

Interval	Range	Rank	Values in interval
Median ± (1/4)IQR	−5.9 to 3.7	12-16	−2.9 to +0.4
(M − (1/4)IQR) to (M − (3/4)IQR)	5.9 to 15.6	1-11	−6.8 to −14.5
(M − (3/4)IQR) to outlier cutoff	−15.6 to −38.0		none
Low outside values	< −38.0		none
(M + (1/4)IQR) to (M + (3/4)IQR)	3.7 to 13.4	17-20	+4.6 to + 10.4
(M + (3/4)IQR) to outlier cutoff	13.4 to 39.3	21-23	+ 15.9 to + 33.1
High outside values	> 39.3	24-25	+ 73.5, + 240.1

we need for some COPC efforts, especially for the larger townships. To locate more precisely the areas of high concentration of the elderly, we show a computer-generated map of the number of persons aged 65 + by census tract in Middlesex County (Fig. 8). (Here, for the large, darkly-shaded area on the left, we will again want to ask, "Are the elderly living throughout the area?") In devising COPC strategies, we might even enhance the value of this map by marking on it the boundaries of the county's five senior citizen transportation districts.

The computerized matching of patient addresses with census tracts involves the use of a Geographic Base File, also known as a Dual Independent Map Encoding File, which is a computerized list of street names, address ranges, and associated census tract numbers. The ADMATCH or UNIMATCH program compares patient addresses with the GBF/DIME File and assigns the appropriate census tract to each (see the diagram in Fig. 9.) This gives the practitioner the possibility not only of identifying the practice catchment area and mapping the patient distribution within it, but also of relating patients to community contexts in some detail.

For both the address-matching activity, and the computerized mapping of community and practice characteristics the practitioner will want to seek collaboration.

However, this step probably should not be considered until you have spent some time with pencil-and-paper-graphics to decide which "community" and which characteristics of its population you want to examine in more detail. You should expect to bring to the collaboration some very specific choices, and you will also be asked to provide in some specified form whatever practice data you want to exam-ine. If you do decide to take this step, your collaborator will be able to provide an estimate of the charge for a program-mer's time and also for the computer time used in running the programs you request.

FUTURE STEPS IN THE USE OF DEMOGRAPHY IN COPC

First Considerations in Data Collection

You will want to give your first attention to a key question that will influence all of

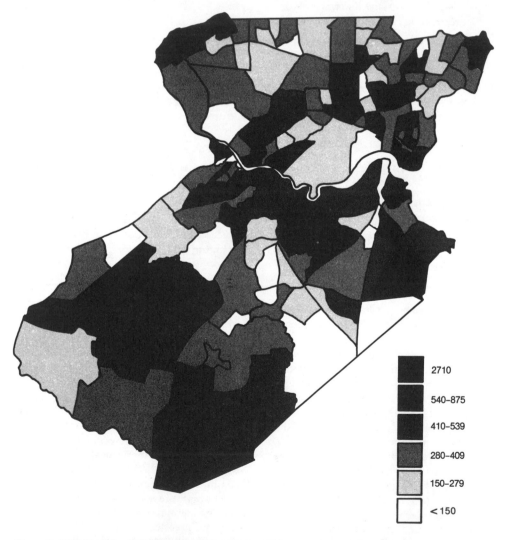

■	2710
■	540–875
■	410–539
▨	280–409
▧	150–279
□	< 150

Figure 8. 1980 Age 65 + Population by Census Tract, Middlesex County, New Jersey.

your data collection activities:

What are the *right* questions to ask about the characteristics of *my* "community" for COPC?

You will then be prepared to ask:

With technical assistance, what are the best data I can get that respond to these questions?

The data on your own practice are under your control, and you will want to make them as accurate as you reasonably can. Much of the secondary data on the community at large will have some limitations. For example, the more removed in time you are from a decennial census, the less the census data will reflect current population characteristics. Projections of population size, based on expected demographic and economic change, may not be available for the smaller geographic areas of interest for COPC in your location. Even the census data on many health-related variables will not be exact counts because the census collects only a limited amount of information for a 100 percent count of the population. For the rest, a sample of the population provides data that are then extrapolated to give estimates for the total population in a census division. The conversion of census tract data on a population sample to census data by zip code also leads to estimates, not actual counts for the total population within zip code areas. Mortality-by-cause data from the State department of health will be flawed by the extent to which the causes listed on the death certificate (often in the absence of an autopsy) differ from the actual causes of death.

The important point is to recognize data limitations but not to let the limitations deter you from looking at the best information you can assemble in response to the right questions. John Tukey (5) has observed, "It is often much worse to have good measurement of the wrong thing—especially when . . . (it will) be used as an

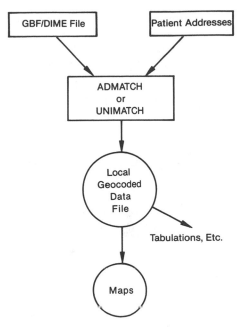

Figure 9. Steps in Mapping Your Practice Community.

indicator of the right thing—than to have poor measurements of the right thing." You may well have to say, "The actual number of persons with the particular characteristic is probably no less than this and probably no greater than that," and then proceed to use this range in your COPC planning decisions.

Next Steps for Practitioner and Demographer

1. To apply these graphic techniques to data for the active patient population, the practice community, other defined communities, and the community at large.

2. To use the techniques to display and examine the pertinent epidemiological and other health-related data for these various communities—e.g. morbidity rates, mortality rates, lengths of hospital stay, utilization of ambulatory care services, indica-

tors of functional status and of socio-economic status.

3. To adapt other exploratory data analysis techniques to COPC uses.

4. To develop a COPC demographic workbook, to be pilot tested by practitioners in a variety of primary care settings.

5. To foster collaboration and networking to aid the practitioner's adoption of a COPC mode of practice.

Practitioners and demographers will need to combine efforts on these steps, recognizing the unique contributions that each can bring to work with COPC data.

SUMMARY

This chapter has focused on techniques for making the readily available demographic information more useful to you as you consider moving into a COPC mode of practice. The age and sex composition of one New Jersey county's population provides the examples of simple pencil-and-paper graphics—age histograms, box-and-whisker plots, stem-and-leaf displays—that draw your attention to similarities and differences. The chapter gives step-by-step instructions for these graphic techniques so you will be able to apply them to pertinent epidemiological and other health-related data for a community of your choice. Computer-generated maps illustrate the cartographic display of the municipality and census tract data to reveal geographic variations within the community that have important implications for COPC planning.

Acknowledgment

David C. Hoaglin, Alfred F. Tallia, and Mona R. Bomgaars reviewed drafts of this chapter. We appreciate their very helpful suggestions. Participants in the February 10-12, 1986 conference "COPC—From Principle to Practice" provided a number of valuable suggestions as well. We also acknowledge the technical assistance of Shirley Robbins, Peter J. Ellis, and Robert A. Beck in preparing the computerized maps and other figures.

REFERENCES

1. Tukey, J.W. *Exploratory Data Analysis*. Reading, MA: Addison-Wesley, 1977.

2. Breckenridge, M.B. *Age, Time, and Fertility: Applications of Exploratory Data Analysis*. New York: Academic Press, 1983.

3. Emerson, J.D., and Strenio, J. Boxplots and batch comparison. In: *Understanding Robust and Exploratory Data Analysis*, D.C. Hoaglin, F. Mosteller, J.W. Tukey (eds.). New York: John Wiley and Sons, 1983, p. 58.

4. Emerson, J.D., and Hoaglin, D.C. Stem-and-leaf displays. In: *Understanding Robust and Exploratory Data Analysis*, D.C. Hoaglin, F. Mosteller, J.W. Tukey (eds.). New York: John Wiley and Sons, 1983, p. 7.

5. Tukey, J.W. Methodology, and the statistician's responsibility for both accuracy and relevance. *Journal of the American Statistical Association* 1980; 74:786.

CHAPTER 17

Building an Integrated Community Health Information Base

Alan Trachtenberg, M.D., M.P.H.
Laura Gardner, M.D.
Jeffrey B. Gould, M.D., M.P.H.
Sylvia Hutchison, B.S.N., M.P.H.

Urban practices have a treasure trove of data available to them in the form of their own practice data, census data, birth and death certificate data, hospital discharge data, as well as many other sources of data that have become available through the advancement of computer and telecommunications technology. The key to aggregating these data in a single data base is to develop a geographic definition of the community that is compatible with that of the other data sources. The combination of data from the clinic's own patients (primary data) and data collected by others (secondary data) can generally advance the ability of the COPC practice to define and characterize the target community.

This chapter describes an approach to defining and characterizing the community using both primary and secondary data. An application of the process in a demonstration project at an urban community health center in Oakland, California is also described. Finally, goals are recommended for community-based practices that are attempting to develop a similar data system from selected primary and secondary data.

There is an advantage to be gained from aggregating data from disparate sources into a single integrated system. The most obvious is that other primary and secondary data can each supply useful information that might otherwise have been inaccessible or too time consuming to obtain. Key questions that should be addressed included: What is the sociodemographic composition of the community? What proportion of the target population is actually using the clinic? How does the health of clinic users compare with that of the nonenrolled members of the target population, the community as a whole, and other similar communities?

A second advantage is that data from two or more different sources may be combined (under certain circumstances) to yield more useful or more easily interpretable data than from either source alone. For instance, the numerator of deaths, births, or hospitalizations for stroke might be obtained from one specialized source while the population denominator from which those incidents came would be obtained from the census. Similarly, live births or total births from birth certificate records could serve as standardization for ectopic pregnancies, abortions, low birthweights, or other specific types of maternal or perinatal morbidity that might be an important target for a COPC emphasis program. The census data is also useful for age adjustment on any epidemiologic data produced by the system, as well as supplying socioeconomic data to help explain differences in health needs of different segments of the community.

CHARACTERIZING THE COMMUNITY THROUGH PRIMARY AND SECONDARY DATA

COPC has been defined as "The provision of primary care services to a defined community, coupled with systematic efforts to identify and address the major health problems of that community through effective modifications in both the primary care services and other appropriate community health programs" (1). The application of epidemiologic methods to the community is integral to the practice of COPC (2). There are two basic types of epidemiologic data obtainable about people in communities: primary data and secondary data.

Primary data are obtained directly from individuals in the community, either by means of a community survey or in an ongoing fashion as individuals obtain services. To obtain primary data the geographic definition of the community does not need to be limited to previously defined microgeographic entities (i.e., zip code areas or census tracts), but can reflect any aggregation of streets, neighborhoods, or cultural definitions that are of interest to the clinic. In another chapter of Part II, Berman reviews the survey techniques available for use in collecting primary data that describe the community.

Secondary data, on the other hand, are data that already have been gathered by other agencies. The most useful secondary data are available on the individual level, with personal identification stripped to maintain the confidentiality of the respondents. When data are available on the individual level, they must include for each individual a data field that allows the individual to be assigned to a particularly definable population. This will almost always be the resident population in a particular geographic area, and may often be subclassified further by ethnicity.

The smaller and more standardized the geographic area assignable (the "Geocode") and the more specific the ethnicity assignment, the more useful are the data in characterizing a defined population. However, the smaller the basic building block, the more difficult is the actual geocoding (i.e., which census block is 9273 Main Street Apt A?) and the more difficult is the process of aggregating the multiple small units into larger and better known areas (i.e., east side of downtown). In general, the two most frequently used basic microgeographic assignments (geocodes) are the census tract and the zip code. Urban census tracts are smaller than zip code areas and have a population of roughly 4,000. Consequently, urban zip codes are more sociodemographically heterogeneous. This heterogeneity tends to offset the zip code's major advantage: most people can tell you their own zip code, while you have to look up their census tract on the basis of their address.

The California Health Facilities Commission, for example, collected and published a discharge data tape that had an entry for each hospital admission in the State of California. Since patients are often hospitalized far from their residence, these data would not be very useful for a population-based description of health needs, except for the inclusion of the zip code of residence of each patient. Any of the individual data contained on the tape can be aggregated and cross tabulated by zip code of residence and race of patient. Thus the hospitalization patterns, by ethnicity, of the residents of any given group of zip codes can be described. The incidence of hospitalization for a specific diagnosis (stroke or major trauma, for example) can then be divided by the census population of that group of zip codes (either total population or by ethnicity) to determine incidences that are comparable across different ethnic groups or zip code aggregations. Such rates could even be age adjusted if that were felt to be important.

Many other types of secondary data with microgeographic assignability can be obtained. For example, birth and death records include zip code and sometimes census tract of residence. Cancer occurrence data, available from the Surveillance, Epidemiology, and End Results (SEER) public-use data tape, includes census tract but not zip code of residence, and are available from the National Cancer Institute for many urban areas.

The next most useful type of secondary data bases are those that have already aggregated the individuals into their microgeographic assignments. Cross-tabulations are limited not only by the data that are originally collected, but also by the cross tabulations and aggregations inherent in the analysis. For example, the United States Census aggregates data at the census tract level or by larger units of combined census tracts such as counties or States.

Unfortunately, zip code boundaries are not congruent with census tract boundaries, nor even necessarily with county boundaries. The former were developed from U.S. Postal Service delivery routes, rather than from sociodemographic or political factors.

The main advantages in using secondary data sources are that they are usually inexpensive, are already in a form that facilitates computerized analysis, and have sampled many more people in the area of interest than most clinics have the resources to include in a community survey. The issue of sample size is further discussed below, but in general, small sample size is a common problem in local surveys that attempt to characterize an urban community. The use of whole-population-based occurrence data, such as that for invasive cervical cancer or hospitalization for stroke, allows the best possible study of these rare events that are important health outcomes and likely targets of COPC intervention. These would not otherwise be available.

There are several limitations in the use of secondary data. First, those who originally collected the data may not have asked the questions of most importance to the COPC effort, or may not have collected the necessary identifying data. For instance, only in the past few years has it become routine to tabulate statistics for Hispanics separately from non-Hispanic whites. Further, access to secondary data may be limited by the parent agency. Analysis may require more expertise than is available at a primary care clinic. Collection and analysis may require access to sophisticated equipment not available to a primary care clinic. Secondary data may not be available in a timely enough fashion to be relevant, as in the case of many vital statistics. Finally, appropriate secondary data may not exist for the community in question.

Nonetheless, there is a great deal of available secondary data of interest for COPC activities. Rapidly advancing computer technology is making more and more data available in a more timely fashion and putting more analytic capability in the hands of smaller agencies and clinics than ever before. Timely analysis of available secondary data might reveal important specific questions that primary data could answer, and would certainly be of use in calculating the size of the sample needed in any community survey sponsored by the urban clinic.

Defining the Community

The question of how to define a community in urban America remains a vexing problem (3). The many different geographic ways to define a community (i.e., the retail market area, police and fire districts, the primary medical care service area, etc.) tend to be fairly consistent in the rural environment. However, as one moves from rural to urban areas the sociodemographic and ethnic compositions often become less homogeneously distributed. This results in more specialized and decentralized services that are more easily accessible to a larger and more diverse population. Consequently it becomes difficult to define precisely the target community and to characterize the community's health needs.

To define a target community we recommend a geographic approach that views the community as the population living within a service area. The service area in turn is defined by the residence of current users of the clinic. In order to utilize secondary data sources that are based on both zip code or census tract aggregations, the creation of two service area definitions from the primary information on clinic users is recommended: one defined by census tracts and one by zip codes.

Describing the Community with Primary and Secondary Data

Primary data can be useful in identifying areas for improving services to current clinic users. First, demographic data such as ethnicity, sex, age, family size, marital status, employment, and income can all be used to characterize the clinic user population. A higher priority can then be placed on diseases and conditions that are known to be more prevalent in the specific age, ethnic, or socioeconomic groups that use the clinic. These entities can then be targeted through special prevention, screening, or treatment programs. Examples include perinatal conditions, hypertension, lead poisoning, iron deficiency anemia, etc. Second, analysis of group-specific prevalences among clinic users can

delineate risk groups that had not been previously defined. Finally, quantification of visits per patient per period of time or per episode of a particular condition can be used to assess the efficiency and appropriateness of current clinic treatment protocols.

Secondary data may be utilized to characterize the service area as a whole, and may be combined with primary data in several ways. First, comparisons between clinic users and the service area as a whole may be used to characterize the particular attributes of those people who are more likely to use the primary care program. This may enable a more effective outreach program to nonusers in the service area. Second, disease incidences and prevalences in clinic users compared to those in the rest of the service area may allow analysis of the effectiveness of clinic programs, both in prevention and treatment of disease. Third, disease prevalence and hospitalization data for the service area may help determine priorities for expanding the scope of services to groups who currently appear to be underusing the clinics. Fourth, when the demographics of the clinic users indicate that this population is approximately representative of the service area as a whole, secondary data from the service area can also be used to determine fruitful areas for enhanced service to current clinic users. Finally, comparisons between the service area (and if possible the clinic users,) and some carefully chosen area might allow incidence and morbidity trends in the service area to be standardized for long-term followup.

Once a clinic's service area has been defined in terms of its geographic boundaries, one can then turn to secondary data sources such as the U.S. Census for sociodemographic profiles, the State vital statistics tapes for natality and mortality information, cancer registries, etc. and build a picture of the service area. It then becomes possible to compare the service area to adjacent geographic areas. With census data it is also possible to identify more distant comparison neighborhoods that are sociodemographically similar to the community-oriented primary clinic's service area, in order to use secondary health outcome data (such as that for invasive cervical cancer or low birthweight rates) to compare the health status of the two communities.

DEVELOPMENT OF AN INTEGRATED DATA SYSTEM— AN EXAMPLE

The system to be described was designed to use all of the data resources available to a two-site urban community health center in Oakland, California. The clinic's planners, administrators, and health care providers are the intended end users of the various data, which are transformed from a multi-machine, multi-database, hard to use conglomeration into a community-oriented clinic information system that will serve the needs of the clinic and the community.

Study Site

Our prototype COPC information system was developed with the active participation of a two-site community health center in Oakland, California. The first clinic was founded in 1971 as a free clinic to serve the unmet health care needs of the East Oakland community (4). It emphasized services to the Spanish-speaking population of Alameda County. With the allocation of revenue sharing funds from Alameda County in 1973 and the later acquisition of State and Federal funds, the clinic quickly grew to become a permanent and vital community institution.

In 1976 a second neighborhood health center was founded in the neighborhood to the north of the first clinic to serve the multi-ethnic population of that area. Although Spanish language services were featured at the second health center, the

emphasis was on outreach to all segments of the neighborhood community, especially the black and Asian immigrant populations. A close relationship grew between the two clinics, and in January 1984 they formally merged.

With the growing scarcity of public funding and the increasing need to compete with the private sector, the merged corporation sought a patient mix that would facilitate a stable economic base. The staff expressed an interest in using computer technology to refine their service area definition and to determine the characteristics and unmet health needs of the population residing in that area. In 1984 the University of California School of Public Health (Berkeley) received a Federal contract through BHCDA to explore the implementation of COPC in existing community health centers. Thus was born a demonstration project that serves as an example of an integrated data system for COPC. The development of this system was a cooperative venture between the Federal Government, a State school of public health, and two community health centers.

In general, the target community receives primary care services from multiple sources as depicted in Figure 1. The heavy black line represents the geographic boundaries of the primary service area for the clinic, based on data from the clinic

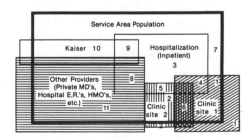

Figure 1. Sources of health information (and medical care) for all residents of the clinic's user-defined service area.

TABLE 1. Sources and Types of Data On Clinic Service Area Population Keyed to Figure 1.

Source or Availability	Type of Data
1) Clinic data system (OPUS)	Users by "Class" (ethnicity, poverty status, language, age, age by sex, payment source.)
2) Clinic data system (OPUS)	Prevalence of selected illnesses, by class.
3) California Health Facilities Commission 1982 and 83 Hospital Discharge Data Tapes	Incidence of hospitalization by diagnosis and zip code of residence, source and type of admission, disposition, and hospital admitted to. Also total charges and DRG.
4) Number and type of clinic users hospitalized not available from OPUS.	
5) Number and type of clinic users hospitalized not available from OPUS.	
6) Overlap of users at both sites (OPUS)	By "Class" (See 1 & 2 above.)
7) a: Medi-Cal Data (Alameda County)	Numbers of clients, and type of eligibility by zip code.
b: 1980 Census data (Summary Tape Files 1 and 3 (STF1 AND STF3), via IPODM-3	Demographics and total population, by age, income, ethnicity, poverty status, sex and marital status of household head, family size, and family density, by census tract.
c: 1982 Birth Cohort (linked Birth-Death Record from State Health Department of IPODM-3)	Maternal and child health data, by zip code and tract, from birth and linked death certificates.
d: 1982 Mortality data from Alameda County death register.	Number and causes of deaths, by Census tract.
e: SEER Public Use Data Tape - all Invasive Cervical Cancer Cases in Alameda County	Ethnicity, age, year of Dx, by Census tract for 1973-1983 (Cancer surveillance data.)
8) California Health Facilities Commission 1982 and 83 Hospital Discharge Data Tapes	Incidence of hospitalization by diagnosis and zip code of residence, source and type of admission, disposition, and hospital admitted to. Also total charges and DRG.
9) California Health Facilities Commission 1982 and 83 Hospital Discharge Data Tapes	
10) Potentially available from Kaiser	Number of clients, by zip.
11) No other provider specific information is currently available.	

for the users of both sites. This Venn diagram is helpful to display and emphasize the areas of overlap that one can expect from different sources of data. The sources and types of data used in the demonstration project for each subset of area residents are listed in Table 1.

Defining the Community

Starting in January 1985, census tracts for all patients of clinic site A were deter-

TABLE 2. Major Census Tracts of an Urban Clinic's User Population, Numeric Cut Point Decision, and Tracts Included in Core Service Area Definition, with Cumulative Percentages, by Number of Users.

TRACT		#	CUM %	TRACT		#	CUM %
4072	*@	647	10.72%	4085	*@	33	78.91%
4062	*@	588	20.46%	4077	*@	31	79.42%
4061	*@	450	27.92%	4272	*@	29	79.90%
4059	*@	363	33.93%	4015	*	29	80.38%
4071	*@	308	39.03%	4221	*	29	80.86%
4065	*@	211	42.53%	4053	*@	29	81.35%
4087	*@	173	45.39%	4011	*	29	81.83%
4060	*@	162	48.08%	4019	*	26	82.26%
4074	*@	155	50.65%	4023	*	26	82.69%
4076	*@	154	53.20%	4055	*	25	83.10%
4063	*@	142	55.55%	4369	*	25	83.52%
4073	*@	142	57.90%	4064	*	24	83.91%
4094	*@	124	59.96%	4010	*	23	84.29%
4070	*@	121	61.96%	4079	*	23	84.68%
4054	*@	96	63.55%	4016	'	23	85.06%
4075	*@	93	65.09%	4251	*	22	85.42%
4058	*@	79	66.40%	4056	*	22	85.79%
4093	*@	68	67.53%	4083	+ +	19	86.10%
4066	*@	63	68.57%	4333		19	86.41%
4088	*@	51	69.42%	4240		18	86.71%
4103	*@	48	70.21%	4284		18	87.01%
4057	*@	47	70.99%	4104		17	87.29%
4095	*@	46	71.75%	4039		17	87.57%
4278	*@	45	72.50%	4018		17	87.86%
4017	*	45	73.24%	4375		17	88.14%
4276	*@	43	73.96%	4048		16	88.40%
4232	*	40	74.62%	4090		15	88.65%
4092	*@	40	75.28%	4220		15	88.90%
4326	*@	39	75.93%	4340		15	89.15%
4096	*@	38	76.56%	4325		15	89.40%
4086	*@	37	77.17%	4273		14	89.63%
4231	*	37	77.78%	4377		14	89.86%
4089	*@	35	78.36%	4049		14	90.09%

* = Tract to be considered numerically for inclusion into service area definition.

+ + = Natural numeric cut point.

@ = Contiguous tracts included in final census tract service area definition (see figure 2).
Total users within this 34 tract area = 4720 or 75.52% of total clinic users for six month period.

mined and entered directly into the computer as each patient was registered. For each census tract the total number of clinic patients in a 6-month period was recorded, and the percent of all clinic patients resident in that census tract during the first half of 1985 was calculated. The census tracts were then sorted by number of resident clinic users, from highest to lowest. A cumulative percentage was calculated for this sorted list. The top

66 census tracts, containing 90 percent of the clinic's patients, are shown in Table 2.

A selection was made of the census tracts in which the highest numbers of clinic patients reside. These were selected to include the smallest number of tracts that contained 80-85 percent of the clinic users, as shown in Table 2. Clearly, the "cut point" is somewhat arbitrary and may be drawn between two tracts that between

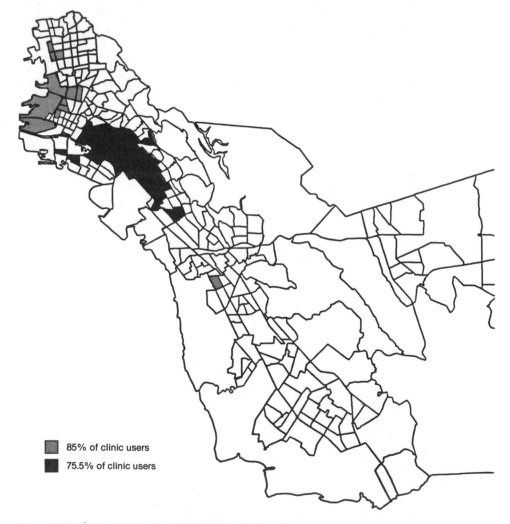

Figure 2. Clinic Core Service Area Definition, by Census Tract.

themselves do not have a statistically significant difference in the number of clinic users (19 vs. 22 in our case).

The high utilization tracts were then mapped and a subjective decision was made as to how to deal with noncontiguous areas. Small outlying groups of tracts, separated from the main body of contiguous tracts, will either be discarded or the intervening tracts of lower clinic utiliza-

tion will be included to finally arrive at one contiguous body of tracts that constitute the defined core service area. The population of this area can then be characterized by the secondary data sources and compared to the actual clinic users. The census tracts that we selected for final inclusion in the clinic service area are demarcated in Table 2. The maps of census tracts chosen numerically and those

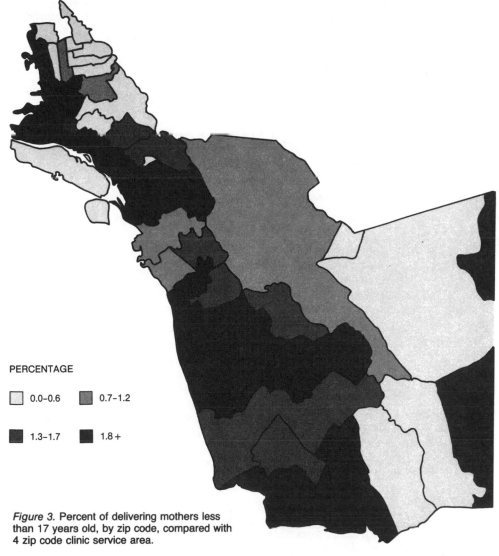

PERCENTAGE

☐ 0.0–0.6   ■ 0.7–1.2

■ 1.3–1.7   ■ 1.8 +

Figure 3. Percent of delivering mothers less than 17 years old, by zip code, compared with 4 zip code clinic service area.

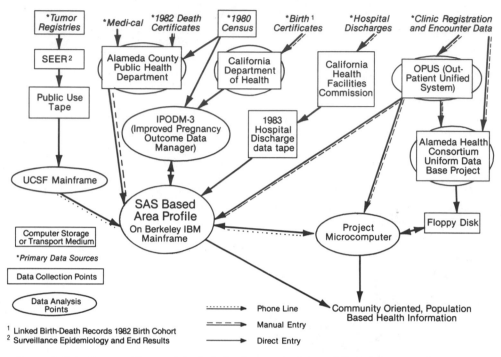

Figure 4. Data Sources, Flow, and Analysis for Community Oriented Clinic Information System.

that are contiguous and therefore retained in the final definition of the service area are shown in Figure 2.

A similar analysis can be made using the zip codes of clinic users. The zip codes, containing relatively large areas, will generally be contiguous and will not require further exclusion or inclusion to make them so. Secondary data drawn from a zip code defined service area, however, will be less specific to the clinic's population.

We further compared the clinic service area to population-based maps showing distribution of median family income, proportion of population of Hispanic origin, low birthweights, and teenage mothers to confirm our impression that the defined service area was related to areas of high health needs. For example, the zip code map showing areas with high proportions

of teen-age mothers (Figure 3) was found to generally correspond to the clinic's service area defined by census tract (Figure 2).

Computer System Configuration

The data system is diagramed in Figure 4, and illustrates the data bases, data flow, and data analysis used by our project. The demonstration project obtained a program (in Pick) from the San Francisco General Hospital Satellite Health Center Computerized System. This program allowed analysis of patient groups by diagnosis, zip code of residence, etc. to be characterized by poverty status, sex, age, sex by age, ethnicity, payment source, and language. Similar analysis of patient data could be performed using commercially available microcomputer database management programs.

118

Any one of several public domain terminal emulation programs (for example, Kermit) can be used to transfer data to a clinic microcomputer from the SAS-based area profile.[1] Some manual reentry into a microcomputer spreadsheet program was originally necessary, but as the project progressed, several proprietary programs came on the market that allowed direct entry of mainframe output or other data into spreadsheet format without manual reentry.

Two additional support systems were appropriate for incorporation into the data system and deserve elaboration. The first (IPODM) is a system that is resident in the University of California, Berkeley computer and was of particular value to us. The second (ADMATCH) is a program that we did not use, but is available from the Census Bureau and would be useful in many settings.

IPODM: IPODM (7) is a collection of computer programs on the IBM mainframe at the University of California, Berkeley.[2] The programs are interactive and designed to create a user-friendly interface with the proprietary statistical programming language.[3] IPODM can access, display, analyze, and map data sets that contain microgeographic (either zip code or census tract) identifiers.

IPODM can also use special data sets that are entered into it, such as the service area data which were entered from the clinic minicomputer. It also contains certain data sets resident in it from two important sources: The 1980 Census (Summary Tape Files 1 and 3, STF1 and STF3) and aggregated birth certificate data for all babies born in 1982 (the 1982 Linked Birth-Death cohort, LBD). Census information is available for all zip codes and census tracts in California as is LBD information for all California zip codes and for the census tracts of six San Francisco Bay Area counties. Other health related data sets will be added to IPODM

in the future, the eventual goal being to create a computerized but user-friendly population-based health data base to be of use to all California health care managers.

IPODM-3 proved extremely useful for the demonstration project and formed the core of our SAS-based, community-oriented small area profile (8-10). Other COPC practices that plan to use computerized, population-based health data on mainframe computers would be well advised to contact the IPODM Project Director or the State of California Department of Health Services' Maternal and Child Health Branch for more information about this system and its future implementations.

ADMATCH: Another mainframe system that may be useful for the definition of a clinic's community is the Admatch geographical matching program available from the Census Bureau. This program uses the information in the GBF/DIME files (Geographic Base File/Dual) Independent Map Encoding, a set of geographic correspondence data bases) to determine the census tracts for 80-95 percent of any given set of local street addresses. This would be useful for a clinic that has not yet coded information for patients' census tracts, but has access to a mainframe computer and wishes to replicate this method using patient addresses.

COPC data analysis can use a wide range of tools, from a large statistical package, such as SAS on an IBM mainframe, to a spreadsheet program such as

---

[1] An excellent Kermit manual is available from the Columbia University Center for Computing Activities. New York, New York 10027.

[2] The system uses CMS, IBM's Conversational Monitor System developed by the Maternal and Child Health Program at the University of California, Berkeley, under contract for the State of California Department of Health Services.

[3] Statistical Analysis System, SAS Institute Inc., Box 8000, Cary, North Carolina 27511.

Lotus 1-2-3 or the much cheaper VP-planner on a clinic microcomputer. The advantage of downloading to a microcomputer is that data manipulation, report generation, and graphics presentation can be greatly facilitated by using mass marketed personal computer applications packages. This relieves the dependency on professional mainframe oriented data personnel, resulting in both lower computing costs and faster turn around times. The total time investment necessary for such a project might be even further reduced by use of some of the newer "integrated" personal computer data programs such as Framework or Symphony. Because of the large size of the commercial markets for such products, most clinics should be able to find some combination of programs that will meet their needs and resources almost exactly. Much of the time-consuming work in this project was manipulation of the primary clinic data on a minicomputer to define the service area, using a nonstandard and unfriendly data system designed for billing purposes. This task would be very easy for clinics that keep their billing data in more standard format on microcomputers and use readily available database programs such as Dbase III or Rbase 5000.

Analysis of Clinic Data

The clinic's computer system was used to define the location of residence of active patients of the practice. This system uses the PICK operating system (5,6), but any type of commercial microcomputer relational database program could be used to define a service are by zip codes and/or census tracts. If sufficient clerical staff time were available, the type of sorting necessary for defining the microgeographic assignments could even be performed by placing index cards in labeled shoeboxes.

Much of the utility in defining a service area from primary clinic data will be found in the comparisons that can be made between the service area and the larger surrounding area, e.g. the remainder of the county. A variety of secondary data sources can thus be tapped to provide information relevant to the clinic's populations and their needs.

The number of visits per patient in a defined period for each diagnostic category at the clinic can be calculated, and more importantly, a period prevalence for any diagnostic category, by any clinic subgrouping, can be derived. This number will represent an estimate of the proportion of any segment of clinic users who are diagnosed with the condition of interest during that period of time. Because the numbers of patients in a particular subgroup may be quite small, and the resultant proportion very unstable between groups or over time, it is advisable to use a measure of the "softness" of the prevalence so obtained. We used a 95 percent confidence interval for our period prevalences. The 95 percent confidence intervals listed for the clinic period prevalence rates thus represent the bounds within which the true prevalence of the illnesses would be found 95 percent of the time, in a theoretical population of which clinic users represent a "random sample." This measure is used as a rough indicator of the uncertainty of a rate based on a small denominator such as that of the smaller subsets of a clinic population. An example of this type of information, in this case for diagnosed hypertension among clinic users, is shown in Table 3. In this table the number of individuals in each subgrouping is shown in the first column, followed by the percentage comprised by that subgroup within the entire clinic population. The third column shows the number of patients in each subgroup with the diagnosis of hypertension, followed by the percentage (group-specific prevalence) of the subgroup who have the diagnosis. Finally, the lower and upper

TABLE 3. Group Specific (6-Month) Period Prevalence of Diagnosed Hypertension in Clinic Users, by Income, by Sex and Age. Similar Arrays Could Be Constructed by Primary Language, by Ethnicity or for Other Groupings.

	All patients		Patients with HYPERTENSION		95% confidence interval	
	#	% (of total)	#	% (of class)	lower bound	upper bound
TOTAL PATIENTS:	4295	100.00%	182	4.24%	3.66%	4.89%
BY INCOME						
< poverty	2695	62.75%	106	3.93%	3.25%	4.76%
1x-1.5x poverty	788	18.35%	46	5.84%	4.35%	7.77%
1.5x-2x poverty	273	6.36%	18	6.59%	4.07%	10.40%
> 2x poverty	539	12.55%	17	3.15%	1.91%	5.10%
no income data	0	0.00%	0	ERR	ERR	ERR
BY AGE*						
< 17 Years	2000	46.57%	1	0.05%	.00%	0.32%
17-24 Years	629	14.64%	3	0.48%	0.12%	1.51%
25-44 Years	1162	27.05%	45	3.87%	2.87%	5.19%
45-64 Years	347	8.08%	82	23.63%	19.33%	28.53%
65-74 Years	102	2.37%	35	34.31%	25.38%	44.45%
> 74 Years	54	1.26%	16	29.63%	18.37%	43.79%
no birthdate	1	0.02%	0	0.00%	10.78%	94.54%
BY SEX by AGE*						
Male	1622	37.76%	57	3.51%	2.70%	4.56%
Female	2673	62.24%	125	4.68%	3.92%	5.56%
Female 0-4	515	11.99%	0	0.00%	0.02%	0.92%
Female 5-9	232	5.40%	0	0.00%	0.04%	2.03%
Female 10-14	174	4.05%	0	0.00%	0.05%	2.69%
Female 15-19	190	4.42%	0	0.00%	0.05%	2.47%
Female 20-34	948	22.07%	9	0.95%	0.46%	1.86%
Female 35-44	255	5.94%	18	7.06%	4.36%	11.11%
Female 45-64	251	5.84%	60	23.90%	18.87%	29.76%
Female > 64	107	2.49%	38	35.51%	26.67%	45.42%
Female no DOB	1	0.02%	0	0.00%	10.78%	94.54%
Male 0-4	548	12.76%	0	0.00%	0.02%	0.87%
Male 5-9	263	6.12%	0	0.00%	0.03%	1.79%
Male 10-14	162	3.77%	1	0.62%	0.03%	3.91%
Male 15-19	95	2.21%	0	0.00%	0.10%	4.84%
Male 20-34	298	6.94%	10	3.36%	1.71%	6.28%
Male 35-44	111	2.58%	11	9.91%	5.29%	17.42%
Male 45-64	96	2.24%	22	22.92%	15.21%	32.83%
Male > 64	49	1.14%	13	26.53%	15.40%	41.34%
Male no DOB	0	0.00%	0	ERR	ERR	ERR

bounds of the 95 percent confidence interval for that prevalence are given, based on the prevalence and the denominator (the first column).

The diagnostic categories for which prevalences are to be obtained can be chosen by counting numbers of visits for each relevant ICD-9 diagnostic code and listing all codes for a given diagnostic category that are both frequent enough to be potentially interesting and felt to be clinically relevant by the providers.

If the practitioner is interested in the distribution of family size among the families of clinic users, the frequency of each number of stated dependents per head of household can be counted. Similarly, if the practitioner is interested in setting up occupational health programs or employer-sponsored group health coverage, a list of all employers with two or more clinic heads of household could be compiled, and those employers could be sorted by number of clinic patients employed. Those firms employing the most clinic heads of household might then be examined for either occupational hazards and/or their interest in sponsoring an employee health program in conjunction with the clinic.

STATISTICAL ISSUES ARISING FROM THE USE OF SECONDARY DATA IN COPC

The most difficult issue that must be faced in small area data analysis is that of small sample size. The need to report confidence limits is paramount, and inferences must be made with caution. One solution is to combine data from multiple years, but even this may not help much when dealing with rare events.

A second problem is the inevitable use of multiple statistical tests. In our project, several hundred chi squares and Fisher's exact tests were used to compare a variety of rates and proportions. In this situaon even the use of a strict alpha of 0.01 or 0.005 would not eliminate the likeli-

hood that some of the statistically significant results will be due to the large number of comparisons tested. The use of multiple comparison correction techniques may help reduce this type of error, but they are difficult and controversial.

Another problem is the frequency of some events in such large populations is very high. Consequently, clinically trivial differences may result in low p-values. It must be remembered that to be important, the difference must still be a difference that makes a difference.

Conversely, events with much lower but increasing rates in smaller populations may be potentially quite important and worthy of intervention, even though the population is not large enough to have produced a significant p-value. In this circumstance, a few individual cases should be investigated to see what, if any, interventions could have made a difference. The bottom line, however, is that data analysis that proceeds without well-formulated hypotheses, must be viewed only as rough indicators of those areas that are worthy of further attention.

OBJECTIVES FOR COMMUNITY-ORIENTED INFORMATION SYSTEMS

In summary, the following operational goals are recommended for the long-term planning of community-oriented primary care information systems in community clinics. These goals should be viewed as specifications that are desirable, and most of them should be attainable at little or no extra hardware cost if proper purchasing decisions are made at the time a clinic computer system is obtained for billing or other necessary uses.

1. The ability to list or map census tracts and zip codes for any given group of patients, i.e., with a particular diagnosis, by race, age group, etc.

2. The ability to develop ethnic, age, and sex breakdowns for any given population subgroup.

3. The ability to link to and access local population-based health and demographic data bases (i.e., Census, SEER, birth and death records, hospital discharge records.)

4. The ability to capture and track clinic patients or family members admitted to local hospitals, whether referred from clinic or not.

5. The ability to record and track major health risk factors of clinic patients.

6. The ability to record and track education, occupation, and place of employment for clinic patients.

7. The ability to count the number of patients, as well as the number of visits with a particular diagnosis, to characterize them demographically and to determine visits per unit time by diagnosis for any subgroup.

8. The ability to link all members of a household as a family unit and record basic demographic data on nonpatient family members, as well as their other regular sources of medical care.

9. The ability to produce basic descriptive statistical formats that tabulate the above data in usable form.

10. The ability to generate regular reports of period prevalence for chronic illnesses and incidence of clinic visits for acute illnesses, by age, race, and sex, with confidence intervals for rates and the ability to easily compare statistically the rates for two different groups or time periods.

ADDITIONAL CONSIDERATIONS IN DEVELOPING A COPC INFORMATION SYSTEM

It is important that clinic staff contact the state and local agencies that can provide secondary data sources before deciding what programs are desirable. Individuals at these agencies often have insight into what programs will be compatible with their computers and data. They will also know exactly what they use for telecommunications, and compatibility with that software will be absolutely essential if the clinic is to make use of their data.

The type of microcomputer to be obtained should be the cheapest and most versatile, both compatible with the software chosen and with enough capacity to hold and process the clinic's data. Generally any microcomputer with hard-disk or other mass storage device will be adequate. A very nice system, adequate for the needs of a small to medium group practice or community health center, should be completed for less that $5,000.00 at 1986 prices. This cost will go down over time.

In addition to the types of software named above, consideration should be given to other resources that may be needed for the development of an information system. There are several reasons to use popular, commercially available software instead of more specialized proprietary packages. They are generally cheaper and easier to use. Once someone on the professional staff has spent several hours setting up and learning how to use this type of application program it can generally be turned over to clerical staff. Most of the commercial applications have support available by phone, some even with toll-free help numbers. Problems with them are generally much cheaper to resolve than with programs that require high-priced consultants or programmers to actually come onsite and improvise individualized solutions.

123

One-half day of professional time and 2 days of clerical time per week for the first few months will be needed to set up the system. Once the system is set up, it will take little extra clerical time to maintain, as long as it is integrated with billing and other essential functions. The amount of professional time it will require will be directly proportional to how much marketing, community health, or other information is desired. It may be desirable to identify one or more staff members who have a particular interest in becoming somewhat computer literate and obtain some extra training for them. They will then become the onsite "expert" with primary responsibility for keeping track of what is going on with the system as well as helping others with it.

Another option exists for small practices that have the capability to define their service area by zip code, but are unable to use secondary data sources. This is the "Market Area Profile" (MAP) service available from the American Medical Association. This service supplies census-derived demographic information for one or more zip codes or for a given radius around a specified street intersection. The AMA also provides information on health care providers and services in the area. This service supplies data that could be combined with a practitioner's own knowledge of the area to generate a rough idea of what COPC services might be needed. The MAP service costs approximately $100-$200 per zip code or other study requested.

CONCLUSION

Community-oriented primary care is an innovative approach to community health that goes beyond the delivery of standard medical services, in order to more fully meet the needs of the community. The first requirement is to define the actual community to be served. This often requires going beyond surveys of the current users, since clinic nonusers may represent a large unmet need for health services.

The methods used to define the service area for the clinic in the examples described involved a combination of geographic, needs-based, and accessibility parameters, that were then correlated with census tract and zip code data to determine the characteristics of the community. Primary data was correlated with secondary data, and a profile of clinic users was developed, with comparison of user and nonuser populations.

The goals of the integrated data system were to refine the service area definition and to determine the characteristics and health needs of the community so priorities could be established for planning emphasis programs. Programmatic recommendations that could be made from the resulting analysis included:

1. Identification of enhanced services for current clinic users;
2. Specification of the health needs of the service area as a whole, which guide outreach efforts to those groups who appear to be underusing the clinics;
3. Assessment of effectiveness and efficiency; and
4. Comparisons among the service area, the clinic users, and other reference areas.

Acknowledgment

The authors wish to thank Miguel Lucero, M.P.H., for his assistance with the mapping functions of IPODM-3 and all of his helpful suggestions. We also gratefully acknowledge the Data Processing Manager of the clinic and all of the many clinic staff who have been so helpful. To Annette Aalborg, Aftim Saba, and the COPC faculty of the University of California School of Public Health we extend our gratitude for their support and contributory efforts.

REFERENCES

1. Nutting, P.A.; Wood, M.; and Conner, E.M. Community-oriented primary care in the United States. *Journal of the American Medical Association* 1985; 253:1763.

2. Kark, S.L., and Abramson, J.H. Community focused health care. *Israel Journal of Medical Science* 1981; 17:65.

3. Warren, R.L. *The Community in America*, Third Edition. Chicago: Rand McNally, 1978.

4. The Clinic's Community Health Center Supplemental Application: Health Facilities Development Project, May 1985 - April 1986.

5. Cook, R., and Brandon, J. The Pick operating system. *Byte* October 1984:177.

6. Cook, R., and Brandon, J. The Pick operating system. *Byte* November 1984:132, 171.

7. Gould, J.B. *Improved Pregnancy Outcome Data Management Project System Manual*. Prepared for Maternal and Child Health Branch, State of California Department of Health Services, Contract No. 84-84088, Maternal and Child Health Program School of Public Health, University of California, Berkeley, June 1985.

8. Bosanac, E.M., and Hall, D.S. A small area profile system, its use in primary care resource development. *Soc. Sci. Med.* 1981; 15D: 313.

9. Bosanac, E.M.; Nottingham, D.L.; and Wyant, W.D. A small area profile system, its use in primary care resource development. *AIIE News* April 1978; 12:1.

10. Bosanac, E.M. A SAS based small-area profile system, its use in primary care resource development. *Proceedings of the SAS Users Group International Symposium* at Las Vegas, Nevada, 1978.

CHAPTER 18

Needs Demand Assessment as a Starting Point for COPC

Robert S. Kohl
Terry Conway, M.D.

The U.S. Public Health Service funds comprehensive primary care health centers through the Bureau of Health Care Delivery and Assistance (BHCDA) Section 330 funding. More than 600 such centers exist in rural and urban areas across the United States. Community-oriented primary care is the stated official clinical management philosophy for these community health centers (CHC's). An essential part of each CHC's grant application is a needs/demand assessment (NDA). The NDA is used for the following purposes: to evaluate the CHC community's continued need for grant subsidized primary care services; to determine number of physicians needed to meet estimated primary care visit demand in the CHC's target area; as a basis for the marketing and strategic planning process; and as a basis for developing a health care plan unique to the needs and resources of the target community.

Near North Health Service Center (NNHSC), a community health center located in Chicago, has attempted to apply COPC for the last 4 years. We see promise in using the NDA as a starting point for COPC. Use of the NDA in this way by all CHC's would increase the volume of practical experience with COPC tremendously. This can be accomplished using data all CHC's have already gathered. This paper reviews how the NDA can be immediately applied for COPC, practical enhancements of NDA that would increase its utility for COPC even more, and recommendations for the Federal granting agency (BHCDA) that would expedite the advancement of COPC even more.[1]

NEEDS/DEMAND ASSESSMENT COMPONENTS AND THEIR IMMEDIATE UTILITY FOR COPC

The NDA, a major portion of the grant application process for federally funded CHC's, forms the basis for a unique health care plan for a given area. Six steps are involved in developing an NDA (see Table 1 for details and Table 2 for suggested enhancements). Some of the steps have immediate utility for the CHC embarking on COPC as discussed below.

---

[1] If a provider without Section 330 Federal support is about to embark on COPC, there may be more appropriate ways to begin than using the NDA alone.

TABLE 1. Needs Demand Assessment for Federally Funded Community Health Centers

	Steps In Current Process	Suggested Enhancements
1. Define Service Area contiguous areas.	a. Conduct patient origin study. b. Plot service areas on map with major hospitals. c. Identify physician/population ratio.	d. Define subcommunities. e. Broaden profile to include sociodemographic characteristics.
2. Describe economic status.	a. Describe income and insurance status of CHC users. b. Describe income and insurance status of service area. c. Describe changing economic indicators (population, Medicaid, unemployment, etc.).	d. Plot economic status by subcommunity.
3-5. Establish and analyze the demand supply capacity of primary care services (physicians).	a. Compare service area age-sex distribution to U.S. Distribution. b. Estimate demand for primary care visits in primary service and contiguous areas. c. Determine supply of primary care physician resources in primary services and contiguous areas. d. Determine surplus or deficit of primary care physicians and number of physicians needed to meet unmet demand. e. Identify physicians currently working at CHC to assist in NHSC physician placement.	f. Identify non-physician resources in primary and contiguous areas. g. Identify potential collaborators among physician and non-physician resources.
6. Identify special health status needs.	a. Examine age/sex distribution, ethnicity, and poverty status to identify population sub-groups which have special needs	c. Analyze health status indicators by subcommunity or subpopulation group.

(Table 1. continued) or require specialty mix due to difference from U.S. norm.

b. CHC identify health status problems by asking providers, checking infant mortality, fertility or % of elderly, prevalence of chronic diseases or document other problems of greater magnitude than state or national norms.

d. At a minimum check neonatality, disability, and cohort/specific mortality by cause.

TABLE 2. Data Sources by Steps in NDA (NDA Steps Plus Enhancements)

1. a. CHC patient records or master file for patient origin study
   b. U.S. census for good census tract maps
   HSA for hospitals in area
   c. HSA for physician/population ratio
   d. U.S. census information plotted on Census Tract map
   e. U.S. census
2. a. CHC patient financial data
   b. U.S. census, local Medicaid agency, Medicare carrier, large employers, HMO's, insurance carriers
   c. Key individuals in hospital administration, HSA, economic development, housing, etc.
   d. U.S. census tract map
3-5. a. U.S. census
   b. BHCDA average visit/person by age cohort

   c. Local HSA, phone survey using yellow pages
   d. Calculation on BHCDA worksheets
   e. Staff roster
   f. Social service directory, yellow pages, community coalitions, community leaders, etc.
   g. Review existing or potential relationships with resources in c. and f.
6. a. U.S. census
   b. U.S. census, Local/State Health Departments, National surveys (see text), well documented prevalence studies for similar population groups, hospital discharge data
   c. Same as b, nominal group methods
   d. Same as b

Note: Some CHC's have a readily accessible data base to compare patient population experiences to service area rates and State and National rates.

Step 1: Define the Service Area of the Site and Contiguous Areas

A patient origin study provides the method for determining the service area, in which a major portion of its patients reside and in which most COPC activities and resources will be located. Depending on the method used in conducting the patient origin study, it may answer several questions. Who is served? Who is not served? Are users of nonclinical services included in the study? If so, are clinical and nonclinical users differentiated to answer whether or not the intended target populations are being reached for various COPC interventions?

Patient origin studies can be compared over time to reveal any shift in program participants. This information may be useful in light of a CHC's overall and COPC objectives.

Step 2: Describe the Economic Status of the Patient Population

A comparison of the income of CHC users to the service area population and patient origin study may reveal substantial numbers of poor who are not being served or are using other primary care services. Other providers may offer potential partners with whom to address particular health problems.

Similarly, the insurance status of CHC users compared to nonusers (if available) can be particularly useful in determining whether financial problems are a barrier to obtaining services. For example, we inadvertently experienced an increase in the number of hypertensive patients when expensive medications were made available at little or no charge. Changing economic conditions, such as the opening or closing of a major employer, can also affect health status and financial ability to obtain health care services.

Steps 3-5. Establish and Analyze the Demand, Supply, and Capacity of Primary Care Resources in the Target Area

The age-sex distribution can be used beyond determining demand to identify substantial variations from the U.S. average. For example, our service area has almost twice the average proportion of youths 17 and under and one-third the expected proportion of elderly. As a result, NNHSC emphasizes maternal and child health services but also addresses the needs of seniors, who are particularly isolated in this service area.

Knowledge of major primary health care providers in the primary service area or contiguous area may suggest potential partners for accomplishing COPC objectives. NNHSC is planning an infant mortality reduction effort with a nearby CHC with a contiguous service area. Knowing the other providers can also highlight potential gaps in primary care services within the target area.

Step 6. Identify Special Health Status Needs

The identification of health status needs is the least structured step in the needs demand assessment process, yet the most critical to COPC. Three indicators for which standards for special need are identified include infant mortality, fertility, and proportion of elderly.

CHC's are free to document unusual age-sex-race distributions that suggest programmatic response. Population subgroups and their particular health needs should be identified. For example, NNHSC serves two major ethnic groups — black and Hispanic. Both are much younger and poorer than average with poor perinatal outcomes and higher than expected cardiovascular disease, cancer, accidents, and violence.

Documentation of health status changes over time can yield valuable information, especially when compared with city, county, State, or national trends to show relative progress or slippage in improving health status within the CHC's target area.

NEEDS/DEMAND ASSESSMENT VERSUS COPC

There are several major differences between the assumptions underlying NDA and COPC. NNHSC has attempted to use NDA for the purposes of COPC and has learned that if left unaltered these assumptions will limit the scope and success of COPC efforts.

The Definition of Need

In the NDA the health needs of the community are mainly expressed as unsatisfied primary care visits, and the solution offered is physicians to meet that need. In preparing the NDA most effort is spent on the tables and schedules to define how many unmet primary care visits exist within the CHC's community. The Section 330 CHC program provides funding to provide for these unmet visits. In communities such as NNHSC's, improving access to primary care is certainly a major ingredient in improving the poor health status. Step 6 in the NDA defines need in terms of significant health status problems that exceed national averages and forms the basis for a community-specific health care plan.

The NNHSC's community population is over-represented by adolescents and young adults. Examples of their health status problems are unintended pregnancy, violent injury and death, sexually transmitted diseases, and substance abuse. CHC funding has allowed us to provide more primary care services of a conventional type such as family planning, prenatal visits, adolescent care, and treatment of sexually transmitted diseases. Certain services such as pre-high school physical exams have been altered to focus on issues such as sexuality, family planning, and prevention of substance abuse. However, the incidence of these conditions would be expected to change a limited amount from this strategy of treatment. This large subpopulation of the community seems to require extensive outreach and case management services. NNHSC feels that pregnant teens can clearly benefit from nutrition behavior change and easy access to nutrition supplement programs and has shown some success at this. This type of health service is defined as "other health" (in CHC funding) and is not included in the NDA. It has been increasingly difficult to obtain funding for "other health" services in recent Section 330 funding.

COPC seeks to improve community health status through whatever strategies seem most effective, and often several complementary approaches are used at once. NNHSC has made efforts in family

life education junior high school students, support for a community coalition on infant mortality, and participation in a gang reduction initiative, and has considered attempts to change the prenatal care content of other health providers in the community. These interventions are difficult to categorize in the CHC grant application process, and it is even harder to secure Federal assistance for them. We have found that the NDA assumption of community health status need as unsatisfied primary care visit demand is limited when viewed from a COPC perspective.

What Is a Successful Outcome?

Data discerned from NDA and other BHCDA documents are gathered by BHCDA at the regional and national level to determine funding levels. Year-to-year trends on these data are provided to each health center and are reviewed at the regional and central offices. These trends are comparisons of performance based solely on the management efficiency of the CHC as reflected in number of encounters, staffing levels, and cost. COPC, however, requires monitoring of health status by health centers. Negative health trends can point to the need for new strategies, and positive trends may be able to show program benefits. CHC's are critically aware of the need for cost efficiency in any health care strategy. However COPC also looks at outcome efficiency to determine if the CHC program is working in the community. The time and effort that the current NDA system requires CHC's to focus almost exclusively on cost efficiency.

Competition versus Collaboration

The NDA and the CHC funding process reflect the current philosophy of competition in health care. However, other community health resources in COPC should be inventoried and looked upon as potential partners in addressing the identified community health status needs. The CHC situated in the community contiguous to NNHSC's service area had been in the position of a "competitor" for sources of funding for years, but the COPC process has encouraged cooperation between this CHC and NNHSC in addressing joint community needs. Nutrition and podiatry personnel currently are shared, and successful programs are replicated in both communities. Cooperation by the centers in a statewide initiative to reduce Illinois' high infant mortality rate has also begun. NDA does not require thought on how to cooperate, and some of the instructions seem to emulate private sector methods in requiring competition against what COPC would regard as partners.

COPC is meaningless if the CHC practice does not survive, but the present call for increased competition may actually do some disservice to a community's health status. It should be remembered that, by definition, CHC's serve populations that the present health care system does not compete to serve. Perhaps some of this competitive orientation is misplaced.

Who Should Be Involved?

The NDA does not include community involvement in any section. However, this is not inconsistent with strong community involvement. CHC regulations do stress strong community representation on CHC boards of directors. COPC, however, requires more than community representation: involvement by the community in needs assessment and program implementation is necessary. In order to use NDA for COPC this dimension will have to be added at several steps throughout the process.

SIMPLE STEPS BEYOND NDA TO PROVIDE GREATER UTILITY FOR COPC

Some CHC's will want to refine their NDA with minimal effort in order to allow greater utility in implementing COPC activities. Several ideas are presented below corresponding to the steps in the NDA process.

Step 1. Define the Service Area

Throughout the entire NDA process it is useful to define subcommunities within the primary service area that have ethnic and behavioral similarities. For example, the NNHSC service area can be divided into black and Hispanic subcommunities, which can be delineated by distinct census tracts. The black target census tracts can be divided into persons who reside in a large public housing development and those who live outside. Further, through discussions with community leaders, the public housing population can be subdivided into three distinct areas with distinct educational, age, fertility, and family structure characteristics. These three areas are separated by gang boundary lines, which form a major barrier to interaction between subcommunities. Knowledge of these subcommunities proves useful in designing programs that are accessible to subcommunities at high risk for particular health problems.

A broader profile including selected population and housing characteristics from the U.S. Census is useful in delineating subcommunities within the target area. Subjective knowledge, perhaps gained through an organized method such as a key informant survey, also provides valuable insights into significant characteristics of the subcommunities that will affect the design and implementation of programs.

Step 2. Describe Economic Status

The economic description of the target area is really an extension of the sociodemographic profile developed in Step 1. Subcommunity analysis allows the CHC to postulate higher relative need for certain subcommunities (either geographic or ethnic) and to target programs accordingly after comparing the sociodemographic profile, economic status, resources, and health status indicators of each subcommunity.

Steps 3-5. Establish and Analyze the Demand, Supply, and Capacity of Primary Care Resources

Primary care resources are defined narrowly in the NDA as primary care physicians. However, nonphysician resources will also have impact on COPC problems. For example, in addressing poor perinatal outcomes, NNHSC considers such resources as WIC sites, public health nursing, schools, head start and daycare programs, churches, and community organizations as essential partners in dealing with perinatal problems, within the limits of available resources.

The NDA process characterizes other primary health care providers as competitors. However, much can be gained in terms of affecting a health status indicator if providers worked together toward common goals. NNHSC provides prenatal care for about one-third of the deliveries in the primary service area. Yet, it is clear that wider impact can be realized if NNHSC cooperates with the teaching hospital that provides another one-third of the prenatal care for target area residents.

Step 6. Health Status Needs

As with the sociodemographic and economic status profiles, the analysis of health status by subcommunity can be very useful in identifying subgroups at higher risk of problems and in planning, implementing, and monitoring programs accordingly over time.

Since health status assessment is an unrefined art limited by availability of data across the range of potential health status problems, some approach for determining the priority issues in a given service area

seems in order. This process is understandably individual to each community due to the number of variables that make each community unique.

There are several sources of data for health status indicators: perinatal indicators (e.g., fertility, birth, teen birth, prematurity) from local or State health departments; reportable disease from local and State health departments; age , race-, and sex-specific mortality rates by cause of death from local and State health departments; and disability rate from U.S. Census.

Health status problems for which there is no local data can be estimated by national surveys such as the Health Interview Survey, Health and Nutrition Examination Survey, National Ambulatory Medical Care Survey, or Hospital Discharge Survey, all conducted by the National Center for Health Statistics. For instance, by knowing the number of persons aged 30 and older by sex and ethnic group, a CHC can estimate the expected number of hypertensives based on national or regional averages from the Hypertensive Detection and Followup Program.

IMPLEMENTATION OF NDA FOR COPC

Adjustments, additions, and reorientation may make NDA a useful tool for COPC. Yet it is only a tool. Currently, NDA is an exercise carried out by most CHC's as a required section of its grant application. Following the grant application it resides in a file drawer. Few staff members are aware of its existence and the data it contains.

The NDA can be a useful tool in a CHC's health plan. However, the health plan cannot remain only a filed document. Its objectives should be applied and achieved throughout the center and within all of its programs. At NNHSC the administrative, medical and nursing, outreach, social services, and nutrition staff are asked to prepare their programs based on COPC (and NDA) data. A consensus on community diagnosis (the leading health status deficiencies and risks within a particular community) should be developed within the health center. It is practical for the community board to be familiar with the community diagnosis if they are to support the policy and the financial decisions that are based on it. COPC partners within the community — whether other health care providers or key organizations or individuals — can help to verify community diagnosis. They can then participate with the CHC in joint efforts to plan and implement strategies for COPC. The NDA as a part of COPC in a community health center is only effective when it is applied and when key persons are involved and invested in it.

SUGGESTIONS FOR THE FEDERAL GOVERNMENT

Several changes at the Federal level would assist in using NDA to encourage COPC:

First, redefine need in the NDA to include health status as well as demand criteria. Spend the same amount of effort in providing methodology, data sources, and technical assistance to assess community health status (community diagnosis) as is currently spent on assessing lack of primary care visits. Remove the disincentives for CHC's to provide nonmedical services in reducing health status problems.

Second, add COPC performance criteria to the database already gathered and computerized at BHCDA's central office. Scrutinize the health status outcome criteria yearly in the same manner as the current financial and productivity data. Provide trends for year-to-year data from a particular CHC and perhaps compare different CHC's. Identify outliers who might require assistance and successful centers that might provide insight into

what elements are necessary for successful COPC outcomes.

Finally, the NDA leads to expansion of primary care visits within a community mainly because that is what is funded. If the BHCDA strongly desires COPC outcomes to come from the NDA process it could expedite such outcomes through funding as well. If funding followed successful assessment of community health status, program planning, and evaluation of health status change, then these results would ensue from CHC's. Recent years have seen the success of funding changes throughout the health care system to change the structure and function of health care organizations. If BHCDA were convinced that COPC is an effective and politically expedient process, then funding changes would do much to implement COPC as the primary CHC health care strategy.

CHAPTER 19

Defining and Characterizing the Community: The Use of Survey Research Techniques and Tools in COPC

Leatrice H. Berman, M.A.

In some practice settings it may be desirable to go beyond the use of subjective data and secondary data sources to characterize the community. The use of primary data, collected to address specific questions, can greatly expand on the ability to describe and understand the community. The initial use of subjective information and secondary data often suggest issues for which more focused data are required—data that can only be obtained from a community survey.

This chapter is based on experience and work conducted by the Department of Community Health, Northwestern Memorial Hospital and Northwestern University Medical School in concert with two freestanding health centers, Erie Family Health Center (1) and the Near North Health Service Corporation (2). The chapter describes an approach based largely on techniques of survey research and introduces the various tools and materials that are available. Survey research methods are not appropriate in every practice setting but have some advantages to be considered. Both advantages and disadvantages will be discussed. This will assist the practitioner in considering ways in which to use basic survey research techniques and negotiate between the social science and statistical requirements and the specific aims of COPC.

COLLECTING YOUR OWN DATA

Why would a practice even want to collect its own community data? There are several reasons.

First, a practice can work up its own patient data in a fairly sophisticated way to get a sense of problem incidence, problem prevalence, or general health care needs, but often practices will not be representative of the total population a practice wishes to serve — both problem-specific (e.g., diabetics, obese children, depressed women) or geographically specific (census tracts, community areas, and zip codes). A practice may not know its market share until it surveys the community, or the market share may be so small that patient data will not provide an accurate picture of health needs within the broader community.

Second, available secondary data such as vital statistics are often not sufficiently detailed to help a practice define the dimensions of community health problems. For example, even in an area in which vital statistics are fairly developed, e.g., infant birth and death data, one cannot get a very clear picture of infant morbidity at birth in relation a defined population. Furthermore, while other secondary data sources such as hospital data sets are increasingly sophisticated in yielding morbidity data by institution, these data sets very often are not geocoded by hospitals to provide geographic profiles on morbidity, and data files that aggregate data from several hospitals are not easily available.

Third, practices concerned with reaching the underserved are essentially reaching out to a population untallied in available health provider or reportable illness data sets. A practice, in this case, is charting its own course.

Fourth, a practice may need a more accurate and current estimate of a specific problem or measure of health status (a baseline data set). This need would occur before the development or modification of a health program for subsequent evaluation, at which point the population would be reassessed to test program impact. Quite frequently, the requirements of such data sets suggest specific and original data collection.

Last, secondary data rarely give a practice acceptable measures of problems that are more health- than illness-related. For example, accident prevalence, alcoholism, family social functioning, child abuse, and obesity are the kinds of concerns for which very little data are routinely collected on populations or patients, but a practice might have a great deal of interest in them.

Data on these problems traditionally come from local or national surveys. However, national survey data are quite difficult to apply to small geographic areas, and one cannot assume that valid comparisons can be made.[1]

Additionally, local survey data are quite often simply not available. It may then indeed be the role of the primary care practice to embark upon its own data collection.

Another basic assumption related to the primary collection of data by a practice needs explicit attention. There are many steps in the transformation of a primary care practice into a COPC practice, but one critical element in COPC relates to the issue of responsibility: a COPC practice takes responsibility not only for assessing, improving, and evaluating the needs and impact of its work on patients, but also takes responsibility for the needs of the community in which it resides and for its own impact on the community. This leads to the premise that a practice can have a wider effect by taking on a broader set of people to serve and problems to address.

Therefore, the collection of primary data or secondary data, or the extrapolation and analysis of a practice's patient data, are driven fundamentally by the assumption in COPC that a practice should look beyond its patients to a target population: to assess the role of the practice relative to other providers in serving a population or treating a problem; to test, validate, or redirect the strategic program focus of the practice to improve health outcomes in a population; or to survey a specific health problem or assess unmet health needs. Collecting data is just a more direct method by which a practice can look at the world beyond its patients.

Questions to Ask in Developing An Approach

As a first step in moving toward data collection, a practice should define a

[1] Personal communications with Norman Hearst, M.D., University of California, San Francisco and School of Public Health, University of California, Berkeley; Ralph Frerichs, D.V.M., Dr. P.H., Professor of Epidemiology, School of Public Health, University of California, Los Angeles; and Eli Zimmerman, M.P.H. (regarding the development of the Community Health Profile Data Base software), Oakland, California.

framework for the inquiry and a problem(s) focus. Several questions can be asked to assist the practice in this step:

- *What do you want to know specifically?* About whom? From whom will you get the information — the target population itself or key informants? How will you use the information operationally? How will it change things? Will it reshape a program? If so, what program? Or will it be used to consider the development of new programs?

- *How can the data be obtained?* What methods might you use? Interviews at agencies, schools, or institutions? Households? Key informants (local leaders or knowledgeable individuals) in the community? Participant observations?

- *What specific test, measures and/or questionnaire items are needed?*

- *How do you want to collect data?* In person? By mail? By telephone? Is the population so small you can sample all of it, e.g., a classroom? If too large, will you interiew people incidentally, e.g., standing at the supermarket or corner and interviewing people who come by, or will you employ some systematic or random sampling techniques?

- *What level of skill is required of your data collection personnel?*

These questions should be discussed within the practice and cast out to a wide net of its providers, community board, or selected patients. At this point, the practice will have a conceptual approach and in many ways will be past the most difficult point.

CHOOSING A SURVEY RESEARCH APPROACH

Survey research approaches lend themselves to both single-problem and broad-based, exploratory inquiries, both of which are appropriate to an initial or repeated excursion into COPC. One can go into a population and collect objective data such as blood pressure, dental caries, or blood sugars, but when one meets a population through a survey tool, the questions fielded quite often broaden the data collection effort. In fact, many clinical problems cannot be fully understood without using questionnaires, e.g., medical histories. Survey tools can be constructed tightly around the exploration of very specific problems, such as accidents among children or functional activity levels among elder adults. Also, surveys can measure many health-related constructs or factors that are relevant when a practice wants to explore overall health needs or the relative importance or health needs in a specific population. Therefore, for broad-based inquiries, survey research is useful. Conversely, however, the use of survey tools can effectively enrich a specific, single-problem orientation.

Survey research is usually accompanied by some form of probability sampling when an entire population cannot be measured. With marginal practice resources available in both time and money, developing a small but accurate and representative data base on a specific problem will serve the interests of a practice well. Therefore, survey research, through its use of systematic statistical sampling procedures, will reinforce rigor in the data collection approach used. Survey research also lends itself to the development of quantitative estimates of a problem and its risk factors, such as frequency distributions or quantitative correlations between one factor and another. If a practice wants to grasp the quantitative dimensions of a problem within the community, survey research would be the logical choice. Survey research can also be conducted by lay staff trained in standardized interviewing and data collection techniques. This method is less expensive than sending technicians or practitioners out to collect clinical measurements.

On the other hand, survey research may not fit many situations. Some problems lend themselves to quantitative assessments, but other inquiries might be best served by using methods other than survey research. These methods are more open-ended and exploratory and lend themselves to inquiries where factors might not be so easily laid out in a predetermined survey-response format. Other approaches, such as interviews with selected individuals or target groups, as reported by Ellerbrock et al. in Part II of this book, are often open-ended (but systematic) and in-depth. Other methods include participant observations and case studies, which can employ both interviewing and observation. These methods, part of a tradition in the social sciences called ethnographic or qualitative research, also have much utility in COPC.

Furthermore, as survey research requires a certain level of sophistication or dedication to mediate between well-developed, scientific survey research methods and the routine, less rigorous data collection needs of clinical practices, it is more time-consuming and therefore more difficult to implement. In contrast, putting a questionnaire together quickly and going, for example, to the local supermarket, local residents, or seniors' apartment complexes to capture data on a "first come, first questioned" basis is not survey research, but it can be quite functional in building good program starts and cases for action in a community. This method is less rigorous than a sample survey research approach. The tradeoff is energy versus rigor.

Also on the cost side, even in the design and implementation of small-scale surveys (100-150 people or households), the cost can be several thousand dollars. Resource constraints in the typical practice may preclude conducting this kind of COPC work. However, practices have been innovative in using surplus resources or institutional subsidies to conduct sur-

veys, and their use in community needs assessments is of interest in select quarters of clinical practice, community hospitals, HMO's, academic medical centers, private foundations, and government.

In essence, choosing methods of inquiry is complex and imprecise. Small samples, even when rigorously studied, may be too small to generalize to the community of interest. Therefore, one might prefer to conduct another type of inquiry, as mentioned. The superiority of one method over another is quite unclear. In summary, a practice does not have to undertake a probability sampling approach to collect original data from the community, but if one is concerned about generalizing and quantitative estimation, then probability sampling is the way to proceed. The most important rule of thumb is to match methods to needs.

SURVEY RESEARCH APPROACH: STEPS, OPTIONS, AND HINTS

To review, in mounting the approach itself, the practice needs to set general parameters related to sampling units (e.g., households, individuals, classrooms); sample size; and whether the interviewing will be done by mail, telephone, or in person. All these decisions have cost implications. Sample location follows from the intent of one's survey, but sample size and methods often derive principally from dollar resources available and how close the practice wants to get to the target community in conducting the project.

The first hint for prospective survey researchers is to get some basic materials, texts (3-8), manuals, and handbooks (9-26). These have been developed in the health and social science communities and often are geared to nonexpert researchers. These materials are invaluable in laying out optimal approaches to community survey research or community needs assessment. Each practice must find its own way through these "how to do" materials,

137

which lay out a stepwise approach to project scope, sampling targets and methods, questionnaire design and layout, training of data collectors, supervision and organization of field work, interviewing, and data analysis and report writing.

The second strategy that can be useful in getting a COPC survey off the ground is the use of local consultants, for example, academic researchers, survey research labs, independent consultants, or technical assistance providers with expertise in community survey techniques. In the Chicago experience upon which this paper is based, several agencies were consulted, and they are illustrative of resources available throughout the country: the Center for Health Administration Studies of the University of Chicago; the National Opinion Research Center; University of Illinois Survey Research Lab; and the Latino Institute (which provides technical assistance to community organizations serving the Hispanic community).

There is much to learn from these consultants. Initial advice is almost always free and rates are not very high. Many of these labs and centers would implement COPC projects for the primary care practice if sufficient resources were offered. However, because COPC means more than mounting a data collection effort, it is not advisable to hire a consultant to direct and implement the project totally. The practice is enhanced by going directly into the community and integrating survey research skills within its own staff so the practice can integrate itself into the life of the community (27). Therefore, the use of consultants should be largely advisory. In this vein, consultations on scope, cost, and timeframe can give a practice a clear concept of how to mount and manage the endeavor (28). Survey research center libraries provide access to lay manuals of the kind discussed above. Without any funds for consulting, a practice could move forward on the basis of these materials alone.

Consultants can also help choose sampling techniques to minimize bias (sample design and procedures), questionnaire wording, and format; link the practice to other local survey research that clarifies the availability of specific data that may be important to the practice (29); train data collectors, develop recruitment criteria, and even recruit experienced, indigenous data collectors who have been used in other survey efforts; and design the supervision of fieldwork, data analysis, and construction of data files.

Finally, short conversations with consultants can provide quick courses in complex methods issues, and these conversations can clarify the difference in objectives between COPC and traditional survey research approaches to the uninitiated.

There is a growing literature in survey research devoted to the efficiency of telephone use over in-person interviews even in inner-city areas. Recent experience in large field studies demonstrates the validity of statistical adjustments in compensating for loss of data anticipated from urban households without telephones (7). Telephones have been used successfully even in small-scale field studies in minority (e.g., Hispanic) samples.[2] However, despite the cost savings reaped through telephone use, having face-to-face contact with one's community is important in COPC. Through such interviews, a practice conducts its "physical diagnosis" in the community and enhances its outreach (public relations), marketing, and case-finding strategies. Furthermore, given the small projected sample size in most routine COPC data projects (as a result of limited resources), compromising the data set by using telephones and relying on

---

[2] Personal communication with Marion Howard, Ph.D., Erie Family Health Center, Chicago, Illinois.

statistical adjustments that have much less reliability in small samples is not desirable. When one becomes clearer about the real differences between traditional survey research — academic or marketing — and COPC data collection, one can be a better interpreter of advice received. This in no way minimizes the utility of consultations, but the process itself educates the COPC practitioner about his or her own particular trade.

Another helpful strategy in mounting a community survey effort is the use of existing survey research tools for the development of a questionnaire. If one lacks confidence to develop a questionnaire, or if one wants to use questions that have been field-tested for their accuracy in capturing a specific set of information, reviewing existing instruments can be quite instructive.

Questionnaire development is the most time-consuming task in a survey research approach. Even after focusing on an area of inquiry, the specific content and scope of the survey may remain fuzzy. Reviewing questions can facilitate ideas about specific content. In addition, questionnaire review not only can assist in making an inquiry more specific but also can broaden one's inquiry by providing ideas about related questions, since many instruments are based on multiple problems.

The review of instruments provides optional ways of asking questions. Slight differences in questions actually do reflect different constructs to be measured, so reviewing several instruments forces one to make choices and become more precise. For example, in Table 1, there are four questions that seem fairly close in their construction, but they get at quite different phenomenona related to what one might generally call self-reported health status. Questions 1, 2, and 3 address most simply the concept of self-reported health and are known in the general literature to be fairly valid and predictive indicators of

good health outcomes. Question 2 adds the dimension of recent change in status, and Question 3 controls for the respondent's perception of the aging phenomenon. Question 4 is both a measure of health status, health consciousness, or health-related stress or fears. This question might very well be sensitive to issues beyond the direct measures of one's health, such as the experiencing of a recent death whereby one might become temporarily concerned about one's own health. Question 5 asks also about health consciousness as reflected in how one cares for oneself, and Question 6 is an attitude question related to one's sense of empowerment over health, or test attitude/motivation regarding potential behavior change.

Tables 2-4 address the measurement of barriers to health care and present several entirely different methods by which one can conduct this inquiry. The source of each set of questions is indicated on the chart. Method 1 (Table 2) creates a long list of reasons why some people do not go to the doctor when they believe they should, and asks fairly directly if people have experienced the situation of not going when they should and why. It also allows the respondent to express an entire cluster of reasons with respect to barriers to access. Analysis of these data can retrieve the frequency with which certain items are listed by individual respondents as well as capture repeated clustering to test patterns in a community syndrome.

Method 2 (Table 3) asks a general question about whether the medical care one gets matches self-perceived need. If problems do exist, then the inquiry is followed by a shorter list of variable. The analysis also focuses on the number of items that the respondent lists to get at some quantitative measure of how large or burdensome access problems are.

Method 3 (Table 4) is unique in emphasizing directly the relationship between

TABLE 1. Health Status Questions

1. Would you say your health is excellent, good, fair, or poor?

_____ Excellent
_____ Good
_____ Fair
_____ Poor
_____ Don't Know

The next group of questions asks your personal opinions about health-related matters.

2. Compared with two years ago, that is, since 1977, would you say that your health is now better, worse, or about the same?

Better
Worse
Same
Don't Know

3. Compared to other people your age, would you say your health is . . . (READ LIST)

Excellent
Good
Fair, or
Poor
DO NOT READ Don't Know

4. Over the past year has your health caused you a great deal of worry, some worry, hardly any worry, or no worry at all?

A great deal of worry
Some worry
Hardly any worry
No worry at all
Don't Know

5. How good a job do you feel you are doing in _taking care_ of your health? Would you say . . . . . (READ LIST)

Excellent
Good
Fair
Poor
DO NOT READ Don't Know

6. How much control do you think you have over your future health? Would you say . . . . . (READ LIST)

A great deal
Some
Very Little
None at all
DO NOT READ Don't Know

Source: National Survey of Personal Health Practices and Consequences (33)

seeing a doctor and both _structural_ (e.g., transportation, hours) and _attitudinal_ factors (e.g., "Shouldn't bother doctors," "I can get over most any disease without medical aid," "Doctors don't tell you enough"). In certain communities or inquiries, attitudinal variables might be critically important to understanding access problems.

Tables 5a and 5b portray Method 4 taken from the 1978 National Health Interview Survey. Two series of questions focus on access in very particular ways while asking episode-specific questions related to an encounter last held with a physician. The subset of questions in Table 5a exemplifies the way one might focus on barriers to getting medication, using physician referrals and consultants, barriers to using one's usual source of care, the difficulty of reaching the doctor by telephone, and the adequacy of time spent on the telephone. Table 5b presents a series of questions why the interviewee might have waited before going to the doctor. This series measures both struc-

TABLE 2. Barriers to Care

Method #1: The following are reasons why some people do not go to the doctor when they should. Please check each reason which explains why your household did not go to the doctor when they should have.

_____ 2. Did not realize that the problem was serious at the time.

_____ 3. Expense of seeing doctor, medicine.

_____ 4. Don't want charity.

_____ 5. Just never have gotten around to trying to find a doctor.

_____ 6. Don't like long waits.

_____ 7. Don't like being in waiting room with others.

_____ 8. They don't take a very long time with you anyway.

_____ 9. Afraid of doctors, shots, etc.

_____ 10. Can't understand their explanations.

_____ 11. They don't explain much to me.

_____ 12. Don't see the same doctor all the time.

_____ 13. Previous bad experience in family.

_____ 14. Doctors are busy and I hate to bother them.

_____ 15. Afraid of being refused service by a doctor.

_____ 16. Don't know how to find a doctor or medical help.

_____ 17. No transportation to get to doctor.

_____ 18. Too expensive to get to doctor.

_____ 19. Was turned away due to full practice.

_____ 20. No one to care for children.

_____ 21. Too sick to travel.

_____ 22. Unable to get there at time service is offered.

_____ 23. Distance to doctor.

_____ 24. Other (Specify: _____)

Source: Community Needs Assessment Survey Instrument, Rockford School of Medicine. (Question 2-24) (34)

tural barriers in the delivery system and respondents' attitudes about physicians and their utility.

In summary, reviewing surveys helps to address both scope and specificity regarding items to be assessed in a survey instrument. From the examples above, one notes that there are multiple resources and a rich history and literature on the design of survey instruments. Particular use can be made of large national surveys that not only provide prevalence and health problem data to be used by a practice for comparative findings, but also provide field-

tested, scientifically validated questions on a variety of health measures.

Although many questionnaire items in these surveys are useful, they also require some adaptation. For example, because they are fielded in such large samples, national surveys can ask about health visits and problems experienced in a 2-week timeframe and come up with reasonably accurate measures of problem prevalence. However, in conducting community surveys with small samples, the number of events (e.g., problems experienced, visits to physicians) would be very few within a

TABLE 3. Barriers to Care

Method #2: Do you have any problems getting all the medical care or treatment you feel that you need?	_____ Don't know where to go.
	_____ Can't get there because of physical condition.
_____ Yes	_____ Can't get a doctor to treat me or my problem.
_____ No	
_____ Not answered	_____ Can't get a doctor to come to the house.
(IF R ANSWERED "YES" TO Q. 68, ASK) What are those problems? (DO NOT READ LIST. CHECK ALL THAT APPLY.)	_____ Other (Specify: _____)
	_____ Not Answered.
	(OFFICE CODING ONLY)
_____ No doctor available in vicinity.	_____ Two or three of above.
_____ Can't afford medical care.	_____ Four or five of above.
_____ Have difficulty getting transportation.	_____ Six or seven of above.
	_____ Eight of above.

Source: Baltimore Seniors Need Assessment Survey. (Questions 68 and 68a) (35)

2-week period. Despite incurring greater recall problems, in smaller surveys one needs to expand the timeframe to 6 months or 1 year to get cogent self-reported problem prevalence or health service utilization data. Several of the national surveys which one can use for questionnaire development are described in chapter 64 of this book.

Local surveys (29-37), special studies (5,38,39), and health risk appraisals (41-46), either university or commercially produced, also can provide useful ideas for questionnaire development. Such surveys may vary in focus and validity, but they provide meaningful items for scope, content, and wording of questions. Their layout and formatting instructions are usually less formidable than national surveys and therefore are quite useful as guides for COPC surveys.

Before the development of one's own questionnaire, and certainly if one is inclined to become just a bit more grounded in this process, there are special "quick and dirty" literature reviews that might assist the COPC novitiate in resolv-

ing several conceptual and methodological problems. For example, a COPC project team (3) had concerns about the effect of culture and male attitudes about physicians on Hispanic male use of health services in a field survey that focused on where and how often Hispanic men and their families went for care. The surveyors thought that perhaps they should assess these attitudinal factors as related to the use of a health center.

Before proceeding, however, a literature review was conducted because the project team knew this had been a question often explored in the health services literature. The literature review attempted not only to find relevant field survey questions but to explain the relationship between attitudes toward physicians and use of services.

The literature review demonstrated that the relationship between attitudes toward physicians and health are so interdependent on satisfaction with prior services and utilization experience that any such question repeated in the local survey would not be easily interpreted (47). As a

TABLE 4. Barriers to Care

Method #3. I will read some reasons that people sometimes give for not seeing a doctor. For each reason, please tell me if you agree or disagree that it would stop you from seeing a doctor?

a. *Attitude toward medical care:*

Most people don't know a doctor to go to.	_____ Agree	_____ Disagree
It is difficult to get a doctor when you need one.	_____ Agree	_____ Disagree
People don't want to spend the money (on medicine, fees, etc.).	_____ Agree	_____ Disagree
The doctor might want to put you in the hospital.	_____ Agree	_____ Disagree
You lose time and pay from work when you go to see a doctor.	_____ Agree	_____ Disagree
Doctors and clinics should change their working hours to suit working people.	_____ Agree	_____ Disagree
You should not bother a doctor unless it is absolutely necessary.	_____ Agree	_____ Disagree
It is better to avoid the doctors or the clinics.	_____ Agree	_____ Disagree
People who attend clinics are put through too much trouble and embarrassment.	_____ Agree	_____ Disagree

b. *Attitude toward illness and health:*

The doctor might find out that you have a serious illness.	_____ Agree	_____ Disagree
As long as you feel right, there is no reason to go to a doctor.	_____ Agree	_____ Disagree
If you wait long enough, you can get over most any disease without getting medical aid.	_____ Agree	_____ Disagree

c. *Quality of care (patient's perspective):*

Doctors usually don't tell you enough about your condition.	_____ Agree	_____ Disagree
Doctor's treatments wouldn't help your condition any.	_____ Agree	_____ Disagree
People are usually not satisfied with the care they receive at their clinic or from the doctor.	_____ Agree	_____ Disagree

Source: Unknown

result, this special component of the local survey was never developed and was tabled for future exploration.

Similarly, a quick review of general articles on health status measurement was quite instrumental in guiding the above project (48-53). In addition, when working in settings serving ethnic minorities such as Hispanics, it is important to review the methods literature regarding special lessons previously learned in field survey work with the Hispanic population (52-57).

In summary, designing one's own questionnaire entails:

TABLE 5A. Typical Sequences of questions from the National Health Interview Survey

18a. During this visit on (date) , did the doctor prescribe or advise you to get any medicine for this . . . ?	1 Y 2 N(19)
b. Did you get this medicine?	0 Y (19) N
c. Why not?	
19a. During this visit did the doctor refer you to another doctor?	1 Y 2 N(28)
b. Did or will you see this other doctor?	1 Y(28) 2 N 3 DK
c. Why not?	
20. Had you ever gone to this doctor or place before this call?	1 Y 2 N
21. How did you choose this doctor or place - through another doctor, a relative or friend, a medical bureau, from a telephone directory, or in some other way?	1 _____ Another doctor 2 _____ Relative/friend 3 _____ Medical bureau 4 _____ Telephone directory _____ Other - Specify
22a. Is this doctor or place you called on (date) the doctor or place you would usually go to for this type of condition?	0 Y(23) N
b. Why didn't you use the doctor or place that you would usually go to for this type of condition?	
23a. How difficult was it for you to reach the doctor by telephone on (date) — was it very difficult, somewhat difficult, or not at all difficult?	1 _____ Very difficult 2 _____ Somewhat difficult 3 _____ Not at all difficult (24)
b. Why was it difficult?	
24. During this call on (date) , did the doctor spend enough time with you or not enough time?	1 _____ Spend enough time 2 _____ Did not spend enough time
25a. During this call did the doctor advise you to come in and see him for the . . . ?	1 Y 2 N(26)
b. Did or will you go in to see him for this condition?	1 Y(26) 2N 9 DK
c. Why not?	

■ Choosing particular categories of interest, e.g., utilization of health services, health status, health problems (general or particular), health behaviors, access to health and human services, emotional well being, neighborhood safety.

■ Reviewing questionnaires to systematically collect questions from instruments which capture the dimension or construct of interest.

TABLE 5B. Typical Sequences of Questions from the National Health Interview Survey

1. Please look at the calendar (HAND CALENDAR) and tell me on what date you first noticed (had) the . . .

2. At that time when you first noticed (had) the . . . , how serious did you think it was - very serious, somewhat serious, or not serious at all?

3a. After you first noticed (had) the condition on (date) , about how long was it before you visited or talked to a doctor about it?

b. We are interested in the various reasons why people wait before going to a doctor. Please tell me whether any of the following statements were reasons why you waited (time) to see or talk to a doctor about this condition.

PROBE IF RESPONSE IS INAPPROPRIATE:

_____   _____
        Month   Day

1 _____ Very serious
2 _____ Somewhat serious
3 _____ Not serious at all
   _____ Discovered by doctor (5)
   _____ Under 4 hours (4)
2 _____ Hours   3 _____ Days
4 _____ Weeks

A. Did you wait because you couldn't get an appointment or the doctor was not available?   1 Y   2 N

B. Because you didn't have the money?   1 Y   2 N

C. Because you didn't have a way to get to the doctor?   1 Y   2 N

D. Did you wait because you felt the doctor couldn't do anything for the condition?   1 Y   2 N

E. Because you felt you could treat the condition yourself?   1 Y   2N

F. Because you didn't want to bother the doctor?   1 Y   2 N

G. Did you wait because you didn't think it was serious enough?   1 Y   2 N

H. Because you feel uncomfortable with doctors or have a fear of doctors?   1 Y   2 N

I. Did you wait for any other reason?   1 Y   2 N(K)

J. What was the reason?
   (1) _____
   (2) _____

If all "Ns" in A-1. Ask: otherwise, go to Q. 3c:

K. Why did you wait (time) to see or talk to a doctor about this . . .?
   Any other reasons?
   (1) _____
   (2) _____

■ Refining the desired information and how to measure it, without being afraid to adapt and simplify questions to fit one's purposes or to use single items out of existing scales in an effort to streamline and construct a most precise question (48).

As the scope of most COPC projects is small, a 30- to 60-minute interview in the field may be all that can be afforded, and this time limitation will be a major arbitrator of how extensively one can pursue any line of questioning. Interview targets, once selected, will determine the number of cases for which one will have data. Especially with regard to household data, a project team must decide if it is going to collect data for single individuals or all individuals within a household and whether such data will be reported by single or multiple parties. Last, in questionnaire design, format and precoding are mechanical but *critical* steps to ease the interviewing and computer entry steps. If one is not experienced in these areas, it is wise to employ or consult with a professional to do this final packaging. One might also wish to pilot test the questionnaire for coherence, sequencing, and flow of responses. Scientific validity and reliability of one's instrument are concerns that can be raised after preliminary data collection or a larger piloting. It is important to state here, that although there is no need to be overly concerned with these issues, as one is not developing a research tool, there still may be reason for concern with accuracy of measurement. Consultations with social scientists and survey research people can guide these concerns.

PRACTICE RESOURCES, SETTING, AND CHARACTERISTICS COMPATIBLE WITH A SURVEY RESEARCH APPROACH

The use of a survey research approach such as that described above requires that the staff of a COPC practice be inclined to conduct more than a quick and dirty, minimalist approach. The approach outlined requires the presence of research-skilled staff either in-house or on loan from an academic environment or agency, and that these people be brought into the project as consultants.

In the developmental stages of such a project that can take anywhere from 6 months to 2 years, senior project staff in the practice will be required to put 4-8 hours of work per week. Even though this does not represent new dollars required, it can represent a direct cost to the proj-

ect related to both staff time and lost revenue. However, this work is usually accomplished in addition to other responsibilities. Certainly, if one had access to institutional grant support, this staff time in development activity should be reimbursed as a legitimate component. Consultation to such projects in early stages usually comes free, but when a project is underway consultants can charge $20-$35 per hour depending upon scope of activity. Costs to the project should not exceed $3,000; the range more likely would be $1,500 to $2,500.

During field operations, which should take from 6 weeks to 3 months to complete, someone administratively skilled is required to spend approximately half-time coordinating field operations and supervising field staff. This assumes that one is conducting 100-300 interviews. Costs for this administrative component will depend on the seniority of staff assigned.

The costs of data collection itself by indigenous field workers — including the costs of training, reimbursement for completed interviews (approximately $1-$2 for eligibility screening, $10 for completed interviews, and a bonus for bilingual interviews), computer entry and analysis, and printing of questionnaires (including translation, if necessary) — can range from $3,000 to $6,000.

The remaining issue to address is the compatibility of a COPC survey research effort, such the one described, with practice setting or type. Because this approach assumes that a practice sees the need to analyze community health data in an effort to broaden its community responsibilities, it is of course compatible with community health centers mandated almost by definition to do so. However, like other practice settings, these centers are continuously under pressure to produce revenue and stay afloat, and the availability of funding and leadership for a systematic survey research approach varies. Special grant funds and subsidies from government or affiliated private institutions such as hospitals, medical schools, or foundations would be required to get this kind of work underway. Also, if community health centers are dominated by traditional medical approaches that limit concerns to patients vs. populations, or are dominated by HMO ventures that emphasize gatekeeping and focus on enrollees vs. communities, then the notion of who the practice has responsibility for and what its priorities are change noticeably. In these instances, not only survey research approaches but COPC itself may take a backseat.

Private practices oriented toward COPC can generate funds to conduct survey research efforts, and the profitability of the practice and its patient mix would be critical variables here. Again, special grants or subsidies often would be required.

Occupational health settings, depending on their financial base, would also be likely places for a population-oriented survey research approach in conjunction with the ongoing surveillance activities of the practice. This work could be built into grant awards or company-sponsored surveillance projects. The focus more likely would be on risk factors, health histories, and overall health service utilization patterns of the workers as related to current or potential exposures.

Many HMO's could take up a survey research approach, but often orient their research questions more to issues in the market. However, perceptions of the accessibility of and need for addition services, expressed by the enrolled community, form the basis of many routine surveys conducted in HMO's. While the concern of HMO's is usually concentrated on the enrolled population, the perceptions of enrollees may reflect composites of many different naturally defined communities (employers, unions, sections of cities), and survey research approaches

could be useful in refining programs concerned with improving utilization and health outcomes, both among enrollees as well as the larger community.

Hospital-based ambulatory care programs would also be able to execute survey research methods in community data collection efforts if such programs developed a COPC orientation. Institutional resources and expertise would be more likely available in hospital settings. Yet, even though hospital programs in an era of competition are very interested in expanding market share, marketing as the priority concern often substantially limits the content of such population-based surveys.

In essence, COPC is generally more likely in settings that have a sense of responsibility for a population beyond clients who walk through the office door. Settings traditionally dominated by a demand-response orientation and limited to patients would not explore methods of original community-oriented data collection. Survey research approaches, in particular, might be more likely to occur in multi-disciplinary and academically oriented practices. Given their utility, however, they could be implemented in any setting that could access the expertise (through libraries and consultants) and the financial support.

SUMMARY

In describing reasons to collect one's own data and the utility of survey research, this chapter raises for the reader's scrutiny the validity of the approach itself. The chapter has described the use of manuals, consultants, existing survey tools, and special literature to assist in the implementation of a survey approach. The chapter has highlighted the core work involved in surveying which is to specify and choose appropriate measures (questions) to retrieve desired information. The chapter has also implied that the use of a multiproblem, broad, and exploratory survey in the conduct of COPC can help a practice assess the degree to which it is on track in addressing priority problems, as they are reported by residents, in an effort to strategically improve health outcomes in the community.

REFERENCES

1. Howard, M.; Berman, L.H.; and Getzenberg, J. Planning a community diagnosis project: The experience of Erie Family Health Center and Northwestern Memorial Hospital's Department of Community Health. Paper presented at the American Public Health Association Annual Meetings, Washington, D.C., November 1985.

2. Berman, L.H.; Conway, T.; Getzenberg, J.; and Kohl, R. Building an urban COPC: Initial forays. Paper presented at the American Public Health Association Annual Meetings, Anaheim, California, November 1984.

3. Bennett, F.D. (ed.), *Community Diagnosis and Health Action: A Manual for Tropical and Rural Areas*. London and Basingstoke: MacMillan Press, 1979.

4. Abramson, J.H. *Survey Methods in Community Medicine*, 2nd edition. London-Edinburgh-New York: Churchill Livingstone, 1979.

5. Haggerty, R.J.; Roghmann, K.J.; and Pless, I.B. (eds), *Child Health and the Community*. New York: John Wiley and Sons, 1975.

6. Dever, G.E.A. *Community Health Analysis: A Holistic Approach*. Germantown, MD: Aspen Systems Corporation, 1979.

7. Aday, L.A.; Andersen, R.; and Fleming, G. Workshop materials: Advances in survey research. Prepared for Association for Health Services Research Annual Conference, Chicago, Illinois, June 1984.

8. Sudman, S. *Applied Sampling*. New York: Academic Press, 1976.

9. Andrews, L. Interviewers: recruitment, selecting, training and supervising. In: *Handbook of Marketing Research*. New York: McGraw Hill, 1975, pp. 2-124-2-132.

10. Atkinson, J., *Handbook for Interviewers: A Manual for Social Survey Interviewing Staff*, 2nd ed. London: HMSO, 1971.

11. Baroux, M. A method for the selection/training and evaluation of interviewers. *Public Opinion Quarterly* 1952; 16:128.

12. Bingham, W.V.D., and Moore, B.V. Selection and training of interviewers. In: *How to Interview*. New York: Harper, 1958, pp. 79-94.

13. Brown, L.H., *Introduction to Community Interviewing*. Minneapolis, MN: Center for Urban and Regional Affairs, University of Minnesota, 1980.

14. Bugher, W., and Duckett, W. *Polling Attitudes of Community on Education: Handbook for Interviewers*. Bloomington, IN: Phi Delta Kappa, Center for Dissemination of Innovative Programs, 1970.

15. Guenzel, P.J.; Berckmans, T.R.; and Cannell, C.R. *General Interviewing Techniques: a Self Instructional Workbook for Telephone and Personal Interviewing*. Ann Arbor, MI: Survey Research Center, Institute for Social Research, University of Michigan, 1983.

16. Macfarlane, and Smith, J. The selection of interviewers (Chapter 3) and The training of interviewers (Chapter 4). In: *Interviewing in Market and Social Research*. London-Boston:

Routledge and Kegan Paul, 1972, pp. 27-38; 39-66.

17. McCrossan, L. A Handbook for Interviewers: A Manual of Social Survey Practice and Procedures on Structured Interviewing. London: Social Survey Division, 1984.

18. Merton, R.K.; Fiske, M.; and Kendall, P.L. The Focused Interview: A Manual of Problems and Procedures. Chicago: Free Press, 1956.

19. NORC. Training and Field Procedures. Appendix B in Hyman, H.H., et al., Interviewing in Social Research. Chicago, IL: University of Chicago, 1954, pp. 361-370.

20. Olson, R.F. Managing the Interview: A Self-Teaching Guide. New York: John Wiley and Sons, Inc., 1980.

21. Orlich, D.C. Designing Sensible Surveys. Pleasantville, NY: Redgrave, 1978.

22. Parten, M. Surveys, Polls and Samples: Practical Procedures. New York: Harper and Brothers, 1950.

23. Phillips, D. Do It Yourself Social Surveys: A Handbook for Beginners. Research Report #4. London: Polytechnic of North London, November 1981.

24. University of Michigan. Interviewers Manual. Revised ed. Ann Arbor, MI: Survey Research Center, Institute for Social Research, 1976.

25. Vamplew, C., and Sharp, G.A. A Manual of Survey Research in Local Government (Laria Monograph No. 3). London: Cleveland County Council, Research and Intelligence Unit, September 1981.

26. Weinberg, E. Community Surveys with Local Talent: A Handbook. (Report No. 123). Chicago, IL: University of Chicago, National Opinion Research Center, 1971.

27. Geiger, H.J. The meaning of community oriented primary care in the American context. In: E. O'Connor and F. Mullen (eds.) Conference Proceedings: Community Oriented Primary Care. Washington, D.C.: National Academy Press, 1982.

28. Howard, M.; Berman, L.H.; and Getzenberg, J. Planning a community diagnosis project: The experience of Erie Family Health Center and Northwestern Memorial Hospital's Department of Community Health. Paper presented at the American Public Health Association Annual Meetings, Washington, D.C., November 1985.

29. Garcia, R.; Saucedo-Gonzalez, I.; and Giachello, A. Access to Health Care and Other Social Indicators for Latinos in Chicago. Chicago, IL: Latino Institute, 1985.

30. University of Illinois. Community Health Planning Needs Assessment (survey instrument). Rockford, IL: School of Medicine.

31. Baltimore County Senior Needs Assessment Survey. Appendix B in Wan T.T.H.; Odell, B.G.; and Lewis, D.T., Promoting the Well-Being of the Elderly: A Community Diagnosis. New York: Haworth Press, 1982.

32. U.S. Vital and Health Statistics, Health Interview Survey Procedures, 1957-1974. Series 1. No. 11. (DHEW Pub. No. (HRS) 75-1311). April 1975, pp. 89 and 91.

33. United Community Planning Corporation and Combined Jewish Philanthropies. Community Needs and Priorities (survey instrument). Boston, Massachusetts. Fall/Winter 1975.

34. Community Health Center, Inc. Health Needs Profile: A Demographic Survey of Health Care, Utilization and Needs of the Midstate

Region of Middlesex County, Connecticut. Middletown, Connecticut, 1980.

35. Fleming, G.V., and Andersen, R. *Health Beliefs of the U.S. Population: Implications for Self-Care* (Series A-11, Perspectives). Chicago: University of Chicago, Center for Health Administration Studies, 1976.

36. Andersen, R. *A Behavioral Model of Families' Use of Health Services.* (Research Series #25). Chicago: University of Chicago, Center for Health Administration Studies, 1968 (reprinted 1974).

37. Medical Datamation. *Health '80's* (a series of health risk appraisals). Minneapolis: National Computer Systems, 1985.

38. General Health, Inc. *The Personal Health Profile.* Washington, D.C.: General Health, Inc., 1982.

39. General Health, Inc. *The Personal Risk Profile.* Washington, D.C.: General Health, Inc., 1982.

40. Well Aware About Health. *Your Health Risk Questionnaire.* Tucson: University of Arizona, 1982.

41. University of Michigan. *Lifestyle Analysis Questionnaire.* Ann Arbor, MI: Fitness Research Center, 1985.

42. U.S. Public Health Service. *Health Risk Appraisal.* Atlanta, GA: Centers for Disease Control, 1981.

43. American Hospital Supply Corporation. *Health Questionnaire*, Good for Life Program. Evanston, Illinois: American Health Awareness Program, American Hospital Supply Corporation, 1981.

44. Department of Community Health, Northwestern Memorial Hospital. Literature review on attitudes, access and utilization of health services.

Spring, 1985 (available from L. Berman).

45. Ware, J.E. et al. Choosing measures of health status for individuals in general populations. *American Journal of Public Health* 1981; June.

46. Brook, R.H. et al. Overview of adult health status measures fielded in Rand's health insurance study. *Medical Care* 1979; 7 (supplement):1.

47. Davies, A.M., and Fleishman, R. Health status and use of health services as reported by the older residents of the Baka Neighborhood, Jerusalem. *Israel Journal of Medical Sciences* 1981; 17: 2-3:138.

48. Stewart, A.; Ware, J.E.; and Brook, R.H. The meaning of health: Understanding functional limitations. *Medical Care* 1977; 11:939.

49. Davies, A.R., and Ware, J.E. *Measuring Health Perceptions in the Health Insurance Experiment.* Santa Monica, CA: Rand Corporation, 1981.

50. Korper, S.P., and Chen, M.K. Self-perceived health status: its utility in epidemiological research. Paper presented at the International Epidemiology Association, Triennial meeting, Vancouver, BC, 1984.

51. Aday L.; Chiu G.; and Andersen, R. Methodological issues in health care surveys of the Spanish heritage population. *American Journal of Public Health* 1980; 70: 2:367.

52. Berkanovic, E. The effect of inadequate language translation on Hispanics' responses to health surveys. *American Journal of Public Health* 1980; 70: 12:1273.

53. Andersen, R. et al. Access to medical care among the Hispanic population of the Southwest United States. *Journal of Health and Social Behavior* 1981; 22:78.

54. Erie Family Health Center. *Research Literature Review: Hispanics and Health Care*. Chicago, 1983.

55. Delgado, M. A grassroots model for needs assessment in Hispanic communities. *Child Welfare* 1979; 58:571.

56. Hayes-Bautista, D. Identifying "Hispanic" populations: the influence of research methodology upon public policy. *American Journal of Public Health* 1980; 70: 4:353.

57. Trevino, F. Vital and health statistics for the U.S. Hispanic population. *American Journal of Public Health* 1982; 72: 9:979.

CHAPTER 20

Defining a Transient Population in an Urban Setting

Mona Ellerbrock, M.P.H.
Lewis Kraus, M.P.H.
Emilie H. S. Osborn, M.D., M.P.H.
Raynald Bujold, M.D., M.P.H.

Defining the community for COPC can present a variety of challenges to the COPC practitioner depending on the setting in which primary care is practiced. If the community is stable, geographically bounded and there is only one primary care provider, the definition of the community is relatively straightforward. However, in many areas of the United States this is not the case. The health service delivery system offers many different options, both in terms of reimbursement and in types of services provided. In an urban setting the diversity of services is compounded by the diversity of the population being served.

In many settings the COPC practitioner will be particularly concerned with that subset of the population that is not receiving services due to any of a variety of reasons. In particular, publicly funded health care programs with a responsibility to serve a geographically defined area are becoming increasingly concerned with care to one particularly difficult to describe group of non-users: the homeless. This chapter describes an approach to defining and describing this transient population. Many of the techniques have be used in a project in San Francisco and elements of

this experience will be used to illustrate the method and its results The homeless pose many difficulties for community diagnosis. Not only are they extremely transient, but they also have no official residence. By definition, the homeless are people who live on the street, in parks or vacant lots, abandoned cars, or shelters provided by community agencies. Besides their mobility, some suffer from chronic mental illness, or abuse drugs and alcohol. They are a population at high risk for receiving health care. As is often the unfortunate reality with providing primary care to an underserved population, those people who are highest risk are those who are the hardest to reach.

APPROACH

Community participation and involvement are essential elements of the COPC concept, and should be integrated into any health project that intends to promote community development. Community development is the process by which members organize for planning and action, so that they may collectively define their needs and solve their problems (1). The community development approach can be combined with the COPC approach so that data collection is used as a tool for community organizing and outreach.

The approach is patterned from the theory of action for a community supportive research, based on Rothman's model of locality development (2). In this model, the researchers, working as community organizers, serve as facilitators in the development of problem-solving skills among community members. Thus, the process of conducting the research becomes an important skill-building device, as citizens participate in defining problems and searching for root causes with the research team. According to Rothman, the themes emphasized in the model include democratic procedure, voluntary cooperation, self-help, development of indigenous leadership and educational objectives. Rothman outlines the model according to selected practice variables as shown in Table 1.

The principles of participatory research are consistent with both the community development approach and COPC, and can be used as the basis for a needs assessment of the homeless. Participatory research focuses on the involvement of those who are being studied in the formulation of research questions, the collection of data and the interpretation of the results (3). The aim of this type of research is to educate the community participants through the research process itself, not just to provide them with results. Since this approach gives authority and control to participants, it can be particularly empowering when used with a disenfranchised population like the homeless.

Two principles are essential to the development of a COPC activity to define and characterize the homeless population using this approach. *Full use of the community's resources*: The project should build on pre-existing resources and work to improve communication between community groups so that when the researchers leave, the community members and service providers will be better prepared to assess needs and resolve problems. The use of "insiders" or community consultants who live and work in the area is important because these people already know how to work within the environment most efficiently. The community consultant can be helpful in identifying key figures for the in-depth personal interviews necessary to characterize the health needs of the population under study.

Involvement of those being studied in the entire research project: A "bottom-up" research design includes using community members and providers to perform data collection tasks, and to participate in the

TABLE 1. Theory of Action for a Community Supportive Research Project.

Practice variable	Model: Locality Development
Goal categories of community action	Self-help, community capacity and integration (process goals)
Basic change strategy	Broad cross-section of people involved in determining and solving their own problems
Characteristic change tactics and techniques	Consensus: communication among community and interests; group discussions
Salient practitioner roles	Enabler-catalyst, coordinator and teacher of problem-solving skills and ethical values

153

decisionmaking process throughout the project duration. The research process is not static, but dialectic, with the researchers facilitating a process of negotiation between experts and community members, providers, and clients.

Through this process, the homeless can be taught skills to aid them in the self-determination of their problems. The training and work experience gained through the project can impart confidence and spur them on to further employment ventures. The homeless seldom have the opportunity to engage in decisionmaking about their needs with professionals, and can develop expertise in communication and gain self-confidence in the process.

The knowledge and acceptance that the researchers gain by becoming part of the community are indispensable. By engaging others in the research process, they build faith and trust in the community towards the project, and all participants become invested in both the process and the outcome. In the words of Howard Nix (4), "Admittedly, this approach is slow and laborious, but when this process is compared to the often abortive efforts when these principles are ignored, the process is very efficient."

METHODS

Both qualitative and quantitative methods are necessary to characterize a community. The quantitative measures are common to all needs assessments and will not be described here. The qualitative methods are more individualized however. They need to be developed to meet the special requirements of the community. Three methods are described here: group discussions, in-depth personal interviews, and surveys. Each method will be discussed separately below, then the advantages and disadvantages of all will be addressed.

Method 1: In-Depth Personal Interview
Interviews of key leaders in the community can provide the COPC consultants

with necessary background information on the history of the community and give a perspective on the current situation of the population under study. These interviews should be from all facets of the community: the population at risk, service providers, health care providers, administrators, and planners. The interviews should be structured in terms of key areas that need to be explored, but they should be open-ended to ensure a free flow of information. Confidentiality should be guaranteed. Leaders can help identify other members of the community to interview, and can even provide entry into offices which may not have been open to the COPC consultants before.

Method 2: Group Discussions
Like the personal interviews, group discussions can also be used to learn more about the community or about the role of that group within the community. These discussions can be with physicians, community service providers, or representatives of the population itself. All will share their perspectives and provide a rich information base on the social, economic, and health needs of the population. The discussions can be valuable for the participants as well. For example, the sharing of information between different agencies providing services to the same population not only can lead to better communication and less duplication of services, it can also help organize the providers to become more effective advocates for the needs of the community. The discussions should be open and free of individualized agendas. The research team should provide a structure in order to obtain the information it needs, and at the same time act as a facilitator so that everyone's ideas can be expressed. It is important to make clear to the participants that the information is being gathered for the needs assessment of the community and that it will be shared with them at the conclusion of the study.

Method 3: Survey of the Population

A community survey of any disenfranchised population becomes a tool for organizing that community. By using community members as interviewers, the COPC team can work directly with the population they are studying and the process becomes one of mutual learning. Community members should be used to conduct interviews because they are more trusted by their peers than outsiders and can obtain more reliable information. Additionally, interviewers can be trained not only to gather data but also to provide information back to the community, thereby becoming community resources. In this framework, the community interviewers become both data collectors and community outreach workers. The most important criteria for a good community interviewer are ability to follow directions, literacy, good interpersonal skills, and a high level of interest. The community interviewers can be recruited from the service agencies in the area and should be representative of the community in age, sex, ethnic background, and language.

Training of the interviewers can take several sessions.[1] A packet containing salient information concerning interviewing and outreach activities should be assembled for assistance during training. For example, this packet could include a copy of the questionnaire, a list of many of the service agencies in the area, a medical resource sheet, a description of the project, interviewer information sheets explaining the use of the neutral probe and hints for reporting, and blank paper for notes. Interviewers should be paid for participating in the training sessions and for their interview time. This payment is extremely important as it means valuable income, as well as a sense of worth and a source of pride.

The interviews are normally carried out in the home or workplaces of the target population. In this case, however, the interviews may have to be in parks, on the street, or in the shelters and meal sites where homeless people congregate at regular times. The sampling scheme should be determined by the survey sites. In some cases a cluster sampling scheme can be used; in others a random sample can be taken. Since all surveys are biased by the nonrespondents, careful attention must be paid to people who refuse to be interviewed, and some demographic information should be obtained to be used in the final analysis. In this project, a systematic random sampling scheme was used. Nonrespondents were tabulated as to basic demographic information and tallies were kept at each site in order to help counteract selection bias.

The questionnaire should include both open-ended and provided-choice questions. While provided-choice questions are the conventional question form in most questionnaires providing easy statistical analysis, the open-ended questions are also important because they allow the interviewee the freedom to speak freely about concerns over personal health, the neighborhood, or health care in the area. In this way, people feel they are contributing, not just being interviewed. In keeping with the community organizing goal, this participation is extremely important in a community where such participation is rare. If other languages are necessary, the questionnaire should be translated by an interviewer, if at all possible, in order to provide appropriate, culturally sensitive, and consistent questions for all the surveys. Questions from the HANES or other well-known household surveys of health status may not be appropriate because of their white, middle-class orientation. However, rephrasing of standardized questions such as these can be useful when comparing results from the survey with

---

[1] An agenda that can be used for training interviewers is available by writing to Dr. Osborn.

155

larger population studies. It is extremely important that the instrument is designed for the target population, not only for it to be received openly and without mistrust, but also to obtain the depth of information necessary.

A COPC staff member should be present at each site where interviews are being conducted to supervise the interviewers and review each questionnaire as it is completed. This not only improves quality control but also serves as a valuable teaching experience in which to strengthen interviewing skills. Interviewers and team members need to meet frequently to ensure open communication and working out of problems as they occur, and also to help build group support. This support system is the least quantifiable but in some ways the most beneficial aspect of this sort of community project.

Strengths and Weaknesses of the Methods

All three of these methods help the COPC team understand the community they are studying. Each method provides validity for information gained from the others. Where there are contradictions, or confusing explanations, more questions can be asked. It is a method that leads to discovering more, rather than less, about a population. It is also a method that empowers the community to learn more about its own health needs and problems. Most important, however, is that it teaches valuable community organizing skills to a population that traditionally has not had a voice. It improves communication between community service agencies so that they can work better together. Finally, it provides an ongoing means for communication. Channels are opened so community members can voice their concerns and community leaders can respond.

The disadvantages of these methods are that they are time-consuming and involve expertise in community organizing. Not all needs assessments of disenfranchised populations will require all of these methods. It is important to note, however, that the survey itself requires a great deal of time and effort. In one recent application in San Francisco the cost was approximately $4,000 for the interviewers and the cost of typing and duplicating the questionnaires. In this case, the cost of the COPC staff time was modest, since the project was conducted using students. Each member of the team received $2,400 for the 3 months they spent on this project. Faculty consultation was available (University of California, Berkeley) and has not been calculated directly, although this would be a real cost in another setting. It took the team 3 months working full-time in the community to conduct all the interviews and survey 449 homeless people, approximately 10 percent of the homeless population in this city. While attending classes, the team spent another 4 months analyzing the data and describing the rich variety of information obtained. Six months after initiation of the project in the field, the students went back to the community and shared the results of their study. Thus the cost of this particular application of the approach is primarily that of staff time.

What about the results? What is the impact of this activity and how useful is the information gained from this kind of survey? One of the more important impacts is perhaps the least quantifiable: the impact on the community participants. At the end of the summer, one of the community interviewers decided that he would use his skills to set up a job-training center for the homeless, a need he had identified not only for himself, a former homeless person, but as a result of his interviews with other homeless people. It is this kind of spin-off that enriches the community and provides it with more resources than it had before.

An important limitation to this kind of

research is its generalizability. Qualitative measures can provide rich data on the population under study but conclusions cannot be transferred to similar populations in other environments. The homeless in San Francisco have particular needs and problems that the homeless in Washington or New York may not have. The survey itself may not even be generalizable to all of the homeless within the same city.

Although random sampling was attempted and care was taken to eliminate bias in the interviews, there will always be sampling bias in face-to-face interviews. Respondents could not be identified by name or social security number because of the need for confidentiality, so there was no way to completely eliminate duplicate interviews. The time frame also engendered bias. The homeless tend to move to warmer climates in the winter and they stay outside more often in warmer weather. Time of the month is crucial because general assistance and social security checks are received at the beginning of the month and many people become "homeless" only at the end of the month when their money has run out. Although attention can be paid to these fluctuations in the population, limitations on resources usually necessitate a shorter time frame than would be desirable.

CONCLUSION

The focus of this chapter has been on describing the methods used to define and characterize the health needs of a particularly difficult population: the homeless. Although many disadvantages and limitations have been described, it is important to emphasize the central strategy of the approach: community involvement. If community-oriented primary care is to move beyond the patterns of primary care, it is incumbent upon the practitioners to keep in contact with other social service agencies and with the people they are trying to serve. Community involvement in the process of the community diagnosis is one way the feedback loop is kept open.

Despite the concern for the generalizability of the results of the survey, the method described should be useful in many other settings. Whether the community is a small coal-mining town in Appalachia, a middle-class suburb with a large health maintenance organization, or an ethnically diverse urban neighborhood, the principle is the same: community involvement builds community resources. This seems to be the essence of COPC.

REFERENCES

1. Anderson, J. N. Community participation in health programs and health planning. *Bulletin of the Public Health Society*, 1975; 9:42.

2. Hall, D. Participatory research: expanding the base of analysis. *International Development Review*, 1977; 4:23.

3. Nix, H. L. *The Community and Its Involvement in the Study Planning Action Process.* Washington, D.C.: U.S. Department of Health Education and Welfare, HEW Publication No. (CDC) 78-8355, 1977.

4. Rothman, J. Three models of community organizing practice. *Social Work Practice.* New York: Columbia University Press, 1968; p. 20.

Defining and Characterizing the Community

Maurice Wood, M.D.

Community-oriented primary care is an idea whose time has come! Traditionally, medicine in the United States has focused on serving those who have voluntarily sought out health care providers and thereby entered the health care system. In the recent past, medicine has been moving towards not just serving those who initiate entry into health care but also those who have unidentified and unmet needs so those needs and some of their demands can be met. Traditionally, these needs have been those of the demographically defined minorities.

This section provides the methods and techniques for developing information systems for COPC models and for defining and characterizing community as well as the active patient population of the practice serving the community. Without such resources, it would be impossible to expand the traditional model of primary health care in the United States to a community oriented approach. Primary care, even in its family practice expression, has limited itself to addressing the needs and demands of individual patients and their household members. COPC, if it is to be effective, must be capable of being applied routinely and pragmatically in a majority of pri-

mary health care settings. These range from communities served by small single-specialty groups to those served by complex, multidisciplinary institutions with variable methods of reimbursement. Until it has been shown that the COPC model can also respond to some of the unmet needs of the medically requited segment of the population, it is unlikely to become the standard of care that is taught universally. Manifestly, until that state of visible presence is reached it will be difficult to instill COPC concepts and practices by teaching forthcoming generations of medical professionals about a model that is significant by its absence.

Health promotion and disease prevention increasingly are being accepted by Americans as important in providing better health. There is growing evidence that prevention is good for health, that is, not smoking, maintaining a balanced diet, and exercise have good effects, not necessarily in terms of longevity but certainly by improving functional status.

In this section, both Zyzanski and Reed make the major point that the marketing of a practice, or an HMO, includes addressing the needs of all of the population in the immediate community. How better to do this than, after identifying the active patient population in the practice as the primary focus of concern, determining the general and special characteristics of the non-attenders in the community and identifying their needs. In U.S. health care delivery, it is axiomatic that yesterday's demands are today's needs, and this apparently insatiable demand has been partly responsible for our present problems in the funding of health care. This fiscal embarrassment has required society to make choices, and one major impact has been a reduction in rates of hospitalization and increasing interest in care in the community as a laudable attempt to find a more cost-effective method of filling the basic health care requirements of the total population. This movement still has a considerable distance to go, and on the national scene the United States still has enormous problems in the area of primary and secondary prevention for the Medicaid and medically indigent sectors of society.

COPC is not a unique or new concept. It is a natural extension of the ideation incorporated in the majority of definitions of primary care that have been produced internationally, including the World Health Organization's concept of "Health for All by the Year 2000." In fact, the idea should be inherent in all primary care physicians' conceptualization of their role in society. Basic to primary physicians' decisionmaking and problem-solving is a pattern recognition that is rooted in an increasing experience of the demand for care made by persons living, working, and interacting in that community in their multiple environments.

Epidemiology is one of the basic sciences of primary care. As clinical epidemiology it requires the recognition of the concept of population medicine with the community being served as "a patient." This is as important as recognizing the place of the social unit of the household

as a significant entity in the causation, management, and recrudesence or resolution of biomedical and psychosocial morbidity, an orientation of vital importance for primary care practitioners. By their use of "time" in patient management, primary practitioners intuitively recognize that their encounter with a patient represents only the beginning of a problem and the beginning of care, and that subsequent encounters may be part of an episode of illness that may either be the effect or the cause of biological or psychosocial malfunction in the household or the community. Change of this dimension has been described by Kuhn as a paradigm shift (1). It enables the practice of clinical care in its fullest dimension, and perhaps the capacity of primary practitioners to undertake this paradigm shift from an encounter- to an episode-based approach to clinical care will identify those who are most willing and able to practice COPC to its fullest extent.

To further this, methods are provided in this section for estimating and defining the practice denominator in the community, of relating the active practice population to the community by developing community information systems to allow community diagnosis. Techniques to be used include survey methods directed towards not only the established underserved members of the community, but also toward the transient populations in urban settings. These techniques enable the need/demand assessments that are the bricks and mortar for building the COPC edifice.

REFERENCES

1. Kuhn, T. S. *The Structure of Scientific Revolutions.* Chicago: University of Chicago Press, 1970.

Part III.
Identifying Community Health Problems

Introduction

The second function in the COPC process is identifying the major health problems of the community, characterizing their determinants and correlates, and setting priorities among them. This function follows logically from the first, and in practice the two often blend together. While the rigor and precision of the methods used are important, it is critical that methods are employed that are consistent with the definition of the target population. For example one should not focus on patients already diagnosed with hypertension in order to study hypertension within the active patient group, nor should one focus on the active patient population if hypertension is to be studied within the larger community. Maintaining consistency between the strategies used and the scope of the community to be addressed is the primary challenge in carrying out the activities of this function.

The most basic approach to this function is to identify the health problems of the community based on the subjective impressions of the practitioner and/or community groups. Such an approach has the advantage of being both inexpensive and continuous, but may lack the rigor of more systematic quantitative approaches and is less likely to identify hidden problems within the community. On the other hand, the practice that uses formal group consensus techniques can approach this function in a more systematic and rigorous manner, with the advantage that consensus techniques can be constructed that do not constrain the range of potential problems to be considered, as is the tendency of many quantitative approaches.

Another set of approaches uses secondary data to identify the community health problems, and must extrapolate from large area statistics that may be available.

The validity of the approach is of course largely dependent on the extent to which the large area corresponds to the target community. The use of secondary data makes it difficult for the practice to conduct further detailed analysis as general problem areas are identified.

The health problems of the community can also be identified and characterized through the collection of original data. While often more expensive, data collection efforts can be carefully targeted on suspected health problems (perhaps suspected as a result of subjective approaches) with a minimum expenditure of resources. In focusing initially on particular health problems, however, one must be aware of the risk of overlooking a major problem simply because it was not included within the scope of the data set. For example, an epidemiologic study of diastolic blood pressure within the community may yield sophisticated data on the distribution, correlates, and determinants of hypertension which, in turn, may lead to highly effective interventions. However, the detail in the data set for hypertension is gained at the expense of a broader scope of the data set. Consequently use of this data to identify the community's health problems may allow the practice to overlook other (and possibly more critical) health problems which also exist in the community.

In addition to simply identifying an important health problem in the community, it is often important to characterize the correlates and determinants of the problem and identify the components of the problem that may be vulnerable to a health care solution. Generally, the components of the problem may be those related to the severity of the problem, those related to the distribution and patterns of health care, those related to health promoting behavior, and those related to environmental variables.

The principles of epidemiology come into play in identifying community health problems. The use of epidemiology, however, will differ somewhat from many of the traditional tasks to which it is applied. Epidemiologic studies usually lead to changes in the manner in which health care is delivered through a rather long feedback loop, in which the data are gathered, analyzed, presented to the scientific community through publications and professional meetings. The findings that have important implications for the practice of primary care will lead to modifications in the standards of care, and eventually will be adopted by primary care practitioners who modify their practice patterns accordingly. In contrast, the applications of epidemiology for this function occur much more locally—usually within the practice—and must be accomplished with a relatively short feedback loop. The primary purpose of this "short feedback loop activity" is not to generate new knowledge about the etiology of the disease, but rather to lead to changes in the local health care program that make it specific to the health needs of the community. Consequently, there is not the same emphasis on the elegance of the design. However, the methods must be sound enough to produce valid results upon which the health program may confidently modify its practices.

In Chapter 21, Kozoll describes a scheme for characterizing a health problem within sequentially smaller subsets of the population. Since any given relevant subset of the community can be used as either a numerator or denominator to express a population rate, it is helpful to maintain clarity on the relationship between subsets with risk factors, subsets predicted to have the problem, subsets with proven problem status, etc. Kozoll also comments on the use of the scheme to decide the numerator and denominator to be used to express a rate that will produce a useful measurement for evaluation of program impact.

The next three chapters describe widely differing approaches to identifying health problems within the community, each successively more focused on the target population. At the first level, local data sets are available from many sources, and in Chapter 22, Stewart, Kozoll, and Rhyne describe the types of secondary data that may be available to COPC practitioners to identify the health problems of a population. The extent to which the secondary data will accurately describe the health profile of the target community will be a function of the similarity of the target community and the larger population from which the data are derived. In Chapter 23, Horowitz and Gallagher describe four group process techniques that should be of tremendous value to the COPC process. Each is a method that permits the experience and impressions of a variety of individuals to be systematically described and analyzed. Use of group process techniques may also offer an important strategy for initiating the collegial relationship among the practitioners and community participants. Finally in Chapter 24, Freeman describes an important approach to using patient-based data in a practice to obtain upper or lower-bound estimates of population-based rates. This approach will be particularly appealing to practitioners, since it is simple and combines gathering COPC data with on-going activities of patient care.

The next three chapters deal with classes of health problems that are often overlooked, but should be considered by every COPC practice. Wagner discusses the identification and response to occupational and workplace related health problems in Chapter 25. He lists a variety of sources of information on occupational health from selected Federal agencies. In Chapter 26, Kamerow describes the data currently available that suggest the growing importance of alcohol, drug, and mental health problems as a concern for the COPC practitioner. He offers suggestions for several alternative approaches appropriate to the COPC practice. In Chapter 27, Maas reviews the range of oral health problems that continue as major problems in most communities. He outlines strategies by which the medical and dental practitioner can collaborate in COPC activities.

In addition to diseases and health problems, the COPC practitioner must be aware of the distribution of services in the community. Viewed largely as an issue of access two decades ago, maldistribution of primary care services continues to be a problem of increased complexity. In Chapter 28, Nutting presents a method for examining the distribution of care and discusses data that illustrate the subtle, but critical, nature of the class of community health problem.

Focusing on a target population that consists of the active patients of the practice, Schlager describes, in Chapter 29, the development and use of an acute illness index to track patterns of illness, treatments, and symptom duration. In addition to providing information helpful to practice management, this approach provides data that are helpful in monitoring acute illness patterns in the larger community.

One of the difficult steps in the COPC process is selecting from among a range of identified health problems those few that can be addressed with an emphasis program. In Chapter 30, Rose discusses the importance of community participation in the process of setting priorities and describes six important elements to consider.

Finally, in the Coda, Arthur Kaufman notes how often we define problems within a medical context. He emphasizes the need to consider health problems from the community's perspective. To the criteria for selecting a health problem he adds two that weigh toward identifying problems that will bring the practitioner and the community together in search of a solution.

CHAPTER 21

A Health Problem
Characterization Schema
Using Sequentially Smaller
Measurable Populations

Richard Kozoll, M.D., M.P.H.

Four community-oriented primary care demonstration (COPC) projects are underway in New Mexico, with technical assistance from the New Mexico Health and Environment Department. All the projects have identified one or more health problems for study in their respective communities. All have struggled with the difficulty of defining a problem by group consensus and linking it to an incidence or prevalence rate appropriate for community or practice measurement. In response to the need for a tool to facilitate this thought process, we have developed and have begun to field test a problem characterization schema shown in Figure 1. It is suggested that the schema be used to answer several important questions COPC practices may pose:

Exactly what is the problem under consideration? A sociodemographic risk factor? A behavioral, exposure, or attitudinal risk factor? An asymptomatic screening finding? A symptomatic disease, condition, or injury? A disease, condition, or injury complication? Death from a disease, condition, or injury?

What is the population at risk for the problem? The entire community? An age, sex, ethnic, or socioeconomic subset of the community? Persons in the community with an adverse behavior, exposure, or belief? Persons with an undetected disease or condition? Persons with a known disease, condition, or injury? Persons with a complication of a known disease, condition, or injury?

If incidence or prevalence rates for a chosen disease, condition, or injury are too small for adequate measurement, can a more common antecedent risk factor or condition be adequately substituted?

The schema, therefore, may prove useful in the community characterization, problem identification and characterization, and health problem modification functions of COPC. It suggests that any of several sequentially smaller measurable populations may appropriately serve as a numerator or denominator for a rate chosen to measure a particular health problem. Its use may best be illustrated by applying it to a common primary care problem, hypertension.

Let us assume that a practice speculates that its community suffers much unnecessary morbidity and mortality from uncontrolled hypertension. A group meets to discuss the problem and propose a measure that can be used to characterize it.

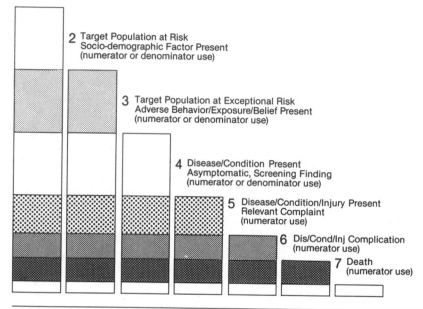

Figure 1. COPC Problem Characterization Schema. Sequentially smaller measurable populations.

They apply the schema as follows:

1. The target population is 5,000 adults over 18 years of age.

2. The target population at risk is 1,500 adult black males.

3. The target population at exceptional risk is an estimated 750 black males more than 20 percent above optimal weight or consuming excessive amounts of salt.

4. It is suspected that blood pressure screening would find that about half of these men (375) have uncontrolled hypertension.

5. Very few of these 375 are expected to have symptoms of hypertension such as headache.

6. It is suspected that 25 of these men

will be admitted each year to the community hospital for complications such as hypertensive encephalopathy, stroke, heart disease, retinopathy, and renal failure.

7. The death rate from complications of hypertension has averaged three black males per year for the last 5 years.

On the basis of this schema the group elects to screen 80 percent of adult black males for the presence of uncontrolled hypertension at practice or work sites. They therefore estimate that for the purpose of characterizing the problem's frequency, its rate will be:

$$\frac{300 \text{ uncontrolled adult black male hypertensives}}{600 \text{ adult black males}} = 0.5$$

166

or

$$\frac{\text{level 4 (asymptomatic screening finding)}}{\text{level 2 (target population at risk)}} = 0.5$$

If the COPC practice estimates it can bring the hypertension of 100 of these men under control as the result of an educational intervention, the prevalence rates before and after the intervention (300/600 = 0.5, 200/600 = 0.33) can be tested for statistical significance. A great likelihood of a difference due to the intervention would be reason for choosing the measure.

Let us suppose that this hypothetical COPC practice had chosen to measure the incidence of annual hospitalization for hypertension of adult black males instead. The rate would be:

$$\frac{\text{25 adult black male admissions}}{\text{750 adult black males}} = 0.033$$

or

$$\frac{\text{level 6 (disease complication present)}}{\text{level 2 (target population at risk)}} = 0.033$$

If the practice estimated a capability of decreasing hospitalizations by 20 percent (20/750 = 0.027) and exposed the difference in rates to statistical testing, they might very well have rejected this measure. Small numbers would have interfered with the ability to measure a difference with desirable significance.

The schema is somewhat flawed in that it regards each sequentially smaller population as a subset of larger ones. This may not be the case for certain problems. In our hypertension schema above, for example, many white males may also have the hypertension risk factors of obesity and excess salt intake. Nevertheless, the conceptual thinking remains the same.

Our problem characterization schema is offered as a potential tool for use by COPC projects. It is hoped that problem-specific schemas developed by various sites can be collected and shared as experience with COPC grows.

CHAPTER 22

Use of Secondary Data: Extrapolating to the Community

Brian Stewart, P.A., M.P.H.
Richard Kozoll, M.D., M.P.H.
Robert L. Rhyne, M.D.

In most settings there is a wealth of health data available to the practitioners from a variety of Federal, State, and private agencies. It is important for the COPC practitioner to be familiar with the available data, its relevance to the target community, and the willingness and capability of the agency to do further analysis. Often secondary data is not easily broken down into data sets that describe the target community and some extrapolation, therefore, is necessary. In New Mexico an Office of Primary Care Epidemiology of the State Health and Environment Department, has been established in conjunction with the University of New Mexico School of Medicine, to serve as the data "intermediary" for four New Mexico COPC demonstration. With many external data sets of potential value to COPC practices, an initial activity of the office has been to perform an inventory of output from various Federal, State, and private agency data systems. Plans include an eventual breakdown of data sets into community or practice level summaries on a routine basis for much of New Mexico, and to this end the four COPC demonstration sites have provided valuable experience. This experience forms the basis for this chapter.

Resources of the Office of Primary Care Epidemiology now include a set of literature and population data files, census maps for the four demonstration sites, a simplified population projection method for use with Lotus 1-2-3 spreadsheet program formats, a list of New Mexico resource people, and COPC planning and measurement "tools."

The literature files include sections on COPC, general epidemiology, general environmental health; New Mexico, U.S., and other statistics; review articles on health problem-specific topics; external data "user" materials and reports; and papers on various statistical, microcomputer, and epidemiologic applications relevant to COPC.

Population data includes a statewide 1980 U.S. Census summary and New Mexico projection reports for counties and incorporated places by race, ethnicity, and occupation. We also have a commercially prepared census on floppy disc. In addition, more detailed 1980 census data for the four demonstration sites includes age-specific and socioeconomic data at the sub-county level.

As an example of the range of data

available in most settings, each potentially useful data source for New Mexico is briefly reviewed in this chapter. It is assumed counterparts exist in most other States.

STATE CENSUS REPOSITORIES AND ANALYZERS

The U.S. Census is a critical demographic base from which New Mexico's primary user agency, the University of New Mexico's Bureau of Business and Economic Research (BBER), does population and economic projections. The BBER, like many State census data repositories, has a data bank available to researchers and provides demographic information necessary for multiple purposes to various agencies. The BBER is also a component of the New Mexico State Data Center, a consortium of user agencies. The State Data Center's goal is to improve the dissemination of census data, assist users in locating and using the data, and coordinate the use of the decennial U.S. Census with other socioeconomic data series.

While four major components of the State Data Center have the census tapes, only the BBER provides the necessary level of access and analysis necessary for the "walk-in COPC practitioner." BBER staff consists of a full-time demographer, two economists, two programmers, two data managers, and several students. All can offer general assistance to "walk-ins," and for a fee they respond to special requests.

STATE VITAL STATISTICS SYSTEMS

The Vital Statistics Section of the New Mexico Health and Environment Department is the State registrar for vital events and collects and analyzes birth, death, stillborn, and abortion certificates. This section and its counterparts in other States aggregate data by county and city and rural areas. Unfortunately, the sub-county geographic units used by the Vital Statistics section do not compare well with those used by the U.S. Census. However, of special interest to COPC practitioners, are monthly and annual statistical reports as well as statisticians and staff available for response to special requests for vital data.

STATE TUMOR REGISTRY

The New Mexico Tumor Registry is a participant in the National Cancer Institute's Surveillance, Epidemiology, and End Results (SEER) program, a national network of 11 population-based registries. They track approximately 4,000 cases of cancer a year to develop incidence, mortality, and survival rates for New Mexico and the Navajo Indian Nation. Their epidemiologist and statisticians have worked extensively on enumeration issues involving both American Indian and Hispanic populations, and have published several papers on survey and research methodology relating these two population groups. The Tumor Registry has also done special projects including cancer incidence in uranium miners and a door-to-door survey in a rural community to assess life-style risk factors and correlate them with lung disease and cancer. The Tumor Registry database, reports, and staff are easily available to those engaged in COPC projects.

TRAFFIC SAFETY

The New Mexico Traffic Safety Bureau of Transportation collects copies of all motor vehicle accidents resulting in police reports and stores the data on magnetic tape for analysis by the University of New Mexico's Institute of Applied Research (IAR). The IAR generates density maps and reports showing motor vehicle accidents and fatality frequencies and driving-while-intoxicated (DWI) citations by an assortment of geographic and sociodemographic variables.

HEALTH DEPARTMENT PROGRAM DATA

The Health Services Division of the New Mexico Health and Environment Department operates, as do all its State counterparts, a number of central programs through statewide field public health offices. All gather and store program data of considerable interest to the COPC practitioner. Family planning and well-child programs provide utilization and risk factor data helpful in characterizing a number of health problems at the local level. Sexually transmitted disease, prenatal care, hypertension, infectious disease, and other data are collected on patient visit reports, which are processed centrally and reported by county and office. The Women, Infant, and Children (WIC) nutrition program collects and analyzes demographic and risk factor data on its participants, and the Emergency Medical Services bureau collects and analyzes ambulance run reports. The Office of Epidemiology, responsible for all acute infectious disease casefinding and control in the State, as well as periodic special projects, stores data of potential use for COPC sites. Staff epidemiologists are available for speedy consultation to practitioners with special interests.

OFFICE OF THE MEDICAL INVESTIGATOR MORTALITY DATA

The Office of the Medical Investigator (OMI), New Mexico's coroner, each year performs postmortem examinations on approximately 4,000 violent, unattended, unnatural, and unexplained deaths, exclusive of those occurring on Indian land. Their data system is a computerized adaptation of the MUMPS programming system used by the Veterans' Administration and enables them to flexibly search their records for patterns and trends. This database is available by special permission to COPC researchers. The OMI annual report analyzes type of death by agent and other key variables.

U.S. INDIAN HEALTH SERVICE

The Indian Health Service (IHS) Program Statistics Branch in Rockville, Maryland develops current service unit population figures by using the U.S. Census decennial figure as its base and projects population growth each year, for the 10-year postcensal period. This projection is then forwarded to each IHS regional Area/Program Office. The Albuquerque Area/Program office, for New Mexico tribal groups, then does periodic age-specific analyses for each tribe within the service unity. Current population data for COPC practices with the IHS are thus readily available. Another function of the Area/Program office is collection of ambulatory patient care reports (APCs), which are forwarded to IHS headquarters in Rockville for preparation of workload and other reports of interest to COPC practitioners. In an attempt to increase load accessibility to APC data, IHS has adopted a MUMPS version of programming for microcomputers at the service unit level. Several service units are already capable of such local analysis.

TRIBAL CENSUS/BUREAU OF INDIAN AFFAIRS POPULATION DATA

Each tribe has its own tribal census office where the certificates of Indian blood are kept by adding new births and subtracting deaths of tribal members. Blood quantity levels may differ by tribe, making population figures difficult to compare with those of the U.S. Census or other geographic surveys or estimates. Additional problems with use of tribal census data are deceased tribal members remaining on tribal roles for years after their death and inclusion of large numbers of off-reservation members that do not relate to a geographic practice catchment area. Bureau of Indian Affairs figures, as well as individual tribal figures, therefore are often considerably higher than those of the IHS.

THIRD-PARTY PAYER DATA

Third-party payer data are available from private carriers such as Blue Cross/Blue Shield of New Mexico or Medicaid/Medicare intermediaries such as Electronic Data Systems, which processes Medicaid payments for New Mexico. The general run reports focus on utilization of services which are often specified by procedure or diagnosis. They may be of value to COPC practitioners if insured populations become or approximate COPC groups. The programming cost of doing a specialized data run, however, can be prohibitively expensive.

SPECIAL SURVEY DATA

Special surveys and studies performed by various agencies of investigators may be of great value to COPC sites. Often, a cooperative venture is undertaken by two or more agencies to merge existing data in new ways. An example is a collaborative effort underway between New Mexico's Traffic Safety Bureau, Office of the Medical Investigator, and the Scientific Laboratory Division to relate blood alcohol levels to age, sex, and location of fatal and nonfatal motor vehicle accidents. Another is a University of New Mexico researcher's study of the epidemiology of Indian suicide.

USING THE CENSUS

Census data forms the basis for characterizing all communities identified by the four New Mexico COPC study sites. Understanding the structure and limitations of census data is critical for most COPC sites and will be further elaborated in this section. The Census is a total population enumeration of the United States performed every 10 years by the Department of Commerce. The data are collected by either a short- or long-form survey of households, either by mail or in person to reach the nonrespondents. Some respondents are given the long form, so supplemental data items can be collected from a randomly selected sample of the populations for a series of estimations in order to reduce the cost and the amount of time to process the census.

The data are then summarized on five magnetic tapes and distributed to user agencies throughout the United States. An additional public use microdata survey tape (PUMSA), a carefully chosen sample of raw questionnaires without the names and local addresses of respondents, is also available for special studies. Of the five standard computer tapes, summary tape file I (STF1) contains the most often used tabulations of 100 percent population and housing items at all major geographic levels (States, U.S. Congressional Districts, counties, minor civil/county Census divisions, incorporated places, census tracts, Enumeration Districts, block numbered areas, and blocks). These data are published by the Department of Commerce in summary form for States, counties, and incorporated places. Published population projections may also be available for intercensal years. For smaller areas, a special computer run will be required at minimal expense to the user agency.

STF2 provides more detailed tabulations of 100 percent data, for example, it contains age by individual year by sex for the above geographic units, whereas STF1 uses for the most part multiple year age by sex "breakouts." This is particularly important for study of populations whose age limits may not coincide with STF1 "breakouts." STF2, as well as STF4 and STF5, also contains data at the Standard Metropolitan Statistical Area (SMSA) level, making these tapes logical choices for urban COPC sites.

Whereas STF1 gives useful summary data on total population counts, age by sex, race, Spanish origin, and numbers of families and households, STF3 gives more useful data on socioeconomic data such as years of education completed and income. STF3 also provides population data by zip code. However, STF3 is an estimation tape using a complex sampling methodology, which may be inaccurate for characterizing a lightly populated rural area. STF3 is also susceptible to the census technique of suppression, the policy of deleting from geographic units containing small numbers of households. An example of the danger of using STF3 is illustrated by one New Mexico COPC site, Carrizozo, where discrepancies of 5-20 percent were found for individual population variables aggregated by zip code from STF3 compared to CCD's from STF1. In fact, our original desire to define primary care service areas by zip code aggregation will have to be abandoned in most rural areas.

In defining a practice's service area with census data, it is usually necessary to aggregate sub-county units and project the population for a postcensal year. County-wide population projections may be difficult to apply to these units because of differential growth experienced within the county. Carrizozo again serves to illustrate this problem as it represents 1 of 5 CCD's in Lincoln County. The BBER estimates that while the Carrizozo CCD population grew only 0.9 percent from 1980 to 1984, the fourfold larger population in the southern neighboring Ruidoso CCD grew at 23.4 percent. In addition much of Ruidoso CCD's new population was Anglo, wealthier, and culturally quite different from that of the Carrizozo CCD. Therefore, use of county projections would have been disastrous for the COPC site. We have found that our sites must choose geographic units carefully and temper standard county population projections by their own insight. The Office of Primary Care Epidemiology is developing simplified projection methodology for future use in COPC

sites such as Carrizozo.

In New Mexico, as well as in other States, confusion over the race and Spanish origin questions has created several problems with both 1960 and 1970 census data and have made 10-year comparisons of these variables unreliable. With the 1960 census, many American Indians claimed to be of "other" race rather than American Indian for various reasons. Self-reporting on American Indian race progressively improved in the 1970 and 1980 censuses, thereby inflating the population growth rate. In many northern New Mexico areas Hispanics also self-reported "other" rather than "white" for race. Census data on Spanish origin are also inconsistent due to a change of the Spanish identifier questions between 1970 and 1980.

In summary, one must recognize that even a "gold standard" data system, such as the decennial U.S. Census, is not without its problems. Bureau of the Census demographers estimate that areas with populations smaller than 5,000 people are enumerated with a range of accuracy of plus or minus 5 percent, while stable populations over 5,000 carry an improved error range of plus or minus 3 percent. Even if accurately enumerated, other problems such as those mentioned in this section must be handled appropriately by practitioners of COPC. Familiarity and methods developed by "small area users" such as our Office of Primary Care Epidemiology should be valuable to them.

USE OF VITAL STATISTICS

Vital events such as births, fetal deaths, stillbirths, deaths, communicable diseases, and abortions are collected and analyzed in every State by a single agency. In New Mexico, as in many other States, they are recorded and filed by year and county of residence. Monthly and annual reports use standard formats including "breakouts" of many events at the level of counties and cities.

For example, births to New Mexico residents are reported routinely in summaries by race, Hispanic origin, age of the mother and father, live birth order, marital status of the mother, birthweight by ethnicity and race, low birthweight by county, low birthweight by weeks of gestation, presence of absence of congenital anomalies, live births in the hospital, and other natality characteristics. Tables of legal induced abortions by county and race are also published.

Mortality is summarized in reports by 11 major causes as both absolute rates and percent of all deaths attributable to specific causes. Age-specific death rates by ethnicity, race, sex, and county of residence are also reported. Infant mortality death rates are summarized by ethnicity, race, and cause, as are fetal and maternal deaths.

Mandatory reports of communicable diseases such as gonorrhea, syphilis, plague, rabies, tuberculosis, measles, and rubella are summarized in the annual statistical report by county.

A number of special studies by the New Mexico Vital Statistics have also resulted in special reports of interest to COPC practitioners including those on level of prenatal care; variables associated with low birthweight; variables associated with infant mortality, and multi-year age-, sex-, and cause-specific mortality. A recent report of cause-specific Years of Potential Life Lost (YPLL) by county provides a different framework for COPC practices to view their major health problems.

All vital data reflect the accuracy with which physicians, hospital staff, and others complete the certificates. Underreporting of suicides in the death certificate or inaccurate reporting of prenatal risk factors and level of prenatal care in the birth certificate are examples of problems.

An important factor to COPC sites is the geographic unit by which a vital event is classified. In New Mexico vital data are generally useful only at the county and city level. New Mexico data reported for many rural areas fall into the classification, "not elsewhere specified." For example, nearly 25 percent of teen pregnancies at one COPC site fall into this category. To match up vital statistics data accurately with subcounty level census units, rural COPC practitioners may need to request or perform a special study in which data are abstracted from individual birth or death certificates. They can thereby select vital events that fall into a particular ED or CCD grouping that best defines their service area. For many rural areas this is far preferable to estimation from total county rates.

SUMMARY

We have reviewed sources of external health or population data that we feel may be useful to practices engaging in community-oriented primary care. Each practitioner will require familiarity with limitations and methodologic problems and may require interaction with a "user" agency and its expert staff. COPC practitioners will want to become familiar with these resources or utilize data "intermediaries" such as the Office of Primary Care Epidemiology.

CHAPTER 23

Group Process Techniques for COPC Practice

Carol Horowitz, M.P.H.
Kaia M. Gallagher, Ph.D.

Community-oriented primary care (COPC) is, first and foremost, a medical practice in which the practitioner treats the community as well as the community's individual residents. Four steps are critical to this approach:

1. Defining and characterizing the community

2. Identifying the community's health problems

3. Modifying the practice in response to community health needs

4. Monitoring the impact of the practice modifications.

For the busy practitioner, the data required for these activities may appear overwhelming. Many, however, will find that through group process techniques, a COPC practice can be initiated with a minimum investment of time. Moreover, group process techniques are a means of involving members of the community in COPC activities.

Data, whether collected from a practice or obtained through secondary sources, provides the practitioner with an objective basis for identifying health needs, modifying the practice, and evaluating the

impact of program changes. The thoroughness with which the COPC process is accomplished will depend on the comprehensiveness and accuracy of the data used.

The absence of data, however, should not stop a practitioner from establishing a COPC practice. Through the group process techniques described in this article, much of the information necessary for COPC can be compiled from the experience of the practitioner, other health providers, and key community representatives. Practitioners are typically familiar with the community that they serve and its most prevalent health needs; the techniques described here are a means of systematically capturing this information for use in a COPC practice.

Practitioners with access to existing data bases may also choose to use these techniques to confirm, enrich, and refine the conclusions of the data analysis. For all practices, group consensus techniques are particularly effective for obtaining input from community representatives whose perceived needs are equally as important as those identified through data analysis.

This chapter briefly summarizes the characteristics of four group consensus approaches and their resource requirements:

1. Brainstorming
2. Nominal Group Technique
3. Delphi and
4. Ringi

The final section reviews criteria for selecting among the group process techniques. Readers are also referred to the bibliography at the end of this article, which lists references on the individual approaches.

BRAINSTORMING

Everyone has brainstormed at one time or another. It is the process by which a group collectively reviews an issue and generates possible solutions. For COPC, brainstorming can be an effective means of identifying a community's health problems and developing new programs in response.

Of all group process techniques, brainstorming is the least structured. The technique places no restrictions on the size of the group or the number of meetings, operating with two guiding principles:

1. The more ideas the better since "quantity of ideas begets quality."
2. Judgment on contributed ideas should be deferred until the brainstorming has ended (1).

Ideally, the group should feel free to explore a wide range of options since the objective of this process is to generate as many ideas as possible. Criticism is to be avoided, but ideas can be modified, combined, and/or expanded upon. One group member should be asked to serve as recorder, writing down the group's ideas on a flip chart or chalkboard, which all of the group can see. In addition to generating ideas, group members may choose to cluster them to facilitate program planning.

One meeting may be sufficient for the practitioner's needs. If alternative issues are being reviewed, however, each might be addressed at separate gatherings. The practitioner may also decide to limit the size of brainstorming session to fewer than 10 participants in order to maximize individual participation, holding several meetings to accommodate all of those who wish to participate.

Brainstorming is particularly useful at the initial stages of the COPC process as the practitioner strives to define the community and its needs. Depending on the mix of participants, a wide range of opinions will surface. The interaction of the group will result in a resolution that is superior to that possible from the practitioner working alone.

Once a brainstorming session has resulted in a list of options (i.e., health problems, alternative programs), the practitioner will need to set priorities among them. Practical considerations may make the priority-setting self-evident. If a more formal decision process is desired, the practitioner may choose any of the alternative group process techniques described in later sections.

NOMINAL GROUP TECHNIQUE

As compared to the unstructured process of brainstorming, Nominal Group Technique (NGT) involves four steps:

1. A group generates ideas by silently writing them on paper.
2. Each group member reports the most important idea on his list in round-robin fashion until all ideas are presented. A recorder lists all contributions on a flip chart.
3. Each idea is clarified and evaluated.
4. Finally, group members vote on the priority order of the ideas and a rating system is used to establish group consensus (2).

The structure of the nominal group technique requires that a skilled group leader guide the process, preferably one who can facilitate the momentum of the

175

group without manipulating it towards overly narrow conclusions. Ideally, an NGT group has eight to ten members, selected for their familiarity with the community and its health problems. The number of meetings required depends on the issue areas to be covered.

The first step of the nominal group technique requires all participants to contribute ideas. The group then works to clarify each option and evaluate them. The ultimate decision regarding priorities is achieved by voting.

After the votes have been received, practitioners can arrive at a consensus ranking by using a weighting system (e.g., lst place = 4 points, 2nd place = 3 points, etc.) whereby the individual item scores are summed across all group participants to derive a group ranking.

For a practitioner interested in COPC, the nominal group technique helps to identify a variety of options and to set priorities among them. As with the brainstorming technique, the nominal group technique can be a means for enlisting community involvement in the COPC process. This approach is particularly useful for larger groups because it guarantees that all individuals will have a chance to participate; it also ensures that a group decision will be reached.

DELPHI PROCESS

In the delphi process, a participant group does not meet face-to-face but is sent a questionnaire(s). The items (or questions) reviewed by the group are predetermined by the practitioner or staff. Moreover, final consensus is derived with no group interaction.

Careful selection of the respondent group is critical to the consensus results. In general, the practitioner should select respondents because of their experience and/or expertise. In general, the larger the group, the less likely group opinion is to be biased.

The critical steps for the delphi process are:

1. Developing a questionnaire
2. Selecting a respondent group
3. Distributing the questionnaire and
4. Compiling the questionnaire results (3).

While more manageable than brainstorming or the nominal group technique, the delphi process presupposes that the practitioner has already identified the issues the group will address. After the initial round of questionnaires is tabulated, additional group input can be sought through followup questionnaires (two to four) that ask group members to assist in priority-setting. This process, however, can become tedious and may be unnecessary if the practitioner can interpret the results without further assistance from the respondents.

The disadvantage of the delphi process is that it takes time. Over a month may be required to develop the questionnaires, distribute them, and compile the results. More time may be necessary depending on the number of respondents and the number of times questionnaires are sent.

Nonetheless, the delphi can be useful with large groups and in environments where meetings are difficult to arrange. Delphi can also be used in combination with data analysis as a means of eliciting community reactions to data regarding community needs and proposed solutions to these needs.

RINGI

This approach is similar to the delphi process in that a written document is circulated in successive drafts among group members who provide comments on the document, but who never meet. This approach is particularly useful if a group statement needs to be developed that represents the consensus of participating individuals. The time necessary to complete the document will depend on the amount of consensus that exists among the group participants (1).

SELECTION OF GROUP PROCESS TECHNIQUES

Each of the group process techniques described in previous sections can be used to achieve consensus among selected groups on issues relevant to community-oriented primary care. The decision as to which technique a practitioner should choose depends on several criteria:

The clarity with which the issues have been defined. Brainstorming and the nominal group technique are most appropriate for generating new ideas. By contrast, the delphi and ringi processes are more effective when practice issues have already surfaced, but need to be ordered according to their priority. Irrespective of the approach chosen, the questions addressed by the group should be concrete enough to encourage the group to develop specific actions for addressing the community problems (4).

The numbers and types of group participants chosen. With a large group, the practitioner may choose to use a more structured approach such as the nominal group technique or the delphi process. Smaller groups may work better through brainstorming, especially if group members are comfortable working with each other. When group members are likely to have differing opinions, group interaction (through brainstorming or the nominal group technique) may be a useful way of achieving understanding of alternative points of view. All group members should have a commitment to working as a group, and should work to prevent any interactions that are destructive of this process.

The resources available to the practitioner. The delphi and ringi processes are more time-consuming than brainstorming and the nominal group technique. Costs include those for developing documents to be circulated, mailing, copying, and staff time, which will vary depending on the size of the group, as well as the number and complexity of the issues.

The level of consensus necessary. For COPC, the practitioner needs to be able to focus on specific community health problems and the ways in which they can be addressed. Hence, complete consensus on the priority of the problems is not always necessary. The intent of the group process techniques will be to establish, from the practitioner and the community's perspective, a starting point for community-oriented health programs. Therefore, although delphi and ringi through their successive rounds of review may achieve a greater degree of consensus than brainstorming or the nominal group technique, this degree of consensus may not be necessary in the early stages of developing COPC activities.

Other objectives of the consensus process. In order for a community-oriented practice to reflect the community's interests, community participation is essential. This chapter has discussed group process techniques as means of collecting data, as well as a means of involving community representatives in program planning. For this reason, the extent to which a group's consensus on the health problems is consistent with secondary data is less important than the fact that a consensus has been achieved. In this respect, group process techniques that bring groups together (brainstorming and nominal group technique) are more effective than the delphi and ringi in allowing groups to acknowledge varying opinions and to reach some compromises as to how priorities will be set.

SUMMARY

Group process techniques can be useful tools for helping people work together. For the practitioner interested in COPC, these techniques offer a means for gathering information not currently available through secondary data and/or confirming the accuracy of data collected. Since community participation is a critical component of the COPC process, a further advantage of the techniques is that they can help to ensure that the community's voice is heard. Practitioners interested in more specific features of the group process techniques described are referred to the following bibliography.

REFERENCES

1. Zander, A. *Making Groups Effective.* San Francisco: Jossey-Bass, 1982.

2. Del Becq, A.; Van de Ven, A.; and Gustafson. *Group Techniques for Program Planning.* Glenview, Ill.: Scott-Foresman, 1975.

3. Linstone, H.A., and Turoff, M. *The Delphi Method: Techniques and Applications.* Reading: Addison-Wesley, 1975.

4. Fink, A.; Kosecoff, J.; Chassin, M.; and Brook, R.H. Consensus Methods: Characteristics and Guidelines for Use. *American Journal of Public Health* 1984; 74:979.

Bibliography—Suggested Readings

Group Techniques for Program Planning, Del Becq, Van de Ven, and Gustafson, 1975.

Problem Solving Discussion and Conferences: Leadership Methods and Skills, Norman Maier, McGraw Hill, NY 1963.

The Planning of Change, second edition, Warren G. Bennis, Kenneth D. Benne, and Robert Chin, Holt Rinehart, and Winston, NY 1969.

Group Dynamics: Research and Theory, third edition, Dorwin Carwright and Alvin Zander, eds., Harper and Row, NY 1968.

Making Groups Effective, Alvin Zander, Jossey-Bass, San Francisco, 1982.

Decision-Making Group Interaction, Bobby R. Patton and Kim Giffin, Harper and Row, NY 1978.

Decision Tables, Marion L. Hughes, Richard Shank, Elinor Svendsen Stein, McGraw Hill, NY 1968.

The Delphi Method: Techniques and Applications, Harold A. Linstone and Murray Turoff, eds., Addison-Wesley, Reading, 1975.

"Consensus Methods: Characteristics and Guidelines for Use," Arlene Fink, Jacqueline Kosecoff, Mark Chassin, and Robert Brook, *American Journal of Public Health.* September 1984, Vol. 74, No. 9, pp. 979-983.

CHAPTER 24

"Piggybacking":
The Selective Use
of Tracer-Conditions from
Patient-Based Data
to Obtain Population-Based
Information Useful for COPC

William L. Freeman, M.D., M.P.H.

Identifying community health problems in COPC usually means *population-based information*, that is, epidemiology. Population-based data are the least available and most expensive to obtain, if obtainable at all. Although patient-based data are more accessible, such data are rightly criticized as being usually inappropriate for COPC. I suggest a method that derives reasonably accurate population-based information from more accessible patient-based data. Patient-based data concerns people who come to a medical care facility (encounters). One usually should not extrapolate from patients who encounter the health care system to total populations, because often the people that come to the medical care system differ in health status from those who do not come.

One can obtain population-based data by "brute-force" methods. These usually involve screening or interviewing a random sample of the population, sometimes including reviewing a random sample of medical charts of the entire population in, for example, a prepaid capitation system.

Brute-force methods are brutal on a small practice that wants to do COPC. The cost in unrecompensed staff time is often too great to be acceptable and may be a major reason COPC is not done.

One solution, suggested by others in this book, is that practices form networks to share the costs and increase the efficiency of obtaining that data. However, this may not be an option in every practice.

Another inexpensive feasible alternative is to collect appropriate *patient-based* data, and "piggyback" the collection onto a useful activity that the practice is doing. I give an example in this chapter. I first describe how a clinic determined the age-specific tuberculosis infection rates and PPD screening rates in a community by examining the medical records of all diabetic patients in the practice. I then suggest some characteristics and limitations of this method.

AN APPLICATION OF THE PIGGYBACK METHOD

The Lummi Indian Health Service Clinic provides COPC to 5,000 American Indians who reside on or near the Lummi Indian Reservation in Washington State. The multidisciplinary staff has special, COPC-based emphases including maternal and child health, general diabetes and diabetic retinopathy, hypertension, immunizations, pap screening, fluoridation, infant car seats, sexually transmitted disease, and prevention and control of tuberculosis.

TABLE 1. Rate of + PPD, Yukon-Kuskokwim Delta, 5-8-year-old Alaska Natives[1].

	1950	1957	1960
No. tested	323	183	379
% Positive	91	79	50

[1] Comstock, G.W., and Philip, R.N. Decline of the tuberculosis epidemic in Alaska. *Public Health Reports* 1976; 76:19-24.

The staff believed its program of tuberculosis prevention and control was effective. It remembered no active transmission of tuberculosis, and only two patients who reactivated. Its clinical impression was that tuberculosis was not a problem. On the other hand, the staff knew that Alaska Natives had suffered a massive epidemic of tuberculosis in the middle of this century. Comstock found that 91 percent of the 5-8-year-old Alaska Natives were positive reactors to PPD in 1950. Because Alaska has no atypical mycobacterium, every positive PPD indicated infection with tuberculosis. With intense programs of preventive chemotherapy, the infection rates declined to 50 percent by 1960 (1). Alaska still needs its effective program of casefinding, treatment, and prevention to control tuberculosis.

Given the difference between its clinical impression and the Alaska experience, the staff decided to evaluate the need for its emphasis on tuberculosis prevention. The evaluation covered the three components of tuberculosis prevention: screen

for tuberculosis infection by applying and reading the PPD skin test; diagnose tuberculosis status for those screened positive by obtaining a history and CXR, and determining presence of risk factors; and treat with INH prophylaxis for one year if at high risk for reactivation. In this chapter, I am concerned with the first component.

Evaluating the first component required population-based data. The staff needed to know the percentage of the entire population that had tuberculosis infection or disease (i.e., a positive PPD) and the percentage that had been screened. The answers to those two questions would let the staff know if it needed to proceed further in evaluating its efforts at tuberculosis prevention and control. The percentage of the population still to be screened, times the percentage expected to be positive, would estimate the unmet need for tuberculosis screening.

There was no information about the rates of tuberculosis infection for American Indians of the Pacific Northwest. Thus the staff itself would have to determine the rates of tuberculosis infection of the local population. Also, the staff itself would have to determine the rates of tuberculosis screening done by the clinic, because they were locale-specific data. What method could the staff use to determine those rates economically and feasibly?

The brute-force method (i.e., standard epidemiology) would develop a list of a random sample of the population, check the charts for screening status and results of the PPD, if any, and then apply the PPD skin test to all in the sample who had not been tested. This method is burdensome to a COPC practice if not paid for by outside funds, and there is no guarantee of benefit worth the effort.

The staff employed a different method. It used "all diabetic patients" as the sample for the population, and determined the infection rate and screening rate for that sample by piggybacking that activity onto an effort in clinical care.

The staff studied diabetic patients because diabetes was another emphasis of the clinic. Part of diabetes care included giving every diabetic patient a PPD test, followed by INH prophylaxis if the test was positive. Diabetics previously infected with tuberculosis (i.e., who have a positive PPD) are at high risk to relapse to active tuberculosis if they had not had INH prophylaxis or full chemotherapy. The staff was able to use "diabetic patients" as a sample for the COPC data because it maintained a list of all known diabetic patients, even if they seldom came to the clinic.

In 1983 the staff reviewed the charts of all diabetic patients for screening status, PPD status if screened, and status of chemotherapy if PPD-positive. The purpose of the chart review was to call in those diabetic patients who had "fallen through the cracks," that is, those who needed a PPD, further workup, or INH prophylaxis under the clinic's diabetes care plan.

Note that the staff did the chart review as part of care to individual diabetic patients. The review was not an epidemiological study to obtain COPC data, but simply a step to identify specific diabetic patients needing medical care. Note also that the review was still a fair amount of extra work. The staff used the chart review to provide the needed COPC information as well. The critical assumption permitting that use was that the rate of tuberculosis infection for diabetic patients was the same as for the entire population.

Being infected with tuberculosis does not predispose a person to develop diabetes, and being a diabetic does not predispose one to be infected with tuberculosis. After the initial infection, however, diabetes does predispose a person to develop active tuberculosis. Hence, the prevalence rate of positive PPDs should be the same for diabetic as for nondiabetic patients.[1]

The clinic's PPD screening, on the other hand, was or should have been related to diabetes, because the staff followed the policy to screen everyone for tuberculosis more conscientiously for diabetic patients than for all patients. The screening rate for diabetic patients should have been at least as high as for nondiabetic patients, if not higher.

Thus ascertaining PPD status among diabetic patients gave for the entire population both a reasonable estimate of the prevalence rates of past tuberculosis infection, and the upper limit of the clinic's PPD screening rate.

TABLE 2. Rate of TB Infection in Diabetic Patients

Screened	66%
Infection rate among those screened	
< 1920	78%
1920-29	87%
1930-39	61%
> 1939	25%

The results of this COPC-study about tuberculosis were fascinating. For the 82 diabetic patients, the clinic had completed the screening component for only 66 percent. Of the 54 diabetic patients

---

[1] Poverty is a possible confounding association between diabetes and TB. Poor people are more likely than nonpoor people to have diabetes (National Diabetes Data Group, *Diabetes in America*, NIH Publication 85-1468). Poor people are more likely than nonpoor people to have been infected with TB. For the Lummi Clinic, almost the entire population was poor in childhood, the time when people would have acquired TB. Thus poverty is not a factor that biased the rates of TB infection among diabetic people compared to rates among nondiabetic people.

who had been screened for tuberculosis, the infection rate ranged from 87 percent for the cohort of patients born between 1920-1929, to 25 percent for the cohort born after 1939. No patients born after 1943 had been infected with tuberculosis. The infection rate for the 1920-1929 cohort in these patients in northwest Washington State is similar to the 91 percent found by Comstock at the height of the tuberculosis epidemic in Alaska![2]

This study illustrates generic aspects of the method of piggybacking a tracer condition of patient-based data onto traditional medical care to obtain population-based information for COPC. One set of attributes concerns the epidemiology of the tracer condition.

TABLE 3. Attributes of a Suitable Tracer.

- Tracer sample is large enough
- Clinic knows most or all people with the condition
- Known relationship between tracer condition and desired information

---

CHARACTERISTICS AND LIMITATIONS OF THE PIGGYBACK METHOD

The tracer condition must be frequent in the population. That is, the size of the

---

[2] Later, I calculated the number of reactivations to be expected if the staff did not improve its TB emphasis program. Using age-specific numbers and rates, and accounting for the shorter life-expectancy of older patients, I estimated that 35 TB patients would reactivate in the next 30 years—or 1.2 per year. The clinical impression that "the TB problem was over" had been faulty memory. Further study showed that in the previous 10 years 11 patients had developed reactivated TB and had infected two new people. The 1.1 reactivations per year matched the predicted 1.2.

sample must be large enough to answer the question. For example, in most practices patients with hypertension would be a potentially numerous sample; patients with systemic lupus erythematosus would be an insufficient sample.

The clinic must see or know most or all of the patients diagnosed with the condition, and must easily and correctly diagnose most cases. If the clinic knows only the patients with the condition who use the facility frequently, differences between frequent and infrequent users may be a confounding bias. Similarly, differences between diagnosed and misdiagnosed patients may be a bias.[3] The tracer disease must be usually diagnosed correctly, and must be severe enough that most people with the diagnosis come to the clinic at least infrequently. Diabetes probably is a better tracer disease than osteoarthritis.

The relationship of the patient-based tracer to the COPC information must be known and useful. As explained above, for the Lummi Clinic the prevalence of tuberculosis infection among diabetic

---

TABLE 4. Attributes of the "Piggyback."

- Keeping track of the tracer condition
- Congruent with traditional care
- Worthwhile in its own right
- Short feedback loop to care
- Less costly than "brute force"

---

[3] For many chronic diseases, fewer patients with less severe symptoms may be diagnosed than patients with more severe symptoms. In many situations, differences of diagnosis vs. no diagnosis (i.e., more severe vs. less severe symptoms) probably does not bias the tracer condition if the clinic has complete ascertainment of all patients *diagnosed* with the disease.

patients was known to be the same as the rates among all patients. The rate for PPD screening among the diabetic patients was known to be as high or higher than that among all patients.

The second set of attributes concerns the piggyback itself. Frequently the tracer condition is one that the clinic has special interest about, maintaining a complete list of all patients with that diagnosis. That is, the facility tracks already, or plans to track, all patients with the tracer condition; the clinic can piggyback a COPC activity onto that tracking activity.

The activity that carries the piggyback should usually be congruent with the staff's customary work of delivering medical care to individual patients. For Lummi Clinic, reviewing the PPD status of all diabetic patients was worthwhile in its own right; it could and would have been done even if there was no need for the population-based data. The review had the shortest possible "feedback loop" to medical care; the chart review identified *individual patients* who needed to be called in for *specific care.*

Piggybacking should be a less expensive method to obtain similar data than other methods, especially the brute-force

---

TABLE 5. Attributes of the Situation in Which to Piggyback a Tracer.

- Appropriate subject
- Range of error is acceptable
- Favorable cost-effectiveness of the method vis-a-vis alternate methods
- Feasible in many COPC settings

---

method. If the information can be obtained elsewhere and less expensively, this method is inappropriate.

The third attribute concerns the context of the study. This method is more relevant for some subjects than for others. For instance, this method would probably not be useful for assessing the need for improved emergency medical services. The method seems most appropriate for "Go/No-go" decisions, i.e., to do or not do components of personal medical care such as screening, preventive medicine, or personally delivered health education.

The range of error must also be acceptable. If a facility wants the results published in the *New England Journal of Medicine* or the *American Journal of Epidemiology*, this method may be too inaccurate. However, the Lummi Clinic's purpose was to make an informed decision, and the accuracy of its data was good enough for that purpose.[4]

Piggybacking should have a favorable cost-effectiveness compared with alternate methods. The method may not be the most accurate, but frequently is less expensive than standard methods. If the added cost of using a more accurate method exceeds the added benefit of the increased accuracy, this method is preferable. "Cost" includes such categories as dollar expenses, staff time, and acceptability to staff. Note that a given COPC practice makes the comparison of the cost-effectiveness of alternate methods; the cost-effectiveness of the same method varies among different practices. This characteristic is differ-

---

[4] For the Lummi Clinic, the rate of PPD screening was expected to be higher among diabetic patients than among the total community. Although "inaccurate," the data was useful because both the direction of the relationship between the data and wanted information was known—the rates among diabetic patients would be higher than among the general population—and the error was acceptable. If the PPD screening rate among diabetic patients were unacceptably low, as it turned out to be, the rate for everyone else would be even lower and more unacceptable. The data supported a decision to improve the emphasis on TB prevention and control.

ent than simply "less expensive"—it is less expensive *without unacceptable loss of accuracy.*

The utility of this approach is not linked to the type of practice. Although the example comes from a federally funded clinic of the Indian Health Service, the study applies to private practice as well. With computerized billing in private practice, both types of practice can identify all patients with diagnoses such as diabetes, to use those patients as valid samples of the population. In both types, there are costs of piggybacking COPC data collection onto a special project for a tracer condition, but usually the costs are much less than by the brute-force method.

The major limitation of this method to obtain data needed for COPC is that many problems cannot be approached this way. The number of legitimate tracer conditions and piggybacked activities seem limited. The question, "What are the rates of tuberculosis infection and of PPD screening," was answered by chart review of diabetic patients in the study described in this chapter. Creative thinking may provide more questions that can be answered by similar methods.

TABLE 6. Examples of the Method.

Study diabetic patients to obtain:

- Rates of tuberculosis infection
- Upper limit of rates of PPD screening
- Lower limit of rates of non-ascertainment blood pressure within the past year
- Lower limits of rates of non-recognition of elevated blood pressure

Study hypertensive patients to obtain:

- Upper limit of rate of diabetes

Study "special care" infants/children to obtain:

- Rate of infant car seat use

THE USES OF PATIENT-BASED DATA: EXAMPLES

A number of questions can be answered by tracer conditions and piggybacked activities, as shown in the following examples:

What are the rates of people who have not had a blood pressure check in the past year, or whose elevated blood pressure was not recognized? Do a chart review of all diabetic patients to call in (or to mark the chart to do for the next visit) those who have not had a blood pressure taken in the past 12 months, or if hypertensive whose elevated blood pressure was not recognized and needs to be treated. Piggyback onto that clinical activity the COPC activity of determining the *lower* limit of age- and sex-specific communitywide nonhypertension screening rates, and the *lower* limit of the rate of non-recognition by the staff of elevated blood pressures.[5] The intent of this COPC activity is to do population-based quality assurance described by Nutting in a chapter of Part V of this volume.

What are the age- and sex-specific prevalence rates of diabetes, to decide if screening for diabetes might be helpful? Piggyback obtaining plasma glucose and random quantitative urine glucose by the Beckman Glucometer (2,3), onto the clinical activity of obtaining yearly urines and electrolytes for all hypertensive patients. The

---

[5] The rates among all known diabetic patients are probably different than among the total population. Diabetics are more likely to come to the clinic, more likely to have a blood pressure reading, and more likely to have elevated readings recognized. However, if knowing the *lower* limits of the rates among the population would help decisionmaking, that is, if the lower limits are still high enough that remedial steps would be instituted, these data are good enough, and are easily obtainable while identifying specific diabetic patients who need specific elements of care. Note that one cannot use this piggyback to determine the prevalence of hypertension itself in the population; 50 percent of diabetic people have hypertension.

prevalence rates of diabetes among hypertensive patients are more than the population's true rates. Answering this COPC question by using hypertension as a tracer condition, and by piggybacking diabetes screening onto routine lab work for hypertensive patients, is most appropriate if one does not know either the number of all diabetic patients in the population served or the population denominator, and if one wants approximate age-specific rates.

Are the rates of infant and child car seat use so low that we should start an educational campaign to increase their use? Many practices have patients who usually come to the clinic by automobile, and have a large number of infants and children requiring special care (e.g., a premature birth, severe congenital defect). Those practices could estimate the percentage of infants and children in the population who are strapped in an infant/child car seat, by having a staff member walk with the parent of "special care" children or infants to the car. That walk could be part of the special care given by the practice; the staff member could discuss the need for an infant car seat when needed. Keeping track of the data on use or nonuse would give an approximation to the rate of use in the total population.

These are a few examples of using patient-based data to develop COPC information that may be accurate enough for decisionmaking. The examples require work beyond "usual care," but remain within the spirit of traditional medical care. Also, the examples are less inexpensive than the usual ways of obtaining COPC data.

DISCUSSION

Some people concerned with the accuracy of COPC epidemiology may argue that this method is too inaccurate and has too many potential biases or confounding factors to be appropriate for COPC.

My opinion follows Kerr White, a well-known leader in community medicine and applied epidemiology, who has said on many occasions, "It is better to be roughly right than precisely wrong." More specifically, there are two answers to that concern.

First, although some COPC problems require more precision than this method allows, some do not. The outline of the characteristics of the method, above, implies that the method is useful for only specific situations. For instance, the staff did not need to know what was the "true" PPD screening rate for its population, because it decided that the upper limit of that rate was too low.

Second, one has to decide if the added precision is worth the added cost of getting it. Conservation of resources is important in COPC. If this method is good enough to answer one's question within budgetary limits, while a more accurate answer would not be achievable due to resource limits, the method can and should be used. Not that the method is cheap. It is more expensive, and its activity (usually chart audits) more unusual, than traditional medical care. But its cost is less than classic epidemiology, and its chart audits also directly help the practitioner give good person-to-person medical care. This method may frequently be more acceptable and desirable than "classic" COPC activity.

SUMMARY

In specific circumstances, population-based data can be obtained easily and economically by piggybacking the effort onto more traditional activities in medical care, and by using a tracer condition as a reasonable approximation of a sample of the population. This method may facilitate doing COPC in a variety of settings in which population-based data are not available.

REFERENCES

1. Comstock, G.W., and Philip, R.N. Decline of the tuberculosis epidemic in Alaska. *Public Health Reports* 1961; 76:19-24.

2. Davidson, J.K. Diabetes screening using a quantitative urine glucose method. *Diabetes* 1978; 27:810-816.

3. Davidson, J.K. Screening for diabetes mellitus. In: *Diabetes*, Davidson, J.K. (ed.). In press.

CHAPTER 25

Community-Oriented Occupational Health Services

Gregory R. Wagner, M.D.

Work and health are inextricably intertwined. Chemical and physical agents in the workplace may pose a direct threat to workers' health. The adverse consequences of shift work, job stress, and unemployment are less obvious but equally significant. Work provides access to health care through the provision of health insurance and wages. Work-related activities consume the largest percentage of awake time for most adults and are central to an individual's self-concept.

Occupational health problems are seen daily in primary care practices. These problems include not only the easily recognized strains, sprains, and lacerations from on-the-job accidents, but also a substantial number of common impairments resulting from workplace exposures, such as decreased pulmonary capacity or auditory acuity.

It is therefore both logical and appealing for primary care practices to use occupation to identify a target population for special services, although few practices have chosen to provide such services for their patients or surrounding communities.

Treatment of occupational health problems though classical individual patient care fails to recognize that these problems have common sources and are preventable. Specialized services that tie together the health problems of a subset of the community and workplace exposures can serve two critical functions: assist in the prevention of future work-related health problems, and help identify previously unknown links between workplace exposures and health.

Community-oriented practices should consider the development of occupational health services in a number of situations. The recognition of work-related problems in active patients within the practice is a natural stimulus. A practice located in an area with a high concentration of a single industry— such as agriculture, mining, or textile manufacture—should develop services to address the needs of people who work in that industry. Sometimes specific hazards such as exposure to asbestos or excessive noise have been common to workers in diverse industries. The commonality of the problem facilitates program development aimed at reducing the impact of these hazards. In some areas public expression of the importance of occupational health problems by workplace or community organizations should encourage a supportive response from a community-oriented practice.

CHARACTERIZING THE POPULATION

Whatever the stimulus, the first step in the development and provision of occupational health services in a community-oriented primary care context is the characterization of the population. The population must be described both demographically and by the nature of work, work-related hazards, and work organization. Questions to answer include:

How many people are in this population? What is their age-sex distribution? How many of them are currently active patients of the practice? Where do they live?

What is the nature of the work? What are its hazards? What are the known or suspected adverse health consequences of these hazards?

How accessible is the working population to the practice? Are there significant employee organizations with a history or interest in health and safety activities with which to work, or is the workforce largely unorganized? What is the history of employment relations in the area—cooperative or confrontational? What kinds of employment-related health services have been provided by the practice in the past that might affect community perceptions of the practice? For example, has the practice served as a "company doctor," closely identified with carrying out an agenda defined by the employer?

What are the current workplace-based or community-based occupational health services available to this group?

What State or Federal disability and benefits systems cover the workers, and what are the roles and responsibilities of health care providers within these systems? Is there special protective legislation relevant to health hazards in local enterprises?

Are the local or Federal regulations giving access to information about substances produced or used at work?

RESOURCES

A variety of resources are available to respond to these questions. Among the most useful are:

1. *Current patients.* By routinely eliciting occupational histories from active patients, one can accumulate a large database of both the substance and context of work. People know a remarkable amount about their work and workplace, and enjoy sharing this knowledge with interested health care providers.

2. *Government agencies.* State and local offices of economic development often gather demographic information concerning employment profiles of relatively small areas. State workers' compensation funds may have information on the size and category of workplaces in an area, as well as the kinds of health problems for which compensation claims have been filed. These data may be useful in attempting to identify significant health problems or risks. Similarly, the National Institute for Occupational Safety and Health (NIOSH) can provide technical assistance to primary care providers interested in occupational health problems. NIOSH, as well as the Occupational Safety and Health Administration (OSHA), the agency that enforces regulations limiting adverse workplace exposures, can provide information concerning potential health hazards associated with particular industries as well as data on risks resulting from specified exposures. There is a Federal hazard communication regulation administered by OSHA that permits access to certain information about chemicals manufactured or used in

plants. Some States and localities have community "right to know" laws, which facilitate access to information. (See Table 1.)

3. *Voluntary organizations.* Chambers of Commerce, associations of manufacturers, as well as trade organizations specific to an area with a high concentration of a particular industry can be of significant help in characterizing employment patterns. Some areas also have citizen-worker "coalitions for safety and health" (often called COSH groups) that have done in-depth investigations of work-related health hazards in the region. Labor unions representing workers at single workplaces as well as district and national organizations have invaluable information they are willing to share. Useful lists of voluntary organizations have been published (1, 2).

Cooperation from these groups may vary. Because of the overt or covert hostility that may characterize the relationship between employers and employees and their respective organizations, primary care providers who attempt to enter this arena in an effort

TABLE 1. Occupational Health Information Sources from the National Institute for Occupational Safety and Health (NIOSH).

Clearinghouse for Occupational Safety and Health Information
4676 Columbia Parkway, Cincinnati, OH 45226, (513) 533-8317

Occupational Safety and Health Administration, U.S. Department of Labor
Third Street and Constitution Ave., N.W., Washington, DC 20210, (202) 523-8151

Regional offices:		*NIOSH*	*OSHA*
Region I	Boston	(617)223-6668	(617)223-6710
Region II	New York	(212)264-2485	(212)944-3426
Region III	Philadelphia	(215)596-6716	(215)596-1201
Region IV	Atlanta	(404)881-4474	(404)881-3573
Region V	Chicago	(312)886-3881	(312)353-2220
Region VI	Dallas	(214)665-3081	(214)767-4731
Region VII	Kansas City, MO	(816)374-5332	(816)374-5861
Region VIII	Denver	(303)837-3979	(303)837-3883
Region IX	San Francisco	(415)556-3781	(415)556-0586
Region X	Seattle	(206)442-0530	(206)442-5930

National resources:

Environmental Protection Agency (EPA), Pesticide Information Hotline, 1-800-858-7378

National Cancer Institute, Division of Cancer Cause and Prevention, Occupational Studies Section, (301)496-9093

National Institute of Environmental Health Sciences (NIEHS), National Toxicology Program, (919) 541-3991

Centers for Disease Control, (404) 329-3534

to improve health status can encounter resistance.

4. *Employers.* Some employers are extremely accommodating to primary health care providers who express an interest in learning first-hand about work in their enterprises. These employers correctly feel that the more the providers know about the work of their patients, the more accurate assessments will be concerning the timing of a return to work following an injury or the availability of light-duty or restricted work for a partially impaired individual. Workplace tours are often of interest not only to the clinicians, but also to other practice staff who have relatives working at the site. Where possible, tours should be supplemented by discussion with knowledgeable representatives of both the employer and the employees who can help highlight jobs or exposures of particular concern because of associated hazards. On request, employers should also provide material safety data sheets detailing health risks associated with exposure to hazardous substances used or produced in their enterprises.

Once work and its associated hazards are described, the target population— the denominator—must be defined. This should be done, to the extent possible, with the formal or informal advice of members of the community and should reflect the goals of the practice. The community can be defined by specific worksite, by employer, by industry, by hazard, or by job. Place of residence may also be relevant. These decisions will reflect local resources, the pattern of local employment, provider preference, current practice, local politics, convenience, and a host of other factors too intricate in their interplay to attempt to anticipate. The complexity of these relationships and their impact on the eventual outcome of a program sup-

port the importance of using the best available advice and maintaining flexibility in denominator definition.

PROBLEM DEFINITION

Although the principles of COPC emphasize the identification of a defined population first and problems within that population later, in reality it is often the identification or recognition of a well-characterized or suspected health problem that stimulates the development of COPC activities, in occupational health as in other areas. Population definition in COPC is not a single step in the process but occurs at various stages as part of an iterative process of refinement, redefinition, and modification.

In some localities, known health risks associated with the dominant industry will allow the practice to target services and develop programs to work toward prevention of known hazards. In other areas, inadequate prior research precludes definition of occupational risks. In these circumstances, the development of methods to document systematically the relationship between certain work or particular workplace exposures and demonstrable health outcomes is the necessary and significant first step that will eventually permit the development of preventive strategies. Occupational carcinogens, asthmogens, and reproductive hazards have been recognized through information generated in the primary care setting. Most areas provide a mix of opportunities, with the ultimate choice of program goals depending upon local interest, information, and abilities.

Problem definition, too, is a process of progressive refinement. For example, a primary health care facility recognized that hearing loss was a significant problem in its industrially employed patients. Exploration of the medical literature and discussion with groups of affected patients indicated that significant adverse exposures existed in the work environment. A population within the catchment area of the health care center was defined and the problem redefined to include the following elements:

1. People did not know that noise exposure threatened their hearing, or, alternatively, there was social acceptance that hearing loss was an inevitable consequence of aging and industrial work.

2. Those who were aware of the connection between noise exposure and hearing loss were unaware that things could be done to reduce exposures or rehabilitate impaired individuals.

3. Motivation towards early identification of problems was limited because of these problems.

4. There had been adverse experience in the community with consumer fraud in the marketing of hearing aids.

Strategies were developed to deal with these problems including: educating the population at risk; working with social and political organizations with potential effectiveness in approaching these problems; screening active patients as well as doing outreach screening for people at high risk who were not active patients at the primary health care center; and developing information and referral for rehabilitation and hearing aids.

Outcomes of the initial efforts led to modification of understanding of the problem. In particular, it became clear that the compensation system for occupational hearing loss was flawed—that it denied motivation to prevent the problem and minimized the motivation to identify early hearing loss. Further, defects in the system had erected barriers to obtaining hearing aids. The focus of activity thus grew to include modification of the system for compensating occupational hearing loss.

The identification and characterization of occupational health problems requires the active involvement of the target community. Problems must be conceptualized in a manner consistent with community understanding if effective strategies for addressing them are to be developed. For example, lung diseases of coal miners can be approached in a variety of ways. If the medical definition of coal workers pneumoconioses (CWP) (x-ray or pathological changes resulting from coal dust exposure) is accepted, a facility would be interested in preventive programs using x-rays as a primary diagnostic modality. However, coal miners interested in lung diseases are concerned about a variety of issues and a variety of conditions. Black lung has been defined both legally and popularly to include the range of lung diseases resulting from coal mine dust exposure. Coal miners (and the medical literature) indicate that coal mine dust exposure contributes to the development of emphysema and bronchitis in addition to CWP. Benefits programs reflect this broader view (3). A health service provider failing to recognize the distinction between the medical and the popular definition would have difficulty developing a program that is likely to meet the needs of the community.

BARRIERS TO PROGRAM IMPLEMENTATION

Because of the complex interrelationships between work and health, worker and employer, and provider and patient, it is important to anticipate the potential barriers to success of a community-oriented occupational health program. Most importantly, primary care providers rarely have access to workplaces in a manner that can control working conditions. Given that the source of work related health problems is workplace exposures and that control of the health problems relies upon control of the exposures, the primary health care provider must work in concert with members of the community who are capable of inspecting, controlling, or eliminating occupational exposures. Further, a community primary care practice must be aware of the nature of the employment relationship, though it has no control over it. Activism around health and safety may result in harassment in the workplace or job loss. Publicly expressed concern about workplace conditions may result in the threat or reality of workplace closure or job loss with reduction in community and individual health.

Confidentiality is a critical issue in developing acceptable occupational health services. If workers fear information resulting from screening programs or other interactions will be shared with current or prospective employers, they may be appropriately reluctant to participate in what otherwise appear to be useful programs. Furthermore, health surveillance that is not tied to specific helpful outcomes (e.g., hazard elimination, job transfer, or potential financial gain) may not be perceived as worth the risk of involvement. Rosenstock (4) has extensively reviewed ethical considerations in the provision of occupational health services.

As with many COPC activities, funding can be problematic. However, because some fee generating clinical services are associated with community occupational health programs, these services may be self-sustaining after an initial investment of time and energy.

Prior research may not be applicable in the primary care setting. Most occupational health research has taken place in industries or universities. The development of services for a specific population reflecting the unique characteristics of the community demands creativity and imagination.

Primary health care providers often lack training and skills in occupational health.

Skills that can be helpful in some settings include the administration and interpretation of clinical tests that can indicate the development of functional impairment, such as audiometry and pulmonary function tests. In some circumstances, familiarity with the method of chest x-ray interpretation developed by the International Labor Organization to provide standardization in the surveillance of people at risk for the development of certain pneumoconioses is helpful (5). Knowledge and appreciation of basic concepts of epidemiology and public health help in looking beyond individual patients toward the occupational group as a whole, and in understanding concepts of risk as well as illness.

One must regard occupational diseases as preventable. Despite the lack of direct control over the workplace, the practice must be willing to be an advocate for prevention of disease through external hazard reduction, rather than concentrating solely on factors thought to be modifiable because they are part of the patient's personal lifestyle, such as smoking or alcohol use. An understanding that most people would rather work in a productive and healthy manner than collect benefits when injured or ill, and an attitude of inquiry resulting from an understanding that what is *not* known *can* be harmful, are both essential for an effective program. It is important to recognize that many significant discoveries in occupational health have resulted from sympathetic and open-minded health care providers taking the concerns and observations of alert workers seriously.

The political and economic issues interconnected with the control of work-related illness and injury generate a dimension of resistance to the implementation of COPC programs that might not be met in other arenas. Hypertension has no advocates, but there are many articulate and persuasive arguments marshalled whenever the elimination of a workplace hazard is considered.

The recognition of these barriers is necessary for the development and implementation of community occupational health programs. Although barriers cannot, in general, be eliminated, they can be met and partially overcome. For example, confidentiality is a key issue in any primary care practice. Practice policies concerning access to and release of patient information can be made explicit and distributed to patients. Health surveillance programs can be tied to helpful outcomes, such as the completion of reports to workers' compensation funds where occupational problems are identified. Easily accessible texts and articles can help overcome some provider ignorance and resistance (Table 2). Finally, a health care practice must recognize that it is in a secondary role in the occupational health arena, and must be content to provide support services for the primary actors—workers, employers, and regulatory agencies.

COPC BY COMPANY DOCTORS

Does the physician practicing part- or full-time within industry have an easier time in the design and implementation of occupational health programs for the workplace community? Surely some barriers are reduced. Demographic information about the workforce is easily available. Detailed information about exposures and conditions may be accessible. The physician is able to consult directly with those with control over working conditions. However, other barriers are even greater. It may be difficult or impossible to convince the target population that improvement in their health status is the primary goal of any program. This is especially true if there is an exclusive focus on lifestyle or habit modification rather than hazard elimination in the workplace—even if the personal factors appear to be of greater consequence to the health of the individual. Such efforts may be seen as a deflection of attention and resources from *occupational* problems, even if they embody

---

TABLE 2. Brief List of Occupational Health General References for Primary Care Practices.

Burgess, W.A. *Recognition of Health Hazards in Industry: A Review of Materials and Processes.* New York: John Wiley and Sons, 1981.

Keogh, J.P. Occupational and environmental disease. In: Barker LR, Burton, JR, Zieve, PD (eds.), *Principles of Ambulatory Medicine.* Baltimore: Williams and Wilkins, 1982, p. 61.

Levy, B. S., and Wegman, D.H. (eds.). *Occupational Health: Recognizing and Preventing Work-related Disease.* Boston: Little, Brown and Co., 1983.

Makison, F. W.; Stricoff, R. S.; Partridge, L. J. (eds.). *NIOH/OSHA Pocket Guide to Chemical Hazards.* DHEW (NIOSH) Publication No. 78. Washington, DC: U.S. Government Printing Office, 1978.

Proctor, N. H., and Hughes, J. P. *Chemical Hazards of the Workplace.* Philadelphia: Lippincott, 1978.

Rom, W. (ed.). Environmental and Occupational Medicine. Boston: Little, Brown and Co., 1983.

Rothstein, M. A. *Medical Screening of Workers.* Washington, DC: Bureau of National Affairs, Inc., 1984.

---

good *clinical* preventive medicine. Physicians are employed by industry to improve the productivity of the workforce, reduce the liability of the employer, and maintain or improve the health status of the workforce. While these roles are often compatible with the best interests of employees, the dual role of the physician can inhibit the development of acceptable community-oriented rather than employer-oriented services.

EXAMPLE OF COMMUNITY-ORIENTED OCCUPATIONAL HEALTH ACTIVITIES

In contrast, employer-independent practices can engage in a wide range of occupational health activities without role ambiguity. The experience of one primary health care center located in a coal mining area is instructive.

The Board of Directors of the Cabin Creek Medical Center in Dawes, West Virginia, a nonprofit community-based comprehensive health care center, decided to make occupational health for coal miners a high priority. Over the last 8 years, Center staff have developed, delivered, and evaluated primary, secondary, and tertiary preventive health care services for and in conjunction with coal miners in the region.

Primary preventive services are those directed toward reducing or eliminating hazards or modifying risk status prior to the development of disease. These include an educational slide/tape program for young miners that outlines health risks of mining; providing personal hearing protection devices; offering smoking cessation literature and counseling; and providing technical assistance to union locals wishing to monitor compliance with dust and noise control regulations. Also, program staff have prepared and presented testimony based on the experience at the Center as it related to proposed regulatory changes that might affect miners' health.

Secondary preventive services are those that may lead to the early identification of health impairment at a point where intervention may preserve functional status. Periodic assessment of auditory and pulmonary function fits into this category, as does some of the educational work raising the association between noise exposure and early signs of hearing loss. Aiding working miners with CWP in their efforts to transfer from high-dust to low-dust jobs also fits into this category.

Tertiary prevention aims to preserve function once impairment is established. The Center offers a comprehensive pulmonary education program as well as the social services and benefits counseling for impaired miners (6).

CONCLUSION

Consideration of occupational health services illustrates both the opportunity and necessity to work concurrently within a practice to modify services and within a community to change conditions that are at the root of health problems. In the proper setting, an occupationally defined community can be rapidly identified leading to health service modification and community service development with beneficial reduction in health risks and potential improvement in health status.

REFERENCES

1. American Lung Association. *Sources of Information on Occupational Health.* Supplement to *Occupational Lung Disease, An Introduction.* New York: American Lung Association, 1979.
2. Frumkin, H., and Hu, H. (eds.). *Occupational and Environmental Health: A Resource Guide for Science Students.* DHEW (NIOSH) Publication No. 80-118. Washington, D.C.: Government Printing Office, 1980.

3. Weeks, J.L., and Wagner, G. R. Compensation for occupational disease with multiple causes: The case of coal miners' respiratory diseases. *American Journal of Public Health* 1986; 76:58.

4. Rosenstock, L. *Ethical Dilemmas Facing Clinicians Who Provide Health Services to Workers.* Tucson, AZ: American Center for Occupational Safety and Health, 1983, (Currently available from the Association of Teachers of Preventive Medicine, 1030 Fifteenth St., Suite 1020, Washington, D.C., 202-682-1698.)

5. International Labour Organization. *Guidelines for the Use of ILO International Classification of Radiographs of Pneumoconioses,* Revised Edition 1980. Occupational Safety and Health Series No. 22 (Rev.) Geneva: International Labour Organization, 1980.

6. Wagner, G.R., and Spieler, E.A. Disease surveillance and health promotion for coal miners utilizing independent community health care centers. *Annals of the American College of Governmental Industrial Hygienists,* in press.

CHAPTER 26

Alcohol, Drug Abuse, and Mental Disorders: Opportunities for COPC

Douglas B. Kamerow, M.D., M.P.H.

Alcohol, drug abuse, and mental disorders (ADM disorders) are common, costly, and poorly recognized in primary care settings. COPC methods, which are usually applied to such problems as hypertension, infectious diseases, and prenatal care, should also be considered for use in identifying community needs for primary care treatment of ADM disorders. This chapter briefly documents the importance of these problems in primary care, discusses approaches for detecting and identifying them in the community, and suggests some specific examples of actions that can be taken.

THE IMPORTANCE OF ADM DISORDERS

A recent paper (1) reviewed the importance of these disorders. They are very common, affecting almost one in five Americans (2).[1] They are also extremely costly; it is estimated that direct treatment and support costs totaled over $50 billion in 1983. When direct and indirect (productivity losses, property damage and the like) costs are combined, a staggering total of $218 billion was spent (3).

Another measure of cost is mortality. Over 100,000 persons per year die as a direct result of an ADM disorder, and this number is conservative. Because suicides are underreported, many more thousands of deaths are not counted. In addition, many ADM-connected deaths are of relatively young persons, resulting in a disproportionately large amount of potentially productive years of life lost (PPYLL) (4). Accidents, for instance, are the fourth leading cause of death in the United States, but they rank first in PPYLL and are responsible for over 20 percent of the productive years lost due to premature death. Because 25-50 percent of accidental deaths are attributable to alcohol abuse (3), a significant percentage of PPYLL is related to this ADM disorder.

Finally, ADM disorders are important because persons suffering from them tend to use up to twice as much general health care services as those without them (5,6). General health care costs for these patients may be decreased, however, by proper treatment of their ADM disorder. Careful reviews of the literature about this so-

---

[1] National estimates were obtained by projecting the Epidemiologic Catchment Area program three-site rates to the U.S. population, after standardizing the rates to the 1980 Census by age, sex, and race.

called "offset effect" (7-9), generally support this finding.

Alcohol, drug abuse, and mental disorders are seen commonly in primary care medicine. A large national survey that used standardized interviews to make psychiatric diagnoses found that more than half of those with ADM disorders received *all* their care from the general medical sector (10). Despite this fact, however, there is good evidence that ADM disorders are not recognized and treated or referred optimally by primary care physicians. For example, several studies have found that only one-third to one-half of patients with major depressive disorder are recognized by their doctors (11-13), and surveys have shown that physicians themselves feel they do a poor job of recognizing and treating alcohol abuse disorders (14,15).

APPROACHES FOR THE DETECTION AND IDENTIFICATION OF ADM DISORDERS

The importance of specific health problems to a community can be determined in different ways, as outlined in the COPC literature (16). With ADM disorders, at the simplest level one can make the gross assumption that they are important in *any* community because they are so prevalent and are generally poorly treated. At the next level, that of health provider consensus, ADM problems that seem important can be selected and targeted for intervention. This is what led the medical providers at the Checkerboard Area Health System in New Mexico to select alcoholism as one of their priority areas (17).

Rarely are specific community surveys made to obtain data on ADM disorders, but other sources of local data may be useful. For alcoholism, high cirrhosis death rates or drunk driving arrest rates might be useful indicators. Similarly, indications of high suicide rates in a community or of

drug use problems in the schools might lead to identification of these disorders as important.

"Community," of course, can mean many different things. Any defined population may be examined for ADM problems. For example, a rash of injuries in a factory might lead to the suspicion that drugs or alcohol are involved. Depression in nursing homes or other facilities is common and could be investigated. The pediatrician's or family physician's position as school doctor might present excellent opportunities for early detection and even prevention of some of these disorders. Like many other problems, ADM disorders often need only to be thought of to be recognized.

EXAMPLES OF ACTIONS TO BE TAKEN

Including the "Missing Patient"

The narrowest definition of a COPC "community," that of the families of all active practice patients, frequently contains persons who need to be brought to care: the missing family member, commonly the father, who has an ADM disorder which is affecting the whole family. Family practitioners, for example, will see the children for school problems, the wife for anxiety or depression, but never actually see the father who has alcoholism. Including this "missing patient" into the practice is the first step toward addressing his or her problem.

Training Practitioners

Physicians and other practitioners can only diagnose and treat ADM disorders if they can recognize them. Better training in the recognition and treatment of persons with these problems is one way to improve community care for them. Practitioners who are sensitized to these disorders can use screening instruments such as the CAGE questionnaire (18) or the Michigan Alcohol Screening Test

(MAST) (19) for alcoholism; the Zung Self-Rating Depression Scale (SDS) (20), the Beck Depression Inventory (BDI) (21), or the Center for Epidemiologic Studies Depression Scale (CES-D) (22) for depression; and the General Health Questionnaire (GHQ) (23) or Hopkins Symptom Check List (HSCL) (24) for general mental distress. All of these screens can help practitioners decide which patients need closer attention.

Treating the Chronically Mentally Ill

Many with chronic mental illnesses have been discharged from institutions and are living in the community. Although they may have ties to outpatient mental health facilities, they frequently get little or no medical care. An aggressive campaign to locate these persons and provide them with a source of coordinated, comprehensive, quality care would certainly help resolve what has become a serious problem in many communities.

Collaborating with Local Alcohol, Drug, and Mental Health Agencies

Another source of access to the community is through local agencies charged with providing care or support for those with ADM disorders. They may serve as a source of referral or as a partner in planning outreach programs into the community directed at those with ADM disorders.

Political Advocacy

Physicians and other health providers can be quite effective in urging public and political action to address ADM problems through testimony before local governing bodies and personal contact with officials. Examples include urging passage of stiffer penalties for drunk driving with stricter definitions of intoxication; advocating increased attention to drug abuse in schools; and publicizing community responsibility for the care of the deinstitutionalized chronically mentally ill.

Using ADM Services in Marketing

Finally, as Garr has pointed out elsewhere in this book, one method of financing COPC activities is the added patient revenues that result from outreach activities. This concept applies to treatment of ADM disorders as well. One need only turn on the television or radio in any large city today to hear advertisements for ADM treatment services. There is no reason that primary care practices with interest and expertise in dealing with these problems should not also use them to attract new patients.

Alcohol, drug abuse, and mental health disorders are common, costly, and poorly treated in primary care. It is hoped that this discussion has drawn attention to these important problems and suggested ways that they can be addressed in a community-oriented primary care setting.

REFERENCES

1. Kamerow, D.B.; Pincus, H.A.; and Macdonald, D.I. Alcohol abuse, other drug abuse, and mental disorders in medical practice: Prevalence, costs, recognition, and treatment. *Journal of the American Medical Association* 1986, in press.

2. Meyers J.K.; Weissman, M.M.; Tischler, G.L. et al. Six-month prevalence of psychiatric disorders in three communities: 1980 to 1982. *Archives of General Psychiatry* 1984; 41:959.

3. Harwood, H.J.; Napolitano, D.M.; Kristiansen, P.L. et al. *Economic Costs to Society of Alcohol and Drug Abuse and Mental Illness: 1980.* Research Triangle Institute Publication No. 2734/00-01FR. Research Triangle Park, N.C., 1984.

4. Perloff, J.D.; LeBailly, S.A.; Kletke, P.R. et al. Premature death in the United States: Years of life lost and

health priorities. *Journal of Public Health Policy* 1984; 5:167-184.

5. Hoeper, E.W.; Nycz, G.R.; Regier, D.A. et al. Diagnosis of mental disorder in adults and increased use of health services in four outpatient settings. *American Journal of Psychiatry* 1980; 137: 207-210.

6. Hankin, J., and Otay, J.S. *Mental Disorder and Primary Medical Care: An Analytical Review of the Literature.* Series D, No. 5, DHHS Publication No. (ADM) 78. Rockville, MD, 1979.

7. Jones, K.R., and Vischi, T.R. Impact of alcohol, drug abuse and mental health treatment on medical care utilization. *Medical Care* 1979; 17 (suppl): ii-82.

8. Pincus, H.A. Making the case for consultation-liaison psychiatry: Issues in cost-effectiveness analysis. *General Hospital Psychiatry* 1984; 6:173.

9. Mumford, E.; Schlesinger, H.J.; and Glass, G.V. et al. A new look at evidence about reduced cost of medical utilization following mental health treatment. *American Journal of Psychiatry* 1984; 141:1145.

10. Shapiro, S.; Skinner, E.A.; Kessler, L.G. et al. Utilization of health and mental health services: Three epidemiologic catchment area sites. *Archives of General Psychiatry* 1984; 41:971.

11. Hoeper, E.W.; Nycz, G.; and Cleary, P.D. *The Quality of Mental Health Services in an Organized Primary Health Care Setting.* Final report, NIMH Contract No. 278(DB). National Institute of Mental Health, Rockville, MD, 1979.

12. Schulbert, H.C.; Saul, M.; McClelland, M. et al. Assessing depression in primary medical and psychiatric practice. *Archives of General Psychiatry* 1985; 42:1164.

13. Nielsen, A.C., and Williams, T.A. Depression in ambulatory medical patients: Prevalence by self-report questionnaire and recognition by nonpsychiatric physicians. *Archives of General Psychiatry* 1980; 37:999.

14. Wechsler, H.; Levine, S.; Idelson, R.K. et al. The physician's role in health promotion: A survey of primary-care practitioners. *New England Journal of Medicine* 1983; 308:97.

15. Sadler, D. Poll finds M.D. attitudes on alcohol abuse changing. *American Medical News* 1984; 27:60.

16. Nutting, P.A. Community-oriented primary care: An integrated model for practice, research, and education. *American Journal of Preventive Medicine* 1986, in press.

17. Institute of Medicine. *Community-Oriented Primary Care: A Practical Assessment,* Vol. 1. Washington, D.C.: National Academy Press, p. 51.

18. Mayfield, D.; McLeod, G.; and Hall, P. The CAGE questionnaire: Validation of a new alcoholism screening instrument. *American Journal of Psychiatry* 1974; 131:1121.

19. Selzer, M.L. The Michigan alcoholism screening test: The quest for a new diagnostic instrument. *American Journal of Psychiatry* 1971; 127:1653.

20. Zung, W.W.K. A self-rating depression scale. *Archives of General Psychiatry* 1965; 12:63.

21. Beck, A.T.; Ward, C.; Mendelson, M. et al. An inventory for measuring depression. *Archives of General Psychiatry* 1961; 4:561.

22. Radloff, L.S. The CES-D scale: A self-report depression scale for research in the general population.

Applied Psychological Measurement 1977; 1:385.

23. Goldberg, D.P., and Blackwell, B. Psychiatric illness in general practice: A detailed study using a new method of case identification. *British Medical Journal* 1970; 2:439.

24. Derogatis, L.R.; Lipman, R.S.; Rickels, K. et al. The Hopkins Symptom Checklist (HSCL): A self-report symptom inventory. *Behavioral Science* 1974; 19:1.

CHAPTER 27

Oral Health Problems in the Community

William R. Maas, D.D.S., M.P.H.

Oral health is an integral component of overall health. Like the major sense organs, the oral cavity is a complex of nerves, muscles, and glands. Unlike them, it is more than a sense organ, performing dozens of physiologic and social functions that place high demand on its unique tissues. Some of the earliest accounts of medical practice describe the diagnosis and treatment of oral diseases as the foundation for better health.

This chapter provides COPC practitioners with insight as to how the community views oral health problems within its overall health concerns, how they might conceptualize their responsibilities, how they might address oral health concerns, and where they might turn for assistance.

In the United States, professional education and training and the business aspects of the organization and financing of health care have encouraged consideration of oral health as something separate from general health. However, most COPC medical practitioners understand through their personal experiences in the practice of medicine that good health is not completely attained without good oral health. COPC medical practitioners, as professionals interested in the total health of their communities, should provide professional leadership to reduce the community's oral health problems.

THE SIGNIFICANCE OF ORAL HEALTH PROBLEMS

Most communities in which COPC providers practice, unless they are very atypical, have serious oral health problems. In the aggregate, dental diseases probably constitute the Nation's most prevalent health problem. The two most prevalent oral diseases are dental caries and periodontal disease (diseases of the gums and tissues supporting the teeth). Other common problems are malocclusions that constrain normal function and increase susceptibility of teeth and gums to disease, traumatic injury treatment, and oral cancer and soft tissue lesions.

Dental caries prevalence has decreased among children in recent years. However, contrary to the belief of some people, this disease remains a major public health problem. By 17 years of age, 89 percent of children have experienced decay in their permanent teeth, and the average child has 11 teeth so affected (1). The proportion of people afflicted by this disease continues to increase throughout life.

Approximately one-half of adults aged 18-79 with teeth have inflammatory periodontal disease, and half of these have experienced irreversible loss of supporting bone. The proportion of the public with periodontal disease increases with age, and it is responsible for a significant proportion of tooth loss in adults over age 35 (2,3).

More than one-third of adults aged 65-74 are completely edentulous. Although 90 percent of persons of all ages who are edentulous have dentures, well over a third require refitting of existing or entirely new dentures (4-6).

Almost 5 percent of all cancer cases in men occur in the mouth or pharynx (7), and 60 percent of oral carcinomas are well advanced when first detected (8). If not detected at early stages, the treatments, although frequently successful in preventing death, may leave the victims with serious cosmetic and functional impairments that make them unable to resume a normal working or social life.

Dental disease costs society much more in social disability (i.e., inability to perform a social role optimally) than it does in loss of life. An expression of the value placed by individuals in avoiding that social disability is reflected in the national expenditures for dental care, which in 1984 exceeded $25 billion and increased at a faster rate than other health care spending (9). The "Closing the Gap" Health Policy Project of the Carter Center at Emory University reviewed the 13 leading health problems of the Nation and concluded that dental diseases rank second in total direct costs (10).

There are also data that reveal the impact of illness from dental conditions on restricted activity and work loss, but these estimates do not fully describe the social consequences of pain, disfigurement, difficulty in tasting, chewing, or speaking, and the contribution of oral dis-

eases to systemic health problems and lowered quality of life. Because they are chronic and progressive, dental caries and periodontal disease, if neglected, advance to stages that are both difficult and expensive to treat. However, perhaps of greatest significance to the COPC provider, these diseases can be prevented (or controlled with minimal expense and consequences) in most people.

OPPORTUNITIES FOR IMPROVEMENT

There is a tremendous gap between the current oral health status of many communities and the oral health that is attainable. Even if members of the community and their leaders do not know what is possible, the COPC provider should.

On the bright side, most communities in the United States have never had better dental health. Dental decay in children, nationally, decreased 20-40 percent in the 1970s and is probably still improving. Oral hygiene and treatment of gingival inflammation, the reversible periodontal disease, have improved. The proportion of people that have no remaining natural teeth is declining.

However, these improvements have not been distributed evenly.

- Twenty percent of children have 60 percent of dental decay (11).

- Almost 40 percent of those on community water systems still do not have access to drinking water containing dentally significant levels of fluoride (12).

- It is suspected that many people with low income or education do not practice adequate oral hygiene or use fluoride toothpaste frequently enough to prevent disease.

- Compounding these problems, access to professional care, even for simple, low cost and effective procedures, is uneven.

Since the mid-1960s, Medicaid, Medicare, community health centers, and related initiatives have all contributed to reduce the differential in utilization of inpatient and ambulatory medical services between the poor and/or nonwhites and the more affluent. However, few States offer adult dental services under Medicaid, many have inadequate fee structures to assure access of children to providers of covered services, and virtually no dental care is covered by Medicare. Consequently, a large gap in utilization, by income and race, remains for dental care (4).

- Black children are 75 percent more likely than white children to have never been to a dentist or to have not been there within the past 2 years, which is the absolute *minimum* interval that could be accepted during these cavity-prone years.
- Seven times as many low-income children as high-income children have never been to a dentist.
- At all ages, people with low income are one-third as likely to have visited a dentist in the past year as people with high income.

As might be expected, low-income people also have fewer total visits than others. The significance of these findings should not be misunderstood. Fewer dental visits is fine, perhaps even desirable, *if one does not need professional dental services.* However, low-income children have about four times more untreated decayed teeth than high-income children. In those without access to acceptable care, dental disease will generally progress to further morbidity and disability.

WHAT THE COPC MEDICAL PRACTITIONER CAN DO

The COPC medical practitioner can influence oral health by providing professional services to individual patients and to the community at large (see Table 1). These services can be provided either personally, through other individuals, or through institutions.

COPC Oral Health Services to Individuals

COPC oral health care services to individuals are those provided to people who present to the clinic for care. On the surface, they are not appreciably different than those provided by primary care practitioners who do not have a community orientation. However, COPC medical providers may approach this care from a more informed perspective. First, COPC practitioners are aware of their community's oral health needs, are more informed about oral conditions, and are therefore more likely to take oral cavities into account. Second, they have knowledge of their patients' environment and can make judgments on the need for such preventive measures as the prescribing of supplementary fluoride. Third, they are interested in helping their patients modify lifestyle or personal care practices to prevent disease. Finally, they are aware of the need for services that are only available from dentists and their staffs and are concerned about their patients' access to acceptable dental care.

Many services, particularly those related to patient education and modification of lifestyle and personal practices, do not have to be personally provided by the COPC medical provider and are often provided by other health workers of the COPC practice. In their leadership of this component of their practice or institution, COPC providers can ensure that consideration of behaviors that influence oral health is an integral part of these efforts.

Educational Services

Among the educational services that might be provided by the COPC institution are including the topic of "baby bottle tooth decay" and appropriate use of

203

TABLE 1. What the COPC Provider Can Do to Improve Oral Health.

	Services To Individuals	Services To Community-at-Large
Services Provided Personally	Observe oral conditions Prescribe fluoride Educate and counsel: -parenting practices -self-care & hygiene -diet Refer for preventive and corrective treatment Provide leadership to staff and other components of COPC institution or practice	Provide leadership to community leaders and institutions to direct their efforts and resources to improve oral health Assist community dentists to be more community-oriented
Services Provided Through Institutions	Education and counseling provided by other health workers of the COPC practice to patients who seek care: -parenting practices -self-care & hygiene -diet	Surveys to determine the oral health problems Education of persons via -schools -workplaces -community organizations -media Protection via community water fluoridation and school-based fluoride programs Inclusion of dental care in employee benefit programs Preventive and corrective treatment provided by community dentists

the nursing bottle in well-child clinic preventive health counseling or emphasizing less frequent ingestion of sweets in dietary counseling. In instruction and encouragement of appropriate hygiene and self-care, attention to the role of proper personal oral hygiene and self-diagnosis of gingival bleeding can have an important influence on oral health among people of all ages. Such education might also include encouraging the use of self-applied topical fluoride, as in toothpaste and mouthrinse, and educating individuals who rely on community water supplies that are not fluoridated as to the benefits they are missing.

Prescribing and Referring

Still other services to individuals are provided personally. For example, COPC medical providers themselves may prescribe dietary fluoride supplements in unfluoridated communities or counsel mothers regarding inappropriate use of the nursing bottle, and this can have a significant effect on the health of individuals of a family. Also included in this category is appropriate referral of patients to dentists. Primary care providers generally have sound referral judgment, but their referrals are usually made for serious dental problems or conditions that are compromising the patient's response to medical care. This is case-finding activity, which is helpful for the individual patient and should be encouraged, but it must be recognized that this activity is not unique to COPC. These referrals are not much different than others made to medical specialists for secondary or tertiary care.

Perhaps a more critical aspect of this issue relates to referral for preventive services that cannot be provided by medical care practitioners, such as pit and fissure plastic sealants to protect the chewing surfaces of recently erupted permanent teeth. COPC providers must understand how to prevent dental diseases and must work to make appropriate dental care or other interventions available *before* the development of the serious problems that are common causes of referral. This requires that COPC providers look in the mouth as part of patient assessment, monitor the personal and socioenvironmental influences on their patients' oral health, and inquire as to whether family members have access to dental care.

Oral Health Services to the Community-at-Large by Professional Influence

The COPC practitioner offers other services to the community that are not dependent on who presents for care. The use of professional influence in providing services to the community-at-large may be the most effective way COPC providers can improve oral health. COPC physicians should be leaders for *health* in their communities, not just for medical care. It is obvious that COPC physicians have a strong influence over the use of the human and financial resources of their practices or organizations and can ensure that consideration of oral health is emphasized by all members of the practice. Active COPC providers also have political influence regarding the resources and activities of the community as a result of their professional reputation.

A hallmark of COPC providers is their interest in getting "upstream" of health problems. They know that there are more opportunities to prevent disease, by affecting personal behavior and altering the physical and social environment, through activities outside of the clinic than within it. As noted earlier, the artificial separation between medical and dental practice, although related to training and financing, is also a consequence of the traditionally different physical clinic settings. When COPC providers orient themselves outside the medical or dental clinics to the community to intervene in a problem, more opportunities for sharing ideas and resources develop. This type of activity can be understood by reviewing three examples.

Protecting the Community by the Services of Institutions

Initiating or supporting water fluoridation in communities with public water systems is the most significant activity a COPC provider can undertake to improve oral health. The fluoridation of community water supplies is the single most important commitment that a community can make to the oral health of its members. The benefits and safety of fluoridation have been firmly established, and it should be the foundation for developing any preventive program. In terms of a community program, fluoridation is the most effective preventive measure because its benefits can be realized without any effort or change in people's habits.

It should also be noted, however, that although individuals can receive the health benefits of fluoridation without individual effort, initiating the measure usually requires action of a board of health, municipal council, or other community leaders. Progress in fluoridating the Nation's water supplies has been spotty. There are politically active organizations whose singular mission is to oppose water fluoridation, who try to put fluoridation decisions up to public referendum. During these campaigns opponents issue a plethora of misleading charges to frighten the public, and unfortunately they have proven to be quite effective. The COPC provider should therefore promote fluoridation with awareness of the political sensitivity of the issue, in concert with others through a thoughtful strategy following consultation with those who have had related experiences.

If community water fluoridation is not possible, the community should look to other effective prevention strategies that do not depend on the initiative of the individual participants. Examples are establishing school-based prevention programs, using self-applied fluorides, providing protection against dental decay and with fluoride tablets, mouthrinse, or toothpaste. It should be noted that although these programs require little initiative by those participating, they require strong professional promotion and continuous oversight.

Modifying Personal Practices and the Utilization of Care

Like other health concerns, great potential for improving oral health also rests with modifying personal behavior, whether it be lifestyle, personal care practices, or obtaining dental care. Examples relate to using fluoride, oral hygiene, avoiding all forms of tobacco, diet, injury protection, and seeking periodic preventive dental care. It is not necessary for a community member to seek care at any particular clinic to benefit from this type of COPC effort. To be effective, however, this strategy requires systematic multiple educational and promotional activities.

Such activities may be directed communitywide, for example, through the use of the media. However, they can usually be more appropriately targeted to individuals with common needs, interests, concerns, or opportunities when provided through institutions serving portions of the community. Examples include schools, workplaces, service organizations, and health fairs. Although the desired behaviors are effective in reducing the risk of oral disease, the effectiveness of educational activities to change behaviors varies. Nevertheless, they should be considered as parallel, or perhaps integral, components of other strategies to modify personal behavior that are promoted by the COPC provider.

Access to Acceptable Professional Dental Services

Although the foregoing activities highlight the activities to improve oral health that can be accomplished independent of dental practice, there are some services that can only be provided by dental professionals and their staffs. Where a community does not have adequate access to acceptable dental services, referral of individuals and education of communities will be of limited value. Many prevention strategies require such care, including application of adhesive pit and fissure sealants to prevent decay and removing accumulations of dental plaque and calculus (tartar) to control gingival inflammation and bleeding. Where prevention was not begun early enough, or measures have not been completely effective, professional treatment is the only option for many in the community to regain oral health.

There are a host of activities that can be accomplished to improve access to dental care, from recruitment and orientation of a dentist to the community, to providing clinic space or subsidizing some aspect of the dental practice, to encouraging community firms and workers to consider including dental insurance in their employment package. When COPC providers stimulate, empower, or support the development of community-oriented primary *dental* care practices, providing both preventive and therapeutic care, they demonstrate to the community an understanding of its health problems and also satisfy an important health need of many in their practices.

DETERMINING THE ORAL HEALTH PROBLEMS OF THE COMMUNITY

Most COPC providers are aware of many oral health problems based on discussions with patients, their personal observations, and information related to them by other community health workers such as school nurses. As with other conditions, it is important to involve people from the community in specifying the oral health prob-

lems. When asked to describe their health problems, communities often mention dental problems as a high priority. For example, a survey of three Boston neighborhoods in 1970-1972 placed the need for dental services *first* in two neighborhoods and third in the other, after general medical and emergency services (13). The interests of American Indian communities were revealed in tribal planning documents in the 1970s, where safe drinking water, round-the-clock emergency medical services, and dental services were virtually always in the top three.

There is no ready source of community or regional dental statistical data, and only limited national data. Since most dental diseases do not have mortal consequences and are not highly communicable, they are not reportable. In some cases, health status and utilization findings from national surveys may be used to extrapolate and predict health status and problems within a community having certain social, economic, and demographic characteristics and to anticipate differences between subgroups of the community.

More appropriately, actual surveys can be accomplished to describe health status, treatment needs, care utilization, personal health practices, knowledge, attitudes, and perceptions of accessibility and acceptability of services in the community. The most useful surveys are those that provide data by methods and criteria comparable to surveys of other populations and thereby offer insight into the unique needs of a community and the potential for health improvement. As has been noted for identification of many medical problems, more efficient methods to acquire oral health data need to be developed that do not detract substantially from the human and financial resources available for health care.

It should be noted that some of the more serious dental health problems can be identified and monitored by simple screening programs. A number of COPC programs have used a "priority" screening instrument that categorizes individuals by the relative urgency of dental care that is needed. This provides one indication of the adequacy of preventive and therapeutic care received. Screening examinations provide a flow of information to individuals and to the community. Findings for individuals can be recorded and explained. Data describing the population can be summarized and provided to local community decisionmakers.

It may be possible to identify individuals and groups at high risk. For example, recent findings that 20 percent of children have 60 percent of the total decay in the population and that 83 percent of the surfaces with decay could be protected by adhesive dental sealants have strong implications for the types of community programs that would be most effective and efficient. When health status and treatment needs of the community are available and appropriate measures for prevention and control of disease are described, they can be implemented and approved by the community.

SOURCES OF ASSISTANCE

Whether oral health problems are clarified and addressed depends a great deal on how the benefits of dental expertise are integrated into the COPC practice. The involvement of the COPC provider should be direct. However, it may not be the best use of a COPC medical practitioner's time to personally assess the situation, develop strategies and monitor the results, unless there is no other option. It is usually more effective and efficient if involvement is directed to providing leadership and acting as nurturer, empowerer, and advocate of strategies that are developed by others.

COPC medical practitioners should collaborate with dentists. They will have no trouble finding dentists interested in pri-

mary care, since only 16 percent of dentists are specialists. However, they may have to look harder to find dentists that share their community orientation. Although the dental profession has a proud history of supporting water fluoridation, a classic primary preventive measure, the character of most clinical practices has been strongly oriented to secondary and tertiary prevention of decay. Some have been slow in implementing adhesive dental sealants as a primary preventive measure for decay, diagnosing early stages of periodontal disease that are amenable to simple professional services, or using systematic behavioral modification strategies for those afflicted. It is possible that COPC providers, by example and assistance, could inspire their dental colleagues to be more fully community oriented. As with COPC, progress to community-oriented primary dental care (COPDC) is made by ever widening the circle of people who understand and are committed to the concept.

Dental Parallels to COPC

Community dentists collaborating with a COPC practice will benefit from advice of other dental experts who can help clarify the community's dental problems and tailor strategies to the needs, resources, and opportunities of the situation. Such experts can assist in formulating goals and objectives and can offer skills and methods for carrying out evaluation to monitor the effectiveness and efficiency of COPDC practice. If COPC providers can identify dentists who share their concern and acceptance of responsibility for a defined community, they can draw on a body of knowledge that has been developing for 50 years that is very relevant to these interests. However, that body of knowledge is *not* called community-oriented primary dental care. It is known as "dental public health." Dental public health is one of eight recognized specialties of dentistry and has been involved with a myriad of efforts to encourage dentists to take a community-oriented approach to their practices.

When incorporated into clinical practice, dental public health *is* community-oriented primary dental care, both philosophically and methodologically. Dental public health is the "science and art of preventing and controlling dental disease and promoting dental health through organized community efforts. It is that form of dental practice which serves the community as a patient rather than the individual. It is concerned with the dental health education of the public, with research and the application of the findings of research, with the administration of programs of dental care for groups and with the prevention and control of dental disease through a community approach" (14).

The body of knowledge encompassed by dental public health provides expertise that is available to any dental practitioner who might be involved with a COPC program. Although many of the operational methods were developed by dental public health practitioners with special training, the professional organizations that offer opportunities for mutual inquiry, information exchange, and promotion of common issues are open to all. There are a large number of dentists who would not consider themselves to be public health dentists who, nevertheless, have significant COPDC experiences and have access to this support network. The COPC provider collaborating with such a dentist will discover a rich cross-over of dental public health applications to current concepts and developments of COPC.

Who to Turn to For Assistance
Because the field of dental public health has so many dimensions, not everyone who is formally trained has the experience to be useful to COPC efforts. In some cases, individuals with experience and interest may be more helpful than someone with public health training. However, individuals who are trained to assist the COPC provider may include staff from county and State health departments and specialists from the nearest school of public health. Other sources of assistance are experienced neighborhood health center personnel, staff from other local health programs, and representatives of State or local dental societies. Eighty percent of dentists are members of their local societies, and the officers of these organizations will know who among their members have the required skills and interest.

SUMMARY

This chapter has not outlined a detailed list of things for COPC medical practitioners to do to improve the oral health of their communities. It has stressed the importance of recognizing need, advocating community preventive practices, and sharing COPC interest and enthusiasm with a community dentist. As noted in Table 1, the best opportunities relate to what can be accomplished by professional leadership within the COPC practice, the institution, and the community to see that the appropriate resources and expertise are brought to bear on health problems. In this regard, dental problems may not be unique.

Oral health needs will not be met by dental care alone. A variety of community and interdisciplinary professional efforts are required. The community-oriented primary care medical practitioner can and should play a leadership role.

REFERENCES

1. U.S. Department of Health and Human Services. *The Prevalence of Dental Caries in United States Children. The National Dental Caries Prevention Survey.* NIH Publication No. 82-2245, December 1981.

2. Douglass, C.W.; Gilling, S.; Sollecito, W.; and Gammon, M. National trends in the prevalence and severity of the periodontal diseases. *Journal of the American Dental Association* 1983; 107:403.

3. Weintraub, J.A., and Burt, B. Oral health status in the United States: tooth loss and edentulism. *Journal of Dental Education* 1985; 49:368.

4. National Center for Health Statistics. Unpublished data from the National Health Interview Survey, 1983. Hyattsville, MD, 1986.

5. National Center for Health Statistics. *Edentulous Persons, United States 1971.* Series 10, No. 89, DHEW Publication No. 74-1516, Rockville, MD, 1974.

6. Ettinger, R.L.; Beck, J.D.; and Jakobsen, J., Removable prosthodontic treatment needs: A survey. *Journal of Prosthetic Dentistry* 1984; 51(3):419.

7. Young, J.C.; Percy, A. et al. *Cancer Incidence and Mortality in the United States, 1973-1977.* SEER-NIH Publ. No. 81(233), National Cancer Institute Monograph No. 57, Bethesda, MD, 1981.

8. Fischman, S.L. Oral health status in the United States: Oral cancer and soft tissue lesions. *Journal of Dental Education* 1985; 49:379.

9. Levit, K.R.; Lazenby, H.; Waldo, D.R.; and Davidoff, L.M. National health expenditures, 1984. *Health Care Finance Review* 1985; 7:1.

10. The Carter Center of Emory University. *Closing the Gap Health Policy Project: Summary of Pre-Consultation Meeting.* Atlanta, GA: Emory University, August 1984.

11. Bell, R.M.; Klein, S.P.; Bohannon, M.M.; Graves, R.C.; and Disney, J.A. *Treatment Effects in the National Preventive Dentistry Demonstration Program.* R-3072-RWJ. Santa Monica, CA: Rand Corp., 1984.

12. Centers for Disease Control. Unpublished data from the fluoridation census conducted by the Dental Disease Prevention Activity. Atlanta, GA, 1985.

13. Allukian, M., Jr. The role of a city dental program in improving the dental health of inner-city communities. *Journal of Public Health Dentistry* 1981; 41:98.

14. American Board of Public Health Dentistry. *Guidelines for Graduate Education in Dental Public Health.* Ann Arbor, MI: ABPHD, 1970, p. 10.

SUGGESTED READING

Many of the ideas expressed in this paper are covered in greater detail by the following:

Allukian, M., Jr. Action programs for community oral health. In: Dummett, C.O., *Community Dentistry: Contributions to New Directions.* Springfield, IL, Thomas, 1974, p. 118.

Allukian, M., Jr. Effective community prevention programs. In: DePaola, D.P., and Cheney, J.G. (eds.), *Handbook of Preventive Dentistry.* Littleton, MA: Publishing Services Group, 1979, Chapter 14.

Allukian, M., Jr. The dentist's responsibility to society. In: Forrester, D.J. et al., *Pediatric Dental Medicine.* Philadel-phia: Lea and Febiger, 1981, p. 666.

American Public Health Association. *Model Standards: A Guide for Community Preventive Health Services,* 2nd Edition. Washington, DC: American Public Health Association, 1985.

Rosenstein, D.I., MacKenzie, L.; and Joseph, L. *Community Dental Programs: A Guide for Development.* Portland,

OR: University of Oregon Health Sciences Center, 1980.

Schneider, D.A. *Dental Caries Prevention in Primary Care Projects*. Rockville, MD: Bureau of Health Care Delivery and Assistance, U.S. Department of Health and Human Services, 1985.

Striffler, D.F.; Young, W.O.; and Burt, B.A. *Dentistry, Dental Practice, and the Community*. Philadelphia: Saunders, 1983.

U.S. Department of Health and Human Services. Evaluation of community involvement in oral health programs. In: *Oral Health Program Guide for the Indian Health Service*. Rockville, MD: Indian Health Service, 1985, Vol. 9, p. 9.

CHAPTER 28

Examining the Distribution of Care in the Community

Paul A. Nutting, M.D.

Achieving the optimal health of a community depends, in part, on the distribution of primary care services among the target population. Two decades ago, this problem was largely one of access to health services, but changes in the health care system, including an impending excess of physicians, have complicated the nature of the problem. Efforts to enhance the community's health now encompass not only the distribution, but also the adequacy of care. Many communities have an adequate or even excessive volume of services available. Yet, it is well known that illness does not distribute evenly across a given population (5); hence, to have maximum impact, health services must be distributed relative to need and to the benefit to be derived. Similarly, primary care must not be provided as a random smorgasbord of services, but must be received by the individuals at risk in the population as a logical sequence of services appropriate to the individual's particular health profile.

Adequacy of care assumes need and presupposes a level of continuity of care necessary for the sequence of services to be effective. For example, an individual who has been screened positive for hypertension (perhaps on several occasions), but has not had the problem recognized, or has been recognized but has not received continuous treatment over a sustained period has not received an adequate pattern of care for hypertension regardless of the volume of disorganized and episodic services he may have received. Problems of this type have been demonstrated in several settings in which there is appropriate access to care (1,2).

Thus, while an adequate volume of services may be available within a community, the distribution of the services within groups at risk may remain as a subtle, but vitally important problem that deserves the attention of the COPC practice or program. Of particular concern is the distribution of services to high-risk individuals or others who most need care.

Over the past 15 years, a great deal of attention has been devoted to methods for assessing the quality of care. Much of the early work on methods development came from major medical centers, with techniques focusing on the care provided to the active patients of a practice during a single visit or during the course of an illness episode. These approaches contribute to an understanding of the technical

212

quality of health care, but can not shed light on the distribution and adequacy of care for a target population. Considerably less attention has been directed to examining the quality of care provided in the primary care setting, and very little work has examined the quality of care received by a population from the multiple practices and programs from which members of the community sought care.

One such method, however, was developed and used widely in the Indian Health Service (IHS). With the responsibility for ensuring comprehensive health services to defined and highly organized communities, the IHS needed methods for examining the quality of primary care services received by the communities served, regardless of the source of care. This method was subsequently tested widely both within the IHS as well as in the private sector. The fundamental tools and techniques of this method may be useful as well for any COPC practice that wishes to identify and respond to that set of community health problems related to the delivery of basic health services within the community.

The practitioner who wishes to examine the distribution and adequacy of care in the community should keep several important principles in mind. First, the study should be designed to examine the adequacy of basic primary care, rather than the technical quality of care. This will have important implications for selecting the health problems to examine and in generating the criteria of care.

Second, the study should examine the adequacy of care for all members of the community, and should not focus only on those individuals who are actively using the health care system. This principle will be an important determinant of the manner in which study cohorts are selected.

Third, the study should examine the distribution of care by risk or priority group and should account for disparities among risk groups in the community. For example, if the study results suggest that 20 percent of the community is not receiving adequate care, it is critical to know if this is a "random" 20 percent, or if it includes most of the high-risk patients and those who would most benefit from health care. If the 20 percent includes a disproportionate share of high-risk patients, modifications in the health program to correct this disparity may have dramatic effects on the overall health status of the community.

Fourth, the study should examine the adequacy of care for a wide range of clinical functions. While most quality assessment methods focus on diagnosis and treatment, the COPC practitioner should be equally interested in the functions of follow-up, long-term management of chronic conditions, screening, case-finding, prevention, and health maintenance. In some circumstances, a problem may be sought in only one clinical function and thus the scope of the study will be narrowed.

Fifth, in order to examine the care received by the total denominator population, the study should examine the care provided by all programs in the community that offer primary care services. This will, of course, require collaboration among community providers.

Finally, the major purpose of the study is to discover remediable deficiencies in the pattern of care received by the community. Application of this approach in the Indian Health Service has suggested that important deficiencies can be traced to impediments to the continuity of the process of care, particularly related to recognition of patient problems during an encounter.

PROCESS STEPS

Conducting a study to examine the distribution and adequacy of care in the community involves nine steps. If the practitioner wishes to focus immediately on a particular health problem, e.g., prenatal care, step one may be omitted, and the subsequent steps are greatly simplified.

Step 1. Define the problem area to be examined.

The first step in the process is to define clearly the problem area to be examined. This may take several forms and each has implications for the subsequent steps. First, the intent may be to take a broad look at the distribution of primary care services within the population. In this case, tracer health problems should be selected which as a group represent all the clinical functions of primary care. In previous studies in the Indian Health Service this has been accomplished with as few as seven health problems. These are selected so each clinical function is examined by at least two conditions. The selected health problems then act as tracers to reflect the care for those functions for a wide variety of health problems. A set of nine conditions are shown in Table 1

in relation to the clinical functions they examine.

More commonly, a practitioner will decide to examine the adequacy of care for certain clinical functions, e.g., health promotion, follow-up, treatment, etc. Two or more health problems should be used to examine each function. If the functions are closely related, the same tracer condition may be used for both. For example, if treatment and follow-up are the clinical functions of interest, two acute conditions such as gonorrhea and nutritional anemia can be used to cover both functions. Alternatively, the study may be designed to focus on a very specific problem area, e.g., the adequacy of prenatal care, the distribution of ongoing management of hypertension among the black males of the community, etc. In this case, of course, the problem itself defines the health problem to be examined. In sum, particular health problems can be selected because they are of interest (e.g., a single health problem such as

TABLE 1. Relationship Between Seven Functions of Care and the Tracers Used to Examine Them

	Seizure Disorder	Hypertension	Prenatal Care	Infant Care	Urinary Tract Infection	Nutritional Anemia	Lacerations	Streptococcal Pharyngitis	Gonorrhea
Prevention			X	X					
Screening		X	X	X			X		X
Health status monitoring		X	X	X					
Diagnostic evaluation							X	X	X
Treatment					X	X	X	X	X
Follow-up			X		X	X	X	X	X
Ongoing management	X	X							

type II diabetes mellitus may be used to examine all the relevant functions) or because they act as a tracer condition and reflect the care received for a broader set of similar conditions.

Step 2. Develop criteria of care.

For each health problem selected, criteria of care should be developed. The criteria should be simple and reflect adequate basic primary care. Unlike quality assurance studies, this effort will not attempt to make judgments of the technical compe-

tence of individual practitioners or provider groups. Rather, the results should reflect the competence of the system itself in providing adequate health services appropriately within the community. Basic criteria that define the essential elements of care for that health condition will best serve this purpose. For example, a basic criterion for treatment of streptococcal pharyngitis might be as simple as treatment with an antibiotic active against the streptococcal organism within 10 days of the positive throat culture result. This cri-

TABLE 2. Standards Used to Judge the Adequacy of Care Received and Reported in the Medical Record.

Function	Task or Condition	Standard
Prevention	Prenatal diet counseling	Pregnant women should receive diet counseling by 26th week of gestation
	Prenatal surveillance	Pregnant women should have fundal height measured 3 times in 2nd and 5 times in 3rd trimester, and FHR measured once in 2nd and 5 times in 3rd trimester
	Infant immunization	Infants should receive 3 DPT and 2 OPV immunizations by 13 months
	Infant diet counseling	Mothers should receive infant diet counseling 3 times before the infant is 13 months old
	Infant care counseling	Mothers should receive general infant care counseling once in 1st 6 months and once in 2nd 7 months of life
	Infant growth surveillance	Infants should have weight and height measured 3 times in 1st 6 months and 2 times in 2nd 7 months of life
Treatment	Anemia	Persons screened positive for anemia (Hct < 33 or Hgb < 11, in the absence of neoplastic disease, acute or chronic blood loss, or anemia previously diagnosed as other than iron deficiency) should contact provider within 3 weeks and start iron therapy within 1 week of contact
	UTI	Persons with positive urine culture (more than 100,000 organisms, in the absence of chronic or recurrent UTI or known abnormal anatomy of urinary tract) should start appropriate antibiotic therapy within 2 weeks

terion specifies an action (provision of an appropriate antibiotic) within a time frame (within 10 days of the culture result). The power of the results would not be enhanced by adding specificity to the antibiotic used, dosing schedule, or duration of treatment. The criteria, however, would be more difficult to generate. Table 2 provides an example of selected criteria for several clinical functions and respective health problems. The practitioner should seek review and endorsement of the final set of criteria by practitioners in the community, but in contrast to the more complex criteria sets developed to examine the technical quality of care, this rarely presents an obstacle.

Step 3. Develop indicators of the adequacy of care.

Indicators of the adequacy of care should be developed based on the criteria developed above. Indicators are generally of two types. *Population-based indicators* are computed from a sample of the denominator population and express the *percentage of individuals* in need of a particular health service who receive that service within the time frame specified in the criterion. They track cohorts of the population through the system of health care and examine the adequacy of the process of care and how it is distributed in the population. *Encounter-based indicators* are computed from patient contacts with the system and express the *percentage of patient encounters* in which a specific need for service is satisfied. These indicators focus on the components of the system of care in order that their contribution to total system performance can be appraised. An example of the combined use of population and encounter-based indicators will be illustrated in subsequent examples.

Step 4. Develop continuity sequences where appropriate.

Most clinical functions can be separated into three sequential events, namely,

contact between an individual and a practitioner, *recognition* of the need for service once contact is made, and *provision* of service after contact and recognition occur. Population-based indicators can be constructed in a similar sequence in order to examine the continuity of the process of care. Figure 1 shows a sequence used to examine the continuity of contact, recognition, and service provision for the functions of treatment and follow-up of urinary tract infections. Although the criteria would vary, the same sequence could be used to examine other acute health problems requiring treatment and follow-up.

Continuity sequences thus measure the extent to which patients pass successfully through sequential steps within an appropriate time frame. Results of continuity sequences provide important information for modifying the primary care program when major dropout patterns are discovered.

Step 5. Define risk and priority groups.

Perhaps the most important information to derive from the study is the distribution of basic health care among the individuals and groups of differing risk or priority for care. For each health problem a simple criterion should be developed that identifies patients for whom the criteria of care are particularly important. For this purpose, the criteria need not be exhaustive, and certainly do not need to identify all individuals at increased risk. For example, age (less than 16 or more than 35 years), gravida (1 or more than 4), and history of adverse pregnancy outcome may not be adequately precise to predict with certainty an adverse outcome in subsequent pregnancies. However, the criteria do define a group of individuals for whom adequate prenatal care is presumed to be particularly important. Similarly, patients with diabetes may define a priority group for urinary tract infections, and pregnancy

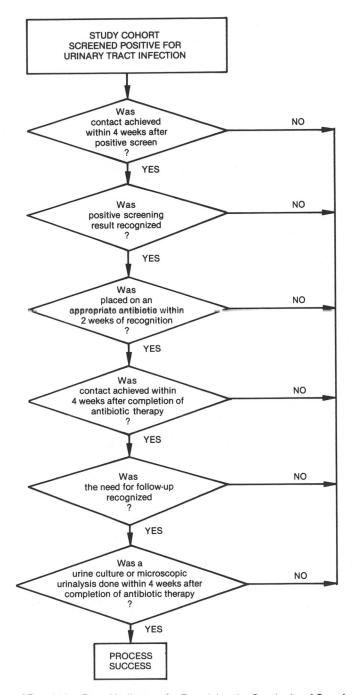

Figure 1. A Sequence of Population-Based Indicators for Examining the Continuity of Care for Urinary Tract Infections.

may define a priority group for nutritional anemia. Similarly, the study may wish to highlight a priority group (such as children under 2 years or the elderly), who, while not necessarily at increased risk for a particular problem, do represent a priority group for which the practitioner wishes to emphasize adequate care.

Step 6. Select study samples.

Selection of the study samples determines the scope of the study, that is, the extent to which the study examines the care received by the entire community rather than by those individuals who are active patients. In studies from the Indian Health Service, the sampling population generally includes all residents of a geographic community usually defined by the boundaries of the reservation. In HMO applications, the community has been defined as all current enrolled members. In both cases, generating study samples is facilitated by a data system, but has also been accomplished in its absence. In private practices, the community from which the sample is drawn has varied from active patients (those contacting the practice in the last 5 years) to the entire geographic community in one rural setting.

The study samples should be generated randomly from the entire community to the extent practical. This is especially important for the functions of screening, prevention, and health promotion. As an example, a cohort of women may be selected for examination of prenatal care by generating a master list from delivery room logs, birth certificates, operating room logs, and laboratory logs (searching for prenatal lab work ordered). When the redundancies are removed from the master list, a standard sampling technique is used to select the study sample. For many health problems, a single type of document may be used to generate an age-and/or sex-specific study sample, e.g., birth certificates alone may suffice for the

generation of a cohort for examining infant care.

Often care will be examined for functions distal to the process of problem identification, e.g., treatment and follow-up of patients screened positive for an acute condition. The study sample will therefore have made prior contact with the health care system and sampling randomly from the total population will not produce adequate numbers to generate an appropriate study sample. In such cases, it is important to sample from the most basic source document available. For example, in generating a cohort of patients with urinary tract infections it is better to sample the laboratory log for patients with a positive urine culture than to generate a sample of medical records for patients who were diagnosed with a urinary tract infection. The latter technique biases the sample in favor of patients who have made contact and for whom the problem potentially has been recognized and treated.

Patients may be eliminated from the study cohort when they do not contribute to the objectives of the study. For example, when examining uncomplicated urinary tract infections, it might be preferable to eliminate patients with chronic urinary tract infections, chronic renal disease, urinary tract anomalies, etc. These characteristics become apparent in the record review and patients thus eliminated from the study cohort may be replaced from the master list. Such conditions will not contribute to the basic purpose of the study, and will require a more complex set of criteria.

Step 7. Identify major sources of care.

Identifying the major sources of health care services in the community and the selection of health records to be reviewed largely defines the scope of the medical care system to be examined. Since medical care systems usually are not clearly delineated, judgment is required to define the system in a way that will produce useful results. Most studies in the Indian Health Service must examine health records at the community hospital and outpatient facility and at one or more field clinics, community health nursing records, health records from tribal health programs, and medical records at one or more referral centers. Studies outside the Indian Health Service have included a similar set of record types. In one rural community, for example, records were examined from two private physicians' offices, the community hospital, the county health clinic, and the county public health nursing program.

Step 8. Develop a data collection protocol.

A data collection protocol must be developed for each health problem for use in extracting data from each health record for each individual in the study cohort. The protocol documents each contact between the patient and any component of the system, and captures the date, location of contact, provider of service, and any of a predetermined list of services required to compute the indicator results for that health problem. When completed, the protocol contains a complete profile for that patient of each contact with the health care system and each of the relevant services provided. An example of a data collection protocol is shown in Figure 2. The results for each of the indicators and continuity sequences can be computed from the completed protocol.

Step 9. Data collection and analysis.

Nonphysician data collectors have been used successfully for both data collection and analysis. Training encompasses approximately a half day per tracer condition. Generally, a set of reference charts have been used to retest the data collectors periodically, particularly where they have been used in very large multi-system

studies. A small set of reference charts can be used to monitor the variation between results obtained by different data collectors, as well as to monitor the variation in a single data collector over time.

In the data collection phase, the same protocol is used to collect all data for a given individual, regardless of the number of different health records examined. Thus, the contents of all contacts with the health care system are profiled on the same data collection instrument (see figure 2), making the analysis and computation of indicator results a simple matter. While the data may by entered and analyzed by computer for large studies, manual analysis is a simple matter for most studies.

EXAMPLES OF ASSESSMENT RESULTS

This assessment approach has been applied successfully in a variety of settings. In addition to over 20 applications in programs of the Indian Health Service, it was tested in three rural private practices and two large health maintenance organizations (2,3). The following will illustrate the range of information produced by the assessment approach on the adequacy of health care received by a denominator population. Data are taken from several relatively large studies and are presented to show the types of problems that may be uncovered. It is not suggested that any practice or program undertake an equally large study as a matter of routine. Although in some settings concerned about the distribution and adequacy of care, this level of effort may be appropriate.

The combined use of population-based and encounter-based indicators will provide valuable information regarding the determinants of care that are found to be inadequate. Table 3 shows data that examine the adequacy of infant immunization in a rural private practice, two programs of the Indian Health Service, and a closed-

PRENATAL CARE

Name ____________________ H.R. No's ____________________

Chart Audited ____________________ Residence ____________________

Study Site: ____________________ Unique Pt. No. ____________________

Audit Phase: 1 2 3 DOB: Mo. 3 Day 14 Yr. 1960

Study Cohort: A B C Sex: M ____ F ____

GR 1 L.C. 0 Date of Delivery: Mo. 11 Day 23 Yr. 1981

PARA 0 A b 0 LMP: Mo. 2 Day 14 Yr. 1981

Date of visit (begin with LMP and include all visits through 8 weeks after delivery)																		
mo.	2	3	4	4	5	5	6	6	8	9	9	10	10	10	11	12	1	1
day	16	2	17	26	20	22	17	18	28	12	14	6	13	21	23	20	28	31
yr.	81	81	81	81	81	81	81	81	81	81	81	81	81	81	81	81	82	82
Week of gestation	0	2	8	9	13	13	17	17	27	29	29	33	34	35	41	—	—	—
Provider Type	MD	MD	MD	PA	MD	PHN	PA	PA	MD	PA	PA	MD	MD	PA	MD	PA	MD	MD
Provider																		
Location	OPD	OPD	OPD	FC	OPD	Home	FC	FC	OPD	FC	FC	OPD	OPD	FC	OPD (H)	FC	OPD	OPD
Evidence of recognition of pregnancy (✓)			✓		✓	✓			✓			✓	✓	✓	✓			
Pap Smear (✓)					✓													
Urine Culture (✓)					✓													
Nutrition Counseling (✓)					✓	✓												
VDRL (or equivalent) (result)					⊖													
Cervical culture (GC) (result)					⊖					⊕								
Hct/Hgb (result) Hct																		
Hgb					11.5					11.0			12.0		12.5			
Evidence of recognition of abnormal Hct/Hgb ( )													✓		✓			
Blood Pressure (result) Syst					116				120			138	130	128	136			
Diast					60				84			94	92	92	98			
Evidence of recognition of elevated BP (✓)												✓	✓	✓	✓			
Fundus (Uterus) (✓)					✓				✓			✓	✓	✓	✓			
Urine protein (0, 1, 2, 3, 4)					0							1+	1+	2+	3+			
FHR (result)					✓				140			136	144	ND	132			
Evidence of recognition of postpartum (✓)																	✓	✓
Evidence that pelvic exam was done (✓)																		✓

Δ1 –Δ2– 20th – Δ3 – DELIVERY + -8W

Figure 2. A data collection protocol for examining prenatal care.

TABLE 3. Data for Infant Immunization From a Rural Private Practice, Two IHS Service Units, and One Health Maintenance Organization (HMO) Illustrating the Performance Patterns Resulting From the Assessment Method

	Private Practice	IHS-A	IHS-B	HMO
Immunization rate (population-based)	52% (26/50)	86% (43/50)	56% (28/50)	58% (29/50)
Immunization rate (encounter-based)	22% (63/285)	46% (179/387)	38% (119/316)	86% (127/147)
Sorted by facility				
Medical office	19% (21/112)			
County clinic	24% (42/173)			
MCH clinic		85% (103/121)		
General clinic		34% (70/208)		
2 field clinics		11% (6/53)		
Inpatient service		0% (0/5)		
Sorted by provider discipline				
Physician			34% (64/189)	
Physician extender			75% (36/48)	
Clinic nurse			50% (6/12)	
Public health nurse			87% (13/15)	
Pharmacist			0% (0/52)	

panel HMO. The population-based immunization rate expresses the *percentage of infants* who had received three DPT and two polio immunizations by 12 months of age. The corresponding encounter-based indicator expresses the *percentage of visits* by infants due for an immunization[1] in which the immunization was provided. In all four sites, the overall immunization rates were found to be inadequate, but the basic causes were different and further explained by the use of the encounter-based indicator.

Among the infant population served by the private practice, only 52 percent had received three DPT and two OPV immunizations by age 12 months and the encounter-based indicator suggested that immunizations were provided on only 22 percent of the visits for which they were

due. This private practice had assumed that infants were receiving their immunizations from the nearby county health clinic. But when the encounter-based indicator was sorted by the physician's office and the county clinic, it revealed that neither location was taking advantage of its opportunities to provide immunizations. In discussing the results, both sites agreed that they had assumed the other was responsible for immunization, and both agreed to begin immunizing more vigorously. An informal follow-up study

[1] The DPT immunization was considered to be due at 2 months of age and to be repeated monthly until three doses had been given. If, at the time of a visit, the infant had a rectal temperature greater than 100.5°F, then an immunization was not considered due on that visit.

by one of the private practitioners several months later indicated that the encounter-based immunization rate had increased threefold at both locations.

In one of the Indian Health Service programs (IHS-A), the population-based immunization rate was 86 percent with the corresponding encounter-based rate of 46 percent. When the encounter-based rate was sorted by location, it was noted that the MCH clinic was performing well at 85 percent, while the hospital outpatient department (34 percent) and the two field clinics (11 percent) were missing many opportunities to provide needed immunizations. Since most of the missed opportunities occurred at the hospital outpatient department, a standing order for immunization was instituted.

In the second Indian Health Service program (IHS-B), 56 percent of the infant population was immunized by 1 year of age. In this case the encounter-based rate of 38 percent was sorted by provider

discipline. These data revealed that the physicians were providing immunizations only 34 percent of the time and were commonly referring infants to the physician-extender for well-baby care. Also 52 of the 316 infant visits made when an immunization was due had been to the hospital outpatient pharmacy, that had recently begun a program providing nonprescription medication directly from the pharmacy. This result and the pattern suggested by other data led to the development of a checklist of potential service needs for prevention and chronic disease surveillance for use by the pharmacist while dispensing over-the-counter medications.

Finally, a contrasting pattern was seen in the immunization indicators for the health maintenance organization. Although the providers were immunizing infants on 86 percent of the visits when an immunization was due, only 58 percent of the infant population was com-

TABLE 4. Results From a Primary Care Program Showing Population-Based Indicators for Prenatal Care

	Total Cohort (N = 50)	High Risk (N = 22)	Average Risk (N = 28)
Contact: the percent of pregnant women who made contact with the health care system by the 20th week of gestation.	64% (32/50)	55% (12/22)	71% (20/28)
Recognition: the percent of pregnant women making contact who had their pregnancy recognized by the 20th week of gestation.	69% (22/32)	50% (6/12)	80% (16/20)
Screening: the percent of pregnant women with pregnancy recognized who had a cervical culture by the 20th week of gestation.	82% (18/22)	50% (3/6)	94% (15/16)
Continuity-of-process index: the percent of pregnant women who had a cervical culture by the 20th week of gestation.	36% (18/50)	14% (3/22)	54% (15/28)

pletely immunized. This pattern suggested that patient contact was the limiting factor in achieving higher immunization rates in the infant community. This was later confirmed by a small study of the utilization pattern of enrolled infants, that indicated that many infants visited the HMO only when they were ill. The study also suggested that a very large proportion of these infants were from the Hispanic subset of the enrolled population.

Results from the assessment can also be used to examine the distribution of care among various subsets of the population. One type of subset of critical importance consists of those individuals at increased risk to a particular health problem. In a study of prenatal care at one of the Indian Health Service programs, 22 of 50 pregnant women in the study cohort were classified as high risk because they were under the age of 18 years, over the age of 35 years, primigravida, with parity equal to or greater than 5, or with a history of miscarriage or spontaneous abortion, while the other 28 women were classified as average risk.

Table 4 shows results for three population-based indicators that constitute a simple sequence to examine the continuity of the process of prenatal screening (using gonorrhea as a tracer condition). Respectively, the indicators examine the proportion of women making contact with the system by the 20th gestational week, the proportion of those with pregnancy recognized by the 20th week, and the proportion of those having a cervical culture by the 20th gestational week.

It is apparent from the indicator results and continuity index of Table 4, that the process of health care favors the average-risk group at each step of the process. The reasons for the differential in care between patients at high and average risk are suggested by the encounter-based indicators for pregnancy recognition and gonorrhea screening disaggregated by site of contact, as displayed in Table 5. Unlike population-based indicators, encounter-based indicators are computed in units of patient contacts with the health care system. Thus, only 43 percent of encounters by high-risk patients compared with 67 per-

TABLE 5. Results for Encounter-Based Indicators of Pregnancy Recognition and Screening for Gonorrhea, Disaggregated by System Component

	Cohort Total	High-Risk Patients	Average-Risk Patients
Recognition rate			
Hospital outpatient department	35% (6/17)	25% (2/8)	44% (4/9)
Prenatal clinic	20% (11/56)	7% (1/14)	24% (10/42)
Field clinic	0% (0/5)	0% (0/2)	0% (0/3)
Home visits by public health nurse	100% (5/5)	100% (3/3)	100% (2/2)
Total visits	27% (22/83)	22% (6/27)	29% (16/56)
Screening rate			
Hospital outpatient department	11% (1/9)	0% (0/3)	17% (1/6)
Prenatal clinic	57% (17/30)	33% (3/9)	67% (14/21)
Field clinic	0% (0/1)	0% (0/1)	— (0)
Home visits by public health nurse	0% (0/3)	0% (0/2)	0% (0/1)
Total visits	42% (18/43)	20% (3/15)	54% (15/28)

cent of encounters by average-risk patients due for recognition of pregnancy resulted in pregnancy recognition. Similarly, only 33 percent of encounters by high-risk patients compared with 71 percent of encounters by average-risk patients with pregnancy recognized and due for gonorrhea screening received a cervical culture. When disaggregated by site of contact, the results suggest that the prenatal clinic performs well in both the recognition and screening functions, the public health nurses perform well in recognition, but the hospital outpatient department and the field clinics contribute substantially less to the overall system performance.

The data of Table 5 show that the average-risk women due for care made a higher proportion of their encounters with the prenatal clinic than did the high-risk women. Specifically, for average-risk women 24 percent (10 of 42) of all encounters when due for recognition were with the prenatal clinic and 67 percent (14 of 21) of all encounters when due for screening were with the prenatal clinic, while for the high-risk women, only 7 percent (1 of 14) and 33 percent (3 of 9) of all encounters when due for recognition and screening, respectively, were with the prenatal clinic. Consequently, the superior performance of the prenatal clinic favors the average-risk group by virtue of the different utilization patterns of the two risk groups. A similar pattern in another Indian Health Service program has been studied and reported in more detail (4).

The assessment approach can also provide important information on the continuity of the process of care received by individuals in the denominator population. Discontinuities can be an important impediment to achievement of the potential impact of health services, and one that is not reflected in measures of access to care or measures of the sheer volume of services provided to a population. In testing the assessment approach in a variety of primary care settings, the continuity of care was measured for uncomplicated urinary tract infections. The study cohorts were generated from the laboratory log at each site by listing those individuals with a screening urine culture resulting in greater than 10^5 colonies per milliliter. Individuals, for whom subsequent chart review indicated the presence of a chronic urinary tract infection, urinary tract anomaly, or chronic pyelonephritis, were eliminated from the cohort.

TABLE 6. Results From Three Primary Care Programs of the Indicator Sequence Designed to Examine the Continuity of Process for Treatment and Follow-Up

	Service Unit C	HMO	Service Unit D
1. Contact for evaluation	92% (46/50)	92% (46/50)	74% (37/50)
2. Recognition of problem	91% (42/46)	70% (32/46)	49% (18/37)
3. Provision of treatment	95% (40/42)	94% (30/32)	100% (18/18)
4. Contact for follow-up	93% (37/40)	93% (28/30)	67% (12/18)
5. Recognition of need for follow-up	92% (34/37)	57% (16/28)	42% (5/12)
6. Provision of follow-up	97% (33/34)	94% (15/16)	100% (5/5)
Continuity index	66% (33/50)	30% (15/50)	10% (5/50)

Table 6 illustrates varying patterns of care in treatment and follow-up in one health maintenance organization and two programs of the Indian Health Service. The data are the results of population-based indicators that express the rate at which patients at a given point in the process of care will pass successfully to the next. Likewise, the rate at which patients pass successfully through multiple steps in the process can be estimated as the continuity index. As shown in Table 6, the data from the three programs express the rate at which patients screened positive for a urinary tract infection will make subsequent contact with the program, have the problem recognized, receive treatment, make subsequent contact for follow-up, have the need for follow-up recognized, and receive the follow-up services. The data of Table 6 suggest that the overall continuity index ranges from 0.66 in one IHS program (IHS-C) to 0.10 in another (IHS-D). Examination of the elements of the continuity sequences for the three programs suggests distinctly different patterns of care. IHS-C with a continuity index of 0.66 appears to have no particular step in the process of care that stands out as a relative deficiency. The HMO, with a continuity index of 0.30, shows a similar pattern except for the recognition steps (indicators 2 and 5), which appear to be the relative weak links. Finally, IHS-D with a continuity index of 0.10 appears to have substantial deficiencies in both contact (indicators 1 and 4) and recognition (indicators 2 and 5). Importantly, the indicators that focus on provider performance for treatment (indicator 3) and follow-up (indicator 6) are quite good for all three sites. Clearly, a quality assessment program that examined the medical records for patients seen with urinary tract infections would have yielded results similar to these indicators, and would have missed totally the important system problems reflected in the population-based indicators for contact and recognition.

DISCUSSION

The examples described are derived from relatively large studies designed to examine the adequacy of care across a broad range of clinical functions. In one setting, data were collected on the time required to collect the data for nine tracer conditions. In this setting, the health care system consisted of a 50-bed community hospital and outpatient department, two separate ambulatory care clinics (each with separate medical records), an active community health nursing program, and a community-based alcohol program. In this assessment, an average of 2.8 health records were examined for each of 30-50 patients per study cohort. The chart audit phase required approximately 12 person-days for collection and tabulation of the data.

The resources required can be much lower for programs that wish to examine the adequacy and distribution of care within their community for a smaller number of health problems. For example the program interested in the adequacy of care for the elderly can do so by examining as few as three or four health problems. In some settings, a single health problem may be used when it is of particular interest. Prenatal care often serves as the focus of such a study. In one study of prenatal care in a community health center, the care of 50 patients was examined by abstracting data from the records of the health center, the county public health nursing program, and the university referral hospital. The time required to collect and analyze the data included 6 hours of physician time for training and monitoring the data collector, and approximately 6 days of undergraduate student time for data collection and analysis.

In many quality assessment activities, generating and endorsing criteria of care consume tremendous amounts of physician time. In this approach, only basic criteria are used and require minimal time for development.

The assessment approach is feasible for application in a variety of primary care settings. It has been extensively tested in health programs of the Indian Health Service (1-4) as well as in fee-for-service private practices and HMOs (2,3). The effort required to apply the method increases geometrically with the number of health programs serving the community. For example, use of the assessment to examine the distribution and adequacy of care in a large suburban population seeking care from a large number of different providers would be difficult.

SUMMARY

In considering the range of health problems affecting a community, the appropriateness of the distribution of primary care among the individuals and subgroups of the population deserves attention. A method is described for examining the distribution of appropriate care among a target community, and data are presented from a variety of primary care settings to illustrate both the importance of examining the distribution of care and the many patterns of care that may be encountered. While not an important problem in all communities, where present, maldistribution of primary care may be one of the most critical problems to be addressed by the COPC practice or program.

REFERENCES

1. Shorr, G.I., and Nutting, P.A. A population-based assessment of the continuity of ambulatory care. *Medical Care* 1977; 15:455.

2. Nutting, P.A.; Shorr, G.I.; and Burkhalter, B.R. Assessing the performance of medical care systems: A method and its application. *Medical Care* 1981; 19:281.

3. Nutting, P.A.; Burkhalter, B.R.; Dietrick, D.L.; and Helmick, E.F. Relationship of size and payment mechanism to system performance in 11 medical care systems. *Medical Care* 1982; 20:676.

4. Nutting, P.A.; Barrick, J.E.; and Logue, S.C. The impact of a maternal and child health care program on the quality of prenatal care: An analysis by risk group. *Journal of Community Health* 1979; 4:267.

5. Starfield, B.; Katz, H.; Gabriel, A. et al. Morbidity in childhood—a longitudinal view. *New England Journal of Medicine* 1984; 310:824.

CHAPTER 29

Acute Self Limited Illness Indexing as a Tool in COPC

Charles E. Schlager, M.D.

The practice of community-oriented primary care in a private practice is a unique and satisfying experience. It generates a sense of adventure. To practice medicine in phase with your community gives you control of your destiny. It increases your understanding of people and their problems, and it cements bonds between you and your community.

In most communities there is little awareness of the possibilities of COPC. The community does not see itself as the foundation of medical practice, and responds to pressures foreign to the practice of primary care. The COPC practitioner must understand the structure and potential for change in the community and use this understanding to establish a practice based on the principles of COPC. The community's perception of the practitioner as an expert and a leader in health issues will be the greatest asset.

Examples of some of the pressures that can develop and then be utilized as a starting point are:

1. Disturbances within a community because a medical delivery system is not responsive to community needs (e.g., inappropriate care of the disadvantaged).

2. Difficulty within the community with the formulation of a system of defining medical practice needs and the location of medical practices (lack of medical manpower planning).

3. Lack of community data regarding primary care problems that present to primary care physicians and are referred to secondary and tertiary facilities.

4. Need of third-party payers to collect practice data in the process of feasibility surveys for developing HMOs, PPOs, or other alternative care delivery systems.

5. The need for residency training programs to document training by demonstrating disease profiles.

As discussed in Section III, the target community can be defined in a number of ways. For many practitioners the most accessible target population to address with the COPC process is that composed of the active patients of the practice. The easiest way to start is to develop an age/

sex description of your practice. This can be done by a check list noting the age categories in one column and the sex in two columns and simply check the list appropriately. Your office staff can maintain and produce monthly summaries. The next step is to create a profile of diagnoses seen in your office. This can be done with any of the many coding schemes available such as ICHPPC-2. The next area of interest should be a survey of the geographic distribution of your practice. This can be done by plotting the addresses of your patient population on an area map. All of these parameters can be compared to nationally reported norms and community census data.

After initial characterizations are performed, additional definition of practice parameters can be done as community needs dictate. It is in this later arena, that we set out to define and characterize the varying patterns of acute self-limiting illness in our practice population. The development of this acute self-limited illness index is only one way of using the product of profiling in a primary care practice. A detailed description of this process is offered as a model to assist in the practice of community-oriented medical care.

AN ACUTE ILLNESS INDEX

We have defined acute illness here as a group of symptoms presenting in a patient for less than 2 weeks which are not related to illnesses previously diagnosed or to an illness of longer duration.

The resource requirements are simple and available to all practitioners:

1. Patient care records.
2. Age/sex data.
3. Symptom data.
4. Followup data.
5. Worksheet grid.
6. Elementary graphing skills.

Patient records are generated in most physician practices. For the purposes of this project, these records must contain the following data elements: age, sex, symptoms ranked in the order of severity as given by the patient, the treatment provided by the physician, the possible contact causing the illness, and an indication of the patient's geographic location in the community. The geographic location can be described by census tract, township, school district, zip code, or whatever seems appropriate.

An age/sex profile for a practice is easily generated at the time of entry into the system. Patients with acute illness can be readily stratified by age and sex and this information compared to the total practice age/sex register, as shown in Figure 1. The differences may be striking, and this set of graphic representations shows that the percent of patients in the lower age groups who have acute self-limited illnesses is greater than the percentage found in the older age groups.

The symptoms presented by patients can be characterized in groups and coded. This process is accomplished by asking the patient what symptoms prompted his visit. The symptoms are ranked from the most disturbing to the least disturbing. A list of codes is provided in Figure 2 as an example. This way of collecting symptom data enables the practitioner to weight the various symptoms so graphic representations of the patterns can be produced. The weighting process is totally arbitrary and can be adjusted to the needs of the individual practice. The most disturbing or prominent symptom is weighted as 4, and the least as 1. Figure 3 shows the type of pattern that results from aggregating the symptom codes and comparing two study periods. Some shifts are evident; these include a relative increase in upper respiratory symptoms and a decrease in abdominal pain.

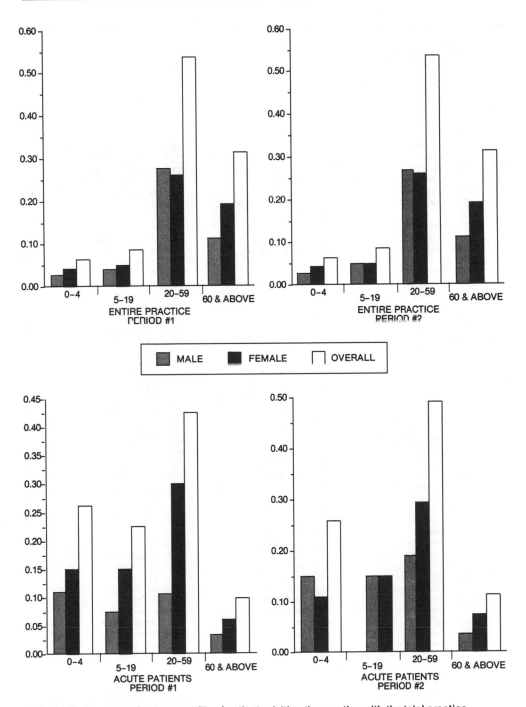

Figure 1. Comparison of age-sex profile of patients visiting the practice with the total practice population during two time periods.

SYMPTOM CODES:

Code	Symptom	Code	Symptom	Code	Symptom
005	chills	347	ears full	647	nocturia
010	fever	350	ear bleeding	650	dysuria
015	tiredness	351	pus from ear	655	incontinence urine
016	fatigue	355	earache	660	can't urinate
025	malaise	360	earwax	700	painful penis
030	syncope	401	bloody nose	714	painful testicle
033	fainting	406	sore nose	719	itching groin
040	weight gain	410	sinus pain	730	amenorrhea
045	weight loss	411	sinus congestion	731	desires contraception
050	chest pain	415	short of breath	735	irregular period
051	chest discomfort	420	allergy problems	736	menstrual problems
052	chest pressure	425	wheezing	740	heavy flow
053	chest tightness	430	breathing problems	741	scant flow
055	rib pain	435	sneezing	742	clots
056	flank pain	440	coughing	745	PMS
057	groin pain	445	headcold	746	dysmenorrhea
058	facial pain	450	flu symptoms	750	menopausal
061	aches	455	sore throat	755	breakthrough
062	cramps	456	lump in throat	756	intramenstrual bleed
063	stiffness	457	scratchy throat	757	post menopause bleed
064	swelling	470	coughing blood	758	postcoital bleed
065	pain	475	chest congestion	759	pain with coitus
067	excessive thirst	480	hoarseness	760	vaginal discharge
068	discharge	500	toothache	765	vaginal pain
096	limping	501	bleeding gums	766	vaginal itch
097	staggering	505	cold sore	775	pelvic pain
100	apprehensive	510	sore mouth	800	breast pain
101	bad nerves	511	dry mouth	805	breast lump
110	crying	512	mouth ulcer	810	nipple discharge
112	sad	520	difficult swallowing	830	acne
114	depressed	525	nausea	840	skin infection
125	restlessness	530	vomiting	845	moles
135	can't sleep	535	heartburn	850	warts
170	personal problem	536	indigestion	855	cyst skin
210	headache	537	belching	856	lump
225	dizziness	546	stomach pain	857	foreign body
226	lightheaded	550	abdominal pain	858	insect bite
227	vertigo	565	abdominal distention	859	bee sting
260	rapid heartbeat	570	increased appetite	860	rash
262	skipped beats	571	decreased appetite	865	ulcer skin
265	pain over heart	580	blood in stool	870	itching
268	dyspnea	581	vomiting blood	875	hives
281	swelling of legs	590	constipation	881	burns
282	leg cramps	595	diarrhea	885	ingrown nail
305	blurred vision	600	mucus in stool	901	neck pain
309	double vision	602	stool changes	906	back pain
311	purulent discharge eyes	603	incontinence stool	916	hip pain
315	pink eye	605	rectal pain	921	leg pain
321	itching eyes	606	rectal bleeding	926	knee pain
323	red eyes	608	rectal itching	931	shoulder pain
326	hayfever	610	jaundice	941	hand pain
335	swelling eyes	640	blood in urine	946	arm pain
340	inflamed eyelid	645	frequency	956	foot pain
346	ringing in ears	646	urgency	960	head problem
				965	face problem

Figure 2. Listing of symptom codes used in developing the acute illness index.

The symptom patterns can be analyzed as well by age and sex. The resulting graphic array will provide the physician with a quick reference when s/he is attempting to characterize an individual patient as one with a usual presentation or that of an outlier.

A system for tracking acute illness makes the physician aware of the course of the current acute syndromes in the practice and enables comparisons to known disease states. This information can then be applied to new patients presenting with similar symptom complexes. A callback system to accomplish this task is easily developed. Three vertical file trays are designated as Days 1-2, Days 3-4, and Days 7-8. Patient records are placed in the appropriate tray so calls can be made in the desired sequence. With each telephone contact, the patient is asked several basic questions: Are you better, worse, or the same? Have you had any side effects from the medication? Are you having any new symptoms? After the call is accomplished the data are recorded on the data worksheet.

The data worksheet can be any standard ruled accounting worksheet, and should be labeled with the codes to be used in order to facilitate comparisons. The coding system also allows weighting to be accomplished quickly. The worksheet concept is adaptable to the data base systems of home computers.

DEVELOPING AND DISPLAYING INDICES

An acute illness index can be calculated by dividing the total number of acute case encounters during the study week by the total number of active patients in the practice. This quotient multiplied by 10,000 then becomes an index, expressing the frequency by which illnesses present to the practice in a measured time period. The suggested time frame for each individual study is 7 days. A longer time frame decreases the usefulness of the information in the decisionmaking process. An example of this index for the two representative time periods is noted below, where the number of visits for a given acute illness is 51 in one time period and 66 in another.

Period one
$51/2{,}025 \times 10{,}000 = 252$

Period two
$66/2{,}025 \times 10{,}000 = 326$

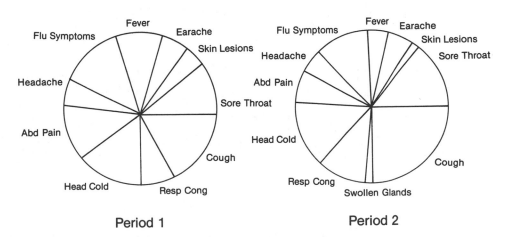

Period 1   Period 2

Figure 3. Comparison of symptom patterns presenting to the practice during two study periods.

These values can be plotted over time to indicate increasing or decreasing trends.

In the confusion of practice, a physician may have difficulty monitoring treatment patterns. In this system such an evaluation can be simply accomplished. Each treatment of interest is assigned a code, and the treatments are weighted. The primary modality is assigned the value of 3, the secondary modality a value of 2, and the tertiary modality a value of 1. Figure 4 displays the patterns for the age group 0-4 and 5-19 years of age for two different time periods. In the 5-19-year-olds a marked decrease in use of penicillin and an increase in the use of narcotic analgesics are readily noted.

The side effects and additional symptoms can also be listed for a specified time frame. A review of this section of the weekly report allows the physician to appreciate the number and severity of the complications and side effects seen in the acutely ill patient group.

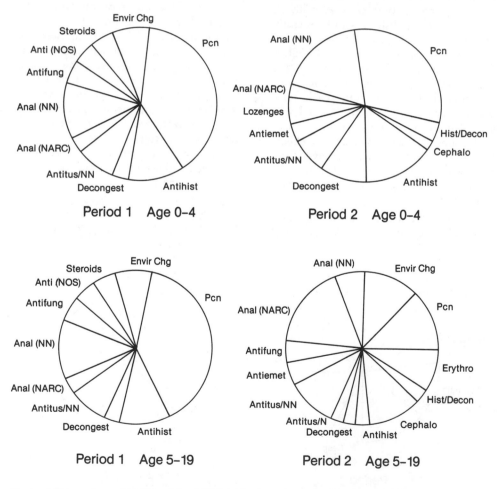

Figure 4. Comparison of treatment modalities in the age groups 0-4 and 5-19 years for two study periods.

232

Figure 5 compares for two study periods the outcomes during the first and second, the third and fourth, and the seventh and eighth days following the visit in the age group 0-4 years. A similar recovery pattern is observed. In the third and fourth

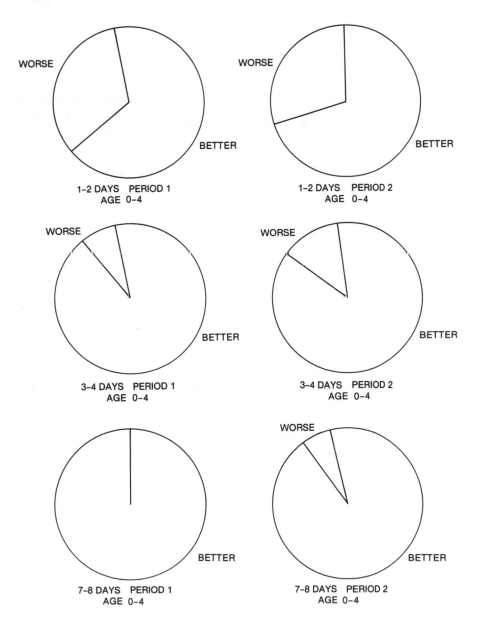

Figure 5. Comparison of the outcomes 0-4 year olds on the first and second, the third and fourth, and the seventh and eighth days following the visit, for two study periods.

day, however, there is a somewhat diminished recovery in the second study period. At 7-8 days all of the initial group have recovered and a small sample of the second group have not recovered.

Contact patterns can be examined as well, and are obtained by asking the patient from what source the illness has come. These responses are displayed in graphic fashion as shown for the 5-19 year age group in Figure 6. Interestingly, in this example non-family contact (school and social) increased in the second time period. Finally, geographic distribution can be examined as shown in Figure 7. This presentation compares visits to the practice for acute illness from different areas of the county.

The evaluation of acute self-limited illness in a patient population has always been within the purview of the practicing primary care physician. Weighted graphic representations of these evaluations are presented as a method to achieve this goal.

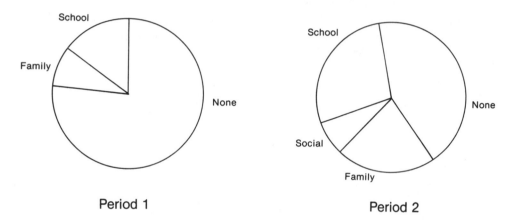

Period 1   Period 2

Figure 6. Comparison of the Alleged Source of the Illness in 5–19-Year-Olds for Two Study Periods.

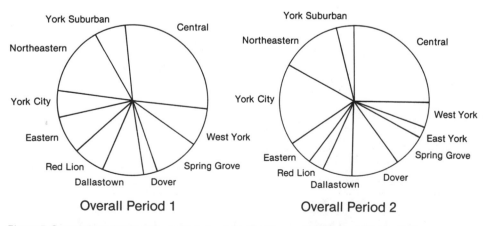

Overall Period 1   Overall Period 2

Figure 7. Comparison for Two Study Periods of the Residence of Patients with Acute Illness the Present to the Practice.

The method described touches only on the larger areas of interest. Separate, but related, subsets can be approached by the same method. For example, the treatment patterns for individual physicians can be compared to outcome patterns. These subset studies can be performed simultaneously with the primary system and add thrust to the information base. The key to the success of this method is the promptness of disseminating the information. The information must be ready for use by the provider within a 7-day time frame to be useful in the decisionmaking process.

A COMPUTER-BASED APPLICATION

In our office indexing is accomplished by using computer-generated patient data obtained from the patient record. We have incorporated an in-house, computerized medical information system into a five-physician, two-office family medicine practice. The five physicians, all board-certified in family practice, have private practice experience ranging from 4 to 27 years. The two offices are located five miles apart, and they have access to the medical information system through a dedicated telephone line and a set of multiplexers. Three clinical pharmacists operate a licensed pharmacy in the same settings. They work in close association with the physicians, and their record-keeping activities have been integrated into all of the individual modules.

All medical, pharmaceutical, financial, and scheduling data are stored in an MAI/Basic Four System 730 (1,2). The medical information system was initiated on September 1, 1980 and over 115,000 patient encounters have been stored in the computer in 5-1/2 years. Five patient-specific reports are printed prior to each visit: physical parameter flowchart; chart summary (active drug list, diagnosis summary, medication summary); health main-

tenance audit; patient history (previous medical history, drug history, immunization history, social history, family history); and examination findings. These reports are used by all members of the health care team. The computer enables the data to be presented to the clerks in a simple report form and therefore does not take the chart out of the main stream of direct patient care. The data are then entered into a data base on a personal computer and analyzed to produce the graphics. This is then merged in a word processing program to produce a report that is circulated for staff and patient information and feedback.

BENEFITS

Some of the interesting spinoffs from this exercise have been office management alterations such as: extension of hours, allowance for increasing numbers of acute care appointments, and personnel scheduling changes during periods where the Acute Self-Limited Care Index is high. These are management decisions made possible by tracking the acute self-limited illness index over time and making the adjustments accordingly. For example, if the index climbs to 450, as would happen in an influenza outbreak, the entire system could plan for the rapid increase in office visits expected. In addition to time management, medical supplies can be purchased according to index trends.

COST CONSIDERATIONS

Timely and easily interpreted representations of this evaluation can be prepared by groups of interested physicians in many settings, although cost considerations may vary. The system described can be developed manually with minimal capital investment, but considerable cost in terms of clerical time. It can, however, be easily adapted to a computer data base and a word processor. In our office, the cost of the project is approximately $50-$70 per week based on processing 150 entries. The major time commitment is clerical, while time is spent primarily in interpretation. A combined physician and clerical time commitment of 8-10 hours a week can be projected.

CONCLUSION

Acute self-limited illness indexing affords the practicing physician contact with his practice and affords the opportunity to compare it with the community experience. Modifications in patient care can be made and then evaluated against this continuing record of experience. Rapid sharing of information allows the medical care team to react quickly to trends suggesting the need to modify practice patterns.

REFERENCES

1. Schlager, C.E., and Schlager, D.D. Computerized patient medical records: A tool for standards of care review. *Proceedings Of The Fifth Annual Symposium On Computer Applications In Medical Care*, November 1981.

2. Schlager, D.D. A comprehensive patient care system for the family practice. *Proceedings Of The Sixth Annual Symposium On Computer Applications In Medical Care*, October-November 1982.

CHAPTER 30

Setting Priorities Among Competing Health Problems

David N. Rose, M.D.

Community-oriented primary care is health planning writ small. A comprehensive health plan addresses all regional health problems and proposes solutions from the practical to the ideal. Community-oriented practitioners cannot and need not address all the health problems identified by their investigations. Along with this advantage, however, comes the dilemma of how to choose which problems the COPC practitioner will address. This chapter proposes a process and raises some considerations to help when the time for choosing comes.

WHEN DOES THE CHOICE OCCUR IN THE COPC PROCESS?

The moment for choosing which health initiative to work on rightfully belongs after the early COPC steps of defining the community and identifying its health problems. Without the benefit of the studied overview, one could easily choose to address a problem of relatively minor importance to the community. The choice then requires some reflection on the reasons for transforming a practice into a COPC practice. If the motivation is to integrate a practice into the social fabric of the community, then the choice must

follow the early steps of initiating and promoting a forum for dialogue with community residents and leaders. Making the choice can itself promote this collaborative process, reinforcing the early COPC step of community involvement. On the other hand, if the reason for the COPC effort is to be responsive to an obvious community need, perceived by either physician or community resident, then the choice is more one of method than goal. It remains important, nevertheless, to study the overview in order to confirm that the perceived need is consistent with the facts. It is also important that the choice of initiative is consistent with the concerns of the target population. Again, this middle step of setting priorities reinforces the early step of involving others in the process.

The principles presented in this chapter are derived from an involvement in community development through health initiatives in East Harlem in New York City. They are really the synthesis of observations of many hard-working people in two neighborhood health centers (NHCs), two satellite health centers, a community hospital, a coalition of hospital and NHC directors with community leaders, and an academic community-medicine consultation team. In many East Harlem COPC efforts in the past 15 years, priority setting was the focus of early collaborations and strengthened the bonds between the participants.

THE PROCESS: INVOLVING THE COMMUNITY IN CHOOSING HEALTH INITIATIVES

The process of ranking priorities for health initiatives by COPC practitioners is characterized by the essential role of community members. COPC is more than primary care modified by an awareness of local demographics, disease epidemiology, health status indices, and health-related behaviors. The personal effort to practice medicine responsive to community needs must be transformed into a collaborative effort that fosters a community striving to improve its health. This requires a dialogue between the practitioner and members of the community. The history of community medicine has shown how the successes of new health initiatives depend not only on understanding the target population's way of life, values, and attitudes, but also on engaging this population in the process of developing health initiatives. Community involvement in the earliest stages of a COPC effort, choosing which problems to attack, is as important as in the later implementation stages.

Several purposes can be served in the process of setting priorities for COPC health initiatives. All should be made explicit. First, the process of making choices can develop the relationship between COPC practitioners and members of the community. Another purpose is, of course, to create a priority list of health initiatives. And finally, the group involved in setting priorities can develop into an ongoing community organization to implement programs, monitor progress, modify priorities, and expand the list of

initiatives when health goals have been met and when new health problems are identified. One must appreciate that any list of priorities is meaningful at only one point in time; populations, disease patterns, resources, and interests change and therefore so do priorities. The process of collaboration, therefore, can and should be experienced as a dynamic continuing process, and the list of potential emphasis programs is a focus for the process.

The process of setting priorities is a natural opportunity for the mutual education of practitioners and community members concerning the two elements that distinguish primary care from COPC: epidemiologic considerations and community input. The education flows both ways between practitioner and community, usually with physicians taking primary responsibility for delineating the epidemiology of disease, health-related behavior, and health resources, and the community members taking primary responsibility for expressing concerns regarding perceived needs. For instance, in the first meetings of community and health leaders who organized to improve ambulatory services in East Harlem, the health providers offered to present pertinent information on disease patterns in subsequent meetings. The presentations, limited to 15 minutes, were intended to stimulate discussion, not detailed analysis. Another provider agreed to organize a description of the hospital-based clinics. The community leaders agreed to poll their community boards for perceived needs. Everyone agreed that learning and teaching was a productive way of getting to know each other. Because each participant was to present something, the tone of the response to the presentations was supportive. The discussions then led to more formal study, which then led to the process of choosing initiatives.

Our experience in East Harlem leads us to believe that an important goal of community development and collaboration is facilitating community participants' individual and group decisionmaking. This requires understanding denominator-based information, group dynamics, and community advocacy.

FACTORS TO CONSIDER WHEN CHOOSING HEALTH INITIATIVES

Participants in the process of reviewing health problems for COPC initiatives can make explicit the factors which they consider important for ranking. Each setting has specific characteristics that make some choices very compelling. It is only important that all participants in the process agree on the factors used in ranking.

1. Foster the COPC Process

Consider the health problems that have solutions that foster the process of collaboration between health provider and community residents and institutions. These are initiatives that promote the dynamics of COPC. This kind of initiative fosters not just community involvement in a medical practice, but also the integration of a practice into the social services of a community. These initiatives encourage the participation of many within the community and have the multiplier effect of many participants' efforts in addition to the practitioner's efforts.

An example of this is a project that the East Harlem Council for Human Services performed with the local school system. Because school health services were deemed insufficient by the school board, the community agency offered to place part-time nurse practitioners and community health workers in each school. This linked the schools with the agency's neighborhood health center. It facilitated referrals for medical care, improved record keeping, integrated preventive and episodic care, and allowed the schools to rely

on a health facility to monitor the progress of a health initiative.

2. Aim for Success

Choose an initiative with goals that can be visibly achieved. People need clear, practical goals and identifiable achievements. Furthermore, community participants can become empowered in the process of community development through a successful collaborative effort. This serves to encourage the ongoing COPC process.

In essence, the first initiative chosen must be successful. An example of this is the first collaboration between an East Harlem health center and a nearby hospital. The health center's community board identified the need for improved prenatal services for the medically indigent. Because of the history of division between the two institutions, the need for a positive experience was expressed by both. As a goal for the first year, they chose prenatal services for 75 women, with the health center's nurse practitioner and nurse midwife providing prenatal care, and the hospital providing labor and delivery services and referral back to the health center. The first-year goal was greatly exceeded, which encouraged further collaboration in Ob-Gyn and other services.

3. Maximize the Products of Your Effort

Get the biggest bang for your buck. Perform an informal cost-effectiveness analysis of the health initiatives highest on your list. (Better yet, find a health planner or policy analyst who will perform a formal analysis. This is hardly essential, often no more helpful than an informal analysis, and invariably time consuming, but it may add a note of authority in any grant application to finance a COPC effort.) Simply ask, given the resources and plans, will people in the community ultimately be healthier with initiative A or initiative

B? This is also the moment when any possible adverse effects from these initiatives should be considered.

Cost-effectiveness analysis is an accounting of all costs involved to achieve a health effect. For each initiative, try to calculate the amount of money and the number of person-hours involved. This budget is the cost. The health effect is more difficult to estimate. A common unit used for comparative purposes is the number of cases of disease avoided by the initiative.

For example, one could calculate the costs for a community drive to immunize the elderly against influenza. This would include the costs of the vaccine and administrative costs for paperwork, transportation, etc. Furthermore, given the available information on the effectiveness of the vaccine and the morbidity and mortality of influenza, one could estimate the number of severe cases of illness averted by the influenza campaign. The cost-effectiveness ratio then is the cost in dollars for each serious case avoided by the prevention measure. This ratio is then compared to the cost-effectiveness ratios of the other health initiatives being considered.

This is not to suggest that cost-effectiveness analysis be used as the sole criterion for making choices. The assumptions of the analysis are usually debatable and the information available is usually not of sufficient certainty to direct decisions. Furthermore, some people are very uncomfortable applying costs to cases of illness. There are many variables that do not fit in well with a formal analysis, such as the costs of anxiety, pain, the time spent by the recipient of the initiative, the cost of bus fare and baby sitting charges. Also, one cannot easily quantify such benefits as the camaraderie of collaborative community service or the pleasure of self-help or exercise.

Cost-effectiveness analysis, nevertheless, forces the examination of time, money, target population, and the effectiveness of the contemplated health initiative. For this reason, even if the analysis never reaches the stage of calculating a cost-effectiveness ratio, it is often helpful to list all the variables and estimates. This serves to clarify the parameters of the initiative for all participants involved in the COPC effort.

4. Keep it Engaging

Address problems that pertain to your interests and skills. This means expressing your own interests and eliciting the interests of participating community residents. This elicitation goes a long way in engaging people in the collaborative process. Since you are not intending to solve all the community's problems, you might as well choose a project that generates enthusiasm.

5. Don't Divide the Pie

Choosing priorities by committee is intrinsically divisive. Because it is so difficult to achieve perspective, the collaborative process may be threatened by the competing priorities of special interest groups. If this occurs, focus on priorities that involve expanding the available resources, rather than "dividing the pie." This may mean applying to public or private organizations for funding.

6. Make Personal Growth a Priority

Remember that you are likely to be involved with this COPC effort for a long time. Choose initiatives that are personally challenging and enhance your skills, such as public speaking, fund-raising, or grant writing. This is as important for community residents as it is for health professionals. The East Harlem neighborhood health centers, like others elsewhere, have many stories of people with little education developing experience and skills

240

that led to further training and advanced careers.

Although I emphasize the collaborative decision process in this chapter, not all COPC efforts involve the community to the same extent as the health practitioner at the time the choice must be made. Some of the factors discussed may help this collaboration. But even if the COPC effort is predominantly the health professional's, the purpose is to be responsive to community need. In this case the health professional must be also the community residents' advocate when the time for choosing arrives. Of course, if the COPC effort is successful, the excitement generated by the process is likely to make the subsequent initiatives even more integrated into the community experience.

CODA:

Identifying Community Health Problems

Arthur Kaufman, M.D.

The chapters of Part III are intriguing in the variety of their approaches, perspectives, and inherent biases. These are born of the very different experiences of the authors. Yet they offer the reader a fruitful mix of diagnostic options. They should provoke useful ideas for the COPC practitioner—from the neophyte to the "old hand," from the solo practitioner to the Federal planner.

I culled important insights from many of the papers. They caused me to reflect and focus on a number of my own experiences in New Mexico. For example, from the introduction to Part III I was relieved by Nutting's suggestion that at times it is more efficient to strive for less rigorous problem identification methods. Simpler techniques that can provide timely feedback to the practice may be far more effective in generating program adjustment to serve the community better. I was reminded of an anecdote recently cited by Dr. Ascher Segal of the World Health Organization.[1] He informally surveyed medical school administrators to determine the impact on their curricular plan-

ning of the educational studies conducted by their program evaluators. To his chagrin he discovered that none of the program research data generated by the evaluators were ever used by medical school administrators to make decisions. Such decisions had to be made within a short time frame—long before evaluators' studies were completed. Thus methods used by the COPC practitioner to identify community health problems must be adjusted to suit the temporal demands of needed program decisions.

The papers made me reflect on the importance of the breadth of one's definition of health. A number of the papers allude to tracer conditions and diagnostic codes that are convenient for identifying and generating data about problems for an office or clinic practice. Yet, in a sense, such definitions have their own constraints and are probably tinged with cultural bias. Patients tend to frame their complaints in terms that are culturally appropriate and acceptable to a given society and its health care system. For example, after visiting a number of hospitals and clinics in China, I was surprised at how few patients carried diagnoses of psy-

[1] Personal communication, September 1985.

chiatric or psychosomatic conditions. In fact, what we in the West would diagnose as stress-related disorders amenable to counseling would in China be attributed by doctors and patients alike to physical causes amenable to drugs and physical therapy (1). In further interviews with Chinese patients they freely admitted to similar emotional stresses experienced by Westerners, but they laughed when asked if they would share those problems with their doctor. "No, no, no, doctors in China don't know *anything* about those problems," said one. In that culture such problems are handled in an entirely different way—usually within the family or by a work supervisor or neighborhood organizer.

I stress this point, because in our quest for clear problem definition and rigor in research design we often overlook our own biases and miss the less quantitative indicators of community illness. Yet these may be far more important to the health of that community. Kamerow's chapter (Alcohol, Drug Abuse and Mental Disorders) touches on this point. He cites a newer public health yardstick of community illness—Potential Productive Years of Life Lost (PPYLL). This reaches beyond the more familiar "leading causes of death" (heart disease, cancer, stroke), which are deceptive indicators for they fail to take into account the age at death. In New Mexico, for example, accidents, suicide, and homicide are among the top four PPYLL killers. Violence, then, becomes one of the key health problems in our community, especially among teenagers and young adults. It is therefore a natural candidate for COPC intervention. Yet while some of the *consequences* of violent behavior are seen by health providers, violent behavior itself does not commonly present to the office or clinic. It is simply not "culturally acceptable." Instead, in our society, we relegate to the police, to the school truancy officer, or to the hall

monitor the "diagnosis" and "care" of these "patients." I wish to thus add my voice to the fine work in this section by calling upon COPC practitioners to keep in mind very broad definitions of health problems. For they will tend to call for intervention strategies that are perhaps less traditional but more effective in diminishing the burden of early death in our communities.

Another point I would like to stress emerges as a thread through the papers by Nutting (Introduction), Horowitz and Gallagher (Group Process Techniques) Wagoner (Occupational Health), and Kozoll, Rhyne and Stewart (Use of Secondary Data). Each admonishes us to listen to the community's own perception of its health problems. Many promising intervention schemes have fallen flat because they were derived more from the perceptions and data analyses of health providers than from the felt need of the community. While the latter is not necessarily an accurate gauge of community illness it is an excellent gauge of the likelihood of a community rallying behind an intervention strategy proposed by the COPC practitioner.

A rather sobering and nearly disastrous experience we had last year illustrates this point. In attempting to implement a COPC model through a full-service clinic in an inner-city high school, we identified the main teen problem (buttressed by State and local statistics) as unwanted pregnancy (2). The clinic's efforts were organized accordingly. But when we later interviewed the school administrators, their main concern was school absenteeism. They had hoped the school clinic would focus more on keeping students in school. When the students were surveyed, on the other hand, they were primarily concerned about peer relationships and an uncertain future. By appreciating those felt needs earlier, we could have obviated resistance by the school administration to our clinic's strong emphasis on sex education and contraceptive counseling—a resistance that later emerged to threaten the very existence of our program.

One step beyond the assessment of felt needs in the community concerns the value one places on community control of the diagnosis and management of its own problems. Maas (Oral Health Problems in the Community), Schlager (Acute Self-Limited Illness) and Kamerow emphasize the strong political and educational role physicians can play in influencing policy and behavior in the community in pursuit of COPC goals. But health providers are easily intoxicated by the leadership role others so easily assign them. The rewards of such control can blind the COPC practitioner to what may be a far more effective contribution to the long-term health of the community: empowerment, encouraging the community's ownership and control of change. This is especially important in communities that traditionally have little power. The skills the COPC provider needs to effectively serve as a community change agent go far beyond the range of community health diagnostic approaches so clearly described in the papers in this section. I wish to call attention to these other useful approaches, for they suggest that in identifying community health problems, one consideration should be "which problems could motivate the participation of the community?" and "which problems could community participation effectively alleviate?"

An important theme that emerges in this section concerns a balance between the range and complexity of available resources and the capacity of the practitioner to marshal needed data in identifying community health problems. Nutting concisely differentiates between population-based indicators and encounter-based indicators. He then illustrates how well they can complement each other in analyzing the adequacy of care for particular health conditions. The approach to data gathering in these two approaches has rather broad implications and raises sobering questions about the availability of resources and the cost of generating the necessary data. For example, in the paper by Kozoll, Rhyne and Stewart, opportunities to obtain population-based data from a range of secondary sources (vital statistics, State census, tumor registries, third-party payer data, etc.) can be, at the same time, awesome and demoralizing. Awesome because they provide such a powerful vehicle for obtaining denominator data. Demoralizing because few practitioners will have the time and skill to develop such information personally out of their own practices. Thus Kozoll, Rhyne and Stewart, I feel, are really calling for the establishment of centralized data resource centers akin to those developed in New Mexico. These could be tapped by busy front-line COPC practitioners needing assistance in obtaining denominator data relevant to their practice populations.

Other authors offer more home-grown schemes—elegant approaches to generating denominator-type data from one's own practice. Schlager has developed an exciting approach to the recognition of acute illness symptom patterns in his private practice population, using a computer. He suggests that a series of interested practices could gather more denominator-type data by having a consortium of practices in a defined geographic area collect and share data. Freeman's work (the Selective Use of Tracer Conditions) provides a marvelous tool individual practices might use in generating population-based from patient-based data. He explores the economy of piggybacking the patient-based data onto an ongoing office audit of patient care activities to derive population data. Though the approach is limited to certain types of conditions, it demonstrates the importance of creatively looking for ways to simplify and harness epidemiologic technologies to office practice.

Finally an unexpected but important byproduct of COPC problem identification emerges from the papers—a new excitement about the practices themselves. In the paper by Schlager, his group is able to find new ways to take a leadership role in the community and to look at their patients' most mundane, acute, presenting complaints in a fresh, investigative way. Freeman's report demonstrates how the entire clinic health team can be a party to an internal audit of the quality of care given by the practice. All participate in the discovery of needs and redirection of clinic services. These approaches to COPC problem identification can thus lend themselves to team-building within the practice and leadership within the community.

REFERENCES

1. Kaufman, A.; Voorhees, D.; Bunch, C.P. et al. Recent developments in health care in China. *Southern Medical Journal* 1980; 73:1621.

2. Gonzales, C.; Mulligan, D.; Kaufman, A. et al. Adolescent health care: improving access by school-based service. *Journal of Family Practice* 1985; 21:263.

Part IV.
Developing an Emphasis Program

Introduction

Once a priority health problem has been identified, the practitioner of COPC should strive to modify the health care program the better to address the problem. In practice emphasis programs generally are of two types. First, the practitioner can initiate an emphasis program by making modifications largely within the primary care program, with only the necessary collaboration with other programs in the community. In this case the emphasis program will consist of varying the mix and array of services provided, by targeting them on high-risk individuals, or by changing patterns of accessibility to services, etc. Second, the practitioner can develop or collaborate in an emphasis program beyond the scope of the practice. In this case the practitioner may retain the traditional role of the practitioner or may assume primarily the role of citizen of the community. The active COPC practitioner will be involved simultaneously in emphasis programs that mix both categories.

The first chapters of Part IV describe emphasis programs that are based in the primary care program and attempt to address the health problem by modifying the mix of services and targeting appropriately on the at-risk individuals. In Chapter 31, Doyle describes the development of an emphasis program that is based on a patient tracking system. Much more than a mere disease register, the process Doyle develops includes selection of a health problem and formulation of specific objectives for the emphasis program. The method emphasizes the need for periodic monitoring of the progress of the intervention and frequent reassessment of the objectives.

Doyle illustrates the six-step process with examples from his rural practice in West Virginia and a general practice in

the Welsh mining town of Glyncorrwg.

In Chapter 32, Rosser emphasizes the importance of disease prevention and the magnitude of the impact that more effective clinical strategies of prevention would have on the health status of the population. Anticipating the increasing use of computers in managing a primary care program, he describes the results of a randomized clinical trial of three different approaches to increasing influenza immunization in high-risk individuals. Each strategy uses computer technology to identify the high-risk individual and track compliance with immunization. The differential impact of the interventions by age group will provide important clues to the expected impact of similar intervention methods in other clinical prevention programs.

Most interventions are not intended to blanket all members of the community, nor are they intended to be limited to those individuals who present for or request certain services. It is common (and far too often a cause of failure of a program to achieve an impact) to simply make a change in the practice and to assume that the individuals at high risk will make contact and receive the emphasis services. A critical specification in the emphasis program is the manner in which to identify and target those individuals who are the intended recipients and who will most benefit from the intervention. In Chapter 33, Nutting details the process for identifying and targeting services on the high-risk individuals within the population. Results are presented that suggest the substantial impact even simple intervention might have when targeted appropriately on specific individuals at increased risk.

Often the at-risk individuals are the most difficult to reach with a primary care intervention and some form of outreach may be necessary. The chapters by Taylor and Nutting both address the use of community members in an outreach capacity. In Chapter 34, Taylor describes an approach to working through "health promoters," the natural health leaders of the community. In Chapter 35, Nutting draws on the experience of the Indian Health Service to describe a stepwise method for integrating auxiliary health personnel into the process of care for an emphasis program.

For many health problems, modification in the primary care program alone would be inadequate to achieve an acceptable impact. In this case practitioners must expand their scope of concern beyond the practice and work toward appropriate modification in other health programs and community institutions. Creating change in the community can be a discouraging undertaking. The medical professional community often looks on the community-oriented practitioner with mild concern, and practitioners who hope to have an impact on the overall system of care must take careful measure of their actions. The community often appears hesitant to make or to promote rapid changes in any of its institutions or behavior patterns. In many cases the community may apparently agree on the need for an intervention, but not on the details of a specific emphasis program. In Chapter 36, Garr offers some important suggestions for the clinician attempting to create change in the programs and institutions that exist within the community. He discusses eleven general principles, and illustrates each by tracing the development of an emphasis program in a small community in the West.

Health promotion and disease prevention (HPDP) is clearly a concept embraced by the general public and represents fertile ground for the COPC approach. Although the medical profession has remained, unfortunately, in the background, COPC offers the substrate for integrating physicians into the health promotion arena. In Chapter 37, Shank describes a strategy that takes physicians into the community as natural leaders in health issues. The DOC (Doctors Ought to Care) approach uses "Madison Avenue" techniques for the purpose of focusing counter-advertising on commercial health hazards such as tobacco.

In Chapter 38, Rivo and Rivo provide a checklist of homework for the practitioner who plans to move beyond the practice to take part in community-based health promotion programs. The last chapter of this section describes an approach to the development of an emphasis program in the Bureau of Health Care Delivery and Assistance (BHCDA) of the U.S. Public Health Service. In Chapter 39, Weaver and Delany describe the Lifecycles concept that forms the basis for emphasis programs in the Migrant and Community Health Centers.

Finally in the Coda, Madison notes that prevention is a common theme that links most emphasis programs. He suggests that COPC is very like the systematic practice of preventive medicine from a primary care base. In reflecting on the history of the role of physicians in preventing illness, he suggests that COPC might be the vehicle that finally provides a context for physicians to combine prevention with their traditional primary care roles.

CHAPTER 31

Patient Tracking Systems in COPC

Daniel B. Doyle, M.D.

The design and implementation of an effective emphasis program is a critical function in the COPC process. While a great deal of attention focuses on the methods for defining and characterizing the community and identifying its health problems, difficulty may be encountered and the entire process falter if the emphasis program to address the health problem(s) is not well conceived and appropriately monitored. This chapter describes an approach to designing an intervention program that is based on a patient tracking system. Applicable in a variety of practice settings, the patient tracking system is a valuable tool for quality assurance and health care assessment. When properly designed, the tracking system becomes the heart of the intervention for a particular at-risk group.(1)

A patient tracking system is a process by which the practice staff, through consensus, organizes its work using a patient register and a specific intervention to protect the health of a particular at-risk group of persons within the community. In this definition "process" is the key word. It is all too easy to think of a tracking system merely as a disease register or a patient list that is periodically checked to see if patients on the list are "in compliance" with some standard of care. "Keeping a list and checking it twice" is part of patient tracking, but only part. The process of tracking requires the active involvement of the practice staff: in deciding what and whom should be tracked, in gathering data for the list, and above all in using the list to evaluate the success of practice efforts and make new plans for the future. Without such involvement, a well-designed and medically needed tracking effort will fail or fall far short of its potential.

The keeping of exact lists is basic to nearly every field of scientific and technical activity. How strange then that until recently the systematic use of patient lists for clinical purposes was conspicuously absent from primary care practice. Recently a number of forces are changing this. The family medicine movement has undertaken a vigorous research program focusing on the content (2) and process (3) of primary care; and the spirit and methods of that inquiry have been carried into practice by a generation of recent family medicine graduates. The growing fields of health service evaluation and quality assurance have paid increased attention to the primary care setting (4,

5). Finally, the interest in COPC stirred by the 1982 Institute of Medicine Conference (6) has had an impact of its own.

Several excellent general descriptions of tracking system principles and methods are available (7-11). Drawing on these works and our own experience at the New River Family Health Center (NRFHC) we identify six essential elements in the development of a patient tracking system.

1. A well-defined health problem
2. Staff agreement on objectives
3. An intervention plan
4. A patient register
5. A record system with uniform notation
6. Periodic audit and review

Each of these elements is described in this chapter. Their application in real situations is also described using the Welsh coal mining town of Glyncorrwg and our own experience at the New River Family Health Center as examples.

A WELL-DEFINED HEALTH PROBLEM

Drawing on information gained from the "community diagnosis" the practice develops a list of health problems facing its defined community. From this list, several problems should be chosen and considered more carefully by asking the following questions. What is the name of the problem? How many people are affected? Does the practice have the needed resources to launch a community-wide attack on this problem? Will there be community support for such an effort? Is there a reasonable chance of success? How will the results be measured?

Finding and discussing answers to these questions is the first step in the development of a patient tracking system. This step requires the participation both of the practice staff and of carefully chosen community members who are affected by the health problems being considered. Together they must choose a problem that fits the abilities of the practice and the needs of the community.

Possibilities for community-based patient tracking systems are almost limitless. The immunization of babies, care of pregnant women, screening for cervical cancer, child development, campaigns against smoking, family planning, malnutrition syndromes, nutrition and social function of the elderly, environmental sanitation, safe food and water, occupational illness, accidents, communicable diseases, and illness-related behavior such as drugs or alcohol abuse have all been suggested as subjects for community intervention and tracking efforts (7, 12).

Glyncorrwg: Dr. Julian Tudor-Hart is the general practitioner for Glyncorrwg, a South Wales coal mining village of 2,000 people (12, 13). Dr. Tudor-Hart came to Glyncorrwg in 1962. He noticed that the death rate in males for ischemic heart disease in South Wales was 70 percent above the national average and was unable to identify any risk factors unique to the South Wales population. In 1968 he found that only half the males aged 20-64 in his practice list had a blood pressure check in the previous 5 years. Dr. Tudor-Hart and his staff decided that the high rate of deaths from ischemic heart disease and the inadequate detection and followup of hypertension was a problem they needed to address.

Since 97 percent of the residents of Glyncorrwg were registered in the practice, the entire community would be the denominator in this effort. The numerator would be those with high blood pressure in need of followup and treatment.

New River Family Health Center: The New River Family Health Center (NRFHC) is a six-provider multi-specialty rural practice serving Fayette County, West Virginia since 1978. The county suffers from high rates of unemployment and poverty. A large portion of the county's Medicaid and medically indigent families obtain care at NRFHC. Thus the practice found itself providing prenatal care to an unusually high risk group of pregnant women.

A pregnancy outcome audit of all 78 NRFHC prenatal patients with due dates in 1981 was carried out. There were 66 live births, 6 spontaneous abortions, 3 fetal deaths, 1 neonatal death, and 2 lost to care. NRFHC providers were stunned to find a practice fetal death rate double the county rate and 4-1/2 times the State rate. The low birth weight rate in the practice was double the State and county rates. They also noted that 21 percent of mothers were under 18 years of age, compared to 12 percent for the State and county, and that 39 percent of prenatal patients were smokers.

The practice staff, the community board, and outside consultants reviewed these findings. It was an easy decision that a special program should be undertaken to improve pregnancy outcome in NRFHC prenatal patients. This decision was reached in 1982 and the program began in 1983. The target group for this effort was determined all women receiving prenatal care at NRFHC.

STAFF AGREEMENT ON OBJECTIVES

The staff must agree on exact definitions of the problem and on the goals of the tracking system. Agreement on definitions is often harder than providers anticipate. While it is easy to agree who is or is not pregnant, it is less easy to agree who is socially isolated, or what levels of elevated blood pressure or low hemoglobin require treatment. Goals are either process goals, e.g., a followup visit every 3 months, or outcome goals, e.g., a reduction in the incident of heart attack. Most tracking efforts have both types of goals.

There are other decisions to be made

at this stage. How will persons be identified for the tracking system and added to it (i.e., identifying the numerator)? Is this intended as a one-year project or a long-term one? What measures will be used to evaluate the effort?

Glyncorrwg: Dr. Tudor-Hart and his staff agreed on the following objectives:

1. All persons age 20-64 should have a blood pressure measurement every 5 years.

2. Persons 20-39 years of age whose blood pressure exceeded systolic 165 or diastolic 100 (mean of three separate readings) were placed in the treatment group.

3. Persons 40-64 years of age whose blood pressure exceeded systolic 180 or diastolic 105 (mean of three separate readings) were placed in the treatment group.

4. Persons in the treatment group should have a followup visit every 3 months.

5. Treatment, in turn, had four specific objectives: no smoking, reduction of pressure to the range below 160-180 systolic and 90-100 diastolic, dietary salt reduction, and weight reduction to within 10 percent above desirable weight.

New River Family Health Center: The NRFHC staff agreed on the following objectives for their prenatal tracking program:

1. Women who were high risk by reason of previous obstetric complications or medical conditions were referred early to an obstetrician for exclusive or co-management of the pregnancy.

2. Women who were high risk for socioeconomic reasons were managed at NRFHC.

3. All pregnant women were to begin

prenatal care within the first trimester of pregnancy with monthly visits through the 32nd week, twice weekly visits through the 36th week and transfer to the obstetrician at 36 weeks for weekly visits until delivery.

NRFHC adopted the same protocol of prenatal care that was used by the obstetricians and nurse-midwives in the referral obstetric practice. All pregnant women were to receive a packet of educational materials explaining nutrition, physical and emotional changes of pregnancy, the birth experience, hospital policies and fees, and family planning.

AN INTERVENTION PLAN

The intervention plan specifies what will be done, when, where, and by whom in order to meet the objectives of the tracking system. Very often, a system to ensure regular followup is part of the intervention plan. Such a system defines a followup interval for each person in the numerator group, notes whether the followup visit occurs, and automatically triggers contact by letter, phone, or home visit with those persons who miss a visit. Providing transportation may also be part of the followup system. Examples of other intervention measures are periodic diagnostic testing, environmental sampling (water, air, building materials), immunization, health education, nutritional programs (Meals on Wheels, school lunches), and home health services.

A critical part of the intervention plan is the delegation of responsibility for various functions within the program to different members of the health care team. Depending on the particular project there may be tasks for the practice receptionist, medical records clerk, nurses, lab technician, administrator, and outreach worker as well as for the providers. Persons outside the practice may also play an important part. Public health nurse, health inspector, welfare workers, children's protective workers, community volunteer, school principal or guidance counselor, journalist, minister, or police officer are all possible partners depending on the project. An individual or a small coordinating committee should assume overall responsibility for the project to ensure that all parts of the project are carried out with good quality and on schedule.

In practices with more than two or three providers, standardized data collection tasks such as obtaining demographic information or blood pressure measurements are more reliably carried out when made part of front desk or nursing routines than when left to a diverse group of providers with varying degrees of commitment to the tracking effort.

Glyncorrwg: First the practice staff planned to ascertain blood pressures of everyone in the village ages 20-64. Since one-half had already had blood pressure readings within 5 years, this left the other half to be ascertained. The plan was to mark the records of all patients needing a blood pressure reading and to obtain these "casually" as patients came in to see the doctor for whatever reason over the next year. At the end of a year those still outstanding would be contacted by letter or home visit.

When screening was complete the population would then be divided into three groups. Those with hypertension would be seen every 3 months and receive appropriate testing, treatment, and education. Those with borderline pressures would have repeat readings at yearly intervals. Those with normal readings would have repeat readings at least every 5 years.

Delegation of responsibility was made explicit. The practice receptionist reviewed the chart when patients arrived to see whether a blood pressure reading was due. The nurse performed the blood pressure readings and recorded them on a graphic flow sheet in the medical record.

The physician saw the patient and discussed treatment including appropriate counseling with regard to smoking cessation, salt restriction, and weight reduction. The nurse noted which patients had failed to keep a followup visit and the receptionist sent them a reminder letter.

New River Family Health Center: The intervention plan of the NRFHC for prenatal patients included the following components. First, the practice would hire a maternal and child health (MCH) coordinator. Her main functions would be coordination of prenatal care and provision of individual counseling, education, and support to all pregnant women, especially those at high risk for socioeconomic reasons. A monthly review of prenatal records would be made to check for completeness and for missed appointments. Monthly meetings of the providers and MCH coordinator would be held to review deficiencies in care, discuss high-risk cases with on-the-spot planning for specialized care or referral, and review pregnancy outcomes.

The health center would become a site for women to register for and pick up WIC coupons (supplementary food vouchers for pregnant women, infants, and children). Prepared childbirth classes would be offered regularly at the health center. This was an effort to improve participation of teenagers, unwed mothers, and indigent couples who tended not to attend the classes offered in a town 15 miles away.

Responsibility for critical tasks was shared among the group. The medical records secretary kept a list of all prenatal patients and made sure records were transferred to the consulting obstetric practice at regular intervals. The MCH coordinator performed the monthly review of prenatal records, compiled statistics on pregnancy outcome, and provided the counseling and education services described above. She also organized the childbirth classes and intensive outreach to encourage participation of high-risk pregnant women often to the point of providing or arranging transportation. The nurses collected uniform data at each prenatal visit (symptom list, weight, blood pressure, urine tests) and recorded this on a standardized prenatal flow sheet. Providers examined and counseled pregnant women at each visit, identified high-risk situations with appropriate referral to the maternal health worker and participated in the monthly prenatal meetings. Practice physicians provided newborn nursery care in the hospital and at the time of the newborn exam collected uniform data on pregnancy outcome.

A PATIENT REGISTER

The patient register is the information system at the heart of the tracking system. It is the most important structural element of the entire system, as noted by Strasser (9):

> The register thus really plays a leading role in the community control programme of hypertension. The whole operation is viable only if there is a smooth and steady flow of information between the community and the register.

The register contains the names of all persons in the at-risk group usually with additional demographic and clinical data about each. The register should be structured in such a way that it can easily be used to generate reports on the status of the entire group or to retrieve information about a single patient. There must be a dependable and nearly automatic system for all relevant data to be gathered, entered, and continuously updated for the register to be effective. Defining these functions and clearly assigning responsibility for each one are important parts of steps 2 and 3 as discussed above.

In setting up a patient register, one of

the first choices to be made is between a manual or computerized system. Even for a small practice microcomputers are affordable and offer major advantages over other systems. Still, manual systems have been used effectively for many years, have minimal startup costs, and may be the best choice in some cases.

There are two types of manual patient registers, the index-card file and the marginal perforated (McBee) card file. The index-card file is the type of register used originally in both the Glyncorrwg and NRFHC practices. Each patient in the system has a 3 x 5 index card with his or her name and limited additional data. These cards are filed alphabetically and according to dates of followup. The disadvantages of the index-card file are the limited amount of data that can be stored per patient, the inability to quickly identify subsets within the tracked group, and its very limited potential for generating reports on the status or outcome of the tracked group.

Patient registers using marginal perforated (McBee) cards also have been used for years in tracking and clinical research (14, 15). Information about each patient is written on a single card and is also coded by using a triangular punch to make appropriate holes in the margins of the card. These marginal perforations allow quick mechanical sorting by inserting a needle through a row of cards. An excellent description of a hypertension tracking system using McBee cards at the Martin Luther King Health Center in South Bronx has been published (16). Figure 1 shows a sample card from that system.

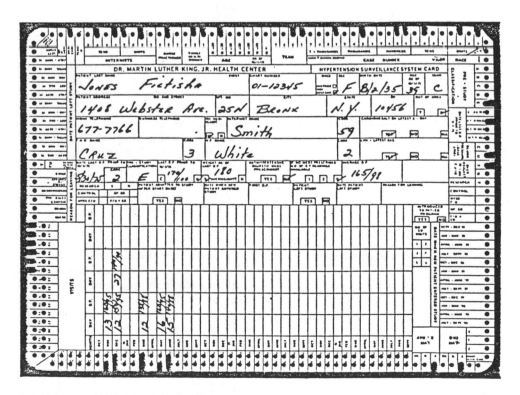

Figure 1. Hypertension Tracking System.

Another report describes a McBee card system for practice-based tracking of preventive measures and chronic diseases (14). The McBee system is far superior to the index card file in the amount of data stored and the ability to quickly identify relevant subsets. There is greater potential for preparing reports, but still this requires manual tabulation of data from each card.

Microcomputers using data base programs are the best choice for patient registers in small or medium size primary care practices. The advantages of a computerized system are the ability to handle large amounts of data quickly, the ability to quickly identify subsets of the tracked group, the rapid preparation of audits on status and outcome of the tracked group, and the ability to prepare lists (even mailing labels) of patients for recall. In 1986 the purchase of such a system ranges from $5,000 to $25,000 depending on the size of the practice and the other functions required of the system. Figure 2 shows the

Last Name
First Name
Account No.
Sex, Race
Birth Date
Address
Phone
Date Last Evaluation
Provider
Pulmonary Diagnosis
Dyspnea Level
Homebound (yes, no)
Pack Years Smoking
Years Mining
Other Occupational Exposures
Pulmonary Hospital Admissions/Days 1985
Pulmonary Hospital Admissions/Days 1986
On Medication ? (regular, p.r.n., none)
PPD (date, reaction)
Pneumovax (year)
Flu Vax (date)
Theophylline (yes, no)
First FEV1 (date, value)
Most recent FEV1 (date, value)
Most recent FVC (date, value)
Clinical Severity Level (I–IV)

Figure 2. File Structure for a Computerized Tracking System of Patients with Pulmonary Disease or Risk Factors.

structure of a single patient file used in a computerized tracking system for pulmonary disease at NRFHC.

Microcomputer patient registers often exist in parallel with other practice record systems. That is, they exist parallel and separate from the written medical records and from the written or computerized patient billing system. The ideal microcomputer system feasible for small practices integrates tracking and billing records. In this way a single register of all persons for whom the practice is responsible is maintained. Each patient file has fields for demographic data (age, sex, ethnicity, address, phone), financial data (procedures, insurance, balance due), and tracking data. Such a system avoids duplication of files, allows calculation of prevalence and case detection rates as well as process and outcome audits for tracked conditions, and gives measures of clinical performance equal status with measures of financial performance in the practice management information system.

There is a crucial caveat about computers. A computer cannot rescue a project that is ill-conceived or ill-designed. "Garbage-in, garbage-out" is always the rule. The health care team should carefully think through its definitions, goals, and methods and write them down in the form of a "Tracking System Protocol." Only then can the advantages of the computer be realized.

Large computer systems, while out of reach for most primary care practices, are also used for patient tracking programs. In Montreal a centralized immunization registry was established for a single health district of 250,000 people and 2,175 eligible infants (17). A large health maintenance organization in Boston with fully computerized medical records experimented with various interventions to improve followup and control of hypertension (18).

Glyncorrwg: The patient register for

hypertension tracking in Glyncorrwg was admirably simple. An index card was prepared with the name, address, and next appointment date of each hypertension patient. These cards were filed in a box by the month of the next appointment, as shown in Figure 3. At the time of the patient's appointment, the date was crossed off, the next date written in, and the card moved to the month of the next appointment (usually 3 months forward).

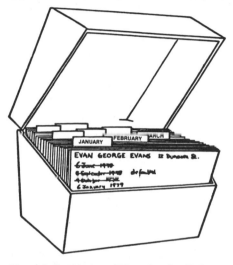

Figure 3. Card Index of Hypertensive Patients.

At the end of each month, the patients who had missed appointments were easily identified. They received a letter or phone call reminding them of the need for followup.

New River Family Health Center: Because pregnancy lasts only 9 months and prenatal care even less, the prenatal register was constantly changing. A simple card file using 3 x 5 index cards was used. For each new prenatal patient, the medical transcriptionist prepared a card as shown in Figure 4. The front side was used to track the patient during pregnancy; the back side was used for entry of information about the birth, the baby's condition, and any perinatal problems.

During the pregnancy the cards were filed by the month of the estimated date of conception (EDC). This made review of overdue patients and patients due in the coming month an easy part of monthly perinatal meetings.

When patients delivered, the NRFHC physician who provided the nursery card completed the back side of the card. These cards were then filed alphabetically for the current calendar year and at the end of the year provided a ready data set for compiling yearly statistics about pregnancy outcomes. The back side of the card was also photocopied for use as the first entry in the newborns NRFHC medical record.

A RECORD SYSTEM WITH UNIFORM NOTATION

The register for a patient tracking system often exists as a duplicate record system parallel to the practice's standard written or typed medical records. The need for uniformity in the register is readily apparent. But a structured format and uniform notation is equally important in the regular medical records. Most clinical information about patients in the numerator group will be stored in the medical record and not on the register file cards. Review of tracking results sometimes requires medical record audit with the register merely serving to locate all patients in the numerator group. Both the efficiency and the accuracy of medical record audit are greatly enhanced by the recording of relevant data in a clear and systematic way.

The practice staff should agree on a system of uniform notation in the medical record as part of establishing a tracking system. For some practices simply adapting a structured problem-oriented medical record (POMR) (19) may be an important step. If child growth and development are the tracking focus, every record needs a growth chart with nurses trained to record and graph their measure-

Front Side

Jane Doe   EDC: 12/11/85
RFD 1, Box   AGE: 21
Oak Hill, WV   G2 P1 ABO
Record No. 016
Phone No. 465-07

Approx. Date:

28 Wks: 9/14/85
34 Wks: 10/27/85

Back Side

NAME/MOTHER: NAME/INFANT:
AGE: EDC:
GRAVIDITY: DOB:
BLOOD TYPE: GA:
SMOKING HX: WT: HC: LN:
PRE-NATAL:
                          APG:
                          BLOOD TYPE:
                          CONSIDERATIONS:
LABOR/DEL: BREAST
                             FORMULA
                             OTHER

Figure 4. 3 x 5 Card as the Basis of Prenatal Register.

ments accurately. If screening for cervical cancer is the focus, providers can agree to record Pap results in a particular place in the chart and to enter "Abnormal Pap smear" on the problem list. Colored markers can be used to flag charts of patients being tracked or in need of a particular test. Structured flow sheets are very useful in tracking programs that require frequent followup visits such as prenatal care, hypertension, or diabetes.

Glyncorrwg: The Glyncorrwg practice used a structured medical record that was a modification of the POMR system. The terms "hypertension" and "hypertension controlled" were not used loosely according to the personal opinion of each doctor or trainee. Rather they had specific

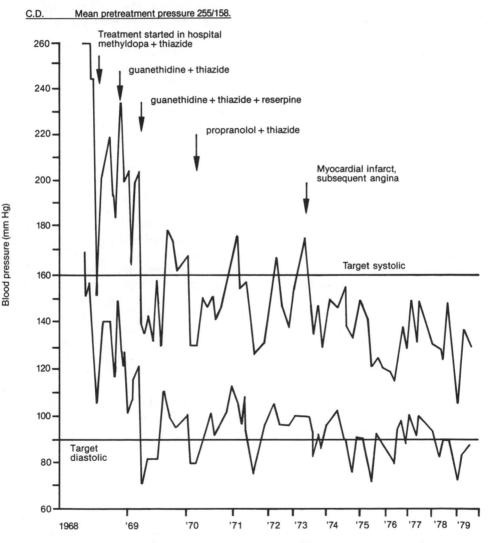

Figure 5. Patient's Record Retyped for Legibility in Reproduction from Hand Written Originals.

quantitative definitions agreed to when objectives were set. A graphic flow sheet of blood pressure readings (Figure 5) served as a powerful tool for synthesizing and highlighting the hypertensive patient's clinical course. Red stickers were used to indicate when the next blood pressure reading was due. For treated hypertensives, the sticker was placed on the outside of their chart indicating a reading every 3 months. For borderline hypertensives or normotensives, the red sticker was placed in the progress notes indicating a reading at 1 year or 5 years respectively.

New River Family Health Center: The NRFHC used a structured problem-oriented medical record. The records of family members (by household) were kept together in a single family folder. The records of prenatal patients had a special prenatal record form with areas for medical history and physical exam on one side and prenatal visit records in a standard flow sheet format on the other side. The second page contained a checklist for education and counseling during the pregnancy as well as a section for dating the pregnancy by history, examination and ultrasound. The third page was a pregnancy weight gain graphic chart with the broad normal curve highlighted.

The charts of pregnant patients were marked with a bright red tag and filed together separate from the other patient records. This facilitated monthly review of prenatal records for completeness and missed appointments. At the conclusion of the pregnancy, the prenatal record forms were filed in the back of the chart with hospital discharge summaries as a permanent part of the patient's record. The record was also returned to the family folder and the red tag was removed.

PERIODIC AUDIT AND REVIEW

On a regular basis the patient register should be used to generate reports about the status of the tracking effort. These reports are distributed to the entire staff and a meeting is convened to consider the following questions. Is the tracking system meeting its objectives? What are the areas of success and failure? What has been learned about the community and about the practice as a result of this effort? Should the program continue unaltered or should it be modified? Should it be terminated because all the objectives have been met? Or should it be abandoned for a different project that is more important or more realistic? All these are legitimate and necessary questions to be periodically and collectively asked about the tracking system. Usually the project is continued, although there may be modification of the intervention strategy, in the data set being maintained on the register cards, or in delegation of responsibility.

A "Tracking System Log" appended to the "Tracking System Protocol" should be kept so that any revisions in the system are carefully and clearly recorded for future reference.

Glyncorrwg: The Glyncorrwg practice held monthly staff meetings. Along with other business, the status of hypertension tracking and ascertainment was discussed. As of February 1982, 80 patients were under treatment for hypertension. Of these 69 percent had a diastolic pressure less than 90 mm Hg and 59 percent had a systolic pressure less than 160 mm Hg.

Figure 6 is a review of ascertainment as of January 1982. The staff concluded they were doing well at followup of untreated hypertensives and normotensives but not of borderline hypertensives. This had clear implications for their future work.

Figure 7 is a graphic summary of the tracking system population from 1968 to 1982. Based on the steady growth of the treatment group, the practice staff concluded they were altering the natural history of high blood pressure in Glyncorrwg; that is, people with high blood pressure were living longer.

Category	Blood Pressure Level		Planned Interval Between BP Readings	% of Patients with Up-to-Date BP Readings
	Age 40–64	Age 20–39		
1	$\geq \dfrac{180mmHg}{105}$	$\geq \dfrac{170mmHg}{100}$	3 Months	85
2	$\geq \dfrac{150mmHg}{90}$	$\geq \dfrac{140mmHg}{85}$	1 Year	45
3	$< \dfrac{150mmHg}{90}$	$< \dfrac{140mmHg}{}$	5 Years	90

Figure 6. Glyncorrwg: Review of Ascertainment as of January 1, 1982.

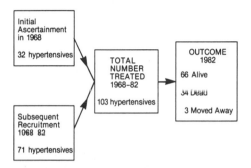

Figure 7. Number of Patients Treated for Hypertension Between 1968 and 1982, with Diastolic Pressures ≥ 105mmHg (40–60yr), ≥ 100mmHg (20–39yr).

Revisions did occur over the years. It was decided that followup visits for treated hypertensives should be organized into special hypertensive clinic sessions rather than spread out randomly over the month's consulting sessions. A computerized system replaced the card file box with monthly reports showing patients who are overdue for blood pressure readings in all three groups: hypertensive, borderline and normotensive.

A research program examining the relationship between blood pressure, dietary sodium intake, and family history of high blood pressure was established with the future goal of primary prevention of hypertension by dietary intervention in families at high risk. The program continues as a respected model that has gained international attention.

New River Family Health Center: The NRFHC providers and MCH coordinator met monthly to review the progress of the prenatal care program. A monthly statistical report prepared by the MCH coordinator served as an agenda for their meetings. Figure 8 shows the report for June 1984.

All cases of perinatal morbidity and mortality were reviewed in detail. Overdue patients or high-risk patients not yet due were discussed in an effort to anticipate and prevent complications. Next, a medical record report was made by the MCH coordinator. The problem of getting prenatal records transferred to the consulting obstetrics practice frequently arose. Presentations of relevant topics such as genetic counseling and gestational diabetes were made at these meetings when time allowed. There were no fetal deaths in 1982 or 1983, two in 1984, and no neonatal deaths in 1982-1984. Practice providers were also pleased that breast feeding rose from 37 percent in 1981 and 1982 to 49 percent in 1984.

In 1983 a grant was obtained allowing the MCH coordinator to expand her activities to include a home visit program to teenage mothers. The prenatal register served as a valuable data source for this effort, which is continuing. In mid-1985 the obstetric practice accepting NRFHC referrals closed. This created a community health crisis and also temporarily reduced the number of prenatals followed by the practice. During this time the tracking system continued but meetings did not.

CONCLUSION

Primary care practices that seek to implement the principles of COPC in developing an emphasis program will find the elements of the tracking system to be useful. The central notions include a

	Jan	Feb	Mar	Apr	May	Jun	Jul	Aug	Sep	Oct	Nov	Dec	Total
New Prenatals	9	7	14	17	10	4							
Total Active Prenatals	42	40	40	42	43	48							
Newborns—NRFHC [1]	9	7	8	7	3	6							
Newborns—Other [2]	3	1	8	2	5	7							
Overdue [3,6]	0	0	0	1	1	0							
Lost to Follow-up	0	0	0	3	0	1							
Perinatal Morbidity [4,6]	1	2	1	0	0	3							
Perinatal Mortality [5,6]	0	0	1	0	0	0							
C Section	1	0	1	2	1	2							
Breast Fed Initially	5	2	6	5	4	6							

1. Newborns whose mothers received care at NRFHC
2. Newborns entering practice whose mothers received prenatal care elsewhere
3. $\geq$ 42 weeks as of first in month
4. Morbidity: any perinatal illness, injury or anomaly of mother or baby. Included prematurity and jaundice sufficient to require photo therapy
5. Mortality: perinatal death of mother, fetus, or newborn
6. All such cases were reviewed in detail at monthly meetings

Figure 8. New River Family Health Center Pregnancy Outcome Project—Monthly Report for June 1984.

multi-disciplinary health care team that considers its community, designs emphasis programs for at-risk subsets, and then carefully evaluates the effect *as a team.* These elements are central to the concept of COPC and allow a practice to go far beyond a traditional notion of "good primary care."

REFERENCES

1. Doyle, D.; Samargo, P.; Vandall, S. et al. Linking epidemiology and clinical practice: Results of a hypertension tracking program in a rural clinic. Paper presented at the National Conference on High Blood Pressure Control, Chicago, April 28, 1985.

2. Geyman, J. (ed.). The content of family practice, a statewide study in Virginia. *Journal of Family Practice,* 1976, 3:1.

3. Green, L.; Wood, M.; Becker, L. et al. The Ambulatory Sentinel Practice Project of North America: Purposes, methods, and policies. *Journal of Family Practice,* 1984, 18:275.

4. Smith, D., and Mukerjee, G. (eds). *Assuring Quality Ambulatory Health Care: The Dr. Martin Luther King, Jr. Health Center.* Boulder: Westview Press, 1978.

5. Hirschhorn, N.; Lamstein, J.; McCormack, J.; and Klein, S. (eds.). *Quality of Care Assessment and Assurance.* Boston: G.K. Hall & Co., 1978.

6. Mullan, F., and Connor, E. (eds.). *Community Oriented Primary Care, Conference Proceedings.* Washington, DC: Institute of Medicine, 1982.

7. Kark S. *The Practice of Community-Oriented Primary Care,* Chapter 2, Community diagnosis and health surveillance. New York: Appleton-Century-Crofts, 1981.

8. Tudor-Hart, J. *Hypertension*, Chapter 17, Organisation of follow-up, compliance, and education; Chapter 18, Data handling. London: Churchill Livingstone, 1980.

9. Strasser, T. *The Uses of Hypertension Registers, in Hypertension and Stroke Control in the Community*. Geneva: World Health Organization, 1976.

10. Owens, R., and Hirschhorn, N. Simplified manual systems for clinical management: Tracking systems. *Journal of Ambulatory Care Management*, 1983, 65:78.

11. *Clinical Data Collection and Retrieval System for Small Primary Care Projects* (Administrative Publication). Rockville, MD: USDHHS, HRSA, BCHDA, Division of Primary Care Services, 1982.

12. Watt, G. Community-oriented primary care in a Welsh mining village. In: Mullan, F., Connor, E. (eds.), *Community Oriented Primary Care, Conference Proceedings*. Washington, DC: Institute of Medicine, 1982.

13. Tudor-Hart, J. The marriage of primary care and epidemiology. *Journal of the Royal College of Physicians*, 1974, 48(4):299.

14. Patient Data Card Systems. Clinical Information Systems Company. PO Box 2850, Evergreen, CO 80439.

15. McBee Systems. Patient Data Keysort Manual. Atlanta, GA, 1981.

16. Smith, D., and Schnall, P. Hypertension surveillance system: An outcome approach. In: Smith D., Mukerjee, G. (eds.), *Assuring Quality Ambulatory Health Care: The Dr. Martin Luther King, Jr. Health Center*. Boulder: Westview Press, 1978.

17. Loeser, H.; Zvagulis, B.; Hercz, L. et al. The organization and evaluation of a computer-assisted, centralized immunization register. *American Journal of Public Health*, 1983, 73:1298.

18. Barnett, O.; Winickoff, R.; Morgan, M. et al. A computer-based monitoring system for follow-up of elevated blood pressure. *Medical Care*, 1983, 21:400.

19. Weed, L. *Medical Records, Medical Education and Patient Care, the Problem Oriented Record as a Basic Tool*. Chicago: Year Book Medical Publishers, 1969.

CHAPTER 32

Strategies for
Clinical Prevention in COPC

Walter W. Rosser, M.D.

Much has been written over the past 15 years about the importance of primary prevention (1). The scientific basis for preventive services was clarified in 1981 when the Canadian Task Force on the Periodic Health Examination developed criteria for appropriate screening procedures and applied the criteria to approximately 150 currently available procedures. The results of the Task Force's work have been widely disseminated to practitioners in North America. The major practical problem with the recommendations, however, is that for each of 10 different age and sex groups, a different list of procedures is required, and each at a different frequency (3).

It would be virtually impossible for the COPC practitioner using manual methods to keep track of the preventive status of a practice and to monitor the frequency with which each procedure should be carried out on each individual. However, this type of tracking and monitoring is a simple task for personal computers, and an important role for the computer in the monitoring of preventive care is for counting, reminding, and tracking people using basic inventory programs. During the past

20 years, only the most dedicated of our practitioner colleagues have managed to maintain age, sex, and diagnostic registers of their patient population using manual procedures. Fewer have been able to consistently maintain those systems for identifying individuals within the community at high risk. For the majority of practitioners, however, the computer when fully exploited can provide the required denominator and numerator data with relative ease. Perhaps one of the most significant impacts of computerization on primary care practices will be the capacity to document the preventive health status of a practice population. Computer software should benefit a practice organizationally and financially while improving patient care and assisting in the provision of preventive care (2).

This chapter presents strategies for clinical prevention programs that will be useful for the COPC practitioner. A clinical trial examining the differential impact of strategies for increasing the provision of effective preventive services is briefly described, the results are presented, and the implications for COPC practitioners are discussed.

THE CLINICAL TRIAL

This line of research has been funded by the Department of National Health and Welfare of Canada, which is seeking the most efficient methods of delivering screening procedures at the recommended frequency to known practice populations. Among the issues being addressed are the most effective and efficient ways to obtain annual blood pressure readings on everyone over 15, how to ensure that all patients have a tetanus-polio immunization once every 10 years, how to assess each patient's smoking status annually, and how to ensure that all women under age 35 have a Papanicolaou's smear annually. In 1985 a clinical trial was completed that examined alternative means for reminding all patients over 65 years of age of the need for the annual influenza immunization.

Defining the Practice Population

Determining the study population in our middle-class teaching practice was a major undertaking. Among the six practices in the Ottawa Civic Hospital Family Medicine Centre, we believed that we were looking after approximately 11,000 patients. Only 8,500 of the 11,000, however, had visited one of our physicians in the previous one-and-a-half years. An algorithm was developed to identify active patients and link them to one of the six practices. The algorithm identified 3,600 persons who either did not meet our criteria of an active patient or did not link to a practice. This was surprising since we had annually contacted all patients who had not visited the practice in the previous two years to maintain an "accurate" denominator.

Letters were sent to each of these 3,600 individuals asking if they still regarded one of the practice physicians as their primary care provider. Only 1,100 positive replies were received. Nonresponders were eliminated from the trial. In August of 1984,

8,508 individuals were judged eligible for the trial. Of these, 1,421 were over the age of 65.

Study Design

Due to our concern for contamination of the control group in our study practices, two of six practices were designated as total-control practices. The *total-control practices* had 482 people over age 65. The four study practices had 939 persons over age 65 who were randomly allocated to four groups. A *randomized control group* was developed for whom no action was taken to promote influenza vaccination. A *physician reminder group* was developed for whom a computer-generated summary of all previous visits by that patient was produced (a sample printout is shown in Table 1). The summary included a reminder to the physician to discuss influenza immunization with the patient. A *letter reminder group* was developed for whom a computer-generated letter was sent stating that the physician recommended a visit to the Centre at a designated time for influenza immunization. Finally, a *nurse reminder group* was developed. Names and telephone numbers of patients assigned to this group were given to the practice nurse to contact by telephone. The nurse was instructed to make no more than five attempts to phone the patient, and the time required to make the contact was recorded. Once contact was made, the nurse would discuss with the patient the need to have the influenza immunization and make appropriate arrangements.

The trial began on October 23, 1984 and lasted until December 31 of that same year. Each influenza immunization was recorded on the computer encounter sheet.

Results

The results of the trial are summarized in Table 2. It was surprising that such a low number of people in the total-control prac-

TABLE I. Sample printout providing the physician with a summary of previous visits and reminder to discuss influenza immunization with the patient.

```
CUMULATIVE                                              Mar  10/09 ( F )(Dr 000 ) 01           (NO 01311
PATIENT                                    OTTAWA       Res:
PROFILE                                    ON           Bus:
                                                        Emerg:
                                                        Pharm:
                                        Ins#: 34152918 Plan: 0  Subsc.name:                    C
```

B.P.		WEIGHT (cm)	WEIGHT (kg)	SMOKING	SCREENING
Dec 16/85	152/ 92			Oct 15/84	does not smk
Nov 25/85	150/ 90				************************
May 07/85	144/ 88				*PATIENT OVER 65YRS OLD*
Apr 12/85	160/ 90				*CHECK FLU IMMUNIZATION*
Nov 14/84	160/ 90				************************
Oct 15/84	120/ 85				
Sept 25/84	190/100				
May 09/83	160/ 80				
Apr 27/83	160/ 90				
Apr 20/83	154/ 84				

DRUG ALLERGIES	IMMUNIZATION	HISTORY/RISK FACTORS

PERMANENT PROBLEMS

OTHER PROBLEMS

Dec 16/85	+ 1	Paresthesias (349)	Dec 16/85	+ 4	401 hypertension uncomplicated
Nov 25/85	+ 6	Elev.bl.(401) pres.(transient)	May 07/85	+ 4	351 peripheral neuropathy
May 07/85		279 metabolic abnormality nyd	Apr 12/85		t#8. cancel - done othr -ver
Apr 12/85	+ 2	447 peripheral vascular disease	Nov 14/84		Non specific dermatitis (709)
Nov 14/84		629 pelvic abnormality n.y.d.	Oct 15/84		does not smoke
Oct 15/84		Osteoarthritis (713)	Oct 01/84		Low back pain (729) without r adi
Sept 06/84		216 pigmented nevus	June 15/83		Immunization (057)
Dec 14/82		300 anxiety			

DRUGS (ACTIVE)		STRENGTH/UNITS	TAKE	FREQ	GIVEN	REPEATS	EXP.DATE
Dec 16/85	Hydrochlorothiazide/amiloride hcl: moduret		1	1	33	12	Feb 18/87

DRUGS (EXPIRED)

May 07/85	+ 1	Hydrochlorothiazide/amiloride hcl: moduret	Apr 02/85	+ 1	Furosemide: lasix
Mar 05/85		Dienestrol: ortho dienestrol	Nov 14/84		Triamcinolone: aristocort,kenacort
Sept 25/84		Hydrochlorothiazide: : hydro-diuril	June 15/83		Tetanus toxoid

tice were receiving the influenza immunization. This did not correspond with the perception of the physicians in the practice who felt that they were doing a fairly good job immunizing their patients with influenza vaccine. Our concern about contamination in the study practices was confirmed; 8.7 percent of people in the study practices received the immunization, a significantly higher percent than in the total-control practices.

The telephone reminder seemed to be the most efficient and effective way of getting people over the age of 65 to have the procedure done; 34 percent of this group received the influenza vaccine. The letter reminder was less well received; only 29 percent of people over 65 responded to the request. Only 21 percent of patients responded to the physician reminder.

When the results were analyzed according to individuals rather than families the overall result was somewhat better, with the physician reminder group having a 22 percent success rate, the letter reminder 35 percent, the telephone 37 percent, the randomized control 9.8 percent, and the total control group 3.8 percent.

TABLE 2. Influenza immunization by families

	Immunized		Not immunized	Total
	N	Percent	N	
Randomized control	18	8.7	172	203
Physician reminder	40	20.9	136	191
Letter reminder	68	29.0	142	231
Telephone reminder	67	34.0	117	197
Total-control[1]	14	3.7	363	404
Total	207	18.2	930	1226

[1] Two of the six practices did not participate in the study in order to control for the potential contamination effect in the control group randomized in the study practices.

Discussion

Several observations may be helpful to move towards the practical application of computerized reminder systems for preventive care in COPC. First, there was a different response by age group in the practice to the three different reminders. Persons over the age 65 responded best to a phone call from the nurse whereas the elderly person receiving a letter was often confused, and phoned the nurse to determine what the letter was for and how should they respond. Some of the very elderly were unable to read the letter and were upset that their physician was contacting them by mail.

Middle-aged (age 45-64) individuals, on the other hand, were difficult to contact by telephone because a high percentage are not regularly at home but are employed and difficult to contact at work. Often five phone calls were not enough to make the contact with the middle-aged group. The middle-aged did respond well to a letter, however. Many patients expressed pleasure about their physician's concern for their preventive health status.

We found that it required an average of 1.2 minutes for the nurse to make the contact with patients over 65 on the telephone. The cost of the telephone contacts was calculated on the basis of the time required to contact and deal with patients and the hourly pay of our nurses. The cost of the nurse reminder was $2.65 per immunization gained. For the letter reminder group it was $2.33.

From the data of Table 2, the physician reminder would appear to be relatively ineffective. Further analysis, however, revealed that during the 9 weeks of the trial, approximately 50 percent of the patients eligible for the immunization attended the office. Of these, 46 percent received the influenza immunization, making this intervention the most effective. It appears that the immediacy of the physician telling a patient that a preventive procedure is indicated and then suggesting the procedure be carried out with minimal inconvenience, may be the most efficient and effective way of reminding people.

One might ask, why was there such a

low response rate? Several other similar studies have been done in Ontario and they have all shown relatively low response rates in the 20-40 percent range even with fairly rigorous interventions (4,5). We surveyed a random sample of our patients who did not receive the immunization to find out why they had declined. Half the group said that they felt fine and were worried that the immunization was dangerous. A small percentage said that they were too sick and were afraid of adding further illness to their already poor condition. Another group was undecided and could not explain why they would not have the influenza vaccine.

We concluded that some form of public education program will be needed to change public perceptions about influenza immunization. With only 3.5 percent of persons over 65 now receiving the vaccine, one can conclude that either definite action to promote the procedure is needed or it should be abandoned. Studies of the non-immunized group, followed by evaluative trials of different strategies to improve compliance, will provide a research agenda for the next decade. We need to understand why people, in spite of being reminded, or in spite of being recalled, are still refusing to have preventive procedures carried out. Whether the problem is lack of education, personality traits, or cultural beliefs, we will have to learn how to address it if preventive medicine is going to be effectively applied to the whole population.

USE OF THE COMPUTER IN COMMUNITY-ORIENTED PRIMARY CARE PRACTICE

The study illustrates the benefits of developing a denominator for a medical practice and the use of the computer to assist in carrying out preventive procedures. It is clear that computer reminder systems significantly improved the rates of preventive procedures being carried out. The study outlined is reasonable in a teaching center, but would be difficult to conduct in a nonteaching practice.

Based on 12 years of experience developing computer software for our practice, we have learned that the only way a computer system will be effective in a practice is if it is cost-effective and if all who use it regard it as a means to make all aspects of patient care and office operation more effective. Individuals using the system have to feel that it is beneficial to them and their work. This may sound like a formidable task, especially in a large office, but in our office where there are six full-time physicians, 30 residents, and a staff of 20 assistants, we have found that the computer has consistently improved the work of all staff members.

The computer is used for scheduling appointments. Once an appointment is registered on the computer system, data summarizing all previous visits by the patient is printed on encounter sheets, which were previously produced manually. The encounter sheets are then completed by the physician. The sheets are also legible for the staff who reenter the data in the computer system. The billing system is also computerized, and this also reduces the workload of the clerical staff. Lists of physician offices are all generated by computer. Patients coming in can be listed according to chart number, which makes it easier for the clerical staff to pull charts.

Much of the difficulty in maintaining a denominator can be overcome by the use of a reminder system in a practice. Our software generates the reminders automatically. We have chosen the patient's birthday as the date to trigger an assessment of preventive activity for the patient in the preceding year and to print a reminder for any procedure not done at the recommended frequency. This kind of software is relatively inexpensive and simple to apply.

In the process of determining the preventive health status of the practice population this system also identifies patients who have not visited the practice for a year. This makes the practice denominator more accurate since inactive patients can be contacted to determine whether they have changed physicians or still consider themselves patients. This may be the most efficient way a practice can maintain a denominator and at the same time provide appropriate preventive care.

The staff have been enthusiastic about the computer. Although our nurses feel that the workload generated by the phone calls is somewhat burdensome they consider it justified and worthwhile. When the results have been completely analyzed, we will probably choose the physician reminder system as the primary reminder, and on each patient's birthday we will scan each chart to determine what appropriate preventive procedures have not been carried out. A letter would be sent to those under 65 and a phone call to those over 65. I believe that this system will achieve a high level of preventive screening in our practice.

The hardware and software required to conduct all of the steps described are currently available for about $7,000, including three monitors, three terminals, a computer, a disk drive, and a printer, adequate hardware for a single-physician office. In our practice there are six physicians and 30 residents. We have a network system of eight screens, three IBM-PC computers, two printers, and three disk drives. The total cost of this system was about $35,000 including hardware and software. The software was developed in our own setting, and is now available for purchase.

The development of this system was financed by convincing the hospital that the approach was more efficient. The hospital has been consistently impressed by the savings in money and staff time and

has continued to fund the system. More efficiency and cost-effectiveness is possible in a group COPC practice. The staff feel more involved in their work with the reduction of boring and redundant components of the workload. Several private practices in Ontario and Quebec have already adopted this system and are very happy with it. It probably is less cost-effective in a single or solo practice than in a larger group practice.

The hardware will eventually become less expensive, but the importance of the quality of the software cannot be over-emphasized. The flexibility of software is exceptionally important in the practical application of computer systems in practice.

IMPLICATIONS FOR THE FUTURE

The application of computers in primary care practice for prevention and case finding interventions has great potential. It has been estimated that in 5 years at least 80-90 percent of primary care practices will be using computers (6). If all primary care practitioners obtain patient tracking and recall systems for both preventive and case finding procedures, the impact on the health care of the nation will be significant. Although the glamor research focuses on artificial hearts and organ transplants, a far larger impact on the health of the population would accrue from effective and widely used methods to improve preventive screening procedures.

It is likely that the major advances in health care research in the next 10 to 20 years will be in prevention. One would hope for vaccines that could prevent cancer, heart disease, and other common conditions. The major breakthroughs are likely to require preventive procedures that will have to be carried out on the whole population or on an identifiable high-risk group. When discoveries are made, the obligation will be on primary care practitioners to get the intervention rapidly out to the appropriate population.

The practice denominator allows identification of high-risk groups according to diagnostic criteria, drug-taking criteria, or other health indices. We will need the capacity to assess people rapidly using reminders and to know what percentage of our practice population has received the procedure. An example from our current study is a process of identifying all the smokers in our practice. Unfortunately, after 8 years of research no effective intervention for smoking cessation has been found (7). Nevertheless, were such an intervention available, we would be in a position to identify and recall all the smokers in our practice denominator.

On the research agenda for the future are the noncompliers in any practice who do not receive preventive procedures. An example is found in the screening for Pap smears. We now anticipate that about 75-80 percent of our patients under 35 will have a Pap smear done annually. There is considerable evidence that those who do not receive the test are the individuals at highest risk for developing cervical cancer (8). The next step will be to determine how to narrow that gap and motivate the noncompliant group to have their Pap smear, since cancer of the cervix is theoretically a cause of mortality that could be eradicated.

CONCLUSION

The great advantage of community-oriented primary care practice is that the target community is defined, its health problems identified, and emphasis programs directed at those individuals in the population at risk. This chapter has proposed a method to both administer and monitor preventive care, to identify high-risk groups and remind them to have procedures done, and to identify those at high risk who are not compliant. This allows us to study improved approaches for giving our patients appropriate preventive interventions.

Critics of this approach have argued that patients should be responsible for their own preventive care. Our experience is that most people are not fully aware of the preventive procedures they should have, and that many appreciate their physician taking the responsibility of identifying their preventive care needs and reminding them. This approach for community-oriented primary care practices appears feasible and is probably cost-effective in most settings. It is likely to have a greater impact on public health than most of the high-profile surgical and chemotherapeutic procedures.

REFERENCES

1. Lalonde, M. *A New Perspective on the Health of Canadians: A Working Document*. Report from the Minister of Health and Welfare, Government of Canada, Ottawa, April 1974.

2. Elmslie, T., and Rosser, W. Computerization of Family Practice. *Canadian Medical Association Journal* 1986; 134:221

3. *Periodic Health Examination: Report of a Task Force to the Conference of Deputy Ministers of Health* (Monograph). Health and Welfare Canada, 1980.

4. Frank, J. W.; Henderson, M.; and McMurray, L. Influenza vaccination in the elderly: 1. Determinants of acceptance. *Canadian Medical Association Journal* 1985; 132:371.

5. Frank, J. W.; McMurray, L.; and Henderson, M. Influenza vaccination in the elderly: 2. The economics of sending reminder letters. *Canadian Medical Association Journal* 1985; 132:516.

6. Rosenblatt, R. (Washington State University), personal communication.

7. McDowell, I.; Mothersill, K.; Rosser,

W.; and Hartman, R. A randomized trial of three approaches to smoking cessation. *Canadian Family Physician* 1985; 31:845.

8. *Cervical Cancer Screening Programs 1982.* Report of a Task Force Reconvened by the Health Services Directorate, Health Services and Promotion Branch, Health and Welfare Canada, Ottawa, September 1982.

CHAPTER 33

Targeting Individuals
at Risk

Paul A. Nutting, M.D.

Efforts to target services on high-risk individuals have been an integral part of primary care for some time. Notions of risk first emerged in obstetrics and were later incorporated into programs of maternal and child health. In prenatal care, programs typically define high risk as the presence of one or more risk factors (gravida, age, and history of adverse pregnancy outcome). Patients are assessed for risk factors as they present for prenatal care, and those with a high-risk profile are offered special services aimed at reducing their risk. This approach allows practitioners to target emphasis services on those among their active patients at increased risk, but does not enhance the ability to identify and target services on those high-risk individuals in the community who do not seek care.

When notions of risk are applied to community-based programs several obstacles generally impede maximum program impact. First, most programs approach the high-risk group in the community as an abstraction, and only identify individuals at risk when they present for care, identifying the risk group in terms of risk factors, but are unable to seek out other at-risk individuals within the population. Often

programs rest on an unspoken assumption that the individuals at increased risk will somehow emerge from the population and present for services. It is assumed that they are out there and if a large enough program is mounted, they will be reached. Further, many programs address a global high-risk group — the high-risk pregnancy and the high-risk infant — as though all were at equal risk to a single adverse outcome. In reality any given infant may be at increased risk for a number of poor health outcomes while at reduced risk for others. While it is clear that some risk factors may predict risk for a constellation of adverse events, all infants at risk for developmental retardation are not at risk for gastroenteritis. Lack of specificity in the predicted adverse event not only makes the prediction more difficult, it also leaves the practitioner at a loss as to the service(s) that should be provided once the high-risk patient is identified.

Community-oriented primary care offers an opportunity to expand the scope of risk targeting to all high-risk individuals within the denominator population. In an ideal world, the COPC practitioner could query his data system for a particular high-risk group. The response would be a listing of all individuals in the denominator population, sorted in order of decreasing risk. Even better, this ideal data system would predict not only risk, but the potential benefit to be derived from one or more intervention strategies, resulting in a more specific priority listing, headed by the individuals with the greatest probability of benefit from the proposed intervention.

While this level of sophistication is well beyond the current state of the art, the COPC practitioner can begin to direct services differentially in favor of high-risk individuals. Doing so is fraught with difficulties, but when successful, risk targeting can have a dramatic impact on the health status of the denominator population. This approach is particularly applicable to programs that can enumerate their denominator population, such as practices that address their active patients, practice communities, enrolled populations, or programs with a defined beneficiary population such as the Indian Health Service.

The following describes the development of a risk targeting effort and provides an example. The process is described as a sequence of activities, but in reality one moves back and forth among the steps, since decisions made in one step influence the variables in the others.

SELECT A HEALTH PROBLEM

A relatively common, yet important, problem should be selected that has one or more adverse outcomes that are preventable through either primary care or community-based health services. Most primary care practitioners are in an ideal situation to generate a long list of such problems, simply by asking after each patient seen, "Could this problem have

been prevented or lessened in severity if I had known before that *this* patient was at risk?"

It is also useful to think of the problem sequence in terms of stages of progression. Each stage represents a potential point of intervention, and proactive preventive strategies may be more appropriate at some stages than at others. For example, gastroenteritis in infants might be viewed as a four-stage process, as shown in Figure 1.

In many settings, it may be impractical or clinically infeasible to impact significantly between Stages 0 and 1. Nonetheless, education of the parents in early recognition and response to mild diarrhea may have an important effect in preventing progression to Stage 2. Early parental recognition of Stage 2 and aggressive clinical intervention may also be expected to prevent progression from Stage 2 to Stage 3.

IDENTIFY RISK FACTORS

Risk factors must be identified that are predictive of the adverse outcomes selected in the previous step. Since risk factors will be used in this effort to identify individuals at risk, the factors selected must be predictive, but need not be causally related to the adverse event. Of course, when causal risk factors can be found that predict outcomes in the relatively near term, interventions can be aimed at removing the risk factor. By comparison, removing a factor that is predictive, but not causal, may be desirable but will not necessarily prevent the outcome in question.

Consideration should be given to risk factors that are stable over time, that can be assessed for all members of the denominator population, and are predictive of outcomes occurring in the relatively near

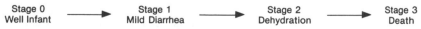

Stage 0   Stage 1   Stage 2   Stage 3
Well Infant   Mild Diarrhea   Dehydration   Death

Figure 1. Staging of Infant Gastroenteritis.

term. Practical considerations related to collecting risk factor data on all appropriate members of the denominator population will usually delimit the final set of risk factors that can be used.

The medical and epidemiologic literature is producing a great deal of information on risk factors, particularly for cancer and cardiovascular disease. While attention should be given to risk factors validated by large data sets, these causally related factors often account for less than 30 percent of the variation in morbidity seen, and may not perform well enough alone. They can be supplemented by other factors, some of which may be unique to the community. Typically, the collective wisdom of the health professionals and community participants can identify a set of risk factors that will perform quite adequately for the community under study.

DETERMINE RISK CRITERIA

In addition to selecting a set of risk factors that predict adverse outcomes, criteria need to be developed that identify the individual at increased risk. Several approaches can be used. The simplest is to set a threshold criterion that distinguishes between high and low risk. For example, if eight risk factors are used, a threshold criterion might define high risk as the presence of factors A or B, or any three or more factors. Another approach is to assign numeric weights to each of the risk factors, based on their presumed predictive power. Thus the risk score for any individual is the sum of the weights of the risk factors present. In this approach, risk can be defined as a score above a certain threshold. The advantage of this approach is the ability to define several levels of risk (e.g. low, moderate, and high) and the ability to rank individuals by their risk score. Both advantages rest on the assumption that the risk scores reflect a real difference in outcomes. A disadvantage is that many risk factors are redundant, such that if one is used the other does not contribute to the predictive power of the criteria. Thus risk scores computed as the sum of several such factors result in an inflated score.

Where possible, it is best to validate the risk criteria with data from the denominator population. Even a relatively small data set can be useful in identifying risk factors with predictive power within the local setting. Where such a data set is available, the "split-sample" technique can be used to randomly sort the population into two groups. The first can be used to generate risk criteria, while the second is used to test the performance of the criteria selected.

In testing the performance of risk criteria, false positive and false negative rates are of particular importance. Generally, the false negative rate, a measure of the percent of patients judged to be at low risk who subsequently suffer the adverse event, should be minimized. Although it is not suggested that, under normal circumstances, services should be withheld from low-risk patients, false negative predictions represent patients who might have benefited from the intervention had they been correctly identified as high risk. While less critical, the false positive rate should be held as low as practical. Emphasis services for the high-risk group generally carry little or no risk, but a substantial false positive rate indicates that the relatively scarce resources that are to be targeted on the high-risk individuals are being used for those who would not have suffered the adverse outcome in the absence of intervention. Thus a high false positive rate decreases the efficiency of the risk targeting effort. In reality, one usually faces a tradeoff between false positive and negative rates. A useful risk criterion will minimize the false negative rate, while running a false positive rate that can be afforded in terms of program resources.

The risk criteria can also be adjusted to identify a particular number of individuals as high risk depending on the resources available for intervention. For example, in a population that produces 2,000 pregnant women per year of which 200 are at high risk, risk criteria that identify 800 individuals at increased risk will be of little benefit (regardless of the false positive and negative rates) if resources are only available to provide targeted services for 300 individuals. Again one faces a tradeoff among the competing demands of the false negative rate and the resources available to target services on the high-risk group.

SELECT FROM A RANGE OF INTERVENTION STRATEGIES

Potential intervention strategies should be considered for each stage of the problem sequence based on their anticipated impact, cost, feasibility, and acceptability to the community. Possible interventions include those that can be implemented totally within the primary care practice and those that require collaboration among other community programs. Intervention clusters aimed at different stages of the problem sequence and implemented by different cooperating health programs are often effective. For example, after a community education effort, targeted through the local media at the entire community, a focused outreach effort may be directed to at-risk individuals by the community health nursing program. In support, the primary care clinicians may be alerted to and target emphasis services on high-risk individuals when they are encountered in the primary care setting.

DEVELOP A "SAFETY NET" STRATEGY

At each decision stage in developing a risk targeting program, one should balance the program design against the resources directed at individuals of varying risk. Risk targeting programs are intended to direct special attention to individuals at risk who might not otherwise receive and benefit from them. This does not mean that resources be *diverted* from individuals or groups currently receiving them on the basis of the risk criteria. In any program, however, emphasis in one area inevitably leads to unintended deemphasis in another. Even when risk criteria have been carefully validated, there will be significant false positive and false negative rates resulting from application of the criteria to the total community. For programs intended to identify individuals at risk for emergent or life-threatening conditions, the false negative rate is of greatest concern, since it reflects those individuals judged at low risk but subsequently experiencing a preventable outcome. For programs that strive to identify individuals at risk for less immediate outcomes, the consequences of errors in predicting risk will be less worrisome. As noted above, the risk criteria are developed to minimize false negatives. Risk criteria are seldom developed and validated with great rigor in the local setting. Consequently, the practitioner should carefully think through the implications of the overall plan to ensure that patients needing or seeking services will not be deprived of them as a result of the risk targeting effort.

At the conclusion of the planning phase, a health problem will have been selected and one or more stages of the problem sequence will have been determined to be appropriate for intervention. The practitioner should also have developed a set of risk factors, the criteria for defining increased risk, and a plan for collecting the risk factor data for all members of the denominator population. All participating programs should help in selecting intervention strategies based on the intervention's potential impact on the distribution of primary care services.

Collecting risk factor data on all appropriate individuals in the denominator population often represents a major cost of the overall effort. Occasionally data will be readily available in either a data system or in the health records of cooperating programs. More often, the data for many of the risk factors must be gathered de novo. Since many risk factors are often subjective in nature, the best and most economical sources of data may be the collective wisdom of those who have worked closely with the health of the community. An approach to collecting risk factor information on the community is described in the following example.

TARGETING INFANTS AT RISK FOR GASTROENTERITIS — AN EXAMPLE

An early effort at risk targeting was developed in the Indian Health Service. Although it occurred several years ago, it was developed in a research and development environment, and thus generated a great deal of information on the design, implementation, and impact of the effort. Consequently, it serves well as an example of the feasibility of identifying specific risk groups, the impact achievable when services are targeted differentially on them, and the ways one might be fooled in monitoring the impact of such an effort if the evaluation does not properly account for the high-risk group.

The Setting

The 10,000-square-mile Papago Indian Reservation in south central Arizona is home for more than 8,000 Papago Indians. The Papagos are one of the few tribes that occupy their ancestral land, and the desert area of southern Arizona has been their home for many generations. The Papago Tribe is highly organized with an elected Tribal Council that delegates all matters pertaining to health to its appointed health board. The board, called the Executive Health Staff, is composed of the directors of the several health programs operated by the Tribe, contracting with and operating closely with the service programs of the Indian Health Service.

Primary health care for the Papago community is provided by the Indian Health Service. At the time of this study the medical staff consisted of five full-time physicians and a full complement of nurses, laboratory workers, and other health care support personnel. Health care services are provided from several sites including a 50-bed hospital and outpatient department in the main town of Sells, a full-time outpatient clinic in Santa Rosa, and two field clinics operating one day a week in the villages of Pisinimo and Chui Chu. Outreach services are provided by community health nurses (working for the Indian Health Service) and several tribal health programs, which include community health representatives who are general health ombudsmen, a disease control program, and a nutrition program.

The health care system is supported by a sophisticated health information system that processes essential health care data from all patient encounters within the total health care program, and provides an on-line integrated patient record available to the provider on each patient visit. This record integrates encounter data from visits made to any of the clinics and the hospital, as well as home visits made by field health personnel. Selected referral and consultation data are also incorporated. While the presence of this data system permitted a number of innovations in the delivery of health services, the COPC emphasis program to be described was conducted largely independent of the data system.

The Problem

For many years the Papago community experienced an annual summer epidemic of deaths among young children due to the combination of a seasonal increase in the incidence of gastroenteritis and a set of adverse environmental circumstances. The combination of desert heat and low humidity, inadequate sanitary conditions, and an incomplete understanding of the importance of early recognition and treatment of diarrhea in infants, took a severe toll in terms of morbidity and mortality, most pronounced among infants in the population.

In 1972 an attempt was made to approach the problem in a systematic manner. From a review of deaths in 1970 and 1971 it was clear that there was considerably more morbidity and mortality than was justified given the etiology (often viral) nature of the seasonal peak, and the sophistication and capability of the health care system. As shown in Table 1, the mortality rate for gastroenteritis, the mean episodes per child, and hospital utilization for gastroenteritis were excessive.

TABLE 1. Indices of infant gastroenteritis for 1970-1971

	1970 (N = 128)	1971 (N = 108)
Infant deaths due to gastroenteritis	10 (7.8%)	12 (11.1%)
Mean episodes of gastroenteritis	2.3	2.8
Mean outpatient visits per infant[1]	3.1	3.4
Hospital admissions per 100 infants[1]	102	126
Hospital days per 100 infants[1]	612	1008

[1] Rates are computed for a 6-month time frame (July-December) representing the peak endemic season for gastroenteritis.

The clinical progression of gastroenteritis in the infant population can be thought of in terms of the four stages shown in Figure 1. Based in large part on the experience of tribal outreach personnel, our initial impression was that episodes of diarrhea in infants generally came to medical attention in the third or fourth day and too often after the child was dehydrated. Parental response to diarrhea was often slow and in many cases inappropriate. We concluded that all deaths could have been averted and many hospitalizations prevented by early recognition and response to the onset of diarrhea and particularly to the early signs of dehydration. Consequently, a risk targeting effort was developed to predict those infants who would develop gastroenteritis with dehydration (Stage 2) during the endemic peak. Services were to be targeted on these infants in an attempt to both prevent dehydration during episodes of diarrhea and to intervene early when dehydration did occur in order to prevent death.

Identification of Risk Factors

Based in part on a study of the diarrhea experience in the previous year, but largely on the insights and experiences of the outreach workers, 11 risk factors were identified that were felt to be predictive of severe gastroenteritis. Of these, shown in Table 2, only a few were readily available in the health record. Clearly, using these risk factors involved a higher cost for collecting them for the total infant population, but the outreach personnel felt that they could readily indicate those risk factors present for each of the infants in their districts, if given a list and ample time to do so.

The list of infants comprising the target population was generated from the computerized data system. The list was subdivided by district and reviewed for accuracy by district outreach personnel. Finally, the outreach personnel made an

TABLE 2. Risk factors and numerical weights for each used for computing risk to gastroenteritis

Risk Factor	Point value
1. Age less than 1 year	2
2. Birthweight less than six pounds	2
3. Principal guardian under 20 years or over 40	1
4. Residence in high-risk village	1
5. Last weight less than 10th percentile	2
6. Last weight less than 3rd percentile	2
7. More than five siblings	1
8. Family tends to child neglect	1
9. Alcoholism in parent/ guardian	1
10. Mental problems in parent/guardian	1
11. Overcrowded home	1

assessment of the risk factors present for each infant, among those infants with whose families they were familiar. In most cases two outreach personnel covered the same district, and duplicate assessments were made for most infants.

Development of the Risk Criteria

Point values (1 or 2 points) were assigned to each of the risk factors (shown in Table 2) based on the presumed predictive power of the individual factors. For several of the factors, an association had been shown by the data from the previous year. An infant's risk score was computed by summing the points for the risk factors present. This permitted risk to be expressed as a

continuous variable ranging from 0 to 13 points.

The criterion for high risk was determined empirically. Data on risk factors were gathered for each infant, and when risk scores were computed they suggested a bimodal distribution — one distribution of infants with 0-3 risk points, and a smaller distribution with 4 or more factor points. Using 4 or more points as the definition of high risk identified about 45 percent of the infant population as the high-risk group, as shown in Table 3. It was felt by the cooperating programs that the resources to target intervention services on this number of infants could be justified without seriously jeopardizing other ongoing efforts.

TABLE 3. Distribution of the infant population on the basis of risk level.

Risk level	Factor points	No. of infants
Average risk	0 to 3	118 (55%)
High risk	4 or more	97 (45%)
	Total	215 (100%)

It is important to emphasize that this process did not define some hypothetical high-risk group that hopefully could be reached by mass action. This process identified specific infants at risk — we knew who they were and where they lived. Consequently, we were able to target specific educational material at the guardian of the high-risk infant. Precise targeting of information to the high-risk group was possible and feasible for two simple reasons. First, we could presumably reach all the high-risk infants by focusing on less than half of the infant population, and second, we knew exactly who they were.

Development of an Intervention Strategy

In conjunction with the Tribal health programs a two-pronged attack was devised. First, we would attempt to reach the guardians of all high-risk infants and provide education in their homes covering the treatment of diarrhea and the recognition and response to dehydration. Second, we would arm the Tribal outreach workers with a means of early recognition and response to gastroenteritis and to the signs of dehydration.

A simple educational task was designed emphasizing five basic points:

1. The importance of diarrhea as a symptom in children;
2. The early home treatment of mild diarrhea, using an electrolyte solution;
3. The critical nature of dehydration;
4. The recognition of early signs of dehydration; and finally,

5. The appropriate response to dehydration.

Outreach workers were trained and provided with graphic material to support and emphasize the message. Having been given a list of the high-risk infants living in their districts, they were asked to visit each twice to provide the educational material and to leave with the guardian a six-pack of prepackaged electrolyte solution.

To extend to the outreach workers an early recognition and response capability, we developed a protocol that guided the health worker through a problem-solving process. At the heart of the protocol was a staging matrix, shown in Figure 2, that specified the items of information required to determine the level of severity of any infant with diarrhea. When the response item appropriate to that child was circled

PROBLEM: DIARRHEA
AGE: BABIES (up to 3 years old)

INFORMATION GATHERING	STAGE 1	STAGE 2	STAGE 3	STAGE 4
Subjective:				
1. Is the baby less than 3 months old?	No			
2. What is the baby's risk level? Average High				
3. Is the diarrhea mushy? for how many days?	1–4	5–7	Over 7	
4. How many in the last 6 hours?	1–3	4–5	Over 5	
5. Is the diarrhea liquid? for how many days?	1	2	Over 2	
6. How many in the last 6 hours?	1	2–3	Over 3	
7. Is there blood in the diarrhea?	No		Yes	
8. Is there mucus in the diarrhea?	No	Yes		
9. Is the baby vomiting?	No	Yes		
10. How many days?	1	2	Over 2	
11. How many times in the last 6 hours?	1	2	Over 2	
12. Can the baby keep down clear fluids?	Yes		No	
13. Is the baby urinating a normal amount?	Yes		Decreased	
Objective:				
14. Rectal temperature	98°–102°	102°–103°	Over 103°	
15. Making tears when crying	Yes		Decreased	No
16. Soft spot (fontanelle)	Normal			Fallen
17. Lining of mouth	Moist			Dry/Sticky
18. Eyes look sunken in	No			Yes
19. Skin tenting	No			Yes

Figure 2. Staging Mechanism for Gastroenteritis in Children Under 3 Years of Age.

for each required item of information, the health worker could determine the stage of severity by noting the highest stage with one or more circled responses. The protocol also included the appropriate response for each stage of severity including instruction in the care of the child, provision of electrolyte solution, referral to a physician, or transport to the hospital. Training and supervision was provided and the health workers, armed with these tools, began their efforts in the summer of 1972.

IMPACT OF THE PROGRAM

Initial evaluation efforts focused on the accuracy of the risk criteria and the methods for identifying the high-risk subset of infants. While the project was not set up as a randomized clinical trial, the absence of health workers in some districts did permit us to examine the gastroenteritis experience of some infants predicted at high risk but not treated with educational intervention. For each of the 95 infants

TABLE 4. Accuracy of risk prediction. Comparison of expected and observed morbidity due to gastroenteritis. Untreated average- and high-risk groups (p < .001)

		Predicted Risk Level	
		Average	High
	Average (less than 5 points)	62	6
Observed morbidity (July thru December)			
	Excessive (5 or more points)	1	26

TABLE 5. Indices of infant gastroenteritis for 1970-1973

	1970 (N = 128)	1971 (N = 108)	1972 (N = 116)	1973 (N = 123)
Infant deaths due to gastroenteritis	10 (7.8%)	12 (11.1%)	0	0
Mean episodes of gastroenteritis	2.3	2.8	2.1	2.4
Mean outpatient visits per infant[1]	3.1	3.4	3.3	3.1
Hospital admissions per 100 infants[1]	102	125	53	67
Hospital days per 100 infants[1]	612	1008	287	325

[1] Rates are computed for a 6-month timeframe (July-December) representing the peak endemic season for gastroenteritis.

who did not receive the educational intervention, morbidity scores were computed to quantify their morbidity experience over the course of the endemic peak. The procedure assigned 1 point for each episode of gastroenteritis and 4 points for each hospital day. There was a natural split in the distribution of morbidity points at 5, and this was assumed to separate infants with (possibly) several episodes of mild diarrhea from those with diarrhea severe enough to require hospitalization.

Table 4 presents data comparing the prediction of morbidity with the observation of morbidity in this group. Of the 27 infants with excessive morbidity, the model correctly predicted 26 for a sensitivity of 96 percent (false negative rate of 4 percent). Of the 68 infants with none or mild gastroenteritis, the model correctly predicted 62 for a false positive rate of 9 percent. This proved to be an unusually accurate risk prediction, and was difficult to reproduce on later applications. Similar programs for other health problems were successful even though risk criteria had false negative rates in the range of 20 percent and false positive rates as high as 40-50 percent.

The impact of the overall program was evaluated in two ways, first by examining the population indices of gastroenteritis over the 2 years after the program. Table 5 expands the indices of Table 1 and includes data for the next 2 years. Clearly, the mortality rate changed, but no changes in morbidity nor in outpatient clinic utilization were observed. Nonetheless, hospital utilization (probably reflecting more severe episodes) did show a decrease, both in the number of admissions and in the total hospital days for gastroenteritis.

A more focused look at the impact of the intervention program examined the morbidity experience of the treated and untreated children and compared the impact in the high-risk and low-risk groups. Table 6 compares the mean morbidity scores for 172 infants for 2-month periods before (June and July) and after (October and November) the intervention was applied for those infants treated. These data illustrate a critically important point. There was no impact of the educational intervention on the average risk group, but there was a substantial, dramatic, and statistically significant impact on the infants identified at high risk.

TABLE 6. Impact of educational task on infants. At differing levels of predicted risk. Morbidity before and after the educational task. (Decrease is statistically significant only for the high-risk group, p < .05)[1]

Group		No. of patients	Morbidity points per infant per month	
			Before	After
Average-risk	Treated	34	0.53	0.08
Average-risk	Untreated	63	0.22	0.13
High-risk	Treated	43	10.26	0.06
High-risk	Untreated	32	3.66	8.00

[1] Morbidity scores were calculated for each infant using 1 point for each episode of gastroenteritis and 4 points for each hospital day caused by gastroenteritis.

TABLE 7: Incidence of severe gastroenteritis in children. There is a significant difference, p < 0.01, between the treated and untreated groups at the high-risk level, but no significant difference in the average-risk group or for all risk levels combined.

	Average risk		High risk		All risk levels	
	Untreated	Treated	Untreated	Treated	Untreated	Treated
None or mild Gastroenteritis only	116 (79)%	42 (71%)	8 (17%)	53 (68%)	124 (64%)	95 (69%)
One or more episodes of severe gastroenteritis	31 (21%)	17 (29%)	39 (83%)	25 (32%)	70 (36%)	42 (31%)
Totals	147 (100%)	59 (100%)	47 (100%)	78 (100%)	194 (100%)	137 (100%)

DISCUSSION

In summary, this program was able to achieve an important impact on the mortality and the incidence of severe morbidity due to gastroenteritis in this community. The intervention was simple and straightforward. The impact was achieved largely by targeting the intervention on specific individuals, identified prospectively at high risk, rather than on mass education or services attempting to reach all members of the infant population.

We learned four important lessons from this experience and went on to apply them successfully in subsequent COPC activities.

First, it is clearly possible and often feasible to identify specific individuals at high risk for a particular problem. While the risk criteria in this effort were extremely accurate, we subsequently were able to implement other successful risk targeting programs with less accurate risk predictions.

Second, we learned that simple, straightforward educational tasks may have an important impact on high-risk individuals. As clinicians we often cast a jaundiced eye on patient education as a truly effective intervention strategy. The lesson we learned and reinforced with later programs is that patient education *may*

have a very dramatic effect when targeted on high-risk individuals.

Third, this impact may not be apparent unless the analysis of impact is directed specifically at the high-risk group. This is an extremely important point and is illustrated by the data of Table 7.

If we had simply compared the experience of the treated and untreated children without regard to risk level (third column), we would have seen no important or statistically significant differences. We might have rationally concluded that the educational task had no effect in reducing the incidence of severe gastroenteritis. However, there is both an important and statistically significant impact on the high-risk group (second column). This is of course due to the lack of impact in the numerically larger low-risk group (first column), which in the aggregate obscures the important impact in the smaller high-risk group.

Fourth, standard population parameters, while readily available and often extremely important tools for monitoring impact, may not adequately reflect the impact on the different risk groups.

The risk targeting program described was an ambitious effort and one that may not be readily duplicated in all primary care settings. The often life-threatening nature of the problem addressed and the critical timing of the intervention during the endemic season dictated that accuracy of the risk prediction be as high as possible, thus increasing the overall cost of the program. On the other hand, the presence of outreach personnel, who knew the communities and their residents very well, greatly facilitated the project. This enabled us to develop a list of the infant subset of the population and collect the risk factor data for each infant.

While in this example, errors in the risk prediction or delay of the educational intervention could have had visible and serious consequences, other programs may not need to meet similar standards of accuracy of the risk prediction model, and consequently will be less expensive to implement. Examples include efforts that target preventive or screening services on high-priority groups, e.g., individuals in need of flu vaccine, mammography, etc.

Risk targeting efforts can be conducted in a variety of settings and with a range of resources, if the basic purposes of the effort are kept well in mind. The important principle is to identify *individuals* with an increased risk to a specific adverse event (relative to similar individuals in the population) toward whom an intervention can be targeted that will prevent or lessen the impact of the occurrence. The key is to identify individuals — not abstract groups — and to target services on those individuals. The accuracy of the risk criteria is critical if either the adverse event is life-threatening or if there is a likelihood that resources used to target the high-risk group will be inadvertently redirected away from individuals previously receiving needed services. Otherwise, concern for the accuracy of the risk criteria need not impede efforts to target high-risk individuals.

The ideal setting would be one that had a data system that included for each individual in the community at least identifying address. The availability of specific risk factor data would be a bonus, and for acute problems difficult to plan into a data system. The kind of risk factor data useful in targeting efforts are difficult to anticipate prior to selecting the health problem, and the data often change for any given individual over time.

Relatively modest efforts to target health promotion and disease prevention services on risk groups could be accomplished in a variety of settings and may be particularly appropriate to practices or programs addressing a "practice community." With the increasing use of practice-based computers, many practitioners could develop a modest data base on all members of the practice community, including such items as age, sex, occupation, major health problems, weight, smoking habits, exercise habits, and height. This data set could be gathered on all household members at the time of registration of the patient and would provide the basic data necessary to identify specific individuals potentially in need of a variety of screening, educational, and therapeutic services. A conditional retrieval of the data base, listing all individuals over the age of 65 years or individuals with cardiovascular or chronic pulmonary disease, would identify a subset of the denominator population potentially at increased risk for complications of influenza. For this subset the physician could compose a letter outlining the epidemiologic patterns of influenza and the relative protection afforded by annual immunization. The letter could further indicate that the immunization is available from the practice or could be requested from the patient's usual source of physician care. Similarly, this modest data base further could be used to identify subsets of the denominator population who would benefit from specific services related to cancer screening (e.g., Papanicolaou smear, mammography, rectal examination, flexible sigmoidoscopy), needed immunizations (e.g., DPT and polio series in children), or health promoting behaviors (e.g., smoking cessation, weight reduction, appropriate exercise patterns).

SUMMARY

A process is described in which the individuals at highest risk within a population may be identified and addressed with emphasis services. The process consists of five discrete steps that include selection of a health problem, identifying relevant risk factors, setting criteria for high risk, selecting an intervention strategy, and developing a "safety net" strategy to ensure that individuals not identified at risk will not receive a lower level of care. The process was illustrated with an example of targeting a subset of the infant population at increased risk to severe gastroenteritis with dehydration. The example demonstrates the feasibility of the approach and the dramatic impact a modest effort can have on reducing the morbidity and mortality of the high-risk subset. Although clinicians do not always show full enthusiasm for intervention strategies based on a health educational strategy, this example demonstrates the dramatic effort achievable from a simple health education task when targeted appropriately on individuals at high risk. Interestingly, the same task had no measurable effect on the larger low-risk population, and an evaluation that had ignored the distinction among high- and low-risk individuals would have concluded erroneously that the educational intervention had no impact.

CHAPTER 34

Health Promoters:
How to Identify and Work
with the Natural
Helpers in a Community

Henry Taylor, M.D.

One important aspect of defining and characterizing the community is to understand the important social networks in the community, how health-related information flows through these networks, and which individuals are influential in each network. One example is the network of individuals to whom others naturally turn for help. These individuals are not always professionals but may be trusted lay persons who are sought for advice, counsel, and support. When these people deal with health issues, I call them "health promoters," although others refer to them as lay health facilitators (1), community health opinion leaders (2), lay health advisors (3), community health advocates (4), community helpers (5), and natural helpers (6). They represent a potential resource for a COPC practice if used appropriately.

Health promoters provide a channel through which the community can express its needs and health professionals can respond with helpful information and appropriate services. Through a "ripple effect," these key individuals reach out to the entire community. In turn, the members of the community respond with their needs and ideas.

Actively collaborating with these individuals facilitates developing the four functions of COPC described earlier in this book; a two-way dynamic is established between individuals in the community and the COPC practice. It then becomes much easier to identify problems, prioritize them, and modify and monitor the health care programs. Program efficiency and integration are enhanced because the community is dealing with individuals it has trusted for years, people who usually give trustworthy information in easily understood terms.

Two similar concepts are interwoven in this chapter: health promoters and informal social networks. *Individual health promoters* are key opinion leaders in the community with regard to health matters who are turned to by members of an *informal social network* (2). The networks can be used to identify health promoters whom the COPC practice can then use to reach target populations. To give a hypothetical example, teenage drug and alcohol abuse prove especially difficult when using the traditional medical model. If, however, the medical system could, by questioning teenaged patients or social contacts, identify and enlist the aid of a teenage opinion leader, a greater impact could be achieved. This individual need not be a teenager; it may also be a trusted teacher, coach, shopkeeper, or parent of a friend.

A growing body of literature in the mental health (7-10), community health education (11-13), medical sociology (14-16), rural health (17), and community development (18) fields provides information helpful in this task. In this chapter, I will summarize examples and methodology from the literature which describe how health professionals can define and work with these natural helpers and the existing informal networks in the community. A few principles and examples will help identify and enhance the natural capabilities of these caring individuals. The overriding goal is to help them do better what they are already doing well.

Social networks have been defined as "a specific set of linkages among a defined set of persons, with the property that the characteristics of these linkages as a whole may be used to interpret the social behavior of the persons involved" (19).

It is important to be aware not only of the relationships between individuals, but the way in which particular individuals may be involved in multiple networks at the same time. It is also important to recognize that while these relationships can be supportive, many are not; a fundamental assumption of this theory is that the relationships can be changed for the better.

DIMENSIONS OF A
SOCIAL NETWORK ANALYSIS

An analysis of social networks needs to consider the following:

The *physical structure* of the network consists of the number, distribution, and density of the relationships of the individuals.

The *dynamic features* of the relationships include many of the qualitative aspects of the interactions between people and the network, for example whether relationships are supportive, how much trust individuals feel towards each other, and whether a particular individual represents a "confidant."

Individuals' perceptions of their networks and the relative importance of individuals within the networks include cognitive, motivational, and affective aspects of the network. Of particular note when considering the role of natural helpers in a network is the observation that people may misperceive whether or not they provide help (5).

Cultural, economic, and political factors affect every relationship and are important in any social network analysis. Many relationships and indeed entire networks can be formed or destroyed as a result of a *single event* that occurs in the community. This was evident in Pendleton County following devastating floods in November 1985. Significant life events such as death, retirement, health problems, or moving, can greatly influence individuals' need for support from a particular network.

The needs of individuals will determine the relationships they form and use. The same person may use different networks to help obtain information, solve problems, or cope with stress. The history of specific relationships can greatly influence all the other factors mentioned. For example, when looking for someone to provide care to an elderly man it would be important to know that he had abused the daughter who has the most time and lives the closest but is unwilling to be involved with her father's care.

IDENTIFYING THE HEALTH PROMOTERS AROUND YOU

The specific way health promoters are defined appears to greatly affect our ability to identify them (20). For example, retired nurses, retired military corpsmen, medical office staff, lay health facilitators, community advocates, natural or spiritual healers, and even experienced mothers are all turned to by other people for health matters, yet they perform different functions.

House and Kahn (21) give a cogent analysis of the problems in defining social networks. The question, "Who do you turn to for advice, counsel, and support?" may be directed to specific problems by adding: "Who do you turn to for advice, counsel, and support when your teenager is pregnant," or ". . . when your child is sick." Alternatively, populations can be identified in the community and one can ask more general questions about members of a specific group: "Who do the elderly turn to for advice, counsel, and support?"

Pancoast (20), working with issues of child abuse and neglect, suggests selecting a "central figure" according to the following criteria: overall program goals and priorities; their stability in the community; their accessibility (I would emphasize access not only in terms of time and geography, but also "psychological access"— their approachability); experience in the problem at hand; and the size of the networks they are central to.

Once these community information sources have been identified, it is useful to consider who they turn to for advice, counsel, and support. These "opinion leaders of opinion leaders" or "bridges" will obviously be very influential. Some call them "head-nodders," those who don't stand at the front during a meeting, but can swing the tide literally with a nod of the head.

SOCIAL SCIENCE METHODS FOR THE COMMUNITY PRACTITIONER

In a small rural community, with a very clearly defined objective (such as providing care for the elderly), informal discussion and observation will be all that is required. For certain sensitive problems, this "depth-first" method (20) is the only practical one, in contrast to "breadth-first" methods (20,22) that survey the informal social networks of the larger community. Surveys are often feared because in academic endeavors they consume excessive time, energy, and manpower. For a COPC practice, such rigor is not always required. A combination of observation, review of secondary data on the community, and key informant surveys as described is a pragmatic compromise.

Four different types of surveys can identify health promoters from four slightly different perspectives:

Key Informants Network Search

The community Health Education program (1) modified the Reputational Analysis Method (23) to create a tool that can be used very quickly with limited manpower (2). Those people most knowledgeable about the community and its interpersonal relationships are interviewed. They include people in prominent occupations such as ministers, shopkeepers, beauticians, postal workers, teachers, and pharmacists, as well as people in service organizations and social agencies. The concept is described to them, and they are asked to provide names of people who might be promoters. Salber has found video "trigger tapes" useful in illustrating the concept. They are also asked to identify others in the community who might know health promoters. By repeating this process over and over, multiple lists of names are developed and compared. Those named most often are health promoters.

Pancoast (20), in identifying informal networks that protect children from abuse and neglect, found it useful to ask: "I am interested in this neighborhood, particularly in its families and children, and was told that you know a good deal about it. May I ask you some questions?" Specific examples of childrearing customs, expectations, and values are solicited. The names of individuals and any comments that reflect their helpfulness are noted. Pancoast also suggests that this is a good time to assess what it would be like to work with these people as health promoters. She cautions that "it is much harder to end a relationship with an unproductive helper, than to decide not to begin it in the first place" (20).

Promoters Network Search

Known health promoters are asked to provide the names of other promoters. A network search then continues as in the key informant search. In fact, many of the key informants mentioned above will turn out to be health promoters themselves. As Salber's program proceeded, health facilitators became a prime source of recruitment.

Users Network Search

In this survey, known users of health promoter services (informally defined at first) are interviewed to determine who they turned to for a variety of problems. In order to fully explore health-seeking behavior, several types of questions are covered:

1. General Questions — about where they turn for advice, counsel, and support.

2. Two-Week Problem Recall — describing who they received advice from for all problems in the past two weeks.

3. Problem Scenarios — asking "who would you call if you wanted to find out about . . . . ?"

Stratified, Random, and Other Sample Surveys

These surveys are identical in format to the users network search, but instead of approaching people through the network process, they use a random cross-section of the community, stratified by geography and other demographic variables.

STARTING TO COLLABORATE WITH HEALTH PROMOTERS

Techniques developed in other sections of this book for effective community participation, particularly in defining and prioritizing community health needs, also apply in this situation:

Learn from those around you. The best information about your community will come from people and organizations who have been successful in your local area. It is particularly important to look at programs that have undertaken a similar process of working with the community. These programs may not necessarily be directed at health, but they may give valuable insights into how your community works. If you are fortunate enough to be part of a practice that has been in existence for several years, you may find a wealth of information in the successes and failures of your own practice. As mentioned above, it is appropriate to be cautious in selecting people, especially at the beginning (20). You must not only observe what others are doing, but talk with the people involved in the program. Often the best insights will come from the field workers or the recipients of the program's services.

Have a clearly defined problem or population that your program will address. Developing the community diagnosis or defining the target population will be much easier if you can involve key opinion leaders from the community. They often have a clarity of insight that comes from years of experience.

Listen very carefully to what opinion leaders are saying. Recognize that they are the experts regarding their community. Even though they may not be able to articulate it in academic terms, they have a depth of awareness that can not be duplicated.

Move slowly. This is particularly important in areas that have not experienced a lot of social change. Many programs take 3 to 5 years to get established. As health professionals we may have biases that work against the true needs of the community. Listening can be time consuming and difficult.

Let the community guide your efforts. This is very difficult for practitioners to do, but vital to program success (5). It seems as though several short discussions are more productive than one extensive discussion. People often need time to ponder the new concepts you are proposing.

QUESTIONS YOU SHOULD ASK YOURSELF

What specific problem or population do I want to start with? You can reach out to include other ones later. A well-defined beginning will become a useful springboard for later expansion. This is reinforced by Pancoast (20) and D'Augelli (5).

What is my agenda? Everyone has one. It is important to be honest about your personal goals. If you are confused about your vision, those you try to explain it to will also be confused. This can easily breed suspicion leading to the program's downfall.

How committed am I to working with individuals in the community?(5) *What level of collaboration do I want?* Don't be afraid to deal with issues of sharing power. There is always a balance of power, even at the extremes.

For example, people can choose to see an arrogant physician, just as physicians and power structures can choose to not work

with too radical a practice.

What effect will I have? ". . . naive intrusions into the social world can unwittingly cause more harm than good, especially if we do not take the individual's view and experience of the network into account" (24).

Do I need to evaluate the program? This may be mandated by funding sources. It obviously appeals to the academic interests of some of us. However, it raises major methodological problems: self-reporting of encounters is unreliable in some situations (20) and followup interviews are unethical if those being helped are not made aware that they may be contacted by someone other than their natural helper (5).

How much can I take on? You will need to know your limitations so you can achieve realistic goals. It may be more appropriate to let another agency in the community work on meeting a particular need. The COPC practice can be instrumental in encouraging efforts by other agencies, or it may be necessary to create a new agency to deal with the problem. In Pendleton County, after the flooding of November 1985, Pendleton Community Care used its resources to work with the local government and other services to develop a centralized relief program.

Am I getting outside my turf? The COPC practice, if it is doing its job right, may find itself in the difficult position of trying to achieve social change without a specific mandate from the community. By collaborating with existing social networks, the COPC practice can often find an appropriate niche. This is essentially a political decision, requiring insight to avoid becoming too closely allied with any one faction. Identifying a problem and mobilizing the community to act on it may require initial involvement by the COPC practice. Once it is started, however, the COPC practice needs a keen sense of timing to decide when to relinquish control. Bowing out too early can weaken support, while staying beyond your welcome can create damaging conflict. The practice needs to constantly assess what its goals are and why.

Do I want my health promoters to be all volunteers? Are there some who should receive reimbursement? In many communities prestige will be all the reimbursement required. If you have identified people who are currently performing a health promoter function in the community, your support and involvement will lend an importance to what they have always been doing. On the other hand, it is important to be sure not to drain their resources. Many times you will need to reimburse expenses, or create financial incentives.

Am I exploiting my health promoters? A program could be designed that would capture talented people from the community and prevent them from further career advancement. The best way to prevent this would seem to be to offer the program as a steppingstone for the health promoters. An example is what happened to the lay health facilitators after the Duke University Community Health Education Program was phased out. Salber provides eloquent individual case studies (24). Several went on to degree programs in nursing, physicians assistants school, public health programs, or hospital administration. However, many facilitators did not change their jobs but returned to the community and situation from which they had come. The overriding principle is to let people choose for themselves.

Is using volunteer and existing informal networks merely a justification for withholding necessary resources? Actually, a well-run program may *increase* the utilization of resources. Pendleton County, West Virginia, was cited by the Physicians Task Force on Hunger in America as being at high risk for hunger because only 30 percent of people eligible for food stamps actually received them (5). If a program

using health promoters were effective in encouraging eligible people to request food stamps, the demand for the local food stamp program could conceivably triple.

Am I trying to reach all the individuals in the community? The health promoters concept is not a panacea. If you have done an effective analysis of the social networks, you should also have defined those individuals who have no support networks. These people will need *additional* formal services. The concept is offered here as one way a COPC practice can take its first steps towards collaborating with the community.

EXAMPLES OF PROJECTS USING HEALTH PROMOTERS

Community Health Workers

Numerous health programs in developing countries have proven the effectiveness of locally recruited and trained Community Health Workers. The World Health Organization emphasized the centrality of the community health worker at the International Conference on Primary Health Care, Alma-Ata, USSR, in 1978:

Primary Health Care is likely to be most effective if it employs means that are understood and accepted by the community and applied by community health workers at a cost the community and country can afford (25).

Newell emphasizes two principles that have relevance to the current U.S. situation: new programs in primary health care can form, reinforce, or recognize a local community organization; and community members can be selected and financed by the community, trained locally for several months, and assume broad responsibilities for promotional, preventive, and curative health (26).

The early U.S. experience with community health aides came from OEO-funded Neighborhood Health Center prototypes such as the Montefiore program in The Bronx (27,28). These aides were shown to be effective, especially in delivering preventive and social services in underserved areas (29-31). However, they are community workers who are hired by the health center to perform certain tasks. Their selection criteria and training may be biased more towards what health professionals feel the community needs, rather than what the community itself perceives its needs to be.

Community Health Education Program (Duke University, Durham, North Carolina)

In a 3-year pilot program in the mid-1970s, 39 lay health facilitators were identified and received training in a wide range of social, economic, environmental, emotional, and family problems, although physical health was the primary focus. The characteristics of the health facilitators and their contacts were evaluated, as were the effects of the training program. Subjective analysis indicated a significant benefit to the community, although the evaluation did not address the program's impact upon health behavior or morbidity.

"The basic aims of the facilitator program remain the same in all situations: (1) to identify those people in a community who give advice, help and comfort to their friends, neighbors, and families; (2) to offer them training which, by increasing their knowledge and skills, enables them to become better advisors and helpers. In this way the natural strengths of a community are reinforced, and natural channels are used for the dissemination of health and health-related information (1)."

The New Mexico Health Education Coalition project was a direct extension that validated several different training approaches in Hispanic, Indian, urban, and rural settings. These projects, pioneered by Dr. Eva Salber, were among the first U.S. programs to work with volunteers. Most of the issues involved in creating an educational program aimed at natu-

ral helpers are well described in a very readable and succinct monograph (1).

Community Health Awareness Training Program[1] (Mountain View Medical Center, Clingman Medical Center, North Carolina Office of Rural Health Services, and The United Way of Wilkes County, North Carolina; Hays, North Carolina)

After 6 months of operation, this program's 60 graduates, with regular supervision and continuing education, are giving health-oriented information and referral sources to neighbors on a one-to-one basis, and have initiated community programs such as walking clubs, blood pressure screenings, distribution of cancer prevention materials, and elderly home-bound visitation. The Program Coordinator is offering weight reduction classes, stress management workshops, and is assisting community groups to set up their own wellness centers. The program is significant for the degree of interagency cooperation, the motivation of its volunteers, its community ownership and community responsiveness, and its relatively low costs. It is becoming an effective channel, not only for educational outreach, but also for collaborating with the community.

The Health and Human Services Project (The General Baptist State Convention, North Carolina)

Implementing the work of Dr. John Hatch in the University of North Carolina-based "Black Churches Project," this program seeks "to create an environment that will be conducive to changing the epidemiological profile of the Black community" (3). It aims to identify and train lay health advisors within their churches and create a formal mechanism within all levels of the church hierarchy that supports health promotion activities. In its first 3 years 200 lay advisors have been

---

[1] This is only one of a burgeoning number of programs applying these concepts to community health education.

trained from 800 churches in 9 counties. Their number of "helping encounters" has almost doubled as a result of the training in how to identify risk factors, recommend preventive practices, refer problems, and practice simple self-help techniques with people from their churches. The training significantly increased the lay health advisors' confidence, prestige, and ability to refer to formal health providers. Most importantly, this program actively involved the individual congregations in the process of selecting people for training.

The Caregivers Project (Pendleton Community Center, Franklin, West Virginia)

The Caregivers Project seeks to enhance the informal community support systems of the elderly in Pendleton County, most of whom have been able to remain in their own homes with the support of caregivers, usually family members or neighbors. This is typical for other areas of West Virginia (22) and for elderly in other parts of the United States (32).

The purpose of the Caregivers Project is to locate caregivers, to describe what they do to help the elderly remain at home, and to have them work with us to enhance their knowledge, skills, and social supports when caring for the elderly.

The project's design is significant because, like the General State Baptist Convention Project, it is attempting to focus on the needs of a target population rather than a specific problem. Like the Community Health Awareness Training Program, it is trying to achieve a high degree of integration with preexisting and ongoing local programs that care for the elderly.

REFERENCES

1. Service, C., and Salber, E.J. (eds.). *Community Health Education: The Lay Advisor Approach.* Durham, NC: Health Care Systems Inc., 1977. Duke University Department of Family and Community Medicine, Durham, NC, 1977, p.58.

2. Bartlett, E.E. Application of the health facilitator concept in four New Mexico communities. In: Service, C., and Salber, E.J. (eds.), *Community Health Education:. The Lay Advisor Approach.* Health Care Systems Inc. Duke University Department of Family and Community Medicine, Durham, NC, 1977, p.58.

3. Hatch, J.W.; Callan, A.E.; Eng, E.; and Jackson, C. The General Baptist State Convention, Health and Human Services Project. *Health and Development*, Winter 1986, p. 12.

4. Callen, W. et. al. MEDEX Program, University of Washington.

5. D'Augelli, A.R.; Vallance, T.R.; Danish, S.J.; Young, C.E.; and Gerdes, J.L. The Community Helpers Project: A description of a prevention strategy for rural communities." *Journal of Prevention*, 1981, 1:209.

6. White, H. Community Health Awareness Training. Mountain View Medical Center, Hays, NC, 1986.

7. Gottlieb, B.H. Social networks and social support: An overview of research, practice, and policy implications. *Health Education Quarterly*, 1985, 12:5.

8. Gottlieb, B.H. *Social Networks and Social Support.* Beverly Hills, CA: Sage Publications, 1983.

9. Erickson, G.D. A framework and themes for social network intervention. *Family Process*, 1984, 23(2):187.

10. Froland, C.; Pancoast, D.L.; Chapman, N.; and Kimboko, P. *Helping Networks and Human Services.* Beverly Hills, CA: Sage Publications, 1981.

11. Israel, B.A. Social networks and social support: Implications for natural helper and community level inter-

ventions. *Health Education Quarterly*, 1985, 12:65.

12. *Health Action! A Medical Self-Help Source.* Kentucky Department of Human Resources, Lexington (undated).

13. *Friends Can Be Good Neighbors.* California Department of Mental Health. Sacramento, CA (undated).

14. Loomis, C.P., and Beegle, J.A. *Rural Sociology: The Strategy of Change.* Englewood Cliffs, NJ: Prentice-Hall, 1957.

15. Rowles, G., personal communication.

16. Cohen, S., and Syme, S.L. (eds.). *Social Support and Health.* New York: Academic Press, 1985.

17. Hassinger, E.W., and Whiting, L.R. (eds.). *Rural Health Services: Organization, Delivery and Use.* North Central Regional Center for Rural Development. Ames, Iowa: Iowa State University Press, 1976.

18. Freire, P. *Pedagogy of the Oppressed.* New York: Seabury Press, 1970.

19. Mitchell, J.C. The Concept and Use of Social Networks. In: Mitchell, J.C. (ed.), *Social Networks in Urban Situations: Analyses of Personal Relationships in Central African Towns.* Manchester, England: Manchester University Press, 1969.

20. Pancoast, D.L. Finding and enlisting neighbors to support families. In: Garbarino, J., and Stocking, S.H. (eds.), *Protecting Children from Abuse and Neglect: Developing and Maintaining Effective Support Systems for Families.* San Francisco: Jossey-Bass, 1980, p. 109.

21. House, J.S.; Kahn, R. et al. Measures and concepts of social support. In: Cohen, S., and Syme, S.L. (eds.), *Social Support and Health.* New York: Academic Press, 1985, p. 91.

22. Rowles, G.D., and Ohta, R.J. (eds.). *Aging and Milieu: Environmental Perspectives on Growing Old.* New York: Academic Press, 1983, p. 117, and personal communication.

23. Hunter, F. *Community Power Structure.* Chapel Hill, NC: University of North Carolina Press, 1953.

24. Snow, D.L., and Gordon, J.B. Social network analysis and intervention with the elderly. *The Gerontologist*, 1980, 20:463.

25. *Primary Health Care.* A joint report by the Director General of the World Health Organization and The Executive Director of the United Nations Children's Fund, about the International Conference on Primary Health Care, Alma-Ata, USSR, 6-12 September 1978. Geneva and New York: WHO, 1978.

26. Newell, K.W. *Health by the People.* Geneva: WHO, 1975, p. 193.

27. Domke, H.R., and Coffey, G. The neighborhood-based public health worker: Additional manpower for community health services. *American Journal of Public Health*, 1966, 56:603.

28. Luckham, J., and Swift, D. Community health aides in the ghetto: the Contra Costa project. *Medical Care*, 1969, 7:332.

29. Cauffman, J.G. et al. Community health aides: How effective are they? *American Journal of Public Health*, 1970, 60:1904.

30. Moore, F.I., and Stewart, J.C. Important variables influencing successful use of aides. *Health Services Report*, 1972, 87:555.

31. Freeborn, D.K.; Mullooly, J.P.; Colombo, T.; and Burnham, V. The

effect of outreach workers' services on the medical care of a disadvantaged population. *Journal of Community Health*, 1978, 3:306.

32. Zarit, S.N., and Summers, T. *Caregivers*, Fall 1985, 10:1.

CHAPTER 35

Integrating Community-Based Health Personnel into the Process of Care

Paul A. Nutting, M.D.

The use of outreach personnel has long played an important role in many community-based programs. Often such personnel are selected from within the community and are expected to provide an important link between the health care program and the community's social networks. While given responsibility for health education, these important components of the health care system seldom take part in direct patient care. The Indian Health Service has a long history of collaborating with village health workers (1-4). The inclusion of these health personnel into direct patient care has, in many cases, substantially magnified the impact of an emphasis program.

One of the challenges of COPC is to target resources on important health problems of the community, by coordinating the efforts of the primary care program with those of other community health programs. Unfortunately, coordination of clinicians and community health programs into an integrated emphasis program has proven difficult. However, if properly structured the work of the outreach worker can play a critical role as a link between the process of health care and the often nonclinical services provided by other community programs.

Auxiliary health workers can be found in a variety of settings and fulfill various roles, many of which are not directly related to health care. They may be called by names that include lay health advisors, community health advocates, and health promoters, among others. In some cases, they are employees of a health program while in other cases they may represent the natural health leaders of the community. For simplicity, the term "health auxiliary" will be used to denote any individual that is a community member and participates in the direct service program, but who may also play a variety of other roles in the community.

The decision to include a community-based health person into an emphasis program is a complex one that is beyond the scope of this chapter. It should be made carefully and should consider the enthusiasm of the individuals, their potential contribution to the emphasis program, the unique skills and insights that they bring to bear on the problem, their other competing activities, and the potential enhancement or damage to their credibility by becoming part of the "system." Key factors to keep clearly in mind are the main role of the auxiliary and the basis of their stature and credibility in the community.

This chapter describes a method for developing the task structure that allows the health auxiliary to function effectively as an outreach member of the primary care team. Guided by a problem-specific protocol, the health auxiliary can extend the process of care beyond the confines of the clinical facility. The activities may reinforce the outreach workers credibility with the community, but will not require so much time as to seriously detract from other important nonprimary care responsibilities. The process of including auxiliaries in an emphasis program can be approached in five steps.

STEP 1: DEVELOP AND DEFINE STAGES OF THE TARGET HEALTH PROBLEM

Defining discrete stages in the progression of a health problem serves several important purposes. First, independent of the use of auxiliary health workers, problem staging supports the overall planning of an emphasis program by identifying points of potential program intervention. Where medical interventions are planned, explicit standards can be formulated for each step of the problem solving process, including information gathering, assessment, and treatment.

Staging the health problem also enhances implementation of the emphasis program by providing a common understanding—one shared by all professional and nonprofessional health care team members—for determining and communicating the severity and appropriate response for a given patient's problem. Depending on the stage involved and its prescribed standard of care, the auxiliary's response may be either direct treatment, referral to a physician[1], and/or followup

activities. Through problem staging, the program's response to any given patient condition will be consistent across the system composed of different health personnel, of differing skill levels, and working in different settings.

Finally, problem staging provides an opportunity to evaluate program effectiveness by measuring patient movement from stage to stage. The rate of transition from one stage to another can be tracked, and the program impact evaluated over time as a reduction in the transition rates of the population (5).

The exact staging scheme for any given health problem will depend on the objectives of the emphasis program and the expected contribution of the health auxiliary. Figures 1 through 4 illustrate staging procedures designed to satisfy four different operational objectives. In all instances, the stage of any given disease case is found after first gathering all necessary items of information and circling a response category for each item, as shown in Figure 1. The stage of the case is then considered to be the highest stage with a circled response.

The staging mechanism shown in Figure 1 is designed to support an emphasis program attempting to intervene early in episodes of gastroenteritis in children under the age of three years. In this case, the staging process defines discrete stages of clinical severity but does not define the etiology of the illness, i.e. bacterial, viral, or parasitic.

The staging mechanism shown in Figure 2 is one of a series in an effort to shift some of the work involved in caring for school children with minor acute problems from a physician to school personnel. In this case, only two stages are

---

[1] Clearly many settings will include certified clinicians other than physicians. For simplicity, however, the term physician will be used to refer to a broad category of clinical practitioners.

INFORMATION GATHERING	STAGE 1	STAGE 2	STAGE 3	STAGE 4
Subjective:				
1. Is the baby less than 3 months old?	No			
2. What is the baby's risk level? Avg High				
3. Is the diarrhea mushy? for how many days?	1–4	5–7	Over 7	
4. How many in the last 6 hours?	1–3	4–5	Over 5	
5. Is the diarrhea liquid? for how many days?	1	2	Over 2	
6. How many in the last 6 hours?	1	2–3	Over 3	
7. Is there blood in the diarrhea?	No		Yes	
8. Is there mucus in the diarrhea?	No	Yes		
9. Is the baby vomiting?	No	Yes		
10. How many days?	1	2	Over 2	
11. How many times in the last 6 hours?	1	2	Over 2	
12. Can the baby keep down clear fluids?	Yes		No	
13. Is the baby urinating a normal amount?	Yes		Decreased	
Objective:				
14. Rectal temperature	98°–102°	102°–103°	Over 103°	
15. Making tears when crying	Yes		Decreased	No
16. Soft spot (fontanelle)	Normal			Fallen
17. Lining of mouth	Moist			Dry/Sticky
18. Eyes look sunken in	No			Yes
19. Skin tenting	No			Yes

Figure 1. Staging Mechanism for Gastroenteritis in Children Under 3 Years of Age.

defined. Stage I describes patients with mild symptoms that could be managed with symptomatic treatment by school staff members, while Stage II includes a category of patients with more serious symptoms, those in which more severe illness should be suspected and referred to the physician.

Figure 3 shows a staging mechanism designed to guide an auxiliary in providing ongoing management for chronic disease patients. Experience from population-based studies suggests that a relatively large number of patients with chronic conditions are often diagnosed, placed on therapeutic regimens, and then lost to followup.

		STAGE I	STAGE II
INFORMATION GATHERING	SUBJECTIVE:		
	Nature of the pain	Mild	Moderate/Severe
	Vomiting more than once in 4 hrs?	No	Yes
	Duration of pain	Less than 2 hrs	2 hrs or more
	Having menstruation or expecting it soon?	No/Yes	—
	Having vaginal bleeding more than normal menstruation?	No	Yes
	Last menstruation?	Less than 2 mos	2 mos or more
	OBJECTIVE:		
	Temperature	Less than 100°	100° or over

Figure 2. Staging Mechanism for a Minor Acute Problem of School-Age Children (Abdominal Pain).

INFORMATION GATHERING	STAGES OF CONTROL			
	STAGE 1	STAGE 2	STAGE 3	STAGE 4
SUBJECTIVE:				
Since last visit has patient developed any of the symptoms or have the symptoms become worse? 1. Nosebleed?	No			Yes
2. Frequent morning headaches (occipital)	No	Yes		
3. Blurring of vision or change in visual acuity?	No	Yes		
4. Fainting	No			Yes
5. Blackouts or lightheadedness on sitting up or standing up?	No		Yes	
6. Chest pain?	No			Yes
7. Shortness of breath?	No		Yes	
8. Skin rash or easy bruising?	No		Yes	
9. Swelling of ankles?	No		Yes	
10. Episodes of depression	No			Yes
OBJECTIVE:				
11. Resting pulse > 100/min or > 40 (record actual #)	No			Yes
12. Resting respirations (record actual #)	< 24		24–30	> 30
13. Weight gain > 4 lb/mo since last recorded weight (actual #)	No		Yes	
14. Swelling of ankles	No	Yes		
15. Presence of skin rash or bruises	No	Yes		
16. Systolic blood pressure (record actual #)	100–200			>200 – < 100
17. Diastolic blood pressure (record actual #)	< 100		100–119	<60 – >120
18. Has patient (under age 45) missed a menstrual period or think she may be pregnant?	No			Yes
19. Is patient following treatment plan?	Yes	No		

Figure 3. The Staging Mechanism for On-going Management of a Chronic Disease (Hypertension).

A potentially important role for the health auxiliary is to follow such patients for set periods of time, referring each back to the physician when followup is needed or when the prescribed therapeutic regimen is no longer adequate. This staging mechanism describes levels of control of the disease process, the presence of drug side-effects, and patient compliance with the therapeutic regimen.

The staging mechanism shown in Figure 4 is designed to help a mental health auxiliary prevent school dropout behavior in boarding school students. Here the staging process defines behavioral problems that are considered antecedents to dropping out of school. In a sense, the process defines levels of risk—how likely a student is to become a dropout—but does not specify a diagnosis, an etiology, or level of severity of the underlying problem per se.

STEP 2: DEFINE THE HEALTH AUXILIARY'S TASKS AND TASK STRUCTURE

The role of the health auxiliary within the emphasis program will be determined largely by the overall program objectives and the stage(s) of the health problem at which intervention is to be attempted. To the fullest extent possible, the auxiliaries should be incorporated into the heart of the emphasis program rather than given an isolated set of activities. Too often health auxiliaries are trained to take blood pressures, for example, and sent off into the community with very little thought as to how the "system" will respond to positive screens that they discover. This creates a situation in which the auxiliary is seen by the community as an isolated (and ignored) appendage of the health care system and may undermine the considerable credibility of the auxiliary in their other roles in the community.

A patient's condition often requires two or more tasks, often separated in time, and the auxiliary must be able not only to select the appropriate tasks, but also to perform them in the correct sequence and at the proper intervals. Therefore, it is necessary to define both task sequences and the functional relationships between the auxiliary and the next level of the health care system. The resulting task

structure defines the pattern of task sequences and relationships and should address six issues.

Who has primary responsibility for performing the task? Within the context of this chapter, this will always be the health auxiliary.

Who has secondary responsibility for performing the task? This is the person who will periodically monitor the auxiliary and to whom the auxiliary can turn if he or she has a question about task performance. In some settings it may be one of the physicians, the community health nurse, or a program manager that is not a health professional.

For what population should the task be performed? The target population and the characteristics of specific priority groups, if applicable, should be defined. For example, if the task is designed to screen for iron deficiency anemia, the target population might include all pregnant women, with a specific priority group including women who are gravida IV or higher.

When and how often is the task to be performed? Specifically, the time to start a task, how often to perform it, and the

		STAGE 0	STAGE I	STAGE II	STAGE III
INFORMATION GATHERING	1. Withdrawal from activities	No	Yes	—	—
	2. Conflict with students (arguments, fights, etc.)	0	1, 2, 3	4, 5, 6	7 or more
	3. Conflict with staff	0	1, 2	3, 4	5 or more
	4. Refusal to do dorm detail	0, 1, 2	3, 4	4, 6	7 or more
	5. Observed phone calls home	0, 1	2, 3	4	5 or more
	6. Upset by news from home	No	—	Yes	—
	7. School non-attendance (class periods missed per week)	0, 1, 2	3, 4, 5	6, 7, 8	9 or more
	8. Frequent complaints about health	No	Yes	—	—
	9. Number of drinking and sniffing incidents	0	1, 2	3, 4	5 or more
	10. Number of incidents of AWOL	0	1	2, 3	4 or more
	11. Visit to School Administration about going home	No	—	Yes	—
	12. Visit to review board or juvenile city court	No	—	—	Yes
	13. Threats or attempts of suicide	No	—	—	Yes
	14. Extremely depressed, upset, or nervous	No	—	Yes	—

Figure 4. The Staging Mechanism Applied to Behavioral Problems of the School-age Child.

time to terminate it should be defined. For example, an initial DPT immunization series should begin at age two months, should continue with immunization every two months, and should end after three immunizations have been given.

What additional tasks should follow on the basis of results obtained with the one performed? In order to promote continuity in the process of care, the action(s) to be taken as a result of each task outcome must be defined. In the case of a screening task, for example, the task structure must specify the rescreening, treatment, or referral tasks that should follow a particular screening result.

How are the results of the task to be reported? It is critical to define the manner in which the auxiliary reports information derived from the task to other parts of the health care system. Reporting may be accomplished by telling someone the result, by filling out a form, maintaining a list, or through a variety of other specific means.

Defining a task and its associated structure requires considerable effort, mainly because one will be forced to deal with small details that are often overlooked. If, however, each of the questions has not been addressed in the planning phase, and if the task structure has not been included in the auxiliary's training curriculum, then the auxiliary will find it difficult to function effectively as an extension of the health care system. The job of defining the task structure, therefore, forces discipline on the planning process.

Once detailed, the tasks and associated task structure form the basis of the auxiliary's training curriculum and provide explicit educational objectives around which the training may be planned and implemented. They also provide the performance criteria against which the auxiliary may be monitored and supervised, as well as criteria identifying the need for refresher training or continuing education.

STEP 3: DEVELOP A PROBLEM-SOLVING PROTOCOL

The protocol is developed by linking assessment criteria and treatment and referral tasks to the staging mechanisms shown in Figures 1-4. When properly designed, the protocol serves several purposes. It provides explicit instructions for the auxiliary by defining the necessary care as a sequence of tasks. It then guides the auxiliary through the problem-solving and treatment process, and in so doing, formalizes functional linkages with the rest of the health care system. The protocol also reduces the documentation needed to show compliance with clinical care criteria to a series of circled items and checked boxes; it thus permits easy monitoring of health workers' compliance with the desired standards of information-gathering, assessment, and treatment. The documentation of staged assessments and planned treatments also provides basic information needed to evaluate the program's impact. A copy of the protocol, which accompanies the patient when referred, makes relevant information available to the physician. Finally, the protocol is a powerful tool and the centerpiece of the training curriculum for both the health auxiliary and those designated to monitor the auxiliary's performance.

Figure 5 shows a protocol for respiratory infections in children 0-4 years of age. Using the staging mechanism described above, the protocol guides the auxiliary through the assessment process by defining stages of clinical severity. For each stage of severity, the protocol specifies a plan of treatment and followup; and for those situations where medication is indicated, the appropriate age-specific dosages of medication are described. By adjusting the staging criteria and the responses linked to each stage, any level of safety can be built into the protocol. Even protocols that appear relatively straightforward

INFORMATION GATHERING	STAGE I	STAGE II	STAGE III
SUBJECTIVE:			
How long has it been present?	(less than 5 days)	5–7 days	7 days or more
Is there coughing?	(Yes) No		
Does he cough so hard he passes out or turns blue?	(No)		Yes
Does he indicate that his ear hurts?	(No)		Yes
Is there pus in his ear?	(No)		Yes
Does he have a sore throat?	No	(Yes)	
Is he throwing up?—After coughing only?	No		Yes
—After each feeding?	No		Yes
OBJECTIVE:			
Temperature: ☐ age 0–6 months	less than 100°		100° or more
☒ age 6 months to 2 years	less than 100°	(100°–101°)	101° or more
☐ age 2 years to 4 years	less than 101°	101°–102°	102° or more
Respiratory Rate	(less than 32/min)	32–40/min	40/min or more
Are there retractions present?	(No)		Yes
Is there flaring of the nostrils?	(No)		Yes
Is there grunting when he breathes out?	(No)		Yes
Is there wheezing present when he breathes out?	(No)		Yes
Is the baby lethargic?	(No)		Yes
Does he have a stiff neck?	(No)		Yes

ASSESSMENT	TREATMENT PLAN
☐ Well Child	Do Educational Task A
☐ Respiratory Infection Stage I	Treat as below; do educational Task A & follow-up in 5 days; Refer to Clinic if not better
☒ Respiratory Infection Stage II	Treat as below; do educational Task A & follow-up in 24 hours; Refer to Clinic if not better
☐ Respiratory Infection Stage III	Refer to Clinic right away
☐ No sickness—Medicine given to be kept on hand	

TREATMENT

1. Fever or Headache (Use Acetaminophen Drops)	☐ 0–6 months—Acetaminophen Drops 0.3cc every 4 hrs.
	☒ 6–12 months—Acetaminophen Drops 0.6cc every 4 hrs.
	☐ 12–18 mos.—Acetaminophen Drops 0.9cc every 4 hrs.
	☐ 18 mos.–2 yrs.—Baby Aspirin 75 mg—1 tablet for each year of age, every 4 hrs.
2. Runny or Stuffy Nose: Saline Nose drops 1 drop in ea. side every 3–4 hrs.	
3. Coughing: (Use Glyceryl Guaiacolate Cough Syrup)	DO NOT GIVE TO BABIES LESS THAN 6 MONTHS OLD
	☒ 6 mos.–2 yrs.— ½ teaspoonful 3 times a day
	☐ 2 yrs.–4 yrs.— ½ teaspoonful 4 times a day
4. Sore Throat:	☒ Throat Culture—Label with name, date, number and village & send to Disease Control Lab within 24 hrs.
5. ☒ Educational Task A	
Other: Encourage fluids	

IDENTIFICATION   Last   First   Middle

Name:_____

B-date: _____ Age: ____ Sex: ____

ID-No.:_____

Residence:_____

Location of Encounter: _____

Date: _____

Signed:_____CHR

Reviewed: _____
                                                    CHR Supervisor

Figure 5. A Protocol for Management of Respiratory Infections in Children Under 4 Years of Age.

should be pretested by a physician on a small sample of patients to assure that they are appropriate to the symptom complexes which most patients present.

STEP 4: DEVELOP A PLAN FOR PERFORMANCE MONITORING

One of the critical weaknesses of many programs that introduce health auxiliaries into a patient care role is the tendency to provide training and send them out into the community without a definite plan for monitoring performance. This results in a sense of isolation, a rapid loss of confidence in the newly-acquired abilities, and a steady withdrawal from the tasks and the patient care role. A systematic plan for monitoring performance and continuing education should be built into the program and should be highly visible to all members of the health care team. It should occur with regularity in order that the auxiliary may be confident of assistance, further guidance, and support in the performance of the tasks assigned.

Because they work in the community, health auxiliaries, whether located in urban or in scattered rural communities, are not readily accessible to standard forms of supervision, a reality that has greatly retarded their utilization. Clearly, a plan for supervision is needed that makes the most of infrequent contact between the auxiliary and their health professional backup and/or supervisor, and that allows the auxiliary to seek help and further guidance when needed. In this regard, the protocol helps to initiate and support the supervisory function when the auxiliary provides a copy of each completed protocol to the supervisor on a regular schedule. The protocols are designed to be easily monitored for completeness of data collection, accuracy of diagnosis by stage, and the appropriateness of the treatment and referral tasks provided. The accuracy of the specific data collected and the ade-

quacy of the educational tasks provided, of course, cannot be assessed from the protocol alone. The latter are judgments of performance that can only be made from direct observation. Frequent review of the completed protocols, however, can provide an indication of the effectiveness of both initial and continuing training.

STEP 5: TRAINING AND SUPERVISION

Once the tasks and task structures have been defined and the protocol developed and pretested, the initial training can usually be accomplished for a single health problem in two to three days. The problem is first introduced by discussing its pertinent features, such as its basic epidemiology and pathophysiology, and the objectives of case finding and treatment. A generic problem-solving protocol is then introduced and is applied, by way of illustration, to a non-health problem. Next the individual tasks are introduced, and once competence has been achieved, the task structure is introduced by way of the problem-specific protocol. A substantial block of time is devoted to instruction in use of the protocol, including role-playing sessions that allow the auxiliary to go through the problem-solving process with "mock" patients. Finally, the auxiliary works with a physician in a clinical setting, applying the protocol to real patients under the physician's supervision. During this phase, it is important to reinforce the auxiliary's strengths as well as to correct any deficiencies. This preceptorship can be mutually beneficial if the physician takes advantage of the rare opportunity to see patients with a community expert who can provide a great deal of information on the community context of the patients seen. It also reinforces the collegial bond between the physician and the auxiliary and supports the image of the auxiliary as an individual with a unique set of skills and insights that can be useful to the overall health care team.

Following the preceptorship, the auxiliaries are given the specific assignment of following two or three patients in the community, using the protocol, returning after the protocols have been completed. Further training, closer monitoring, or several home visits with a professional may be appropriate depending on the completeness of the protocol and the auxiliaries' confidence in their abilities. Even after the auxiliary is fully competent and confident in his or her abilities, it should be apparent to both the physician and the auxiliary that the training opportunity has not been terminated. The auxiliary should continue to feel confident that assistance is available from their preceptor as needed.

Based on the needs of subsequent emphasis programs and the individual auxiliary's skill and interest, additional problems and problem-specific protocols can be added over time. As further training is completed, the auxiliary keeps the protocols and the tasks learned in a notebook for future reference. These items thus become the task inventory, to which new tasks and protocols are added in conformity with his or her progress and the needs of the community.

POTENTIAL IMPACT

This approach has been used widely in the Indian Health Service through the Community Health Representative (CHR) program. CHR's are health workers selected by the individual communities to receive two weeks of basic training and are subsequently employed by the tribal government to live and work in their community in a variety of health related roles (1). In many cases the CHR program has collaborated with the health program of the Indian Health Service in emphasis programs using the approach described. Emphasis programs have also included school and other non-health personnel in a direct patient care role with equal success. In the early stages of the development of this approach, the process and outcomes were carefully studied and described (5-11). From these early studies, several important types of impact were observed.

In all studies, the auxiliary's level of compliance with care criteria was consistently high (5,6) and exceeded those of the health professionals in some cases (5). In no case was an adverse patient outcome observed that was linked to the care provided by an auxiliary.

The effectiveness of the emphasis program was often enhanced through a case-finding and early intervention effect that led to earlier contact with the physician by patients with serious illness. Using protocols for respiratory infection, CHR's were able to detect and refer patients with early pneumonia to a physician usually before the onset of severe respiratory distress. In a population served by these auxiliaries, only 43 percent of all pneumonia cases showed clinical respiratory distress when first presenting to the physician, compared to 95 percent in a similar population with no auxiliary (6).

In the case of less serious illness, this approach enabled CHR's to provide direct primary care and followup. For example, in remote communities served by CHR's using the respiratory disease protocol, patients were found more likely to receive needed care in their communities, and thus the primary care services were made more accessible (6). Similarly, protocols for minor acute illness in school-age children enabled school health workers to achieve a 22 percent reduction in physician visits (7). Furthermore, the health outcomes of cases managed by health workers were indistinguishable from those treated by physicians.

The health workers also made a measurable impact on the health status of the target population. In one emphasis program, a primary prevention strategy resulted in a dramatic reduction in morbidity and mortality from gastroenteritis in children, particularly when services were targeted towards a high-risk group (8). Significant secondary prevention was also achieved through casefinding, staging of severity, and referral to the physician (5). A similar impact was achieved by school health workers using protocols designed to permit early detection of emotionally troubled children and intervention on their behalf (9-10).

DISCUSSION

Use of auxiliaries as outreach workers can greatly increase the effectiveness of an emphasis program in reaching the at-risk members of the community who may not otherwise present to the physician for care. In addition to providing a means of targeting an intervention on the high risk subset of the community, use of this approach results in additional portals of entry into the health care system and improves the accessibility of health care. Continuity of care is also maintained by ensuring that the system gives a consistent response governed by standards of problem-staging and clinical problem-solving that are mutually agreed upon by the practitioners within the system. Most important, the health status of individual patients is improved.

Adaptation of this method for use in a given location requires consideration of several issues. First, the functional integration of the auxiliary into the primary care system must be assured. Care standards and explicit task structures must be devised and agreed upon by a variety of practitioners at several levels and sites within the system. Both the standards and task structures for auxiliaries must be based on the resources available for the total emphasis program, taking into account communications and transportation constraints. It is reasonably easy to provide health auxiliaries with basic training and equipment and to place them in a community, but continuing interaction is necessary to assure that they will function effectively as a member of a health care team.

Second, the mechanism by which the auxiliary can refer patients to the physician, have them seen in an expeditious manner, and receive feedback on their condition, must receive serious attention. When the physicians are operating on a strict appointment system, provision must be made to accommodate patients referred by the auxiliary.

Third, supervision of the auxiliary, however well planned, is often impeded by the realities of distance, health professional availability, and barriers to communication. The protocol approach does, however, provide a basis for objective and task-oriented supervision. This can be performed either concurrently, through observation of an auxiliary's performance, or retrospectively through a review of completed protocols. The actual monitoring of completed protocols for compliance with the standards of care can be done by nonprofessionals, who then provide tabulated results to a physician or supervisor responsible for interpretation, supervision, and continuing education.

The cost of incorporating health auxiliaries into an emphasis program will vary considerably with the setting. In general, the method described is relatively inexpensive, particularly where auxiliary health workers are already in place as in the Indian Health Service and in some community health centers. Volunteers could be used if available through voluntary health related organizations within the community. Major cost components include the time spent by professionals in planning the program and designing and testing the protocols. The cost of the onsite training for both auxiliaries and supervisors, while modest, must also be included. Equipment costs will vary with the type of health problem, but will be relatively minor in most cases.

SUMMARY

A method is described for incorporating health auxiliaries into an emphasis program in a direct patient care role. Staging of the target health problem is a central feature of the method and allows all members of the health care team to describe and communicate levels of severity of patient problems in a consistent manner. When stages of severity are linked with the appropriate responses by the auxiliary, a protocol can be developed to guide the auxiliary through the problem-solving process. The details of the five developmental steps required for this approach are described along with the impact of the approach on carefully studied applications in the Indian Health Service. Important issues to be considered for applying the approach to different settings are also discussed.

REFERENCES

1. Uhrich, R.B. Tribal Community Health Representatives of the Indian Health Service. *Public Health Reports* 1969; 84:965.

2. Eneboe, P. The village medical aides: Alaska's unsung, unlicensed, and unprotected physicians. *Alaska Medicine* 1971; 7:124.

3. Harrison, T.J. Training for village health aides in the Kotzebue area of Alaska. *Public Health Reports* 1965; 80:565.

4. Shook, D.C. Alaska native community health aide training. *Alaska Medicine* 1969; 5:62.

5. Nutting, P.A.; Shorr, G.I.; and Berg, L. E. Process and outcome measures of tribal health workers in direct patient care. In: *Advanced Medical Systems Issues and Challenges*, CD Flagle (ed.). New York: Stratton Intercontinental Medical Book Corp., 1975.

6. Nutting, P.A.; Manuel, S.; Lopez, P.; and Pancho, M. *Management of Respiratory Infections by Community Health Representatives.* Office of Research and Development, Indian Health Service, USDHEW: Tucson, Arizona, 1976.

7. Nutting, P.A.; Reed, J.C.; Shorr, G.I. Non-health professionals and the school age child: Treatment of minor acute health problems. *American Journal of Diseases of Children* 1975; 129:816.

8. Nutting, P.A.; Strotz, C.; and Shorr, G. I. Reduction of gastroenteritis morbidity in high risk infants. *Pediatrics* 1975; 55:354.

9. Nutting, P.A.; Price, T.B.; and Baty, M.C. Non-health professionals and the school-age child: Early intervention for behavioral problems. *Journal of School Health* 1979; 49:73.

10. Price, K.B.; Baty, M.L.; and Nutting, P.A. An intervention process designed to recognize and prevent school dropouts in an American Indian boarding school. *BIA Education Research Bulletin* 1977; 5:15.

11. Nutting, P.A.; Tirador, D.F.; and Pambrun, A.M. An approach to utilizing health auxiliaries in direct patient care. *Bulletin of the Pan American Health Organization* 1978; 12:283.

CHAPTER 36

How to Facilitate
Change in a Community

David R. Garr, M.D.

In many cases an effective approach to a community health problem requires the practitioner to go beyond the confines of the practice itself. Often the development of an emphasis program involves changes in the larger system of care for the community. Consequently, the practitioner must have, in addition to sound clinical knowledge and skills, an understanding of political and social factors that affect the health care of people in a community (1). In addition, COPC requires the ability to build effective alliances without alienating patients or others in a health professional community.

This chapter presents perspectives on facilitating change in a community. A brief case study is presented, and used to illustrate strategies for being an effective COPC change agent. Potential problems to be anticipated when designing a COPC project are then examined. The chapter concludes by proposing when and how to teach physicians to be change agents.

AN ADOLESCENT PREGNANCY PREVENTION PROJECT

This community of 15,000 people is located in the Intermountain West, 40 miles from the nearest urban area. Four young physi-

cians, all graduates from family medicine residency programs, had recently moved from other states to set up a practice in this community. Soon after their arrival, they became aware of a very high adolescent pregnancy rate within the community. Over a period of months they worked with adolescents, community residents, other health professionals, and representatives from local agencies to identify contributing factors. The young physicians first thought that more teaching about sexuality and contraception should be provided within the school system. During the many discussions, however, it became apparent that there was considerable resistance to such education in the classroom. This was based in large part on social and religious beliefs in the community. The emphasis program that eventually developed was one that worked closely with representatives from the adolescent community, their parents, concerned community residents, and church and political leaders to provide educational programs and resources in the community.

STRATEGIES FOR BEING EFFECTIVE CHANGE AGENTS

The following suggestions have been distilled from the experience of the author (2) and from the references cited at the end of this chapter (3-6). After each item, an example is given which refers to the case study of the COPC Adolescent Pregnancy Prevention Project.

1. Seek to understand why things are being done a certain way in the community. Explore the sociopolitical factors that gave rise to the present health care system.

   Example: Soon after our arrival, members of our practice met with leaders in the community who were familiar with the history of local health care. We learned about the development of the local hospital and about the growth of the community's health services. We sought to understand the influence of religion on local health care practices. These perspectives helped us as we sought to address the adolescent pregnancy problem.

2. Acknowledge the good that has occurred in the past before suggesting changes for the future. Provide positive feedback to those who have been working in the community. There are always opportunities to do this in a sincere way.

   Example: There had been prior initiatives in the community to address the adolescent pregnancy problem. Since a new task force had been formed to address the present concerns, it met with those who had already devoted time and energy to the problem before it considered any new proposals. We acknowledged the good work they had done, and we invited them to join the task force. They appreciated our positive feedback and their input proved to be of great value throughout the planning process.

3. Enlist input and support from other health care professionals in the community when selecting a COPC project focus. Prepare the COPC project well, incorporating as much outside input as possible.

   Example: A subcommittee of the task force organized a meeting and invited representatives from all health care groups in the community. The discussion at the meeting revealed a high level of concern about the adolescent pregnancy problem. The subcommittee solicited and received a commitment from most physicians in town to collaborate with and support the work of the task force.

4. Identify key people within the community whose guidance and support will increase the likelihood for a successful COPC project.

   Example: From our initial discussions, we learned who were the key people in the community. Fortunately, they were supportive of our efforts and helped remove some of the obstacles that arose along the way.

5. Work closely with community groups and local agencies, integrating them closely into the COPC project. Better yet, have them carry the COPC project to the community.

   Example: The physicians from our practice suggested that the task force should have a broad base of community representation. When the specific projects were developed and initiated, the community members of the task force took the lead, and our practice served simply in a supportive, advisory role. This strategy worked because opponents could not discredit the

COPC Adolescent Pregnancy Prevention Project as simply being our practice's project. It was, in fact, a community-wide effort.

6. Work behind the scenes to acquaint people with new suggestions before they are introduced to groups in communities or in other formal settings.

   Example: When the physicians in our group became aware of the adolescent pregnancy problem, we considered asking the local school board to place the issue on the agenda at its next meeting. We discussed the adolescent pregnancy problem with the chairperson and two other members of the school board. They suggested that a grassroots effort would be a better first step. Then, if the community group wanted to present a proposal to the school board, there would be a broader base of support for a new program. This advice was very useful and helped us avoid a potential mistake early in the development of the COPC project.

7. When introducing new ideas, expect them to be viewed with suspicion and realize that acceptance of new ideas comes slowly.

   Example: One of the first steps in the COPC project was the formation of the Adolescent Pregnancy Task Force. This group had broad representation, including some people who were skeptical of the advisability of a community-wide initiative to approach the adolescent pregnancy problem. The first several meetings were devoted totally to informing the group about the causes, contributory factors, and implications of adolescent pregnancy, looking first at the national and then at the state and local data. This process resulted in the broad-based task force making a commitment to address this problem.

8. Define goals clearly and develop a realistic timeline for attaining the goals. Generally, multiply by a factor of 2 or 3 the amount of time you expect a COPC project to take, then include this more realistic estimate in your timeline.

   Example: By the sixth task force meeting some of the members were eager to move forward with the specific community initiatives. A consultant from the state health department cautioned us to clearly define our goals and projects, then move slowly. She had seen well-meaning efforts in other communities fail because enthusiasm was not combined with effective planning. By moving more slowly than we would have liked we were able to broaden the support for our efforts in the community and thereby be more effective.

9. Avoid the tendency to get into a win/lose posture. Use a compromise approach when introducing change.

   Example: Some community residents were absolutely opposed to including any sex education in the schools. It became clear that this was a highly charged emotional issue for these people. The task force had included classroom education as only one component of its multi-faceted intervention program. The group decided to emphasize other and less controversial interventions first and to address classroom education later. When the in-school education issue was finally addressed, the decision was to provide very general sex education in the science classes. Students and parents could attend classes after school or in the evenings that would provide instruction in greater detail.

10. Recognize that personality clashes will arise and do not let them obscure your goals and objectives.

Example: Effective leadership is the key to most successful COPC projects. The leader of the COPC Adolescent Pregnancy Task Force was a highly respected person who was skilled at negotiation. He was able to keep people focused on the goals for the project, and on several occasions he was able to arbitrate very different points of view. He kept reminding people that the central focus was the welfare of the young people in the community. That perspective helped ensure the success of the effort.

11. Work within the system. Do not ignore the rules, but do question them when appropriate.

Example: The task force learned that sex education in the classroom had been quite helpful in other communities when addressing issues that lead to adolescent pregnancy. Yet we realized that the introduction of this teaching in our community's schools would not be easy. We chose to ask questions about why this teaching did not occur, but we did not push to introduce changes immediately. By asking questions of the right people, we served notice that the task force was studying the issues and might provide recommendations to the school board in the future.

POTENTIAL PROBLEMS WHEN INTRODUCING A COPC PROJECT

Those who attempt to introduce a COPC project must expect problems to arise. If these problems are not anticipated, the entire project may fail. First, the emphasis program may be viewed as being motivated only by a desire to market a particular practice or service. Similarly, the project may offend community residents or health care professionals if those implementing the project are perceived as being critical, self-righteous, or meddling in community affairs. The project may result in an over-extension of the practice and its providers. The providers may try to accomplish too much too fast. The result could be too little attention to important details of the project or overlooking other important clinical issues which, if left undone, could jeopardize patient care in the practice. If the physicians involved with the COPC project are overextended, they are likely to become exhausted and lose their enthusiasm for the project. Finally, although a community may say that it wants and needs a particular COPC project, it may not be ready to fully support the details of the proposed intervention.

WHEN AND HOW TO TEACH CHANGE AGENT STRATEGY

The skills required to be a change agent can be taught, and they are best taught during medical school and residency years. If physicians do not learn them during this formative period, they are likely to make tactical errors that could have been avoided.

Small group meetings provide an excellent forum for exploring strategies for change. Role playing and group problem solving can provide opportunities to identify issues, to find solutions to problems, and for group members to learn from one another's experiences and perspectives. Strategies for introducing change can apply to common situations such as: how to make a change in a medical school or residency curriculum; how to provide feedback to a less-than-effective teacher; or how to introduce a new patient care service. The group leader should be able to provide guidance to the group, drawing from the literature and personal experience when appropriate. Much of the teaching about change strategies can be found in writings related to the fields of sociology, political science, education, and business. This type of information is less common in medical literature.

Practicing physicians who are effective leaders in their communities can provide a rich resource for teaching change agent strategies to medical students and residents. Many physicians are successful community leaders because they have followed many of the strategies presented above, either knowingly or intuitively. If we identify such physicians, gather them together in groups, and help them see clearly why they are successful, then they may become teachers of physicians. When students and residents are seeking preceptorships with community responsive physicians, we can direct them to these physicians who are fine clinicians and effective change agents who have developed COPC projects. Such preceptorship experiences should have very specific goals and objectives that the preceptee and preceptor pursue together. They would emphasize these areas and assure that the learners receive both clinical instruction as well as teaching in the areas of community leadership and change agent strategies.

The practitioners who serve as preceptors can meet regularly to provide support for one another and to share what they are doing in their respective practices. Thus a network of community oriented physicians could emerge that could initiate new COPC projects and teach medical students and residents.

CONCLUSION

A practice rarely becomes an excellent practice spontaneously. Rather, hard work and interpersonal skills are necessary to create the environment for excellence. To excel as clinicians and community leaders, practitioners need to be effective change agents and need to be taught how in our medical education system. By doing so, we will prepare young physicians to bring about effective changes in their own practice settings. If some of these physicians are interested in initiating COPC projects, the likelihood of success will be enhanced. By offering training and experience in change agent strategies, in conjunction with clinical training, it is likely that physicians will improve the quality of health care in their communities and thereby derive considerable personal satisfaction.

REFERENCES

1. Kark, S. L. *Community-Oriented Primary Health Care*. New York, Appleton-Century-Crofts, 1981.

2. Garr, D. R. Idealism vs. realism: Reflections on primary care practice and training. *Journal of Family Practice* 1980, 10:911.

3. Zaltman, G., and Duncan, R. *Strategies for Planned Change*. New York: John Wiley and Sons, 1977.

4. Lippitt, R.; Watson, J.; and Westley, B. *The Dynamics of Planned Change*. New York: Harcourt Brace and World, Inc., 1958.

5. Nutt, P. C. *Planning Methods for Health and Related Organizations*. New York: John Wiley and Sons, 1984.

6. Bennis, W. G., and Benne, K. D. *The Planning of Change*. New York: Holt, Rinehart, and Winston, Inc., 1976.

CHAPTER 37

"Doctors Ought to Care": A Model Utilizing the Physician as Community Health Promotion Specialist

J. Christopher Shank, M.D.

Community-oriented primary care offers a challenge to physicians to engage more aggressively in a variety of health promotion and disease prevention activities. Despite the growing interest of the public in health promotion and wellness, the medical profession has been slow to fully embrace the health promotion and integrate it into the practice of medicine. In addition to emphasizing health promotion in the examining room, physicians can draw on their role of health leaders and have an important impact on activities beyond the office setting as well. One strategy for exercising the leadership role in health is offered by an organization of physicians called Doctors Ought to Care (DOC). This chapter describes that strategy as a model for those physicians and other health professionals seeking a broader role in promoting the health of the community.

DOCTORS OUGHT TO CARE: THE ORGANIZATION AND THE APPROACH

Doctors Ought To Care was founded in Miami, Florida, in 1977 by Dr. Alan Blum. He and fellow family practice residents were very interested in promoting healthful life styles and speaking out against harmful health habits. They developed a lively pro-health campaign and were the first physician-led group to purchase advertising space in which to counteract the images created by the makers of cigarettes, alcohol, and other adverse products. Dr. Blum was soon joined by Dr. Rick Richards, another family practice resident from South Carolina, in the national leadership role, and both knowledge and understanding about DOC subsequently spread (1-8). The organization has grown to include several hundred physicians with efforts currently existing in over 25 States and several other countries. These physicians have given health promotion presentations to over a half million students in their school classrooms and to over 50,000 physicians.

DOC is a nonprofit, incorporated organization with three objectives: to educate the public about the major causes of preventable disease; to increase dialogue on the effects of smoking on medical costs; and to train and motivate physicians to be effective health promoters.

The philosophy of DOC has a central concern with the power, economics, and influence of anti-health advertising on both the local and national level in the United States. It is ironic that tobacco, the number one killer in America, is also the most advertised product. Cigarette smoking and alcohol consumption are responsible for many more preventable deaths than any other risk factor, yet efforts to curtail them are often regarded as moralistic. The tobacco industry now spends over $2 billion annually to promote the imagery and illusion of smoking-associated sophistication, beauty, and athletic prowess. In contrast, the Federal Government and all voluntary agencies spend less than 0.1 percent of this amount on counter-advertising.

Table 1 summarizes the unique features of the DOC approach. First, there is a consistent effort to raise the community's awareness of subtle, "socially acceptable" anti-health efforts and messages bombarding both youth and adults. Twelve-year-olds no longer memorize commercials for sugared cereal, but instead know every word and every superstar in the commercials for Miller Lite beer or Skoal smoke-

---

TABLE 1. Unique Features of the DOC Approach

---

1. Raise the community's awareness of subtle, socially acceptable, anti-health advertising.

2. Emphasize preventive health topics in proportion to relative impact on U.S. morbidity/mortality.

3. Parody "Madison Avenue" advertising techniques: Image-based.

4. Use humor to ridicule and entertain.

5. Focus on youth, both as target and collaborator.

6. Physicians lead purchase of mass media time and space.

---

less tobacco. Adults too easily accept regular full-page cigarette ads in their newspaper, and teenagers regularly see tobacco ads on sidewalk placards and at the checkout counter of the convenience store.

Second, DOC places its energy and health promotion emphasis on preventive health topics in proportion to their relative impact on U.S. morbidity and mortality. Thus tobacco, which is associated with 350,000 premature deaths per year, and alcohol, associated with 100,000 deaths per year, receive the major emphasis. Accidental death, the leading killer of children and teenagers, is also emphasized, whereas such topics as lead poisoning, toxic shock, and acquired immunodeficiency syndrome receive very little emphasis.

Third, because "Madison Avenue" advertising works, this same type of "image-based" advertising is utilized to promote the good health product. Irwin Braun, president of a New York-based advertising agency, has correctly observed that "doctors are unrealistic about the power of advertising" and "they don't understand the role of marketing, creativity, media selection, repetition, continuity, and timing of a campaign" (9). DOC accepts this observation and seeks to teach physicians how to use advertising for good health.

Fourth, DOC uses color, humor, and the unexpected to ridicule, satirize, and entertain its audience for the purpose of effective counter-advertising. Figure 1 illustrates a DOC poster used in presentations to community audiences.

Fifth, DOC focuses on youth, both as a target and as a collaborator, to create unique approaches. Image-based advertising has proven successful for stimulating behavior change in youth (10-13). Although the tobacco industry endlessly states that cigarette advertising is not targeted to young people, teenagers do buy the most heavily promoted cigarettes, and 80 percent of children consider advertis-

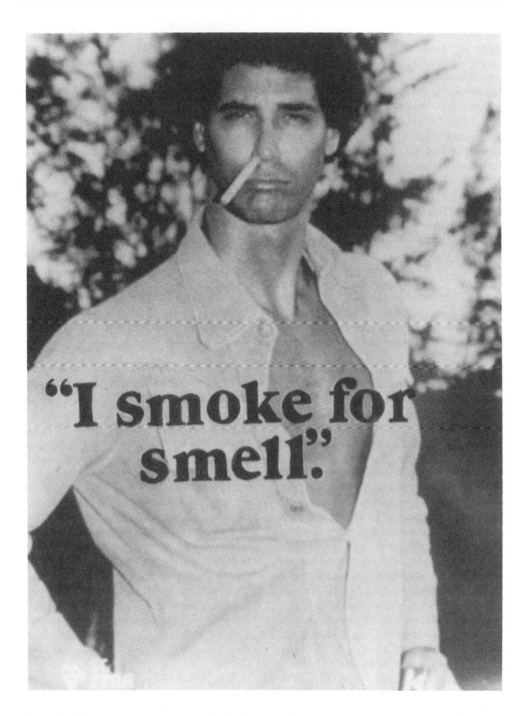

Figure 1. DOC Image-based Counter-ads for Good Health.

ing influential in encouraging them to begin to smoke (14). Recent DOC research has found a dose-response relationship between high school students' smoking levels and cigarette advertisement recognition. Regular cigarette smokers recognized 62 percent of advertisements seen compared to 33 percent for nonsmokers (15). Students smoking as few as one cigarette a week were found to identify a preferred cigarette brand. As Bartlett has discussed, community-oriented physicians can coordinate programs to reach both school students and the adult community, using both school-based and media-based techniques (16).

Lastly, DOC emphasizes physician-led purchase of mass media time and space for good health advertising. Typical public service announcements are well intentioned and can be used, but they are subject to manipulation. For example, they may not be run frequently nor at predictable or ideal times, unlike prime advertisement time and space which is purchased. The major reason cigarette advertising is no longer on television is the success of the health promotion counter-advertising effort in 1967-70. Government-mandated counter-advertising that ran in only a small fraction of the time allotted to cigarette commercials succeeded in cutting the expected sales of cigarettes by nearly 30 percent in 3 years (17). With tobacco companies now the leading advertisers in magazines, newspapers, and billboards, DOC believes counter-advertisements are desperately needed in these media too.

The philosophy and approach of Doctors Ought To Care was considered unorthodox in 1977. By 1981, however, the American Academy of Family Physicians (AAFP) cited DOC as one of the most innovative and outstanding health promotion efforts in the United States. The 1985 AAFP meeting included a Doctors Ought To Care health promotion lecture, workshop, and exhibit. To date several hun-

dred DOC physicians have talked with approximately 500,000 students and 50,000 physicians. Surgeon General Koop has been highly supportive of the DOC approach (18). Although initially reticent to speak out about the problem of tobacco advertising, the American Medical Association has recently called for a total ban on such advertising, to focus the American public's attention (19). While advertisers in all media around the country are concerned with this physician-led recommendation, they are encouraging physicians to do exactly what DOC has been recommending for the last 8 years (20).

Blum has characterized the philosophy of DOC as "medical activism" (21). By virtue of earned respect and credibility, the community-oriented physician has both the power and the pivotal role to educate, motivate, mobilize, and coordinate community health promotion efforts.

DOC AND THE COMMUNITY ORIENTED PRIMARY CARE MODEL

The strategies of Doctors Ought To Care represent one model for practicing community-oriented primary care (22-23). According to the operational definition of COPC, the first component is a practice or service program actively engaged in primary care. DOC activities originated from practicing and teaching family physicians with a defined active practice. The qualities of accessibility, comprehensiveness, coordination, continuity, and accountability are particularly intrinsic to the specialty of family medicine. The DOC approach can be activated in practices ranging from one physician in a small town to a large group in an urban setting. The latter, in turn, can range from a residency teaching practice to a multi-specialty clinic.

Regarding the second component of COPC, a defined community, DOC practitioners clearly relate to a community. Consistent with Nutting's report (22), there is considerable variation in the denominator population served. Although the philosophy and attitudes of DOC can be used with patients personally in the office setting, this approach to health promotion functions primarily in social or geographic communities.

The third major component of the COPC model, attention to major health problems of the community, fits perfectly with the DOC approach. As noted above, DOC particularly focuses on the major lifestyle risk factors of youth, namely tobacco abuse, alcohol abuse, and risk-taking behavior.

Research by Doctors Ought To Care practitioners to date has involved working through the stages of the third component of the COPC model (24-25). Referring to the process by which major health problems are identified and addressed, questionnaires have been used to quantitate the knowledge, attitude, and behavior of students' lifestyle habits, thus consistent with Stage III of the COPC model. DOC attempts at modifying the health care program of the community, although in their infancy, have approached Stage III also. Research to date with the function of monitoring the effectiveness of program modifications has been at Stage III of the COPC model. Prospective design has primarily been used. Farquhar, a leader in the field of community-based lifestyle intervention trials, has outlined both the benefits and the limitations of this type of community intervention (26).

STRATEGIES FOR COMMUNITY INVOLVEMENT

As noted, DOC activities have spread across the United States and into other countries. Although often with a lot of enthusiasm, DOC activities generally start on a small scale. Typically the first step in organizing a DOC chapter involves assessing what already exists in the community regarding health promotion. Care is taken to avoid duplicating existing services. The community's problems, and specifically the needs of the youth of the community, should guide the initial DOC efforts. Typical early activities include: publicizing the availability of the DOC chapter as a health promotion consultant; offering regular health contributions to the local newspaper; staffing educational booths at health fairs; and establishing dialogue with the local school curriculum directors regarding status of health education (specifically concerning tobacco, alcohol, and risk-taking behavior). Depending on the number of physicians involved, regular meetings may be held and specific duties assigned.

One of the most active community services provided by DOC has been the development of speakers bureaus in various locations around the country. The DOC chapter in the Family Practice Residence Program in Cedar Rapids, Iowa, has been exemplary with this approach. A total of 14 different 30-45-minute slide presentations have been prepared. These are available at no charge for group presentation to both adult and youth audiences in the Cedar Rapids area. The presentations are colorful, humorous, and image-based. They stress the importance of peer pressure, advertising, lifestyles, and thinking for oneself. Audience participation, questions, and suggestions for health promotion ideas are always invited. From 1979-1986 nearly 400 presentations have been given to 19,500 individuals in eastern Iowa. Occasionally a DOC representative is asked to provide specific consultation with the school system on emerging problems such as teen pregnancy or smokeless tobacco use.

Another very typical DOC activity has been the sponsorship or co-sponsorship of family and youth oriented community fitness events. Five- and 10-kilometer races are quite common across the United States. However, unique "family fun runs" which include 25-yard "dashes" for toddlers, and 2-kilometer "health walks" for those out of shape, are more typical of DOC runs. Prizes are offered in unusual categories such as youngest finisher, oldest finisher, fastest mother and child, fastest father and child, and most members of one family. Rather than co-sponsorship with a beer or soft drink company, DOC fun runs are co-sponsored by such groups as the dairy industry. Rational and nutritious use of dairy products, with an emphasis on calcium intake, is enthusiastically promoted along with exercise.

While tobacco and alcohol companies have sponsored tennis tournaments, racing cars, and jazz festivals, DOC has offered an alternative with its "Emphysema Slims" celebrity tennis tournament. The hypocrisy of associating bad health habits with sporting events and risk-taking behavior is emphasized, and role model athletes are associated with good health products.

Perhaps the ultimate DOC activity is effective advertising in the local community media. This was initially done by buying space on bus benches and bus posters. An annual elementary school good health poster/billboard contest in Cedar Rapids has generated student created health posters for display in community retail stores, shopping malls, newspapers, and even on billboards directly juxtaposed to anti-health advertisements (Figure 2). This type of effort truly bridges the gap between school health education and community health promotion as discussed by Bartlett (16). The ultimate advertising media, television and radio, have been used initially in Seattle, Washington with great success. Efforts are now underway to coordinate student-created radio and television counter-ads with modern music and video images. Finally, DOC physicians have regularly appeared on radio and television talk shows.

Both in the spirit of the traditional family physician and of the DOC medical activist, DOC physicians have made "house calls" to cigarette company-sponsored film festivals on college campuses, cigarette company-run tennis tournaments, and to the headquarters of news media that relentlessly accept advertising dollars from tobacco and alcohol companies.

Finally, DOC physicians have been involved in legislative efforts on both the local and State levels. Concerned DOC members have devoted time, energy, and money to deal with such issues as "look-alike" stimulant sales, child restraint/seat belt/helmet laws, drunk driving laws, clean indoor air laws, fire-safe cigarette laws, convenience store/drug store sales of cigarettes to minors, and cigarette sample distribution on public property.

RESOURCE REQUIREMENTS

As with any COPC model, the DOC approach requires one or more dedicated physicians. Although physicians can be effective alone, there is an advantage to having a critical mass of 3-10 individuals. This allows cross fertilization of ideas, more time for community service, and a nurturing environment in which to share the fun of DOC.

Most DOC activities are provided voluntarily to the community. Time for providing a school talk or stimulating a poster contest must be carved out of an otherwise busy schedule. This time resource is one of the biggest challenges. However, the time spent can be considered a step in "marketing" one's practice, and many physicians to date feel this pays benefits in the long run.

The second major challenge is fundraising to support local community pro-health advertising. The budget for a typical family fun run may be $1,000. A poster/billboard contest costs $3,000-$5,000 (12 billboards shown for one

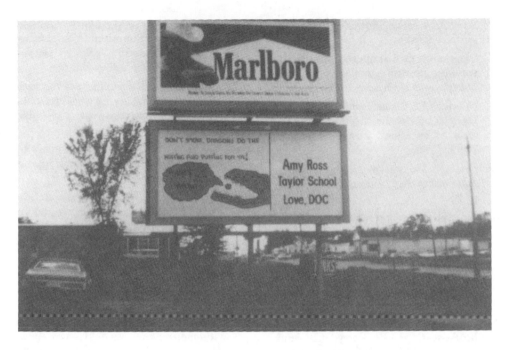

Figure 2. Student Poster Enlarged on Billboard, Juxtaposed Below Cigarette Billboard.

month). DOC activities have been sponsored by generous donations from local businesses, medical societies, hospitals, auxiliaries, and service clubs. Initial research has been sponsored by the Family Health Foundation of America (25). Larger grants and a truly national commitment will be needed to refine this exciting approach.

CONCLUSION

The philosophy and unique features of Doctors Ought To Care clearly offer a variation on the theme of community-oriented primary care. While originating from within the discipline of family medicine, Doctors Ought To Care is gaining increasing notoriety and respect across the United States. In the final analysis, DOC physicians care about their community, and quite simply have fun in providing modern health promotion advertising to the community.

REFERENCES

1. Check, W. A. Doctors, let's stop dragging our feet. *Journal of the American Medical Association* 1979; 242: 2831.

2. Mansur, L. What's up doc? *AAFP Reporter* 1980; 12:6.

3. Blum, A. Medicine vs. Madison Avenue: Fighting smoke with smoke. *Journal of the American Medical Association* 1980; 243:739.

4. Blum, A. The family physician and health promotion: Do-gooding or really doing well? *Canadian Family Physician* 1982; 28:1620.

5. Blum, A. Cigarette smoking and its promotion: Editorials are not enough. *New York State Journal of Medicine* 1983; 83:1245.

6. Richards, J. W. A positive health strategy for the office waiting room.

New York State Journal of Medicine 1983; 83:1358.

7. Chapman, S. Competing agenda in smoking control agencies. *New York State Journal of Medicine* 1985; 85:287.

8. Shank, J.C. Cedar Rapids DOC: An integral part of the community medicine curriculum. *Family Medicine* 1985; 17:96.

9. Braun, I. Doctors are naive about ads. *Advertising Age*, February 3, 1986, p. 18.

10. Federal Trade Commission Report to Congress, Pursuant to Cigarette Smoking, October, 1978. Document AO 11345. "An Action-oriented Research Program for Discovering and Creating the Best Possible Image for Viceroy Cigarettes." Ted Bates Advertising, March 1975.

11. McAlister, A.C.; Perry, C.; and Maccoby, N. Adolescent smoking: Onset and prevention. *Pediatrics* 1979; 63:650.

12. Edger, G.; Fitzgerald, W.; Frape, G. ét al. Results of large scale media anti-smoking campaign in Australia: North Coast "Quit for Life" programs. *British Medical Journal* 1983; 287:1125.

13. Flay, B. R.; DiTecco, D.; and Schlegel, R. P. Mass media in health promotion: An analysis using an extended information-processing model. *Health Education Quarterly* 1980; 7:127.

14. Fisher, D.; Codde, J.; and Armstrong, B. *Primary Schools' Smoking Prevention Program.* Report I, National Heart Foundation of Australia, 1981.

15. Goldstein, A. O.; Fischer, P. M.; and Richards, J. W. The influence of cigarette advertising on adolescent smoking. *Journal of the American Medical Association* 1986, in press.

16. Bartlett, E. E. The contribution of

school health education to community health promotion: What can we reasonably expect? *American Journal of Public Health* 1981; 71:1384.

17. Warner, K. E. The effects of the anti-smoking campaign on cigarette consumption. *American Journal of Public Health* 1977; 67:645.

18. Koop, C. E. A smoke-free society by the year 2000. *New York State Journal of Medicine* 1985; 85:290.

19. Lundberg, G. W., and Knoll, E. Editorial: Tobacco: For consenting adults in private only. *Journal of the American Medical Association* 1986;255:1051.

20. Editorial. A second opinion for the AMA. *Advertising Age*, December 23, 1985, p. 9.

21. Blum, A. Medical activism. In: *Health Promotion, Principles and Clinical Applications*, R. B. Taylor (ed.). Norwalk, Conn.: Appleton-Century-Crofts, 1982, p. 373.

22. Nutting, P. A.; Wood, M.; and Connor, E. M. Community-oriented primary care in the United States. A status report. *Journal of the American Medical Association* 1985; 253:1763.

23. Nutting, P. A. Community-oriented primary care: An integrated model for practice, research, and education. *American Journal of Preventive Medicine* 1986; 2:140.

24. Shank, J. C.; Erickson, R. A.; and Miller, G. The effect of DOC talks on seventh grade students in rural Iowa. Submitted to *Family Medicine*, 1985.

25. Shank, J. C. The community impact of a family physician-led, elementary school good health poster/billboard contest. Paper presented at NAPCRG, Baltimore, April 1986.

26. Farquhar, J. W. The community-

based model of life-style intervention trials. *American Journal of Epidemiology* 1978; 108:103.

CHAPTER 38

Physician Participation in Community Health Promotion Efforts: Planning for Success

Marc Rivo, M.D., M.P.H.
Karen T. Rivo, R.N., M.S.P.H.

For many practitioners, COPC offers a framework for moving beyond the practice itself, and joining a community-based emphasis program. Doing so may be particularly appropriate for the practitioner who has incorporated some health promotion activities into his or her practice, such as encouraging proper dietary habits, use of seat belts, smoking cessation, and other healthful habits. This chapter briefly outlines some of the considerations that will prepare the practitioner to make a positive contribution to a community-based emphasis program.

The community-oriented primary care model (1) should have a natural appeal to the physician interested in health promotion. Broadening the target population from one's practice to the community presents an opportunity for greater impact. In addition, multifaceted preventive interventions, ranging from public education campaigns to public referendums, are possible. Coalition building with schools, civic organizations, city government, private business, public health departments, and medical institutions can create a powerful health promotion team.

Ambitious community health promotion efforts, such as the North Karelia Project (2) and the Stanford Three Community Study (3), or national studies, such as the Multiple Risk Factor Intervention Trial (4), represent one approach. If evaluated against the COPC criteria, they represent highly developed, carefully targeted and monitored health promotion trials. They are worthwhile reading for those interested in large-scale community health promotion interventions.

However, this paper is directed towards physician participation in less ambitious, although equally important ways. Many physicians want to help teenagers resist smoking, alcohol, and drugs or get the elderly and at-risk populations immunized against the flu. Yet, resources may not appear readily available. Furthermore, the physician may have time constraints. One must recognize, however, that any level of involvement, if well planned, can have a positive impact on a particular health issue.

GETTING STARTED: ASSESS THE PROBLEM

Before getting involved in a community health promotion project, do your homework. Learn about the health issue of concern and the population you are targeting.

Most health problems invite several potentially effective interventions. Knowing the unique attributes of those involved or affected may suggest an approach that has the greatest chance for success.

Problem assessment involves detective work. Information gathering may be guided by asking the following questions:

What is the extent of the health problem?

Who is affected?

What do those affected feel about it and want done?

What intervention strategies are being considered?

Who is for and against it? Why?

What has been tried? Did it succeed or fail and why?

What is currently being done or planned?

Busy clinicians must maximize their detective time. While it may be ideal to perform a thorough study of the target population, it may not be feasible. Instead, identify and question knowledgeable people. Use existing data sources. Depending on the health issue, resources may be available through the public health department, local government, hospitals, community groups, voluntary agencies, and medical and other professional schools.

While assessing the problem, compile a list of local resource people and involved organizations. If the issue has political implications, determine the position of the local government, affected individuals, institutions, and community groups. Do your homework well. A few brief yet thoughtfully placed phone calls may provide a wealth of data and important insight into the problem.

With time at a premium, collaboration is essential. Your problem assessment will identify individuals or organizations sharing common interests. For example, the school board and parent-teacher groups may share a common concern about teenage smoking; employer and employees may rally around a worksite health and fitness initiative; senior citizen groups and the public health department may support an influenza immunization campaign. As you are assessing the problem, look for individuals and groups with whom to join forces.

BECOMING INVOLVED: COMPARE INTERVENTION OPTIONS

Problem assessment will often uncover a number of organizations and individuals addressing the same health problem. For example, community groups, the medical society, city government, and public health officials may all simultaneously sponsor initiatives against drunk driving. Their methods may take several forms, involving educational programs, new legislation, fund-raising, volunteer services, and media campaigns.

Carefully consider these different intervention strategies when determining how you might participate. First, analyze the program's strengths. Ask yourself: Is the effort addressing a significant health problem? Is the emphasis on promoting health and preventing disease? How carefully was the intervention strategy selected? How is it being received?

Then consider your own strengths when determining how you might contribute to the effort. Often, a physician's medical knowledge and technical expertise may be called upon when developing or modifying a health promotion program. A physician's credibility and respect may enhance community presentations, fund-raising and lobbying efforts.

In addition, be cognizant of your limitations. Recognize the amount of time required to lead, rather than join, a cause. Volunteer for what you can realistically provide. Once you do volunteer, be certain to produce. By knowing your limitations, you will avoid frustration. By carefully choosing how and with whom you will become involved, you can find a level of participation that yields both important community health benefits and much personal satisfaction.

Finally, recognize that urban and rural strategies for community health promotion may differ. The community's size, composition, and location may influence the level of interest in the problem, quality of available resources, and cultural attitudes towards change. While large metropolitan centers provide abundant sources for information, those from small communities may have to look elsewhere for resources and expertise. On the other hand, the well known and respected small town physician may carry much more influence to bring about change.

SUMMARY

For the physician with an interest in health promotion, COPC provides an opportunity and rationale for moving beyond the practice and joining a community-based emphasis program. Physician participation in community health promotion efforts involves several steps: assessing problems; identifying intervention options; and determining how one might be able to contribute. By adhering to such an approach, both community health benefits and personal satisfaction are tangible outcomes.

REFERENCES

1. Mullan, F. Community-oriented primary care: An agenda for the 80's. *New England Journal of Medicine* 1982; 307: 1076.

2. McAlister, A.; Puska, P.; Salonen, J. et. al. Theory and action for health promotion: Illustrations from the North Karelia project. *American Journal of Public Health* 1982; 72:43.

3. Farquhar, J. W.; Wood, P. D.; Breitrose, H. et. al. Community education for cardiovascular health. *Lancet* 1977; 1:1192.

4. The Multiple Risk Factor Intervention Trial (MRFIT): A national study of primary prevention of coronary heart disease. *Journal of the American Medical Association*, 1982; 235:825.

CHAPTER 39

Life Cycles:
A COPC Strategy for Community and Migrant Health Centers

Donald L. Weaver, M.D.
Carol A. Delany, M.S.S.

This chapter discusses life cycles as a community-oriented primary care strategy to be implemented in Community and Migrant Health Centers (C/MHC's). It focuses on combining Federal requirements with COPC elements in a life cycles framework to develop a plan for a comprehensive primary care delivery system.

Over 600 C/MHC's, providing primary care services to approximately 6 million medically disadvantaged and underserved populations, are funded by the Bureau of Health Care Delivery and Assistance (BHCDA). The Bureau has always sought ways to ensure the delivery of high quality, comprehensive health care in a community-based setting.

C/MHC's have been community-oriented from the start. They were established to serve definable communities rather than individuals. Each project is required to have a community-based governing board; the majority of its members must be users of the centers' services. A quality assurance program must be in place including a health care plan, a tracking system, periodic assessment, and clinical indicators. Health promotion and disease prevention activities are expected to be incorporated into day-to-day care.

The life cycles concept provides the framework needed to weave these components into a coherent clinical strategy recognizing that people progress through five cycles of life: prenatal, pediatric, adolescent, adult, and geriatric. It incorporates the concepts of COPC and stresses that quality assurance and health promotion/disease prevention are integral parts of a health service delivery system.

A comparison of basic COPC precepts with Federal requirements for C/MHC's in Table 1 shows obvious, if somewhat oversimplified, similarities. In comparing the lists it is tempting to say, "We always did community-oriented primary care!" However, that is far too simplistic.

As each center develops its plan for the provision of health services it must consider the five life cycles. A health care plan, based on the needs of the community, must be developed that sets measurable goals, objectives, and action steps for each lifecycle. Services can then be targeted to ensure that those life cycles with the greatest needs are provided appropriate services. The plan should be developed and shared with the entire staff so all members of the health care team are involved in the setting of goals and objec-

TABLE 1. Comparison of the elements of COPC and Federal requirements for Community/Migrant Health Centers (C/MHC's)

COPC elements	Federal requirements
1. A defined community.	1. An unserved or underserved population to be served.
2. Identification of community health problems.	2. A need/demand assessment of the service population.
3. An emphasis program to deal with community health problems.	3. A health care plan for the population to be served.
4. Patient and community involvement.	4. A community board.
5. Assessment of the impact of the emphasis program and development of a revised plan, if needed.	5. A quality assurance program that incorporates health promotion/disease prevention, tracks patients, and reviews clinical indicators on immunizations, hypertension and Pap-smear followup, and adolescent family planning counseling.

tives. This promotes the likelihood of active staff participation in ensuring compliance with the quality of care standards.

The community board needs to be a partner in understanding and implementing these goals and objectives. The members should participate in planning, implementing, and evaluating the program. Board members are a valuable resource for C/MHC review and assessment.

By using life cycles as a framework for developing a clinical strategy, community health centers should be able to:

1. Incorporate positive ideas from the past.
2. Avoid a "disease of the month" approach to health service delivery.
3. Have a community-appropriate health service delivery program.

The general concepts of quality assurance have been well documented for centers in various editions of *A Guide to Quality Assurance and Primary Care Effectiveness in BHCDA Projects* (1). The basic quality

assurance principles of accessibility, acceptability, availability, affordability (cost effective and cost efficient), and medical standards are integral parts of life cycles. It must be noted, especially in the current health care environment, that cost containment and quality assurance must be balanced to ensure the delivery of cost-effective health care. The four basic elements of a quality assurance program in C/MHC's are the health care plan, a tracking system, periodic review, and compliance with Federal reporting requirements.

THE HEALTH CARE PLAN

This plan should be a document that is simple, usable, and based on the needs of the community served. It should be developed by and shared with the entire staff. It should address appropriate goals, objectives, and methodologies for prenatal, pediatric, adolescent, adult, and geriatric life cycles. Finally, it should be shared with the community board.

TRACKING SYSTEM

A center must be able to track patients in order to practice prospective medicine and perform many aspects of community oriented primary care. The complexity of the tracking (management information) system will vary according to many factors including time and costs, but, ideally, centers should be able to identify their patients by age, sex, and major disease entities. This would facilitate such communications as notifying people who need flu vaccine, contacting patients who are on a drug that is recalled, and notifying patients about a new treatment for their condition.

PERIODIC REVIEW

The objectives set in the health care plan should be reviewed systematically. Whenever possible, this should be outcome-oriented, although structure and process reviews also have their place. Creativity is important here. Reviews can consist of exchanges between clinics or the use of a visiting professor, as well as more traditional review methods.

FEDERAL REPORTING REQUIREMENTS

Twice a year C/MHC's are required to report on a set of clinical indicators which relate to basic standards of patient care. This set of indicators is necessarily selective, not comprehensive. C/MHC's are encouraged to go beyond this list in developing patient care goals and review procedures in areas of special importance to the population they serve. The required clinical indicators are as follows (percentages shown are those required for compliance):

1. Immunizations of 2- and 6-year-olds (90%)
2. Adolescent family planning counseling (90%)
3. Pap smear followup (100%)
4. Hypertension followup (80%)

5. Anemia screening in 2-year-olds (90%).

The final component in the development of a comprehensive and effective clinical strategy is the integration of health promotion/disease prevention into day-to-day care. Nationally, basic guidelines are well laid out in *Healthy People* (2) and *Promoting Health/Preventing Disease: Objectives for the Nation* (3). Although these are national in scope, they can serve as a useful starting point for developing community-specific goals and are arranged according to the life stages.

The BHCDA regularly introduces special clinical initiatives. The use of the life cycles framework facilitates the incorporation of these initiatives into a continuum of care rather than viewing them as isolated efforts. A major example is the perinatal care initiative which was launched in the spring of 1984 to help each center review its role in the perinatal system of care in its community. For the purposes of the initiative, the definition of "perinatal" included preconceptional care through the first year of life. The three elements of review are outreach/casefinding, care provision, and referral linkage.

Outreach/casefinding requires obtaining information on the needs of the population served. It should include facts about available community resources, the number of births in the community, the projected number of expected births, information on low birth weight and infant mortality, and other pertinent statistics. In this way, the remaining need, if any, can be assessed.

Care provision requires that centers use the standards of the American College of Obstetricians and Gynecologists and the American Academy of Pediatrics in their care delivery. They must do continuous risk assessment to assure that mother and infant received risk-appropriate care.

Referral and linkage require that centers have appropriate arrangements with community organizations (including the health department, WIC, social services, and other appropriate groups) as well as with Level I, II, and III hospitals.

The initiative emphasizes that a health center should be part of a perinatal system of care to avoid duplication of effort and to use its resources effectively. This model for perinatal care can also serve as an outline for review of pediatric, adolescent, adult, and geriatric services.

For any clinical system to produce quality care it must have effective clinical and administrative leadership. In a survey of "best practices" carried out for the BHCDA in 1984, representatives from health centers were asked to list positive and negative factors affecting the quality of care. The three major areas that surfaced included well-trained providers, administrative and clinical leaders working together, and active community interest. These ideas are not new to this study; they were enumerated, all or in part, in the Rural Practice Project.[1] Center administrative and clinical leaders need to work together to deal with the current health care environment, as well as to plan and implement community-oriented primary care. Consultation with and training for administrative and clinical leaders may be provided to maximize their effectiveness and efficiency in working together.

Any review of health center implementation of COPC would be remiss if some potential problems were not mentioned. Three potential problem areas are the need/demand assessment, the community board, and other factors which inhibit the implementation of COPC.

Need/Demand Assessment. The need/demand assessment is a document, produced each year, which describes the current provider to population ratio and some health indicators in the population proposed to be served. The current document may need additional epidemiologic data to be more helpful in health planning. This may include information such as cervical cancer rates as indicators of Pap smear testing, and stroke rates as indicators of hypertension control.[2] Another potential problem is that the excellent information gathered in the need/demand assessment may not have been shared with both the administrative and clinical staff.

Community Board. The existence of a community board does not necessarily mean community involvement. A good community board that is broadly representative of the divergent aspects and interests in the community can provide the basis needed for community involvement. But there must also be continual interaction with other community institutions, organizations, and agencies. The danger for C/MHC's is in thinking that community involvement ends, rather than begins, with the establishment of a community board.

Other Factors. A variety of other factors may inhibit the practice of COPC. Physicians are not trained to look at the community as their patient. This, combined with the realities of dealing with individual patient management and illness on a day-to-day basis, creates a powerful negative bias against COPC. Additionally, requirements placed on care providers by funding sources often work against COPC. The current movement toward prepaid programs forces providers to consider their community of patients and may be a positive factor for implementing certain aspects of COPC.

[1] The Rural Practice Project, Robert Wood Johnson Foundation, School of Medicine, University of North Carolina at Chapel Hill.

[2] J.M. Newman, personal communication.

In conclusion, the congruence between Federal requirements and COPC precepts, while not automatically leading to COPC, provides a positive base upon which to build a community-oriented practice. C/MHC's have a real potential to build on this base, using a life cycles strategy, to increase their ability to provide community-oriented primary care.

REFERENCES

1. *A Guide to Quality Assurance and Primary Care Effectiveness in BHCDA Projects*. U.S. Department of Health and Human Services, PHS, Health Resources and Services Administration, September 1983.

2. *Healthy People, The Surgeon General's Report on Health Promotion and Disease Prevention*. Washington, D.C.: U.S. Department of Health, Education, and Welfare, 1979.

3. *Promoting Health-Preventing Disease: Objectives for the Nation*. U.S. Department of Health and Human Services, Washington, D.C., 1980.

CODA:

Developing a COPC Emphasis Program

Donald L. Madison, M.D.

The intent of most COPC emphasis programs is prevention. So central, in fact, are preventive ideals to community-oriented primary care that one could almost define COPC as the systematic practice of preventive medicine in and from a primary care setting. To stretch the point further, if we accept Leavell's "levels" of prevention (health promotion, specific protection, early diagnosis and prompt treatment, disability limitation, and rehabilitation), then virtually every clinical act performed in a COPC practice, or any primary care practice, can be termed preventive medicine (1). However, while COPC is mostly prevention, the converse is not true: most of what is called preventive medicine is not COPC. Until it is organized into an emphasis program—implying that the practice has defined one or more health problems to address and determined precisely how it intends to address them—preventive medicine in medical practice will strike most observers as an idealistic phrase: easy to repeat, but difficult to see and impossible to measure.

Yet, merely proclaiming that COPC is a systematic approach to the practice of preventive medicine from a clinical setting will not bring it applause. There are many other workable approaches to preventing disease that have been around far longer than COPC and have little or nothing to do with medical practice. In fact, a central question about preventive medicine, "Leavell's levels" notwithstanding, concerns its relation to the usual work of physicians. Specifically, how can the medical practitioner (the dominant healer) and the medical practice (an organization dominated by the healer) carry on effective disease prevention?

I should note here that the COPC assumption—that medical practice and prevention are naturally linked—is by no means universally held. Recalling that the medical profession's traditional task is healing and not prevention, some even question whether practicing physicians should attempt prevention of disease at all. For example:

Longer lives and a healthier population are definitely good things, but achieving them is not the function of the medical profession and never was. Historically, doctors have cared for sick people. Dealing with healthy people (and) populations is not agreeable to them. . . . Keeping people healthy is important. To a limited extent it is even

328

feasible, but giving the job to doctors is foolish (2).

Such critiques are not, I think, directed at the kinds of activities that show where physicians' sympathies lie. The medical profession's endorsement of the *idea* of prevention or the participation of public efforts are not being questioned. Rather the critics are addressing another issue: whether practicing physicians should themselves attempt programs of prevention within their own practice organizations alongside their usual tasks of responding to the pain and discomfort of individuals who come seeking medical attention. Can such attempts succeed? Might they not promise more than they can deliver? And won't they dilute what has always been seen as the central purpose of the medical profession and the source of its greatest successes? (3)

While the practicing medical profession may not have emphasized it, prevention of disease has always interested society, and whatever attention society asked its physicians to give to its preferred methods of disease prevention was, with minor exceptions, given willingly. These methods changed over time along with the diseases that evoked greatest public concern. In the history of Western Europe and North America five main patterns of preventive action stand out as the dominant responses to diseases that were seen as the most significant public health problems (4).

The first pattern, characterized by the response to leprosy and plague, dominated preventive thought and action during much of the medieval era. Prevention was mostly by isolation—banishment, actually—and quarantine of ships. The practicing physician's role was to pronounce suspected victims "clean" or "unclean."

The next pattern lasted nearly 400 years, from the late fifteenth to the early nineteenth century. By now society was taking a more active approach to prevention, with measures carried out through the mercantilist state by "medical police" (regulation and administration of public health matters). They included, for example, removal of miasmas (cleaning up sources of foul-smelling air) and inspection of prostitutes. Such preventive measures were legally enforced government responses to, mainly, typhus and syphilis. Practicing physicians, of course, were obliged to cooperate with the civic authorities, but they otherwise had no major role in disease prevention.

The third pattern came during the middle decades of the nineteenth century and was characterized by the public response to epidemic gastrointestinal disease, especially cholera and typhoid. Prevention now was largely a matter of urban sanitation—removal from the streets of accumulated filth and, later, construction of sewers and purification of water and milk. In this pre-germ theory period medical practitioners once again played no central role, although some notable physicians, for example, John Snow of London and Stephen Smith of New York, carried out important investigations that led to preventive actions, while others advocated a broader preventive mission for the medical profession including medical advocacy of improved working conditions, housing, and wages for industrial workers. Notable among these physician activists for health related social reforms were Jules Guerin, editor of the *Gazette Medicale de Paris*, (5) and Rudolf Virchow, who expressed his "social medicine" views as a columnist for the weekly journal, *Die Medizinische Reform* (6).

The fourth pattern of prevention was a response to tuberculosis and the communicable diseases of childhood during the late nineteenth and early twentieth centuries. Prevention was by improved nutrition and specific immunization, the latter probably the first effective linkage of a dominant, publicly sanctioned preventive action with medical practice—although most immunizations during the early part of this period were administered through public health programs rather than by physicians in the course of medical practice.

The fifth and final pattern covers approximately the last half-century. It includes the preventive responses to the most prominent diseases of today—cardiovascular-renal disease, malignant neoplasms, and accidents. Today's prevention is a matter of self-imposed lifestyle (including persuasion of individuals to adopt a healthful lifestyle), state regulation of personal and corporate behavior (control of individual safety practices and environmental pollution), and early diagnosis and treatment.

There were, of course, many other diseases as well as other modes of prevention in each historical period, but these five characterize the major patterns of public response.

It is notable that in this chronology one finds the clearest natural connection between medical practice and a large part of the dominant pattern of preventive response in the fifth and last period. The reason is that, with the exception of accidents, the most important diseases of our era tend to run a chronic course and are therefore observable in all their stages by practicing physicians, especially primary care physicians. They are the experts in caring for people afflicted with the disease throughout its course, and they are able to recognize and come in frequent contact with many others who are at risk of developing the disease. Most importantly, the nature of that contact, the context of the modern doctor-patient relationship, makes preventive interventions by the practicing primary care physician not only possible, but potentially very effective.

This is so because of the dominant place that their physicians now occupy in people's lives. Despite frequent criticism of them, physicians are generally held in high con-

fidence by the public, especially in terms of their honesty and ethical standards (7). The information that the medical profession offers is trusted more than that from any other major organized source (8). The public, therefore, generally esteems the medical profession; but the trust and confidence placed by people in their *own* physicians is, by all accounts, much higher than that placed in the profession as a whole (9). Physicians, who are visited frequently by both healthy and unhealthy people, are seen by their patients as knowledgeable experts and powerful commanders of opinion and motivators of behavior. Their potential as effective agents in disease prevention is, therefore, substantial (10).

This potential by the practicing physicians of the modern era is generally agreed to. Yet the styles of preventive action that are most often suggested, and that are in fact followed by most prevention-minded practitioners and the practice organizations in which they work, fall far short of reaching this potential. These styles of action are of two main types:

Clinical Primary Prevention. This term was suggested by Peter Morgan (11) and is discussed at length in a W.K. Kellogg Foundation-sponsored analysis (12). I use it here to describe the style of the primary care physician who in the course of practice is conscious of preventive medicine ideals, *thinks* prevention, presumably sticks in a word or two with each and every patient when the occasion arises, understands the epidemiologic basis for preventive procedures, and schedules them whenever appropriate. It is essentially an integration of "preventive medicine" with the rest of clinical practice at the level of the individual physician's work.[1] Clinical primary prevention stops short, however, of altering the practice at the organizational level by creating formal programs of emphasis that imply some explicit recognition of (a) denominators of people at risk, and (b) observable, attainable goals.

The Preventive Medicine Unit. This is the style followed by some larger practice organizations that have established or proposed special units to carry out preventive activities. Such preventive medicine units administer emphasis programs and preventive activities of various types, such as patient education classes, a video tape library, a multiphasic screening program, and a weight control group. The special unit's activities exist in parallel with the usual clinical functions of the practice. The clinicians know of the unit's programs, are presumably supportive of it, and refer their patients there, but may not participate directly themselves.

Either of these two styles of preventive medicine has limitations. The separate unit, with its enormous advantage of being able to initiate organized actions readily, is, of course, limited to practice settings that are sufficiently large and organizationally complex to support it. A further limitation may come from moving "prevention" into a separate organizational niche, and thereby lessening the primary care physician's sense of responsibility for the emphasis programs and his or her immediate interest in their results.

Yet clinical primary prevention has never really taken hold either. Physicians give several excuses: patients don't want the services—they seldom ask for them, nor do they usually approach the medical practice with disease prevention in mind; preventive services are of questionable effectiveness; detailed explanations of the consequences of harmful habits consume too much of the physician's time and are therefore too costly, and in any case cannot be billed for; and most third-party payment sources exclude preventive services from their list of benefits. Even when such excuses are not offered and a physician is doing an exemplary job of clinical primary prevention, it is difficult to validate from personal experience what effect these efforts may have.

The immediate empirical evidence that reinforces most clinical actions (there is usually some visible cause-effect relationship between a treatment action and the subsequent clinical course) is not usually available for the preventive measures a physician can offer an individual patient. As a result, the importance physicians attach to prevention is probably less than it otherwise would be. To see results from personal preventive measures, the point of reference can never be the individual patient, it has to be the *group* of individuals at risk. Yet defining and following patients as a group at risk is not normally done in medical practice—not because physicians lack the requisite epidemiological skills (although some epidemiology is needed), but simply because most of the *curative* modalities that are the customary products of medical practice don't require it; the needed feedback is visible anyway, if not immediately then usually at the next visit. On the other hand, the empirical evidence needed to reinforce *preventive* measures does require such a denominator or "community" orientation, yet the notion of clinical primary prevention fails to incorporate it.

Without a denominator orientation, the practitioner necessarily sees preventive medicine merely as good works, whose payoff will come at some indeterminate future time in a nonvisible form. This is why in most of medical practice the concept of prevention has become a platitude, full of well-meaning but often gratuitous actions—unorganized. If it is to be effective, prevention in medical practice must be seen by the primary care clinician in a programmatic dimension. It must be turned

---

[1] This was also the ideal preventive role envisioned for the practicing physician by the "preventive medicine" textbooks that appeared from about the late 1940s to the mid-1960s, the high-water period for preventive medicine's place in the American undergraduate medical curriculum (13).

into one or more emphasis programs.

All COPC practices and all emphasis programs depend on the group or community view. Even before they have defined it as such, the clinicians in a practice must *sense* that they are serving a denominator population and one or more subpopulations that correspond to the health problem(s) the practice intends to address with an emphasis. They then define the population at risk according to both problem-specific criteria and community-specific criteria.

The problem-specific criteria come from clinical and epidemiological insights. They might include, for example, an agreed-on level of diastolic blood pressure or body weight, a certain age group, a particular family configuration, the presence or absence of some selected social characteristic, a specific diagnosis, the history of a previous clinical incident of some kind, and so on. These kinds of criteria, alone and in combination, are used to define the population at risk of the problem.

The community-specific criteria define how widely the practice intends to search for and intervene on behalf of its problem-specific population at risk. Unlike the problem-specific criteria, the community-specific criteria are likely to be peculiar to the individual practice organization. In organizations that serve a group of people defined by entitlement or contract—like a staff model health maintenance organization, a university health service, or a military dispensary—that defined group is usually the *only* community from which the problem-specific subpopulation is defined. However, most practices have several possible "communities" to choose among. First is the geopolitical community where the COPC practice is located, within which most or many of its patients live. It may count among its clientele nearly all of the citizens of this community or only a small fraction of them. In either event, the practice must decide whether it in-

tends to direct its emphasis program to this largest of its communities and when. The main criterion the clinical staff will use in making this decision is level of concern. How concerned are the clinicians with the health problem in the community-at-large? Enough to mobilize the practice's own resources along with those of the larger community for a community-wide emphasis program? Enough to collect or locate the data that can serve as the necessary empirical evidence of the program's effectiveness? Or only enough to respond favorably should a request for help come from some other community agency that has already taken the lead?

A second, smaller community is the one made up of people who have used the service of the COPC practice or who are members of families that have, and are, therefore, known to it. This is normally an easier group to reach and to design a program for. But the most convenient community the practice can select is one limited only to its *active* patients, those who have recently been seen by the practice and are likely to visit again soon. Obviously, designing an emphasis program for this group is much easier, mobilizing resources is also easier, and the data needed are already available or can be readily collected.

Ideally, the COPC practice will direct its emphasis program toward all of its communities simultaneously, in which case the components of the program will probably vary according to the community being targeted. These different program components, directed to different communities, can also be expected to reinforce each other. An excellent example is found in the program of teenage pregnancy prevention described by Garr in Part IV of this book.

This account of lessons learned through trial and error while attempting to mobilize support for an emphasis program initiated by a COPC practice, deals only with the program component that was directed toward the geopolitical community served by the practice. What Garr's description does not include, but what must have been vitally important to the launching of such a community-wide effort, was the other part of this emphasis program, the part that focused on the smaller community made up of the practice's own teenage patients, who were at risk not of pregnancy (they were already pregnant) but of an untoward outcome because of their relative social and emotional immaturity. Obviously, at any one time this must have been a very small community indeed. Yet it was large enough to prompt an organized emphasis program within the practice, consisting of group prenatal visits with peer discussion and counseling by the nurse-midwife, educational sessions in the basic skills of motherng and, of course, the usual series of medical checkups at regular intervals. It was the practice's experience with this small subpopulation of adolescent girls that generated its wider concern. The experience was the source of the anecdotal and social data that prompted the wish to expand and redirect the emphasis program toward the prevention of teenage pregnancy in the community-at-large.

Just as starting with the community of active patients may stimulate a wider program, starting with a shared concern for a health problem in the larger community, perhaps participating in an existing community-wide prevention program, might also prompt the practice to intensify its own clinical activities and design a COPC emphasis program targeted to those of its active patients who are at greatest risk.

The first step in launching a COPC emphasis program is, of course, selecting a problem to address. Often, as in many of the experiences reported in this book, this selection will flow out of the clinical experiences and impressions of the practi-tioners. The next step is to decide on the problem-specific criteria that will be used to define the subpopulation at risk. Third is deciding which of its communities the practice will target first with the emphasis program, keeping in mind that the strategies selected will necessarily follow this choice. The actual design of the program is the last step. Here, there are many and varied possibilities: using computers and other novel tracking systems; recruiting and training lay people to assist; forming alliances with community organizations; planning screening programs and followup procedures; writing new clinical protocols; organizing patient education forums, scheduling group care, and running peer support groups; and so on.

Probably the single most important part of the design is making sure that the record of the program is compiled in a way that allows the clinicians to see the empirical evidence that the emphasis was effective (or the reasons why it wasn't). It is this part of the design more than any other that makes COPC work, that allows the practicing physicians to see that the emphasis on preventive medicine can yield results, and to see the community grow healthier.

REFERENCES

1. Leavell, H. R., and Clark, E. G. *Preventive Medicine for the Doctor in his Community—An Epidemiologic Approach*, Second Edition, New York: McGraw-Hill, 1958, p. 17.

2. Oppenheim, M. "Healers." *New England Journal of Medicine* 1980; 303:1117-1120.

3. Inglefinger, F. "Editorial—The Physician's Contribution to the Health System," *New England Journal of Medicine* 1976; 295:565.

4. Anderson, O., and Rosen, G. An *Examination of the Concept of Preventive Medicine*, Research Series #12,

New York: Health Information Foundation, 1960.

5. Galdston, I. *Social and Historical Foundations of Modern Medicine*, New York: Brunner/Mazel, 1981, pp. 74-78.

6. Ackerknecht, E. *Rudolf Virchow: Doctor, Statesman, Anthropologist*, Madison: University of Wisconsin Press, 1953.

7. Shriver, J. (ed.) "Honesty and Ethical Standards," *Gallup Reports* 1983; 214:4-29.

8. National Science Board. *Science Indicators — 1980*, Washington, National Science Foundation, 1981, p. 167.

9. Lance Tarrance and Associates. *Public Opinion on Health Care Issues: 1983*, Chicago, American Medical Association, 1983, pp. 1-25.

10. Holcomb, B. "Doctors Could Do More to Promote Health: Poll," *Health Care Week*, December 4, 1979.

11. Morgan, P. "Health Education and Risk Assessment: A New Role for Physicians in Primary Prevention," *Canadian Medical Association Journal* 1980 120:623-642.

12. DeFriese, G., et al. *Health Promotion/Disease Prevention in the Clinical Practice of Medicine and Dentistry*, Chapel Hill, NC, Health Promotion/Disease Prevention Program, Health Services Research Center, University of North Carolina at Chapel Hill, 1981, pp. 6-18.

13. Clark, D., and MacMahon, B. *Preventive Medicine*, Boston, Little Brown, 1967, pp. 7 and 8.

Part V.
Monitoring Impact of Emphasis Programs

Introduction

Those who have struggled with implementing the principles of COPC in their primary care practice will quickly recognize the many difficulties inherent in monitoring the impact of emphasis programs. The initial decision to be faced is the extent to which limited effort and resources should be directed to examining and documenting the impact of a previously implemented emphasis program rather than directing that effort to identifying and addressing another important health problem. Perhaps the greatest challenge facing the COPC practitioner lies in making the tradeoff decision between the feasibility of the evaluation and the rigor of the design. The practitioner should keep in mind that every program evaluation will not be subjected to the same critical review as a study submitted for journal publication. On the other hand, the results need to be credible within the practice and the community if locally important decisions are to be made regarding continuation, modification, or discontinuation of an emphasis program.

In reality, all programs are evaluated at a subjective level. Practitioners and patients alike form opinions of new programs and both are often vocal in their views. Often decisions to continue, modify, or discontinue an emphasis program are made on a subjective basis.

As a strategy for program evaluation, the strength of subjective impression can be increased by being systematic in collecting, analyzing, and describing the impressions of practitioners and consumers. For example, simple and targeted questionnaires can be used to gather practice impressions of the practitioners as well as those of relevant subsets of the community. Similarly, a variety of structured group consensus techniques can be used to systematically derive valuable, inexpensive, and highly informative data on program impact. These techniques are reviewed in the chapter by Horowitz and Gallagher in Part III.

In some cases program impact can be estimated through the use of secondary data. Several authors in Parts II and III offer strategies for using secondary data to identify and describe community health problems. Using the same data sources for a time frame following program implementation permits a before-after comparison of the extent and severity of the problem. While this approach may be useful, three issues should be kept clearly in mind. First, the results obtained will be in part a function of the "fit" between the population upon which the data is based and the community being served. Where the secondary data are drawn predominantly from one's target population the fit may be quite good, although often such data have been drawn from a much larger and more diverse population than that served by the practice. Next, secondary data provide measures of morbidity and mortality that may not be particularly sensitive to or specific for the changes in the health problem sought in the evaluation. This may be due to lack of sensitivity of the measures themselves; for example, cardiovascular mortality rates are not very sensitive to the impact of a weight reduction program. Similarly, sensitivity may be lost if the reference population is much larger than the target population. For example, the impact of a prenatal care emphasis program within a single practice would not be expected to alter the infant mortality data for an entire urban area. Finally, before-after designs in general do not distinguish well between the impact of the program and the many other potential causes of differences in the data. Nonetheless, comparing secondary data for time frames before and after the emphasis program may be of considerable value in many settings.

Where more formal evaluation and primary data collection are needed, the evaluation plan should be simple enough to be realistically implemented, but rigorous enough to provide information that is locally useful in determining the future of the intervention effort under study. The design considerations in formal evaluation studies are beyond the scope of this book, but are well covered in a number of useful texts on evaluation research (1-5).

Despite the choice of evaluation strategy and the selection of data to be used, several considerations deserve particular attention. First, the evaluation question itself should be carefully stated. A poorly stated question will inevitably lead to a poor evaluation, regardless of the volume of data collected or the cost of the overall effort. It is particularly critical to frame the evaluation question in the context of the entire denominator population that comprises the community. Too often emphasis programs are designed to address an important problem in the community, but evaluation efforts focus only on those individuals who emerge from the community as active users of the program services. In any effort to monitor the impact of an intervention program, it is critical to derive measures and information from the appropriate denominator population.

Second, in most primary care practices the energies and attention of the clinicians are nearly saturated by the demands of routine patient care. Thus, an emphasis program aimed at one particular problem will inevitably draw attention from another, and may result in an unintentional and unrecognized deterioration in care for a range of health problems not addressed by the intervention program. Reduction of individual effort can create "opportunity costs" even when program modifications do not involve the reallocation of funds from one effort to another. For example, a program to screen for hypertension may result in less aggressive

follow-up for diabetes, or, a strategy to improve the immunization rate in children may result in less attention to care for the elderly. Regardless of the rigor of the evaluation design, or the use of subjective, secondary, or primary data, evaluations should consider not only the impact on the target health problem, but also the impact of potential competition for resources on a variety of other problems which were not addressed.

Third, the evaluation should also provide information that will suggest both positive and negative effects of the emphasis program as well as pinpoint its relative deficiencies. Gaining an understanding for the reasons that the impact was less than anticipated forms the basis for further modifications to refine the program.

In Chapter 10, Walker outlines the fundamental principles of evaluation in the COPC practice. He suggests an approach to evaluating the impact of an emphasis program that is simple and realistic relative to the competing time and energy demands on the COPC practice or program.

In Chapter 41, Nutting stresses the importance of framing the evaluation question in the context of the total denominator population. He presents data that illustrate the extent to which "numerator-based" evaluations can lead to erroneous judgments of program benefit.

In more complex evaluation designs, the practitioner is often confronted with the problem of small sample sizes. Where statistical analysis is to be used to determine the statistical significance of differences observed, small sample sizes can lead to evaluation results that are ambiguous, even after a considerable effort has been expended to collect and analyze data. In Chapter 42, Kozoll, Rhyne, Stewart, and Skipper introduce and discuss power curves to assist practitioners in determining an adequate sample size to achieve statistical power and thus justify the expense of a formal quantitative evaluation.

REFERENCES

1. Weiss, C.H. *Evaluation Research: Methods of Assessing Program Effectiveness.* Englewood Cliffs, NJ: Prentice-Hall, 1972.

2. Rossi, P.H.; Freeman, H.E.; and Wright, S.R. *Evaluation: A Systematic Approach.* Beverly Hills, CA: Sage Publications, Inc., 1979.

3. Rutman, L. *Evaluation Research Methods: A Basic Guide.* Beverly Hills, CA: Sage Publications, Inc., 1977.

4. Suchman, E.A. *Evaluative Research.* New York: Russell Sage Foundation, 1967.

5. Drew, C.J. *Introduction to Designing Research and Evaluation.* St. Louis: C.V. Mosby Co., 1976.

CHAPTER 40

Evaluating Impact in COPC

Robert B. Walker, M.D.

This chapter discusses evaluation as a major component of COPC. Reasons to evaluate, some practical methods of evaluation, and application of results are discussed.

REASONS TO EVALUATE

Evaluation of any kind often has a low priority in providing health care to a community. It is apparent that resources expended in evaluating one activity could be used to begin another. There are, however, several good reasons to include evaluation as a fundamental step in organizing community-oriented health care projects:

Evaluation is vital to the development of community-oriented primary care. Implementation of community-oriented primary care in North America has been rarely, and only partially, accomplished. Applying the concept requires careful evaluation at all stages. Evaluation will help to identify the most effective methods of improving health as well as those areas most amenable to improvement.

Evaluation is necessary for the most efficient use of resources. The resources available to a community-oriented practice are usually severely limited, but there is no limit to the number of problems to be considered. Evaluation is necessary to set priorities and make the best use of community and practice resources.

Evaluation is necessary to provide feedback. There are many ways to participate in a community-based primary care project. Clinicians, consultants, research support staff, employees, and those providing financial support may reasonably expect to be informed of the outcome of a project. Funding is easier to obtain when it can be shown that accurate evaluation is available. Documentation of past achievement, even when limited, makes future requests for support easier to justify.

Evaluation is necessary to manage projects in progress. It is difficult to predict the success of a project. Activities that are using resources at an unforeseen rate should demonstrate probable benefit or be stopped. Activities that are unexpectedly successful can sometimes be expanded. Only through ongoing evaluation can such decisions be made.

The process of evaluation may identify new areas and methods for future intervention. Every project yields valuable lessons for future projects. Methods that are particularly successful in a community may be reused to good result. It may be found that methods described as useful elsewhere have limited use with a different population. Research usually generates more new questions than answers.

Evaluation is necessary to justify expenditure for research. Research, like all phases of health care, must be justifiable. Those responsible for the allocation of resources may question these activities, especially since they are relatively new in community health care.

A concept central to community-oriented primary care is the potential for positive impact of a project on the population participating in it. Evaluation is necessary to demonstrate this "closing of the feedback loop."

MISCONCEPTIONS ABOUT EVALUATION

There are common misconceptions about evaluation, each of which is regularly used to avoid project evaluation:

Evaluation must be complex and expensive. Evaluation of a community-based health care project is most helpful when it is simple and straightforward. The evaluation design should certainly be no more complex than that of the project itself. Evaluation of a well planned project should be inexpensive and understandable by all researchers.

Evaluation requires complex statistical methods. Statistics is a valuable tool in the performance and evaluation of a project. All statistics used should be readily understood by the researchers. This generally means simple statistical methods, or sometimes none at all.

Evaluation begins after the completion of a project. A plan for the ongoing evaluation of a health care project should be part of the initial design. It is true that impact may be delayed and evaluation may extend well beyond the planned activity, but evaluation that begins only after completion of a project is seriously flawed.

Evaluation means repeating much of a study. One rarely needs to repeat portions of a study to evaluate impact. The careful selection of indicators of impact usually makes repetition unnecessary.

PLANNING THE EVALUATION

It is important to establish an evaluation plan. This should be done as part of the original project design. The plan should include evaluation of both project implementation and impact. Evaluation of project implementation is important in improving the ability of the practice to carry out research. This chapter deals only briefly with evaluation of the implementation. The elements of establishing an evaluation plan are listed below, with comments.

Establish a Schedule for Evaluation

A schedule of activities related to evaluation should be established. This schedule should be as specific as possible. It should specify "who, what, and when," i.e., who will complete what specific task by which completion date.

When establishing a schedule for evaluation of project implementation, the schedule should be linked to each project task or component. Often, these correspond to a project objective. For example, for the following task: "Fifty subjects will be identified and informed consent obtained," the evaluation schedule could be as follows: "By October 1, 1986, the project director will have identified 50 adult subjects and will have obtained informed consent from each one."

Evaluation of impact should also follow a specific schedule. This schedule will define the specific tasks related to estimating the impact of some health care intervention. An abbreviated example of a schedule for evaluation of impact follows:

1. By September 1, 1985, the total sales of smokeless tobacco for the period of January 1, 1986 to June 30, 1986, in three local convenience stores nearest to West High School, will be filed with the project director.

2. By September 1, 1987, similar sales figures for the same interval in 1987 will be filed.

3. By September 1, 1987, enrollment of males and females, by age and grade, at West High School for the periods of January through June, for 1986 and 1987, will be filed.

4. By September 1, 1987, a report will be filed with the project director, containing the following information: alternative local sources of smokeless tobacco, changes in regulation or enforcement, changes in cost or availability, changes in local advertising, local educational programs relating to the use of tobacco, all subsequent to June 30, 1986.

5. All of the above will be the responsibility of Jane Smith, M.S.W., clinic social worker.

Establish a Review System

It should be the specific responsibility of the project director or a designee to review the schedule at each completion date. If an activity has not been completed as scheduled, a reason should be noted and filed, and a revised schedule defined.

As the project progresses, regular evaluation sessions should take place. This will probably not occur unless previously scheduled. Interim evaluation should consider budget, expected and unexpected difficulties, areas for future research, weakness in design and planning, and consideration of project modification.

Choose Indicators of Impact

Evaluation resembles a statistical sampling process. The true impact of a project can rarely, if ever, be determined. An accurate estimation of impact is sought, with the expenditure of a carefully allocated amount of resources. One or more indicators of impact are chosen. These usually represent compromises between variables that reflect basic goals of the project and those that can be realistically determined.

For example, a program to encourage smoking cessation may have a goal of a long-term decrease in the number of smokers and cigarettes smoked within the defined community. Realistic indicators may include cigarette sales within the community one year after the program and responses to a survey of randomly selected households. Neither indicator perfectly reflects basic project goals, but both are reasonable.

A project intending to improve rubella immunity within a population is ultimately concerned with the prevention of congenital rubella syndrome. This condition may be diagnosed so infrequently that a reasonable indicator might be the number of women with serologic immunity to rubella entering local family planning and prenatal programs. Using rubella serology to estimate protection from congenital rubella syndrome and generalizing those entering special programs to the entire childbearing population are obviously significant compromises. However, this indicator is accessible, cost effective, and plausible.

EVALUATING IMPACT

The impact of a health care project on a

community can be estimated in many ways, as discussed below.

Surveys

The survey is probably the most common method of evaluating impact. Proper methods for determining sample size, sampling, and interviewing are available in many texts. Consultation is available at a local university or medical school.

Ideally, identical surveys are performed before and after intervention. Often, however, baseline studies have already been completed by another agency. These may include national or multi-State surveys, the U.S. Census, and surveys by State or local agencies such as by home extension services. Identical postintervention surveys may not be possible, but parallel studies may be reasonable.

Some consideration should be given to performing a master survey of the defined community as a project in itself. In addition to providing valuable primary information, this survey may serve as an evaluation baseline for many future projects.

Highly sophisticated surveys are difficult and expensive, but reasonable data can be gathered at a smaller scale. Local high school students can conduct interviews after a few training sessions to promote accuracy and standardization. Local graduate students or undergraduates can be hired. There are advantages to local interviewers, including knowledge of local geography and easier entry. Disadvantages concern confidentiality and competition for positions.

Federal Sources

United States Census data for specific localities are available through computer networks and on reasonably priced microcomputer disks. National surveys in nutrition, housing and education, as well as health, can be helpful, especially when they have included the practice community.

State Sources

Much vital statistics information is in the public domain and can be very helpful, especially in infant mortality studies. State health department laboratories usually have extensive data by county on infectious diseases and reportable diseases. Immunization divisions of State departments of health usually carry out intermittent surveys.

Programs administered by a State, such as EPSDT and WIC, can often give valuable pooled information.

Local Sources

Local health professionals, including physicians, dentists, mental health professionals, and public health and home health nurses may provide surveillance or other anonymous pooled data. The local board of education may provide attendance figures and pooled immunization information, and may allow classroom surveys. Local merchants, sanitarians, and law enforcement personnel may all be valuable sources of information.

Local institutions, such as hospitals, may be valuable sources, if permission and access can be obtained.

Other Sources

There are many other sources of information potentially helpful in evaluating impact, such as telephone books, tax rolls, tax revenues from listed specific sources, attendance figures from local health activities, and graduate research studies from local colleges and universities. The identification of available data is often the key to cost-effective evaluation.

USING THE INFORMATION

It is easy not to use evaluation results. Pressure to "wrap up" a project is often heavy in the final stages. Either group fatigue or a desire to start something new can predominate. It is wise to anticipate this, and approach the analysis and application of the evaluation as a necessary and worthwhile activity. The following are recommendations concerning analysis and application of evaluation findings.

Hold a meeting dedicated to review of evaluation findings. Evaluation can often be a "foster stepchild" in the completion of a project. The consideration of evaluation results should be considered separately, if possible. Several meetings may be necessary.

Consider the broader aspects of the project. It is easy to focus on the most recent problem or the most time consuming or exciting aspect. To ensure the best feedback it is important to consider a broad overview of the project.

Look at the project both optimistically and critically. The project should be considered in both positive and critical terms. Virtually all projects have some positive features. It is important to enumerate even minor positive aspects. It may be helpful to assign positive and critical orientations to separate evaluators for group presentation.

Note the limitations of the evaluation. During the analysis session, compromises reached in estimating impact should be noted and discussed. These should be clearly stated in writing.

Consider the general implications for future projects. The design, methods, and timing of the project should be considered for general application to future projects. Would better planning have been helpful? Was the evaluation plan too costly or too ambitious? Were schedules followed? Did the activity interact negatively with the normal provision of health care? Was the general project design effective?

Consider the implications for specific future projects. Should future projects be undertaken in this area? Should this project be extended? Did areas emerge that call for future study?

Consider the implications for current and future health care. What are the implications of the project for the community? Is some specific action called for in education, improved or increased technology, manpower, funding, or change in priorities?

Prepare a summary. It is important to prepare an evaluation summary as soon as possible. Delay will result in an effort of afterthought and some content will be lost. The summary should be detailed enough to be understandable to future readers who did not participate in the study.

Inform supporters and participants. Some information concerning the relative success of the project should be shared with participants. In a community-wide effort, this may be most reasonably accomplished through the local media. With fewer participants, individual contact is best. Groups providing financial or logistic support deserve to be informed about project completion and outcome.

SUMMARY

Evaluation is an important component of community-oriented primary care. It is best accomplished by integrating evaluation into the research process.

Methods used to estimate impact of a health intervention on a defined community involve considerable compromise of scientific rigor because of limited resources. Once completed, evaluation of both implementation and impact should be reviewed to improve future efforts and to ensure maximum positive intervention in community health.

CHAPTER 41

The Evaluation Function in COPC: Quality Assurance for the Community

Paul A. Nutting, M.D.

The fundamental purpose of evaluation in COPC is to determine the extent to which modifications made in the program are having the desired impact on the target health problem of the community. The evaluation activity is, in part, an exercise in discovering remediable deficiencies in the way an emphasis program has been designed and implemented. Thus, there is an important relationship between the evaluation function and the quality assessment activities that are becoming routine in many primary care programs. The standard methods of quality assessment, however, must be modified in order to fully accommodate the needs for monitoring impact in a COPC practice. While the rigor of the evaluation design may be adjusted to the resources and needs of the local situation, the development of the evaluation question must be rigorous, since it determines both the kind of results that will be obtained and the effectiveness of the monitoring activity. This chapter expands on the relationship between quality assurance and the evaluation function of COPC. Two fundamental principles will be emphasized and illustrated with examples from the Indian Health Service. They will emphasize the pitfall

awaiting the practitioner who carelessly incorporates the monitoring activities of COPC into the quality assurance program.

The fundamental danger of careless evaluation design is well illustrated by the story of the man who is feverishly crawling around on his hands and knees under a street light. When a passerby asks him what he is doing, he responds that he lost his watch and is looking for it. Offering to help, the passerby asks where he lost his watch. The man shrugs and says, "I don't know exactly, but somewhere on this street." The passerby asks why, if he was unsure, was he looking in this particular spot. The man responds, "Because this is where the light is." Evaluation activities are very much like this street light— they will reveal only that which is within their scope to examine. Further, the poorly focused evaluation question may not simply provide a poorly focused answer, indeed it may give precisely the wrong answer.

In 1961 Kerr White published a classic paper (1) that emphasizes a point that should shape our approach to evaluation of program impact in COPC. As shown in Figure 1, he suggests that of 1,000 individuals in an adult population, 750 will

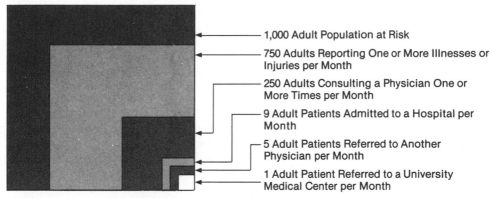

- 1,000 Adult Population at Risk
- 750 Adults Reporting One or More Illnesses or Injuries per Month
- 250 Adults Consulting a Physician One or More Times per Month
- 9 Adult Patients Admitted to a Hospital per Month
- 5 Adult Patients Referred to Another Physician per Month
- 1 Adult Patient Referred to a University Medical Center per Month

Figure 1. Monthly Prevalence of Illness in the Community.

report one or more illnesses over a one month period. Of these, however, only 250 will consult a physician one or more times, only 9 will be admitted to a hospital, and 1 will be referred to a tertiary care center.

While granting that evaluation of the care in the hospital is important, quality assurance activities that focus on hospital care do not provide information on the health issues or the health care that affect most of the people most of the time. The COPC arena includes those individuals who seek care not at all when in fact they should. Unfortunately, most established methods of quality assessment emphasize the care provided for well-defined conditions in patients that actively seek care. To appropriately assess the impact of a COPC emphasis program, we must examine the impact on the entire community, not simply on that subset of the population that has made contact with the health care system. For example, evaluating the care provided to patients under care for hypertension will provide no information on the health or health care of all individuals in the community with elevated blood pressure. To be useful in the evaluation function of COPC, quality assessments must look beyond the adequacy of care in any given patient visit and begin to examine the process of care over a series

of visits, across all practitioners, and for health problems that may not yet be firm diagnostic entities.

Fundamental Principle: There is an important difference between the impact of a program on the program users and the impact on the entire denominator population. This is a critical point for the program that plans to expand its quality assurance mechanism to evaluate the impact of a program modification. Quality assurance activities typically examine a series of medical records selected on the basis of a particular diagnostic category. A typical chart audit procedure involves pulling the charts of the last 25 patients in the clinic with a urinary tract infection and tabulating the compliance of the practitioner with a set of predetermined criteria for the diagnostic workup and treatment of urinary tract infections. Several years ago I participated in just such an audit from which we concluded that as a group of clinicians we were delivering good quality care, at least for urinary tract infections. Feeling that such an audit somehow was looking under the wrong street light, we did a second study of the quality of care for urinary tract infections using the same time frame. Instead of looking at charts of patients already diagnosed with a urinary tract infection, however, we went back to the laboratory log and found the chart numbers of the last 100 people with a positive urine culture. We then reviewed these charts and constructed an algorithm to ask six basic questions about the care they received:

1. Did the patient make contact with a practitioner within 4 weeks after the positive urine culture?

2. If so, did the practitioner recognize the positive result?

3. If so, was the patient given an appropriate antibiotic within 2 weeks of problem recognition?

4. If so, did the patient make contact with a practitioner within 4 weeks of completing the course of therapy?

5. If so, did the practitioner recognize the need for followup?

6. If so, was a urine culture or microscopic urinalysis done?

We then constructed the flow chart diagram shown in Figure 2 to describe the sequence of care and to identify the points in the process where major problems occurred. From these data we concluded that only 36 percent of the patients with positive urine cultures were receiving timely treatment and followup. The major causes for patients dropping out of the process of care were related to failure of the patient to make contact with the provider and failure of the provider to recognize the problem when not the patient's chief complaint.

These data taught us two important lessons that were to be reinforced many times in our subsequent COPC activities. First, important problems in health care programs will be discovered only if the evaluation question is properly framed. Second, the measured quality of care provided by the program and the measured quality of care received by the population may be two entirely different things. When looked at from this perspective, we clearly had problems in the quality of care for urinary tract infections. Specifically we had problems that derived from patient behavior (failing to make contact with the clinic) and problems of recognition on the part of the practitioners. In fact, the only aspects of the care that were acceptable were those on which our original chart audit had focused.

Fundamental Principle: Inappropriately focused evaluations may suggest that a program modification is having the desired effect, even though the modification may be making the problem worse. Evaluating the impact of a program modification must also be geared to examining the problem in the way it presents — not in the way an evaluation is designed to examine it. This principle is illustrated by a maternal and child health program we developed and evaluated in the Indian Health Service several years ago (3). In this particular program, an evaluation had been done looking at certain key parameters of the quality of prenatal care. The results are shown in Table 1.

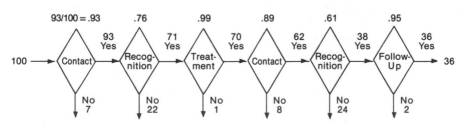

Figure 2. Continuity of the Process of Care.

TABLE 1. Baseline Indicators of Prenatal Care

MEAN WEEK OF GESTATION IN WHICH PRENATAL CARE WAS STARTED	24.6
MEAN NUMBER OF PRENATAL VISITS	5.8
PRENATAL WORKUP RATE: Percent of first prenatal visits with VDRL, Pap smear, cervical culture, and clinical pelvimetry.	23.5%
PREGNANCY ASSESSMENT RATE: Percent of first prenatal visits with assessment of risk.	11.8%
ANEMIA SCREENING RATE. Percent of first prenatal visits with HCT/HGB.	43.1%
POSTPARTUM FOLLOWUP RATE: Percent of delivered women making a postpartum visit within eight weeks of delivery.	28.4%

Based on these data the prenatal program was redesigned to provide extensive patient education, risk identification, and medical and social intervention for identified problems. A special high-risk clinic was established within the outpatient department of the hospital, staffed by physicians, public health nurses, and tribal nutrition personnel. All prenatal patients from the three remote ambulatory care facilities were to visit the high-risk clinic in their first trimester for initial evaluation and assessment of risk and again in the last trimester for reevaluation and delivery planning. All women identified at increased risk, using accepted risk criteria (2) were to be followed in the high-

risk clinic throughout the pregnancy. No attempt was made to discourage use of the special clinic, however, by women not considered at high risk. Initially the clinic was scheduled to operate for a half day each week, but a rapidly increasing patient load led to operation for 1-1/2 days a week.

After a full year of operation, the impact of the special program was evaluated. Comparison of "before" and "after" time frames using the measures employed at baseline suggested that the emphasis program had been successful. As shown by the data in Table 2, the mean gestational week in which prenatal care was started improved from 24.6 to 21.8, the mean number of prenatal visits made increased from 5.8 to 7.4, and several measures of the adequacy of prenatal care also improved.

Cognizant that the care provided and the care received are not necessarily the same, we developed a set of population-based measures of the adequacy of prenatal care. Rather than collecting data only for those women who received prenatal care, we sampled randomly from all women in the community who subsequently delivered during an appropriate time frame.

The results of this population-based evaluation are summarized in Table 3.

While showing general improvement, these data do not suggest a dramatic impact of the program on the adequacy of care received by the overall prenatal population. For example, although the mean gestational week for starting prenatal care had improved, only 55.9 percent of the pregnant women in the community started prenatal care by the 20th gestational week. Further, most of the other criteria of adequate prenatal care were met by less than half of the prenatal population. Nonetheless, the data suggested statistically significant improvement, and based on these data we might have concluded that the program had in fact im-

TABLE 2. Assessment of Program Impact: Comparison of Indicators of Prenatal Care Before and After Program Implementation

	BEFORE	AFTER
MEAN WEEK OF GESTATION IN WHICH PRENATAL CARE WAS STARTED	24.6%	21.8% *
MEAN NUMBER OF PRENATAL VISITS	5.8%	7.4% *
PRENATAL WORKUP RATE: Percent of first prenatal visits with VDRL, Pap smear, cervical culture, and clinical pelvimetry.	23.5%	37.2%
PREGNANCY ASSESSMENT RATE: Percent of first prenatal visits with assessment of risk.	11.8%	57.8% *
ANEMIA SCREENING RATE: Percent of first prenatal visits with HCT/HGB.	43.1%	64.7% *
POSTPARTUM FOLLOWUP RATE: Percent of delivered women making a postpartum visit within eight weeks of delivery.	28.4%	48.0% *

*Differences statistically significant, $p < 0.05$

proved the quality of care received by the prenatal community.

The impetus behind the prenatal program, however, was to improve the care to the high-risk women in the community and these data, while showing that care had been improved in general, did not focus specifically on the high-risk group. Consequently we disaggregated the population-based data by risk group, where the high-risk patients were defined using standard criteria of age, gravidity, and previous pregnancy experience. These data are shown in Table 4 and suggest that the entire benefit of the special prenatal program went to the low-risk group. Care for the high-risk group did not improve significantly on a single parameter, and on three indicators may actually have deteriorated. Based on these results, we made additional changes in the program to target outreach services more specifically on the individuals at high risk, and to incorporate them into the prenatal care pro-

cess early in pregnancy. From this experience, however, we learned another important lesson — improving the care received by the overall community does not necessarily improve the care received by those individuals who most need care.

These examples show that the evaluation function in COPC must move from concern for the quality of care *provided* to those patients who present for care, to the care *received* by the entire denominator population, and finally to the care received by those in the denominator population *who may most benefit from care*.

In summary, four points deserve emphasis. First, evaluation efforts will examine only the issues for which they are designed. Inadequacies in the quality of care received by the community will not be uncovered unless the techniques used are capable of discovering and describing this class of problem. Second, measurements of the quality of care provided by a practitioner or program (e.g., through stan-

TABLE 3. Assessment of Program Impact: Use of Population-Based Indicators of Prenatal Care

	BEFORE	AFTER
PRENATAL CONTACT RATE: Percent of pregnant women who made contact for prenatal care by the 20th gestational week.	56.9%	55.9%
PRENATAL WORKUP RATE: Percent of pregnant women who had documentation of a VDRL, cervical culture, culture, Pap smear, and clinical pelvimetry by the 20th gestational week.	16.7%	31.4%*
NUTRITION COUNSELING RATE: Percent of pregnant women who received nutritional counseling by the 26th gestational week.	8.8%	34.3%*
BLOOD PRESSURE MONITORING RATE: Percent of pregnant women who had their blood pressure documented at least 3 times in the second and 5 times in the third trimester.	26.5%	46.1%*
PREGNANCY MONITORING RATE: Percent of women who had fundal height recorded at least 3 times in the second and 5 times in the third trimester, and had the fetal heart rate recorded at least once in the second and 5 times in the third trimester.	22.5%	32.4%
POSTPARTUM FOLLOWUP RATE: Percent of women making a postpartum visit within 8 weeks of delivery, who had documentation of an exam of the uterus, blood pressure recording, and weight.	66.7%	74.1%
FAMILY PLANNING RATE: Percent of women who either began family planning or for whom their intention not to was documented within 8 weeks after delivery.	41.2%	61.8%ᶜ

*Differences statistically signficant, $p < 0.05$

dard chart audits) are not necessarily reflective of the quality of care received by the community. Third, improving the care received by the community at large does not necessarily improve the care received by those at highest risk. Most priority health services are intended for the high risk members of the community and should be targeted appropriately. You will not know if you are achieving this unless the evaluation question and subsequent methods distinguish between the care received by the high and low risk subsets of the population. Finally, the component activities of community-oriented primary care are essentially community-based quality assurance activities. While standard chart audits will continue to serve an important purpose, there are a number of problems in providing community-oriented primary care that will never be discovered by simply reviewing the charts of the last 10 patients seen with the problem. The application of epidemiologic principles to the quality assurance process, even in fairly nonrigorous ways initially, are required if a program is to identify and address the important health and health care problems within a target population.

Concern for the care received by the denominator population is the basis of community-oriented primary care. The four functions of COPC are 1) defining the community, 2) identifying the com-

TABLE 4. Impact of Program by Risk Group: Use of Population-Based Indicators Disaggregated by Risk Group

	AVERAGE RISK		HIGH RISK	
	Before	After	Before	After
PRENATAL CONTACT RATE: Percent of pregnant women who made contact for prenatal care by the 20th gestational week.	61.0%	66.7%	54.1%	48.3%
PRENATAL WORKUP RATE: Percent of pregnant women who had documentation of a VDRL, cervical culture, Pap smear, and clinical pelvimetry by the 20th gestational week.	31.7%	59.5%*	6.6%	11.7%
NUTRITION COUNSELING RATE: Percent of pregnant women who received nutritional counseling by the 26th gestational week.	7.3%	57.1%*	9.8%	18.3%
BLOOD PRESSURE MONITORING RATE: Percent of pregnant women who had their blood pressure documented at least 3 times in the second and 5 times in the third trimester.	26.2%	69.0%*	26.7%	28.3%
PREGNANCY MONITORING RATE: Percent of women who had fundal height recorded at least 3 times in the second and 5 times in the third trimester, and had the fetal heart rate recorded at least once in the second and 5 times in the third trimester.	21.4%	52.4%*	23.3%	18.3%
POSTPARTUM FOLLOWUP RATE: Percent of women who made a postpartum visit within 8 weeks of delivery with documentation of an exam of the uterus, blood pressure recording, and weight.	71.4%	82.9%	62.5%	57.9%
FAMILY PLANNING RATE: Percent of women who either began family planning or for whom their intention not to was documented within 8 weeks after delivery.	43.9%	78.6%*	39.3%	50.0%

*Before-after differences statistically significant, $p < 0.05$

munity health problems, 3) modifying the health program, and 4) monitoring the program impact. These are easily recognized as the analogues of the basic steps in quality assurance, and in fact COPC can be viewed as a community level quality assurance mechanism. It is the logical extension of quality assurance for programs that have made the commitment to address the health and health care of defined populations or communities. The critical point, however, is that evaluation activities should maintain a population-based perspective and that care is given to appropriately framing the evaluation question. While methods for examining the quality of care for the denominator population are not well developed, it is probably better to maintain an appropriate evaluation perspective with less rigorous methods than to be very precise and get the wrong results — as was the inevitable fate of the man looking for his watch under the streetlight.

REFERENCES

1. White, K.L.; Williams, T.S.; and Greenburg, B.G. The ecology of medical care. *New England Journal of Medicine* 1961; 265:885.

2. Wallace, H.M.; Gold, E.M.; and Lis, E.F. *Maternal and Child Health: Problems, Resources, and Methods of Delivery.* Springfield, Ill.: Charles C. Thomas, 1973, p. 243.

3. Nutting, P.A.; Barrick, J.E.; and Logue, S.C. The impact of a maternal and child health care program on the quality of prenatal care: An analysis by risk group. *Journal of Community Health* 1979; 4:267.

CHAPTER 42

A Graphic Method to Depict the Relationship Between Health Problem Frequency and Frequency Reduction After Intervention

Richard Kozoll, M.D., M.P.H.
Robert L. Rhyne, M.D.
Brian Stewart, P.A., M.P.H.
Betty Skipper, Ph.D.

P ractitioners designing an evaluation of the impact of an emphasis program face a number of difficult questions. Among these are the decisions to evaluate impact with a formal evaluation design using primary or secondary data, the rigor that is required in the design, and the sample sizes that may be required to yield results that may have statistical significance. We have begun to develop a tool to assist primary care providers in planning community or practice measurement through independent sampling activities before and after an intervention or practice modification. The graph shown in Figure 1 may be used to choose sample sizes, determine feasibility of using a particular sample size to measure a problem, or determine the significance of a difference between samples.

This graph is one of several we are developing for different levels of significance (alpha, type I error) and power (1-beta, 1-type II error). We are in the process of refining the following graphs, which reflect varying degrees of rigor:

1. Alpha 0.05, Power 0.7
2. Alpha 0.1, Power 0.7
3. Alpha 0.05, Power 0.8
4. Alpha 0.1, Power 0.8
5. Alpha 0.05, Power 0.9
6. Alpha 0.1, Power 0.9

The sample size curves are developed from a program adapted from Miettinen and detailed by Rothman and Boice (1). It should be noted that this program is inaccurate for use with very small sample sizes (n < 20). It assumes that first and second samples are independent and equal in size. It also assumes that the second sample, if reflecting a change, will do so only in one direction (recall that incidence or prevalence can be unaffected, or can go up or down as a result of an intervention). We expect these assumptions to be valid for most problem measurement at our COPC demonstration sites.

USING THE GRAPHS

Steps for use of the graphs for three purposes are listed below.

Choosing Sample Size

1. Select desired alpha and power, refer to appropriate graph.
2. Estimate frequency of health prob-

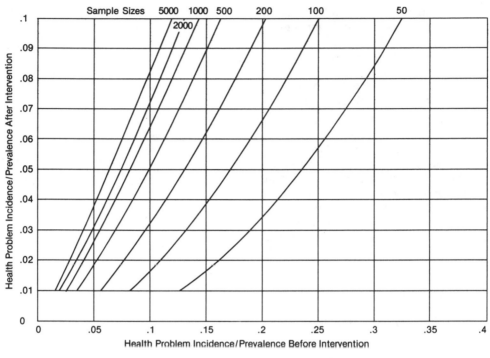

Figure 1. Power Graph—Equal Sample Sizes. One-tail Alpha = .05 and Power = .90.

lem in the community, locate on x-axis.

3. Estimate reduction in frequency achievable through an intervention/program modification, locate on y-axis.

4. Select sample size between appropriate curves.

Determining Feasibility of Statistically Significant Measurement with a Sample Size

1. Select desired alpha and power, refer to appropriate graph.

2. Estimate frequency of health problem in the community, locate on x-axis.

3. Select a curve with a desirable, feasible, or known sample size.

4. Locate needed reduction in frequency of the health problem for

significant measurement on the y-axis.

5. Determine feasibility of achieving this reduction.

6. If not feasible, consider a larger sample size or different alpha and power and repeat process.

Determining Significance of a Difference between Samples

1. Select desired alpha and power, refer to appropriate graph.

2. Select *actual* health problem frequency found on first sample and locate on x axis.

3. Select *actual* health problem frequency found on second sample and locate on y axis.

4. Plot a point and determine position in relation to sample size chosen:
   a. Consider rejection of statistical

353

significance of differences if point located far to left of nearest sample size curve.

b. Consider acceptance of statistical significance of differences if point located far to right of nearest sample size curve.

We do not offer the power graphs as a substitute for biostatistical consultation or definitive statistical significance testing. Rather, they are suggested as a tool for use by COPC practitioners to estimate the feasibility of statistically significant measurement of the efficacy of an intervention before greater effort is devoted to designing COPC interventions and measurement plans.

REFERENCE

1. Rothman, and Boice,. *Epidemiologic Analysis with a Programmable Calculator*, Epidemiology Resources Inc., 1985.

Monitoring Impact

Joyce C. Lashof, M.D.

Evaluation of COPC as a whole and/or specific emphasis programs within a COPC practice presents a number of difficult problems. Yet COPC advocates are challenged to respond to the question: What evidence is there that COPC is an effective model? We could counter with the question: What evidence is there that individual practice directed only to the seekers of care is better? Before attempting to answer such questions, we must ask: A more effective model to do what; and better for whom? Thus, the most important question to come to grips with is: What do we want to evaluate? Are the goals of the models we are comparing the same? I think not.

If we want to know whether a particular practice delivers care to its patients that is in keeping with the best standards of medical practice, then we can set up a quality assurance program based primarily on chart audits. There is an extensive literature dealing with the various aspects of quality assurance including methodologies for implementing quality assurance programs in different settings. If we want to know whether a specific treatment for a certain disease is effective, then we need to set up a rigid research protocol. The

literature on research design is even more extensive and includes discussion of how to determine the most appropriate research design dependent upon the questions to be addressed and the setting in which the research is to be undertaken. All of this literature is helpful in addressing various components of COPC.

But if we want to determine whether a particular form of practice improves the health status of a defined population, we find little to help us. To determine the health status of a population, we have generally depended on basic vital statistics: infant mortality, post-neonatal mortality and, more recently, the incidence of low-birthweight infants, age-adjusted life expectancy, death rates, and incidence of preventable diseases. Health indices designed to measure functional ability and quality of life have also been developed in an effort to further refine our ability to evaluate health status. All such measures are helpful in comparing large population groups such as cities and countries, but are much more limited in value when comparing practice populations which may vary from 1,000 patients in a single practice to 25,000 or even 100,000 for large group practices. In addition to the problem of population size, we are faced with defining the denominator. Except in isolated rural areas where there is only one source of care, one cannot define the denominator by geography. For closed panel HMOs, the enrolled population is the denominator, but then the availability of the appropriate vital statistics is problematic. As if such problems were not enough, we have the further difficulty of knowing what role medical care let alone the practice organization plays in determining health status. Faced with such obstacles, how do we address the question of the value of COPC as a whole or of individual program modifications? I submit that some of the answer lies in dissecting the elements of COPC, identifying values, and selecting sub-goals that can be measured. If we place value in making care available to a specific segment of the population and set up a method for doing so, then we monitor the process and determine whether or not we have succeeded. If extensive studies have shown the value of specific interventions such as the identification of and special care for high-risk pregnant women, and the practice develops a methodology for implementing those interventions, then the monitoring may be directed toward the implementation plan. Thus, when specific values can be agreed upon, when specific interventions are known to give specific results, and when there is congruence around goals, then monitoring the process should be sufficient to enable us to draw conclusions about the likely outcome. But when a COPC program wishes to implement a program which has not been previously evaluated, then it is necessary to develop a research protocol. Evaluation should be rigorous and outcomes must be measured. But the responsibility for proving that providing health care in general improves the health of a population need not be laid upon the back of COPC.

Thus we return to the earlier question:

What do we want to evaluate? If one of the major goals of COPC is to address the needs of the non-utilizers as well as the utilizers of care, then monitoring how well that part of the mission is accomplished may be the most important addition one needs to make to a quality assurance program for a COPC practice.

Part VI.
Patient and Community Involvement

Introduction

Of the elements of community-oriented primary care, participation of the community is the most difficult to characterize and to describe precisely in the context of the U.S. health care system. Involvement of the target population in the COPC process is a major feature and a central strategy of COPC. It is widely held that the COPC process will be more effective—will have a greater impact on the health of the community—through appropriate involvement of the target population in the activities of each of the four COPC functions described in Parts II through V. However, for many primary care practitioners the strategies for accomplishing appropriate community participation are confounded by the diversity of the community or population to be addressed. Clearly the nature of the involvement will be quite different in a program of the Indian Health Service, an HMO, and a private practice of general pediatrics.

In the past, the primary care practitioner maintained a relationship with the community that was a logical extension of the patient-physician relationship. The ability to understand patients in the context of their sociocultural and physical environments was taken for granted by both physicians and patients. With the preoccupation on specialization and its technology, the relationships between the physician and patient (and its extension to the community) has been nearly lost. Fortunately, primary care is making a definite comeback in the United States, and in our zeal to define COPC we must remain cognizant that mechanisms to heighten the awareness of practitioners to the social and cultural values of the community are central components of the primary care model, rather than a special domain of COPC. It is the active involve-ment of patients and community members in the process of identifying and addressing their health problems, however, that is unique to COPC.

Consumers can participate in COPC in a wide variety of ways, and in general, forms of community involvement can be categorized in terms of its organization, the level of involvement, and the focus of attention. The three dimensions of community participation are virtually independent of each other, and varied combinations can occur.

ORGANIZATION OF COMMUNITY INPUT

Frequently community participation suggests the presence of health boards or health action groups, although many other forms of community input are possible. While boards are often associated with a particular facility or program, participation may also occur through the formal organizational or political structure of the community. Practitioners in the Indian Health Service are familiar with working with communities that are active and well organized political entities. Community input can also be obtained from routine canvassing of the community such as through surveys or hearings on health issues. Community outreach workers are believed to be an effective means of incorporating community values into the operations of the health program. Perhaps most important in the long run is the less formal community input gathered by the conscientious practitioner who becomes involved in a variety of community-based and health-related activities.

Understanding the organization of community input in large communities is a more complex problem. The multiple organizations and mechanisms for dealing with health matters that characterize urban communities offer a bewildering assortment of organizations, many of which will not agree on any given issue.

LEVEL OF INVOLVEMENT

From nearly any organizational structure, the role of the community can range from primarily advisory to governance of the program. There is not universal agreement on the importance of either extreme on this spectrum. Arguments have been made that COPC is an important strategy for community self-determination and that community control of the health program should be a central feature of COPC. Others argue that the central purpose of COPC is to tailor the health program to the needs of the community, and while patient and community participation is an important strategy for accomplishing this, it is not in itself a central purpose. Clearly, the level of involvement will be determined by the individual practice setting, and will be determined in part by the financial or legal structure of the practice or program.

The issues of control of the health program have assumed new proportions with the advent of corporate medical care programs. In a sense the "for-profit" ventures in medical care remove a critical element of control from both the practitioner and the patient. Yet, the overall effect that corporate medical care will have on the ability to tailor the program to the health needs of the population remains to be seen.

FOCUS OF ATTENTION

Patients and other community participants can vary widely in the way they define the "community" that they represent. Of particular importance in the context of COPC is the extent to which community involvement is directed to the full range of health issues that affect the target community for which the practice has accepted responsibility. Often, community health boards are formally constituted around a particular program or facility, and limit their attention to political and administrative issues surrounding daily program

operation. Clearly such issues affect the "numerator" of users of the facility rather than the community as a whole. While producing results that may improve the primary care program, such activities do not contribute to the broader objectives of COPC. To be effective in the COPC context, community participants (however organized and at any level of involvement) should adjust their focus to consider health issues of the entire target community, whether this is defined as the active patient population, the practice community, an enrolled population, or the surrounding geographic community. The challenge to the community participants is, therefore, to adopt a "denominator bias" in identifying and addressing the health problems of the target community. It is this dimension of community participation that is most critical to the principles of COPC.

With a focus of attention compatible with the definition of the target community, and with an organization and level of involvement appropriate to the specific setting, involvement of the patients and community can add a distinctly new and vitally important dimension to the COPC process. In particular, community participation can be invaluable in setting priorities among a range of health problems and in allocating constrained resources among competing emphasis programs.

Previous chapters have dealt indirectly with issues of patient and community participation. The reader interested in involving consumers in the activities of characterizing the community should refer to the chapter by Ellerbrock, Kraus, Osborn, and Bujold in Part II. In Part III, Rose discusses the problems of setting priorities among competing health needs and stresses the role of the consumer in this process. Horowitz and Gallagher describe several group consensus techniques that allow the practitioner to use the perceptions of community participants to identify health problems of the community. In addition to supporting this important COPC function, the use of group consensus techniques offers a strategy for engaging community participants in the COPC process. In Part IV the chapter by Taylor discusses the use of "health promoters," the natural health opinion leaders of the community, in the COPC process.

The chapters of Part VI cover a range of topics in community participation. In Chapter 43, Lukomnik provides a reconnaissance of the general terrain of community involvement in primary care. She summarizes the varying roles that patients and community participants can play, and the variation on these themes appropriate to different health care settings. She also reviews the variety of effects that derive from community participation.

In Chapter 44, Freeman examines some of the ethical issues implicit in the COPC model. He explores the implications of the assumption that the COPC practice "assumes responsibility" for the health and health care of a defined population. He identifies three fundamental conflicts in this assumption, and from an ethical analysis he derives two critical roles for community participation.

Finding appropriate avenues for patient and community participation has been problematic for many clinicians in private practice. In Chapter 45, Seifert describes an innovative Patient Advisory Council that he developed and has used for over a decade in his solo family practice in suburban Minneapolis. From a rural practice in West Virginia, Taylor describes, in Chapter 46, a program designed for maximum collaboration among the practitioners and the community that eliminates some of the problems with the more traditional structure of health boards.

In Chapter 47, Nelson, Kreuter, Watkins, and Stoddard describe a community-based approach to identifying and addressing a health problem of importance to the community. Supported in part by the Centers for Disease Control, the program starts with a committed base of community support and involvement. This approach differs from those described in Part IV in that it draws leadership from the community itself, rather than building on an assumption of physician leadership in the development of the intervention. In Chapter 48, Robinson writes from the perspective of the community organizer. He points out that community participation must involve those people at risk, not merely representatives of the organizations and institutions that wield power in the community.

CHAPTER 43

Patient and Community Involvement in Different Settings

Joanne E. Lukomnik, M.D.

Community involvement is an essential component of community-oriented primary care. The actual and potential advantages of community participation are enormous in all types of communities. The essence of COPC is the acceptance by a practitioner or a practice of responsibility for the health of an identified community beyond the immediate patients seeking cure or relief from acute and chronic diseases. Since developing a COPC practice depends on identifying health problems within a community and planning programs to intervene systematically in specific health arenas on a community level, some order of community participation is a prerequisite for developing a successful practice. This chapter will discuss the rationale for and describe examples of the variety of roles that patient and community involvement can play in primary care.

BACKGROUND

The call for community participation came into vogue in the late 1960s and early 1970s. From antipoverty programs to school board elections, community participation and community involvement seemed implicitly to promise a democratization of control and management that had previously been lacking in local institutions, agencies, and programs.

In contrast, many critics have objected to the principles as well as the operational regulations that attempt to implement community participation in federally- and State-funded programs. Pointing to selected failure and half-successful examples in which community participation failed to deliver on the implied guarantee that community involvement would ensure successful programs, these critics consider community involvement a wasteful effort.

For the majority of professionals, however, community participation has never been a fundamental issue. Even while supporting the notion in the abstract, many are unsure how community participation could operate in the here and now. Citing a lack of sophistication, education, and management skills within most communities, most professionals shy away from the politically and socially sensitive issue of community participation.

Since much of the discussion about community participation and community medicine derived from organizing principles of the civil rights movement and equal opportunity programs, for many health professionals "community" has become synonymous with poor, blighted areas of urban decay or rural outbacks that qualify as medically underserved. Professionals, especially health professionals, generally are of different class backgrounds than many community residents and may not share values, priorities, or even language with large segments of the community.

Except for a few medical schools and residency training programs, there is minimal didactic teaching, and less experiential learning, around concepts of community or population-based medicine. Even potentially interested doctors leave training without a conceptual basis from which to approach complex issues like how to identify a cohesive community, recognize various types of leaders, or involve representatives of the community in health programs.

While the debates about community participation continued, a tradition of community participation became incorporated into programs. The principle was written into the regulations for most federal health programs (community health centers, migrant health, Title X, National Health Service Corps sites), and consumer representation on health planning bodies came to be standard. The involvement of community members, patients, and their families (a criterion for funding under certain State and Federal programs and conspicuously absent in most other arenas of health service delivery) has added to the success and survival of many of these programs.

DEFINING COMMUNITY

While the problems of choosing and identifying a community as a denominator for epidemiologic purposes have been discussed elsewhere in this book, analogous issues arise in trying to define community participation in COPC practices. What constitutes a community? Who speaks for the community? What is the role of other community organizations beyond identified health programs boards?

Communities vary in character, structure, history, culture, economic relations, degree of homogeneity of its residents, and even the degree to which members of the community self-identify with the community (1). The identified and defined community in COPC may take various forms, from residential communities to workplaces to schools. All communities, even those that seem at first glance to be relatively simple and homogeneous, represent a series of complex networks with individuals assuming roles (e.g., a woman can be a worker, patient, mother, wife, daughter, consumer, and head of the P.T.A. simultaneously). Each role not only brings with it its own expected behavior, status, and values; in each role the definition of community might shift slightly (the community identified as "neighborhood" may differ from the community with which one identifies as a worker). Multiple formal and informal organizations and networks with partially overlapping membership exist within the community. And each network and organization will have its own leadership.

DEFINING COMMUNITY PARTICIPATION

Community participation may mean very different things to different groups and individuals within the same community. For some, it may mean simply having access to a service. Others may want an advisory voice or see themselves as a sounding board for professionals to test ideas. For many groups, as a direct result of shifts in the understanding of community participation in the 1960s, community participation has come to mean minimally a voice in decisionmaking processes that control local institutions. This may take the form of complete community control, e.g., total governance or a partnership model (2).

Rather than abstractly discussing forms of community participation, we present several examples of different ways in which segments of communities have interacted with varying health service delivery models to illuminate some of the issues involved. Not all of these examples were self-consciously attempting to create COPC practices. Many examples of community participation are limited to some phase of the development of a practice or to a particular short-lived outreach effort of an isolated health promotion/disease prevention campaign. However, these examples may add to the discussion of how to build COPC practices.

COMMUNITY PARTICIPATION IN GOVERNANCE

All federally funded community health centers are governed by a community-based board of directors that represents the population of the catchment area, with health center users comprising a majority of the membership of the board. The governing board not only controls the budget and resource decisions, it also sets priorities and policies. Migrant health centers are not required to have governing boards but must provide for community representation. Many other local health delivery systems, as well as some nonprofit health maintenance organizations (HMOs), are also governed by boards of directors that represent patients and other elements of the community. These governing boards vary in the extent to which they get involved in specific policy decisions and program planning. In many community health centers, however, members of the board will initiate discussions about particular health-related issues or will question the effectiveness of certain programs.

At a community health center in North Carolina, board members expressed concern over the increasing numbers of teenage women having babies and dropping out of school. They questioned whether the health center was doing all it could to help reduce the rate of adolescent pregnancy in the county. The health center initiated a coordinating network with the county department of health, local school officials, church leaders, and some private practitioners within the area. Using the vital statistics for the county as a measure of the extent of the problem, the network attempted to assess which teenagers within the county were most likely to get pregnant. After determining the subpopulation most at risk, some selective modifications were made in existing programs to try to intervene with the teenagers thought to be at risk for early unplanned pregnancies. Only after the repeated urging of the health center's governing board was ongoing surveillance introduced to assess how well the network's activities dealt with the problem. The individual and collective enthusiasm of the board provided the energy to keep the network functioning until all its constituent members were able to perceive the value of continuing program coordination and surveillance.

Especially interesting in this example are the multiple ways in which community interests became involved. Not only did the impetus for the network originate with board members, but many of the individuals who became involved with the network represented other segments of the community, from certain traditional organizations (e.g., churches) to governmental agencies (e.g., department of health) to individuals with professionally-dictated interest (private practitioners whose concern extended beyond their own patients). Although teenagers (the target population of the intervention effort) were not initially represented in the network, they became involved during the implementation phase through peer groups comprised of both pregnant and nonpregnant teenagers. The initial formal network was able to incorporate and exploit informal networks among the teenagers to draw increasing numbers of teenagers to participate in some discrete activities (1).

ADVISORY BOARDS

Some solo practitioners and private group practices as well as larger health delivery systems have instituted advisory boards with consumer and community representatives. These advisory boards may sometimes function for a special project, or they may be ongoing boards helping a practice to refine its services. Members are recruited onto advisory boards in a variety of ways and may represent a spectrum of the community or a narrower group drawn together through concern over a particular interest.

Dr. Milton Seifert's private fee-for-service practice in Minnesota has had a patient advisory council (PAC) for the past 13 years. Membership is open to all patients and their families. The PAC and its several committees serve to "insure a good working relationship between the practice staff and the patient group" (3). Although the community for which the practice assumes responsibility is limited to registered patients, the PAC is involved in all areas of decisionmaking including those related to practice management, financial administration, and the creation of special programs to meet the health care needs of the practice's patients. Partially through sampling of medical charts to collect diagnostic data and through nonquantified impressions of members of PAC and of the practitioners, several programs not generally seen within private practices have been established. These include a well-child care program, marriage health education, parenting, body weight management program, alcohol education program, etc. The practice has been expanded from a single full-time physician to an additional part-time physician, a

health educator, and a Living Problems Counselor.

Adding an advisory council did not expand the community for which the practice assumes responsibility beyond the registered patients. The advisory council has, however, allowed the practice to expand beyond traditional curative services and to identify some nontraditional arenas in which the practice could focus on health promotion and disease prevention. The patient advisory council, in this case, additionally helps to guarantee quality comprehensive services for a defined patient population.

The Hudson Headwaters Health Network (HHHN) serves a large remote and mountainous area characterized by indigenous poverty, with the highest unemployment rate in New York State and substantial geographic barriers to care. HHHN operates five health centers served by a team of physicians, physician assistants, health educators, a nutritionist, nurses, and ancillary personnel. The Network operates with a Section 330 grant from the Federal Government and several State grants and therefore has a governing board for the entire network. This board is the grantee and is legally and fiscally responsible for the operation of HHHN. In addition, both the board and the management realized that each of the five centers, separated by miles of roads and mountains, served hamlets and communities with different histories, resources, health profiles, and needs. Each health center therefore developed an advisory board that was able to offer a distinct and additional viewpoint to the operation of the network. The priorities identified by the local advisory boards, while overlapping some of those of the management of HHHN, also brought into sharper focus major health concerns of each local community.

The advisory boards identified treatment of accidents and occupational injuries (for example, chain saw injuries) as a major concern of local residents whether or not they were active users of the centers. Trauma was a chief cause of adult morbidity within the region and, for some of the communities served by the health centers, the nearest hospital was over an hour and a half drive over often treacherous roads. HHHN ensured that each health center was well equipped to stabilize trauma victims. In each community, the health centers joined with local organizations such as the volunteer firemen to sponsor emergency medical technician (EMT) courses and to raise money for ambulances. Individuals within the service communities volunteer for training as ambulance drivers. The advisory boards, as well as project management, actively continue to monitor the EMT program, often bringing to management's attention perceived problems in the performance of this program.

Noteworthy in this example was the way in which community participation, in the form of advisory boards, identified a problem and suggested an intervention program that affected a wider community than that of active users. Perhaps because HHHN is virtually the sole provider of health services in the geographic area, the governing board, advisory boards, and project staff and management accepted responsibility for this problem once it was identified. Looking to cooperate with other elements of the communities involved, HHHN was able to plan and implement an intervention which required broader support than could have been provided by HHHN alone. Continued surveillance of the success of this effort is understood to be the responsibility of several groups in each of the participating communities.[1]

COMMUNITY SERVICE AS A BASIS FOR COPC ACTIVITIES

Physicians are often involved in community service projects. Many donate time to schools for physical exams for team sports. Others are asked to give lectures or advice on a regular basis or to serve on advisory boards for local campaigns. In many communities, the collective expectation is that the physician's role includes assuming a degree of community leadership. This ascribed status can be useful if the physician (and other health practitioners) chooses to consciously attempt to identify health problems within the community and wants to elicit support from other members of the community. From identifying toxic waste problems or other environmental hazards to developing community-based screening programs, health practitioners can inspire community-level efforts to deal with health-related issues. This community service can easily be extended into COPC activity if the physicians and community organizations began to systematize the collection of data so that education and programs can be designed and evaluated to meet epidemiologically determined needs.

In many instances physicians have participated in such nascent COPC efforts. Many years ago, pediatricians in a small community in upstate New York were asked to give lectures as part of a series to volunteer firemen. In preparation for this, they reviewed samples of their own charts and hospital admission data. Startled to find that a large percentage of childhood emergencies were injuries sustained in relatively minor auto accidents, they enlisted the firemen and subsequently other groups in an educational campaign to get parents to "buckle-up." Realizing that many parents within their community couldn't afford baby car seats, they established a lending library of car seats. Beyond educating the parents within their practice, they took their educational campaign to

---

[1] Information on Hudson Headwaters Health Network comes from several reports written by the project staff during 1984-1985 and from a site visit made in September 1985.

schools, newspapers, and community organizations. Even before New York State passed a law making it compulsory for children under 5 to be in appropriate car seats, these doctors knew they had aided in reducing injuries due to trauma.[2]

WHEN THE COMMUNITY IDENTIFIES THE NEED

The processes in the development of COPC have been defined in detail elsewhere (4,5). In a simple form, the process can be described as follows:

- Preliminary steps
- Community health diagnosis and health surveillance
- Planning of intervention
- Implementation
- Evaluation
- Decisionmaking for future action

One of the many advantages of community participation in COPC is that often different groups within a community will bring different perspectives to identifying priorities and problems. Although difficulties might develop by their identifying competing priorities, more frequently the addition of a perspective beyond that of the professionals involved adds to the appreciation and identification of health problems.

In the late 1970s, community health activists in a Chicago slum had, after a long campaign, succeeded in gaining access to, and a voice in the control of, the two local hospitals serving the area. Despite winning the battle for access to services, the major health problems within the community were not ameliorated. Changing medical services was not the answer to health problems which required major changes in "individual, social, economic and environmental relationships"

(6). By reviewing hospital records and sampling emergency room charts, the frequency of problems which brought people to the hospital was determined. The seven most common reasons for hospitalization, in order of frequency were: automobile accidents; interpersonal attacks; accidents (non-auto); bronchial ailments; alcoholism; drug-related problems; and dog bites.

Because these community activists were interested in attacking a problem they had hopes of solving, they chose dog bites, which accounted for 4 percent of the emergency room visits. They used community block clubs to advertise a finder's fee for every stray dog identified. During a one-month period, 160 of these wild dogs were captured and cases of dog bites seen in the emergency rooms decreased dramatically.

Buoyed by success in the dog bite campaign, they identified automobile accidents as their second campaign. Using data on location of automobile accidents, they were able to map where accidents were occurring most frequently. Discovering that one parking lot entrance accounted for a disproportionate number of accidents, they were able to negotiate with the owners to create a safer entrance. Simultaneously, they were able to document that a traffic routing pattern had contributed to excess accidents, and joined by other community organizations they were able to tackle Chicago's bureaucracy to redirect traffic flow.

Without the community activists' involvement neither of these health problems (nor their ultimate solution) might have been recognized by the health professionals within the hospital. Indeed, neither of the problems might have been seen as "health" or "disease" problems, despite the frequency for which they accounted for hospital admissions, by professionals trained to recognize pathophysiology.

Some health problems go unrecognized, not because they fall outside of the tradi-

---

[2] Private communications with physicians in Columbia County, N.Y.

tional purview of medicine, but because individual physicians may not see enough of the problem to recognize and identify a pattern. Workers at a chemical plant in New Jersey, through talking with each other, discovered that many were deeply upset by periods of impotency, by an inability to conceive in some cases, by miscarriages, and by offspring with congenital malformations. Convinced of a problem by the frequency with which these problems were arising, the workers concluded that these events must be related to each other and to some exposure at the work site. The Oil, Chemical, and Atomic Workers Union took their suspicions seriously enough to pay for an appropriate work-up of all individuals working within the plant. When the results of the exam indicated that man of the men had problems with spermatogenesis, OSHA was called in and dichlorobromopropane was found to be hazardous. This community of workers had accurately identified the existence of a problem that would not have been discovered by health professionals alone.

Even when health professionals have been able to identify a pattern of diseases, they may not be able to identify the issues that impede or thwart efforts to prevent or treat. At El Rio Community Health Center in Arizona, elderly members of the community approached the governing board asking that pharmacy policies be modified. Physicians treating the elderly for chronic diseases had assumed that lack of compliance in medication taking was a result of language barriers or educational lacks. Instead, the elderly identified the high cost of medicines not covered by Medicare as the major obstacle in complying with the doctors' instructions.

Community participation has been essential in many situations in accurately assessing barriers to care. The William Fitz Ryan Health Center in upper Manhattan had been providing excellent comprehensive primary care for over a decade when a group of elderly residents in the neighborhood requested a meeting with the governing board. These elderly, concerned that many of their peers did not have personal physicians or waited until they were severely ill before seeking medical aid, helped the center identify ways to increase the Ryan Center's attractiveness to the elderly.

The Center, used in an old clinic building, was waiting to build a new facility. The elderly felt that many of the architectural features of the building made it difficult for relatively frail elderly to use the facility. The Center, stymied by an inability to renovate, welcomed the suggestion by the elderly of establishing satellite clinics in day care and housing projects for the elderly.

Even with Medicare, the copayments, deductible, and pharmaceutical costs of ambulatory services are prohibitive for many elderly living on fixed incomes. Working with the elderly advisors, the Ryan Center was able to derive optional payment mechanisms that made services financially feasible. Working with sympathetic health providers, including nurse practitioners, health promotion and nutritional programs targeted at the special needs identified by the elderly were developed.

The Ryan Center's elderly satellite clinics working with other social service agencies serving the elderly have become a model for ambulatory services to this age group. The Center's administration is quick to point out that the impetus arose from the elderly within the community and that the creation of programs was through joint planning by the center and community representatives (7).

Su Clinica Familiar (SCF) is located in a largely Hispanic, rural, medically underserved area on the Texas-Mexico border. Among the most severe health problems confronting the community were extremely high infant mortality, maternal morbidity, and low birthweight rates. In trying to discover why more women failed to use the existing prenatal services, the SCF staff needed the help of community members. Through meetings and by fostering a "coalition of commitment" among community groups, providers, and patients, SCF was able to develop a birthing center that met the distinctive cultural needs of the community.

Using traditional midwives working alongside midwives and obstetricians trained and licensed though conventional American medical schools, the birthing center was able to attract women who had never before sought prenatal care. Older women who had already raised children and who shared the new mothers' culture and language became partners throughout the pregnancy and after childbirth. Su Clinica Familiar's collaboration with other community groups and with its own patients led to a dramatic decline in the infant mortality and maternal morbidity rates. The continued refinement of the maternal-child health programs through constant surveillance and evaluation of birth outcomes allows SCF to feel confident that the initial success of this program will continue. (8)

The inability to pay for care is too frequently the greatest barrier to seeking care in this country. Yet, even in financially more stable communities, other barriers to care exist including cultural, educational, traditional, and social barriers. In the Midwest farmbelt, the recent increase in suicide among farmers has led to the establishment of hotlines and support groups. Physicians, psychiatrists, and social workers have been asked for help by farmers' organizations in designing surveys to assess how many farm families have members with severe depression who are reluctant to seek help, either because asking for help is foreign to the farmers' tradition of self-reliance or because admitting

to feelings of despondency is culturally forbidden. Knowing the extent of families at risk may help in creating successful intervention programs.

The farmers' organizations seeking the aid of the health professionals recognize that a "health" problem exists whose origins are economic, political, and social. They know the solution to the problem is outside of the health arena. Recognizing these limitations has not discouraged them from trying, with professional help, to create an intervention that depends on a coalition of farm groups and professionals.

Neither the farmers nor the health professionals are aware of the conceptual framework of COPC, yet they are taking the initial steps by identifying a problem, trying to quantify the extent of the problem within the community, and trying to create an intervention program that involves the community in the promotion of its own health. While this effort attacks a single problem and fails to place it within the framework of primary care, it illustrates (along with other examples) that community participation in identifying health problems often brings an energy and perspective that would be lacking if health professionals try alone to identify problems and determine priorities for a community.

COMMUNITY PARTICIPATION IN PROGRAM DESIGN AND IMPLEMENTATION

In many of the examples already cited, community involvement in identifying health problems led directly to involvement in creating the epidemiologic base for evaluating the severity of these problems. Since some segment of the community was already involved in identifying the health needs, community participation in program design and implementation followed naturally.

At times, the practice or the physicians will identify a problem independently of direct community input. Frequently, elements within the community will have expressed concern with related issues. Involving the community in program planning and implementation is a necessary step to ensure success. Since implementation needs to take into account existing resources, social and behavioral mores, and health-related beliefs and behaviors of community members, implementation of a health intervention program will be doomed unless practitioners seek community cooperation.

Many implementation programs require also that multiple service agencies coordinate their efforts. Other implementation programs are relatively straightforward and require little more than aid from other organizations in the form of publicity, manpower, or physical space. Yet no matter how simple or complex the intervention appears initially, some form of community participation is a prerequisite. Not only will community participation during implementation bring a different perspective to the activities, future cooperation will be much more forthcoming if groups and individuals have been intimately involved through the whole process.

The planning and implementation process may call on groups of individuals who have not previously been involved. Several family planning clinics, concerned that male teenagers were not being reached, systematically attempted to include teenagers in the planning of campaigns to reach them. The inclusion of teenagers in the planning process generated innovative methods for recruiting new patients. Sports teams and social clubs became central to several of the family planning centers' drives. The Spectrum Center in Philadelphia used spot announcements on local rock stations and was able to get a rock star to record messages for family planning. Spectrum Center registered over 900 new male family planning users and will be continuing to monitor the impact,

both by counting users of its services and by following the teenage pregnancy rate in its community (9).

In Bolivar County, Mississippi, community participation in the development and implementation of community health programs starting in 1966 has led to the transformation of the entire community. It would be naive to argue that the health center alone transformed one of the poorest counties in the country. Certainly a combination of historical factors, economic programs, and legislation helped. But the point of entry for much of the social intervention was the creation of the North Bolivar Health Council. Rooting this program in viable community institutions and ensuring policymaking and program creation was always seen as directly responsive and responsible to community needs led to the successes of this legendary program (10,11). Dr. Geiger states that "every black household in the poverty population in all of northern Bolivar County has at least one (and often more than one) adult member actively participating in decision-making, program planning and program operation. . . ." (11).

Beyond providing primary care, the Health Center became the center of enormous numbers of health and health-related programs within Bolivar County. Many families' only water source was contaminated water from drainage ditches. Crumbling surface privies were used for disposal of human excrement. Well-digging and hand-pump installation and the construction of sanitary privies became priorities for the health council. Children and adults were often hungry and showed signs of malnutrition. There was not enough food. The North Bolivar County Farm Cooperative, an outgrowth of the health center and health council but ultimately independent, began to grow food.

Perhaps the largest accomplishment of the Center is the encouragement and support it gave to more than 100 community residents, in providing for pre-professional and professional training in health-related fields. Many of these individuals have returned to Bolivar County and continue to work for the community's health. The tradition of community participation built into every phase of program development continues even while individuals from the community assume new roles as health providers.

COMMUNITY ROLE IN EVALUATION AND DECISIONMAKING FOR THE FUTURE

Evaluating the relative success and failure of any program is very difficult. Participants who have sweated over programs, stayed awake through many meetings, and invested their energies may find it extraordinarily difficult to step back and ask the tough questions: Are we accomplishing what we set out to accomplish? Have we evidence, quantifiable or nonquantifiable, of the effect of this program on the health status of the community? What could we have done differently? What should we do in the future?

Here again community participation can add another dimension, a different point of view. Expectations of what could have been accomplished may have differed from the start or the intimacy of living or working within the community may lead to differing perspectives on what actually was accomplished. Since evaluation is an essential part of "closing the loop," of developing a systematized approach to providing care, evaluating the health status of a community, creating programs in response to documented needs and modifying these programs on the basis of informed decisions, community participation is as essential at this stage as in any other.

CONCLUSION

Community participation in any health program is inherently difficult. Problems abound—defining community, deciding who speaks for the community, functioning around the shifts in local power bases, coping with the different cultural expectations of different groups within the community and the potential class differences between health care providers and community members (12). Yet community participation is essential for the success of any exercise in community medicine and, certainly, for the development of COPC practices.

Many of the examples of community participation chosen here are taken from community health centers and other organized systems of care. Perhaps because community health centers, migrant health centers, family planning clinics, etc., have acknowledged their responsibilities for a community wider than that of their patients alone, these examples may be closer at hand. Or the author's professional experience may have led her to look more closely at community health centers and their close relations. Certainly community participation is possible, and has been achieved, in a variety of settings.

None of these practices are the full-blown model of COPC as outlined in the Institute of Medicine study, *Community-Oriented Primary Care: A Practical Assessment.* Each has some elements of community medicine combined with a service delivery model that responds to problems beyond its own walls. Each is answering to the health needs of a known population and is a richer practice for involving the community. While none may have yet created the synthesis that is the conceptual model of COPC, each is somewhere on the way.

The benefits of community participation in creating COPC practices do not only accrue to the practice. Community members gain in experience and in self-confidence and collectively the community gains in coherence and self-definition. Community participation serves to strengthen the commitment to the community. As community health projects and community-oriented primary care practices evolve, communities will be healthier not only as a result of the measurable outcomes but as a result of the process. Community participation and involvement is a central premise of COPC.

REFERENCES

1. Susser, Watson, and Hopper. *Sociology in Medicine*. New York: Oxford University Press, 1985.

2. Salber, E. Community participation in neighborhood health centers. *New England Journal of Medicine* 1970; 283:515.

3. Seifert, M.H. The patient advisory council. In *Community-Oriented Primary Care: New Directions for Health Services Delivery*, Connor E. and Mullan, F. (eds.). Washington, D.C.: National Academy Press, 1983.

4. Connor, E. and Mullan, F. *Community-Oriented Primary Care: New Directions for Health Services Delivery*. Washington, D.C.: National Academy Press, 1983.

5. Institute of Medicine. *Community-Oriented Primary Care: A Practical Assessment*. Washington, D.C.: National Academy Press, 1984.

6. McKnight, J. Community health and a Chicago slum. *Health/PAC Bulletin* 1980; 11(6).

7. Lukomnik, J. *Ambulatory Services and the Poor Elderly*. Report to the United Hospital Fund, 1986.

8. Fish, S. COPC in the Texas Valley. In *Community-Oriented Primary Care: New Directions for Health Services Delivery*, Connor, E. and Mullan, F. (eds.). Washington, D.C.: National Academy Press, 1983.

9. *Report from the Executive Director*, Regional Cluster Training Center Meeting, July 1985.

10. Geiger, J.H. A health center in Mississippi—a case study in social medicine. In: *Medicine in a Changing Society*, Corey, L.; Saltman, S.; and Epstein, M. (eds.). St. Louis, MO, C.V. Mosby, 1972.

11. Geiger, J.H. The meaning of community-oriented primary care in the American context. In *Community-Oriented Primary Care: New Directions for Health Services Delivery*, Connor, E. and Mullan, F. (eds.). Washington, D.C.: National Academy Press, 1983.

12. Hochbaum, C.M. Consumer participation in health planning: Toward conceptual clarification. *American Journal of Public Health* 1969; 59:1698.

CHAPTER 44

Responsibility in COPC: An Analysis in Medical Ethics

William L. Freeman, M.D., M.P.H.

T he COPC model includes a "defined community for which the practice has accepted responsibility for health care" (1). There is an unanswered question in that definition: when, and how, did the community *accept* that a COPC practice had responsibility for its health care?

Do members of a community accept the offer by a COPC practitioner that "I will be responsible for your health care?" Do they reciprocate by responding "You are responsible for my health care" or "Dr. X is responsible for my personal health care, but you are responsible for my community health care?" Do all staff of COPC practices accept that the practice has responsibility for the health care of community members who are not patients of the practice? Do all, or most, physicians feel comfortable with COPC's responsibility?

In my experience, the answer to all four questions is no. What, then, are the limits of responsibility in COPC?

In the COPC model, a practice provides care to an identified group of people. The assumption of the model seems to be that all members of the community either come to the practice as patients, or are nonattenders but would come to the prac-

tice except for difficulties such as access or ignorance. Yet people encounter the health care system in more varied ways than COPC implies.

For instance, when I review charts to identify and call in all patients needing Pneumovax immunization who have not received it, I encounter grey areas that are puzzling. Some people have charts (i.e., have assumed the patient role at least once), but I am not sure they are patients in the usual sense. They have come to the Indian Health Service (IHS) Clinic for only limited services, for example, dental care. What are the parameters and limits of responsibility for COPC-linked personal health services, such as Pneumovax, to these "limited patients?" Other community members either go nowhere for care, or go elsewhere for all their personal care. What are the parameters and limits of COPC responsibility to intentional nonattenders?

In relationship to COPC, there are eight categories of patients. At least five types are problematic for COPC practitioners:

1. *The intentional nonattender who goes elsewhere.* This is the otherwise full member of the community who goes elsewhere

for all personal medical care. For example, in a family that considers itself enrolled in the COPC practice, one member goes to another practice, or a member of the Indian Reservation goes to a non-IHS clinic.

2. *The intentional partial attender who goes elsewhere.* This is the full member of the community who uses the practice for limited care and goes elsewhere for major care. For example, a member might go to the practice for lacerations but to other physicians for hypertension and diabetes treatment.

3. *The intentional partial attender who is a partial- or noncommunity-member.* This is the intermittent user of limited services provided by the practice who is not a full member of the community, for example, the yearly summer vacationer.

4. *The intentional nonattender who goes nowhere for care.* This is the full member of the community who refuses medical care by anyone.

5. *The patient who accepts all personal care, but refuses COPC intervention.* This is the full member of the community who thinks, states, or complains that he or she does not want to receive any COPC intervention, or even feels that the practice should not do COPC activity.

Other types of patients are less problematic.

6. *The nonintentional nonattender.*[1] This is a full member of the community who does not attend for reasons such as poverty, access problems, or ignorance—the type of person the COPC practitioner hopes to influence by outreach, community programs, etc.

7. *The patient who is not a community member, accepts all personal care, and wants to receive COPC intervention.* This is the patient from outside the community who

wants the community-based COPC interventions. Often it is a patient who followed a physician who moved to the COPC practice, or who believes that the COPC practice offers the highest quality personal care available.

8. *The patient who accepts all personal care and COPC intervention.* This is a full member of the community who accepts and wants full personal and COPC care.

What is a COPC practitioner's responsibility to those kinds of patients? Many physicians understand the doctor-patient relationship as a mutual "contract" (2). The patient asks the physician for help or care, and the physician responds by accepting responsibility to provide that care. Most physicians seem comfortable doing an active outreach, for example, calling in patients needing Pneumovax, so long as they have a "contract" with the patient to provide care. Many physicians wanting to do COPC are uncomfortable doing an active outreach with a patient who intentionally has no "contract" with the physician (types 1 and 4 above), or has a "contract" on which the patient has placed limits (types 2, 3, and 5 above).

The problem is a conflict between two values: improving people's health, and needing a "contract" to have legitimacy for active intervention in a person's life. It is a conflict in ethics and in acceptable role behavior. I discuss the details of this conflict and propose an analysis to resolve it.

---

[1] "Intentional" and "nonintentional" are not dichotomous categories, but are ends of a continuous spectrum. The categories may not help one analyze the situation. Rather, the variables *attendance to care elsewhere* vs. *no attendance anywhere*, and if no attendance anywhere, the *degree of commitment* to nonattendance if factors external to the person were changed, are most helpful in analyzing the situation.

A METHOD TO ANALYZE THE PROBLEM: MEDICAL ETHICS[2]

Although most medical ethicists are content to analyze case studies, Robert M. Veatch (3) provides a thoughtful method to develop an ethical system for analyzing specific cases or conflicts.

Veatch's method is to ask what would be the system of ethical principles agreed to by members of society who had the "moral point of view," that is, a view that *gives other people's interests the same weight as one's own.* Veatch's method is close to John Rawls' method (4) of asking what would be the system of ethical principles adopted by rational people coming together "under the veil of ignorance," i.e., not knowing their biases and the special interests of their specific role in life.

My purpose is not to describe the system of ethics that Veatch derives by his method, but to use a method similar to his to analyze the ethical problems of COPC. However, because I will use his system of ethical principles in the discussion that follows, I give a brief outline of the system he proposes.

People with a moral point of view, that other people's welfare is of equal value to one's own, would chose three levels of medical ethical principles:

The first level is *the basic social contract of the total community*—the fundamental ethical principles, the content of the ethical system, that apply to all, not just to lay and medical people (e.g., "agreements freely entered into should be kept").

The second level is *the contract between society and the profession,* which gives the role-specific duties of laymen and medical people when they interact with each other (e.g., "medical confidences will be maintained, except when the professional obtains knowledge of danger to another person").

The third level is *contracts between laymen (singly or in groups) and professional people,* which govern mutually desired specifics of their relationship (e.g., people who feel strongly about abortion might go to physicians with similar feelings).

The second level is compatible with the first, and the third with the second. *Medical* ethics involves primarily the second.

Veatch states that people with the "moral point of view" would choose a contract between society and the profession with the following basic ethical principles of *primary* importance: keep and honor contracts including confidentiality within specific limits; respect the autonomy of patients, guardians, and professionals within specific limits; maintain truthful relationships within specific limits; the killing of human beings is in severe conflict with the role of the healer; with specific exceptions, physicians giving personal care are exempted from the obligation to distribute resources justly when that obligation conflicts with the rights and responsibilities of the doctor-patient relationship.

Once these primary ethical principles are met, the contract follows the general principle of producing benefit to the patient.[3]

Returning to the analysis of COPC, there are at least nine different interests concerning COPC's responsibility:

1. Community members and patients of the COPC physician(s) who want full personal and COPC care;

2. Nonmembers of the community and patients of the COPC physician(s)

[2] For most of what follows, much of my analysis is derived from R.M. Veatch's A *Theory of Medical Ethics* (New York: Basic Books, 1981). Henry Taylor introduced it to me. My unfamiliarity with Veatch's approach and method of analysis, despite my having taken both advanced ethics courses in the Department of Philosophy and medical ethics in medical school and residency, illustrates that in medical ethics, as in medicine, advances are made, and that keeping up with the advances requires knowledgeable and guided effort.

who want full personal and COPC care;

3. Members of the community and nonintentional nonattenders of medical care;

4. Members of the community and intentional nonattenders of all medical care;

5. Members of the community and partial or complete attenders to providers other than the COPC practice;

6. Community members and noncommunity people who want personal care only, not COPC intervention;

7. The community as a group;

8. Non-COPC physicians who care for members of the community;

9. The COPC physician(s).

My adaptation of Veatch's method is to ask what would people who adopted the moral point of view agree to about COPC as they discuss these nine interests. The discussions would distinguish concerns or interests that are ethical (e.g., to have one's autonomy respected) from concerns or interests that are not ethical (e.g., about a physician's share of the market).[4]

As I see it, there are three problems or conflicts concerning responsibility in COPC. The first concerns personal health care linked to COPC activities, such as an immunization initiative to have all people over age 60 get influenza vaccine every year. The second concerns community health programs linked to COPC, such as establishment of an emergency medical system in a rural area by the initiative of the COPC practice. The third is the time or resource allocation between giving personal care and doing COPC. I adapt Veatch's method to discuss each of them.

PERSONAL HEALTH CARE LINKED TO COPC ACTIVITIES

A practice with active outreach to do COPC-related personal medical care, for example, to promote immunization with Pneumovax for appropriate people, is compatible with all nine interests if it has certain characteristics.

All lay members of the community, irrespective of their relationship with the

---

[3] The reader may wonder about the lack of reference to the formal statement of professional ethics by organizations such as the American Medical Association, or the extensive involvement of lay people in the method of determining the principles of medical ethics. Veatch gives the history of both points, and argues well why the historical facts should be accepted. I strongly recommend his book.

The reader may also question the artificiality of conducting a thought experiment, involving an imaginary discussion by people with a "moral point of view" as a method to derive a system of medical ethics.

This is in the tradition of the "social contract" of Thomas Hobbes and John Locke. Their method is a sophisticated application in the tradition of the Golden Rule. Hillel (d. 10 A.D.) gave the Rule's Jewish version (Babylonian Talmud Shabbat 31a): "What is hateful unto you, do not do unto thy neighbor. That is the whole of the Torah. The rest is commentary." A few years later, Jesus gave the Christian version (Matthew 7:12 RSV): "So whatever you wish that men do to you, do so to them; for this is the law and the prophets." Many philosophers have stated nonreligious versions of the Golden Rule.

For instance, in Veatch's method to derive the system of medical ethics, lay people with a moral point of view respect physician autonomy: "If I were a physician, I would want . . . ." Similarly, physicians with a moral point of view respect the autonomy of lay people: "If I were a patient, I would want . . . ." In fact, many physicians are a patient or family member at one time or another, and write commentary and critique about medical care from that perspective (e.g., Feinstein, A.R. The state of the art. JAMA 1986; 255:1488).

People who disvalue or disagree with our mutual interdependence in a community, or with the reciprocity of the "moral point of view"—that one should consider other people's values and interests equal to one's own, are unlikely to agree with Veatch's method because they do not agree with Veatch's fundamental values, nor mine.

---

[4] "Legitimate" or "not legitimate" are not dichotomous classes but two ends of a single spectrum.

375

COPC physician(s), have two interests relevant to the discussion. One is that the COPC practice respect their autonomy by permitting the community members to refuse the COPC care without being ridiculed or pressured, even if they are patients of the COPC practice. The other is that the COPC practice offer care to all community members and inform all community members about the availability of the care.

Specific types of community members and patients have additional interests. Nonmembers of the community who are established patients of the COPC practice want the COPC-linked care to include them; they want the same attention as patients of.the same practice who are community members. Community members who are partial or complete attenders to providers other than the COPC practice want their choice of personal physician to be respected (i.e., not be forced to reject their relationship with a non-COPC physician in order to receive the COPC service, and be informed that they can go to their own physician for similar service if that physician offers it). The interest of members of the community who are nonintentional nonattenders of medical care want the outreach because they would be the major group benefitting by the outreach as part of a just distribution of resources.

The total community's interest is that the COPC practitioners respect its values and autonomy by delivering the service with minimal community disruption. That is, the COPC-linked personal care should be offered in a positive manner, without being negative toward nonresponders.

COPC and non-COPC physicians have similar interests in one respect: both support the delivery of COPC-linked personal care by the COPC practice because both want to respect the autonomy of the provider to decide how care is delivered. The non-COPC physicians have two addi-tional interests. Non-COPC physicians are concerned that COPC physicians not actively interfere with the relationship between non-COPC physicians and their patients, and that COPC practices not handicap possible participation by non-COPC practices (e.g., by arranging that only the COPC practice get Pneumovax free from the Health Department). (These latter two activities are aggressive competitive marketing, not community-oriented primary care.)

COPC physicians have ethical interests in configuring their outreach in ways that do not make it a weapon against non-COPC practitioners in the competition battle. Using COPC to obtain a marketing advantage will elicit passive-aggressive resistance, if not active sabotage, by non-COPC physicians against a program beneficial to the entire community. Also, the involvement of the non-COPC practitioners will likely increase the total number of people who accept the COPC service.

COMMUNITY HEALTH PROGRAMS LINKED TO COPC PROGRAMS

Activities in COPC-linked community health programs, such as improving the community's emergency medical system, are compatible with all nine interests if they have certain characteristics. Most of the comments about COPC-linked personal health care apply here as well.

Established patients of the COPC practice who are not community members have only a peripheral interest—that all communities have improved health care.

The total community has strong interests that COPC practitioners respect its values and autonomy by planning and doing COPC programs with minimal disruption or controversy in the community, and that they recognize the community's legitimate and legitimizing role in community-oriented primary care.

Non-COPC physicians have an interest that they be allowed to participate in the COPC program if they desire—that the program be inclusive rather than exclusive concerning physician participation.

Most people dislike self-appointed community spokesmen who exclude the community from decisionmaking, and most physicians dislike a community program that excludes them. Lay or professional people who are excluded from participation may resist or sabotage an otherwise beneficial program. The COPC practitioners' practical self-interest is to comply with the community's and non-COPC physicians' interests. The COPC practitioners' ethical interest is to work in a way that elicits maximum possible acceptance of these benefits by both lay and professional community members.

TIME OR RESOURCE ALLOCATION BETWEEN GIVING PERSONAL CARE AND DOING COPC

Potentially contradictory interests are more obvious in this subject. On the one hand, both established patients of the COPC practice and the total community have an interest that the physician provide personal care. Providing such care is the societal role of the physician, and society gives the physician special rewards and dispensations for being in that role. If that role is abandoned, no one else will fill it for the physician's patients.

On the other hand, the total community, the nonintentional nonattenders of medical care, and the attenders of medical care irrespective of physician involved, would potentially benefit by a COPC program. An important aspect of COPC is its positive impact on distributive justice.

Veatch states that, when the physician's responsibility to a patient collides with his responsibility to a nonpatient with greater need, only "in *extreme* cases

the principle of justice overrides considerations of the existing contractual promise between physician and lay patient" (3) (my emphasis).

The COPC situation is not a direct conflict between the two obligations. (An example of a direct conflict would be if a physician interrupted a patient encounter by saying, "Sorry, I have to interrupt your exam to study a computer printout of a COPC report.")

Rather, doing COPC presents an *indirect* conflict between the physician's role as healer and the role of benefitting large groups of people with need. The number of hours a physician is available for patient care is reduced by the number of hours devoted to COPC. People with a moral point of view, and considering the nine interests listed above, probably would conclude that physicians can do COPC if there is reasonable evidence that doing COPC would benefit the practitioner's patients and the total community; that the indirect conflict should never become direct, i.e., no patient should be presented with a severe interruption of service due to COPC; that the COPC practice's primary responsibility is to provide medical care to its patients; and that the COPC practice should see that its commitment to COPC does not cause so much loss of patient care time that the quality of personal care is reduced.

DISCUSSION

The involvement of the community in planning and doing COPC is critical for resolving potential ethical conflicts. As shown in the foregoing analysis, the COPC practitioners must accommodate eight interests beyond their own.

There are many reasons for involving the community, such as a more accurate assessment of community needs and enlisting active and interested people to improve the community's health.

The ethical analysis above implies that community involvement should meet two, even more fundamental, needs. The first is to legitimize the community-oriented primary care program by including the community's values and viewpoints in planning, doing, and assessing COPC. The second is to have a group with community legitimacy discuss ethical conflicts in COPC, by people who try to adopt the moral point of view.

These needs must be met while acknowledging that "the community" in reality is composed of people with at least nine differing interests. Because COPC involves conflicts among values, roles, interests, and responsibilities, and because COPC practitioners are one of nine groups in the conflict, COPC practitioners should explicitly ask for help from people knowledgeable about those other interests, values, roles, and responsibilities.

More explicitly, the analysis above implies that the community board, or group of interested patients, or any other form of community involvement, explicitly consider and discuss these differing interests, values, roles, and responsibilities.

SUMMARY

Many physicians feel uncomfortable with possible ethical conflicts from doing COPC. Using a method of analysis derived from Robert Veatch, I conclude that if the COPC program has certain characteristics, COPC is fully compatible with the basic principles of medical ethics. However, because there are potential ethical conflicts of legitimately different interests and values, a COPC program should discuss those ethical questions related to COPC with appropriate local people.

REFERENCES

1. Institute of Medicine. *Community-Oriented Primary Care: A Practical Assessment*, Volume I. Washington, DC: National Academy Press, 1984, p. 28.

2. Magraw, R.M. Social and medical contracts: Explicit and implicit. In: *Hippocrates Revisited*, Bulger, R.J. (ed.). New York: Medcom, 1973.

3. Veatch, R.M. *A Theory of Medical Ethics*. New York: Basic Books, 1981.

4. Rawls, J. *A Theory of Justice*. Cambridge, MA.: Harvard University Press, 1971.

CHAPTER 45

An Incremental Patient Participation Model

Milton H. Seifert, Jr., M.D.

General physicians have a natural interest in the health of their communities. Awareness of community health comes from contacts with individual patients and individual families. Practitioners know that community medical practices are an efficient listening post. Given this experience base it is easy for a practitioner to imagine a concept that would start with identifying the health needs of individuals and families and lead to the identification of community health problems. In the same way, practice programs would develop in response to individual needs and lead to programs responding to community needs. But then practitioners would want to know if these exercises were practical, useful, and worthwhile. This would lead the community practitioner to thoughts of how this might be measured, i.e., how to monitor the impact of modifications. Finally, it is also easy to imagine the practitioner discussing these ideas with a professional researcher who would point out that measurements must be made against some standard, some denominator. The practitioner would then see the wisdom in defining and characterizing the community.

The foregoing is a description of the heart of COPC. It may not be a conscious concept but it is internalized in the experienced community practitioner. In addition, it is both natural and conscious for the practitioner to understand the need for clinical skills, for availability and accessibility, for comprehensive care, and for continuity of care. Similarly, it is extremely rare for a general physician not to understand the need for interdependence and team functioning. These characteristics then, complete the COPC concept.

The practitioner in a small, personal, and relationship-oriented practice is more likely to understand the concept early on, but is overwhelmed by the lack of resources, namely, time, money, and expertise. Busy general physicians cannot get their mind around the idea of taking on the whole community in addition to so many other responsibilities, but they do understand the value of patient participation in health care delivery. One needs only to see that it is neither wise nor necessary to assume the whole responsibility of bringing the concept of COPC to reality, and that it can be a manageable task if it is done with the help of patients and in an incremental fashion.

The small office that must practice economy of purpose, time, and economics, and by its nature is small and personal, is in a unique position to adopt the incremental patient participation model. It is in this setting that practitioners and patients understand the value of their ongoing relationship. As familiarity increases, they assume the roles of co-examiners and co-therapists. When diagnosis and treatment is unclear they adopt the processing method wherein each contributes what each can until a negotiated consensus is achieved. The better the quality of the relationship dynamics, the better will be the quality of the health care outcomes. A practitioner begins to move from COPC principle to COPC practice by seeing himself or herself as a research investigator and the practice as a research laboratory. The practice can move from COPC principle to COPC practice when it realizes and then adopts a patient participation model. Patients now become co-developers and co-researchers. The practitioner/patient partnership can now begin some simple data collection, and the process has begun. In time, this partnership of practitioner and patient will begin to see the community as its patient and the community as its laboratory.

The first steps that an interested community medical practice can take are as follows:

1. For the first month ask various patients their opinion on the medical practice and its services. Record these opinions.

2. The second month ask various patients their opinion of community health needs. Record these opinions.

3. Begin to think of a way to formalize the relationship between the practice staff and the patient group.

RELATIONSHIP ENHANCEMENT

The dynamics successful in the health care services can now be extended and applied to the patient group/practice staff partnership. Some practical next steps are as follows:

1. Start a folder labeled: Patient Group/Practice Staff Cooperation.

2. Construct a patient satisfaction questionnaire to be completed by patients in the waiting room. Choose questions from the information gathered in the first 2 months. Write your own questionnaire, then ask a research professional to critique it and help you refine the questions.

3. Start a patient grievance committee to resolve patient complaints and preserve relationships.

4. Ask your malpractice insurer to give you a 10 percent discount for your grievance committee (1), since it is actually a form of risk management.

5. Meet with patients identified in months one and two and see how they might help you to help your practice or help you to help the community. Adopt the processing method used when practitioners and patients find themselves with an unclear medical situation, perhaps focusing on what they could do to help you meet a specific need.

ORGANIZING THE PRACTICE STAFF/PATIENT GROUP PARTNERSHIP

Start a Talent Bank Registry

The first step in organizing a partnership with the patient group is to start a file of individuals possessing desired skills and talents—a Talent Bank Registry. Make a list of people who might come to mind as helpers to others, for example, Alcoholics Anonymous and Alanon members, or a support person for a body weight management problem or for grief management. Design a postcard questionnaire for these individuals. When the cards are returned they can form a basis of a card file. Ask one person to be chairman and help you develop a larger committee.

Develop Special Committees for Special Needs

Several specialized committees will need to be formed, including: a committee to look at business, financial, and practice management issues; a committee to study increasing obstetrical safety and decreasing malpractice risk; a support group for general problems (a local AA member might be willing to act as a facilitator); a research committee, which might study seatbelt use, patient satisfaction, or the number of patients seen on an acute and episodic basis compared to the total number of patients seen. Eventually develop an age/sex register.

Formalize the Development of a Patient Advisory Committee

Choose a membership chairman, using the method described on page 16 of the booklet, *Starting Your Own Patient Advisory Council*, by Early and Seifert (2). The principal thing to remember here is that the membership chair must get the people together in order to have regular meetings.

Call a meeting of previously active patients and organize committees to address one or more of the issues outlined in Table 1.

DISCUSSION

Our Patient Advisory Council in Excelsior, Minnesota, has been cited in *Megatrends* (3) as an example of the response to one of the current trends in society. People are weaning themselves from dependence on community institutions and relearning the ability to take action on their own. For health care, this means that patients are more ready and willing to take more responsibility for their own health.

When we began in 1974, there were some misconceptions among our patients of their potential role. At first some believed participation in a patient advisory council would be disrespectful to their physician. Other patients questioned the value of the contribution of a lay person to the complex world of medicine. Finally, once our patients could believe that we wanted their participation and could see that they had something of value to contribute, the final concern surfaced: "Isn't this an awful lot of responsibility for us to take?" The answer to this was that we would share the responsibility just as we do when we meet in the examining room to negotiate medical care.

Someone wishing to initiate physicians into this sort of partnership should be prepared for a negative physician response. Cree, et al. (4) reported on a negative physician response when a patient participation group was attempted in a California family practice residency program. An educational program was developed and a favorable attitudinal change was achieved.

Our council has been meeting regularly since 1974 and much has been accomplished. Patients participating in the management of their own medical practice have increased production, decreased costs, and achieved a 10 percent discount on their malpractice insurance premium. Hundreds of good deeds have been done by and through the Talent Bank Registry. Eleven annual health fairs have been offered to the community. A how-to-do-it book has been written, and the council has protected and supported their physician in the face of heavy competition from the HMOs. But what is probably most important is that these people have become empowered to better care for their own health as well as the managerial and financial health of their medical practice.

Income for our Patient Advisory Council comes from annual dues of $8.00 per person, from fees collected from support group members, and from direct contributions. The costs to the medical practice include about 6 hours a month of physician time and about 4 hours a month of secretarial time.

Council members were once asked in an interview if they thought this idea could work in an urban area (5). One member answered, "I don't think it's the size of the community that matters so much as the continuity of physicians and patients in the practice and the lasting relationships." Another answer is that the council is constructed in such a way that all issues are negotiated. This should mean that each council would adapt to the needs of its particular setting and thereby become an appropriate ally of the community in the achievement of quality health care. A final reflection is that practice with multiple distinct populations might have separate practice management committees for each population.

CONCLUSIONS

At first the small, personal relationship-oriented community medical practice seems at a disadvantage because it lacks

---

TABLE 1. Areas of Council and Practice Cooperation

Patient Advisory Council: Milton H. Seifert, Jr., M.D. and Associates, Ltd.

A. Organization
    1. Membership . . . . Assistance of Staff Secretary
    2. Treasury
    3. Meeting Arrangement
    4. Recording Secretary . . . . Assistance of Staff Secretary

B. Accountability
    1. Policy Development & Assessment . . Assistance of physician and whatever staff is appropriate, e.g., Bookkeeper, Nursing, Services Coordinator, etc.
    2. Services Improvement . . . . Assistance of appropriate staff to acquire Practice version of a patient complaint.
    3. Support Services . . . . Physician, Accountant, Practice Manager, Bookkeeper, and Services Coordinator attend all meetings of this Committee.

C. Patient Services
    1. Talent Bank Registry . . . . Referrals provided by Practice staff.
    2. Health Education Forum . . . . Staff assistance in program development.
       (also, see attached)
    3. Patient Education . . . . Staff assistance in developing group and educational formats. Usually physician and nursing staff.

D. Liaison . . . . Assistance of Staff Secretary.

E. Research . . . . Staff assistance in refining a research question, and to aid in issues of human subject use.

---

resources such as time, money, and expertise. However, a small office that must be economical in terms of purpose, time, and economic resources is not likely to do anything inappropriate or unnecessary. The small practice status is a strength rather than a weakness.

While practitioners and patients already understand their roles as co-examiners and co-therapists, they need to also understand their roles as co-researchers and co-developers of an organization that would form a partnership between the patient group and the practice staff. Simple strategies have been suggested, and these first manageable steps can lead to the implementation of a practical pathway to achieving the concept of community-oriented primary care.

The practice staff/patient group partnership model described above will lead to appropriate programs in the local medical practice. Perhaps in 5 years, as medical practices begin to form an association of these partnerships, redesign and reorganization of the system can begin from the grassroots. However, in the beginning it is necessary to form partnerships with patients and to add to the idea in an incremental fashion.

REFERENCES

1. Seifert, M.H. Patient advisory council cuts malpractice costs. *Patient Education Newsletter* 1984; 7:1-2.

2. Early, F., and Seifert, M.H. *Starting your own patient advisory council.* Spring Park, MN: M.D. Publishing Co. 1981.

3. Naisbitt, J. *Megatrends.* Warner Books, Inc., 1982, pp. 138-139.

4. Cree, J., et al. Negative physician response to patient participation in a family practice residency program. *Family Medicine* 1982; 14: 4-7.

5. Early, F. D. Sharing practice management with patient. *Patient Care* 1981; 15: 141-162.

CHAPTER 46

Use of a Cooperative Board Structure to Enhance Community Support

Henry Taylor, M.D.

Building community participation into a primary care practice can be difficult. The traditional means by which this has been accomplished is through community boards, yet even with the best intentions, community board members are not always full partners in a practice. Limits on the extent of community participation narrow the range of a community-oriented primary care practice, and ultimately, restrict its effectiveness. This article describes one practice's efforts to increase community participation through forming a cooperative, a membership structure designed to enhance ongoing community involvement in practice management.

HISTORY OF THE COOPERATIVE

Residents of Pendleton County, West Virginia, have traditionally been very self-reliant, suspicious of outsiders, and willing to reject "Federal projects" such as the Rural Health Initiative. Hence, from its inception, designers of Pendleton Community Care worked to create a board structure that would ensure maximum community involvement. The solution was a cooperative board structure, a membership-based corporation where providers and community representatives could collaborate in identifying and solving priority health problems.

In 1976, Pendleton Community Care, a primary care practice in Franklin, West Virginia, established itself as a tax-exempt 501c3 corporation. The practice offers a prepaid membership: an annual fee of $10.00 for an individual and $25.00 for a family provides access to a number of health promotion, health education, and other preventive care benefits. Acute care services, however, are reimbursed on a fee-for-service basis.

GOALS OF THE COOPERATIVE

Pendleton Community Care operates with four guiding principles:

1. Attitudes of Service and Commitment on the Part of the Providers

Provider attitudes are critical to the establishment of a community-oriented primary care practice, particularly one with active community involvement. Providers interested in COPC generally start with a commitment to service. To initiate COPC, however, a provider must channel this commitment into a willingness to be part of a community, to understand its needs, and to work to ensure that the community's sense of priorities is reflected in the practice's goals.

Pendleton Community Care providers have found that there is no substitute for hard work in developing a personal relationship with the community. Their goal has been to become sufficiently integrated in the local subculture to understand the community's language, its life styles, and its priorities. In addition, cordial relationships with other local practitioners are maintained. These physicians have a commitment to the community and its overall health, and while not actively supportive of the program, have been tolerant of its efforts.

2. Broad-based Community Involvement

Pendleton Community Care has tried to bridge the gap between the health care system and the different elements that comprise the community. A majority of the board (five out of nine) members are community members elected annually by the practice membership for three-year terms. The board also includes two independently appointed technical experts, the clinic administrator, and an elected staff representative. Officers are elected only by the community board members.

Continuing efforts are made to ensure that all segments of the community are represented on the board, yet full community representation has not yet been achieved. Moreover, the practice has had difficulty retaining representatives from historically poor and disenfranchised neighborhoods. The board's attitude is to strive for better representation, recognizing that achieving this goal will require time.

3. An Ongoing Collaborative Relationship Between Providers and Community Representatives

The different members each bring a distinct perspective to the Pendleton Community Care board. The community board members articulate perceived health needs, program impact, and community acceptance of and resistance to new initiatives. The experts on the board bring skilled advice regarding the planning and administration of the practice, while the staff recognize the practicality of implementing specific programs in light of institutional resources.

The unique feature of Pendleton Community Care as a cooperative is that the board seeks direct feedback from its members, monitoring membership enrollment trends, and the relative popularity of specific services.

4. A Problem-solving Approach to Practice Management

The commitment and energy of Pendleton Community Care Board members can not always overcome their cultural differences, yet, the board remains committed to the goal stated in its bylaws:

> To conduct a continuing assessment of community needs, to identify inefficiencies, inadequacies, or gaps in human care services, and to promote the expansion, development, modification, and reduction of services to meet the existing human needs and community needs of Pendleton County and surrounding areas.

SUMMARY AND CONCLUSIONS

Community physicians traditionally used informal social contacts to obtain patient feedback. More recently, however, these contacts have been replaced by "the invisible hand" of the market—doctors learn that patients expected a different type of service when they leave to use other doctors. In some practice settings (e.g., the neighborhood health centers funded by OEO), community boards were established to give power back to the health care consumer. These boards have ranged from informal advisory committees to powerful and controlling managers of center activities.

Nonetheless, experience suggests that community involvement in primary care practices is an elusive phenomenon, difficult to establish, and even more difficult to maintain.

The Pendleton Community Care practice has sought to give all its patients a stake in how the practice is run by making them members in the organization. A cooperative has been established in which the membership elects a board consisting of a majority of community representatives.

The principles used by the practice to maximize community involvement are: provider attitudes of service and commitment, broad-based community involvement, a collaborative relationship between providers and consumers, and a problem-solving approach to community-oriented primary care.

At Pendleton Community Care, community members have a majority of the power on the board. Their knowledge of the community is balanced by the technical expertise of experts and the programmatic perspective of the staff. A truly balanced partnership has been hard to maintain, but the ongoing investment in creating community self-reliance for health care has been the cornerstone of a community-oriented primary care practice at Pendleton Community Care.

CHAPTER 47

Planned Approach to Community Health: The PATCH Program

Charles F. Nelson
Marshall W. Kreuter, Ph.D.
Nancy B. Watkins
Ronald R. Stoddard

While some may quibble over what are often microscopic differences, most people unanimously recognize that behavioral and environmental factors are major links in the causal chain leading to the major causes of premature death, disease, injury, and disability. Because so many of the behavioral and environmental factors associated with unnecessary loss of health are modifiable, it is not surprising that considerable worldwide attention is being given to community-based prevention activities targeted at those factors.

In this chapter we describe the methods used in carrying out one of those efforts: PATCH. PATCH is an acronym for Planned Approach To Community Health. PATCH is a programmatic response by the Centers for Disease Control (CDC) to create a forum through which citizens, local level health workers, and the local and State health departments plan and carry out health community-based health promotion programs.

The philosophy and spirit of PATCH have been captured accurately by Halfdan Mahler, Director-General of the World Health Organization (1):

Health is not a commodity that is given. It must be generated from with-in. Similarly, health action cannot and should not be an effort imposed from outside and foreign to the people; rather it must be a response of the community to the problems that the people in the community perceive, carried out in a way that is acceptable to them and properly supported by an adequate infrastructure.

Imagine a neighborhood or community where the incidence of teenagers and children injured or killed as a result of auto accidents is twice the rate at the State and national level. Imagine that the citizens in this community become aware of this alarming situation and express outrage at such unnecessary carnage. They form groups to study the problem and find out what can be done to correct it. Their inquiries lead them to the conclusion that there are many resources in the community with the potential to contribute to the resolution of the problem. They make plans to put that potential into action. As a result, the highway maintenance agency takes steps to improve street lighting, repaint roadways, and put up better signs, and local stores put signs on the shopping carts and shopping bags urging people to use seatbelts. The local health department starts an infant/children restraint loaner program, and the State legislative representative introduces legislation that makes seatbelt and child restraint use mandatory. The police reinstate their support of the local youth athletic groups, and church groups do the same. Schools add health-related content and activities to their curriculums. Businesses provide support via poster and media campaigns that urge safety. Local taverns offer free soft drinks to drivers to help ensure sobriety after the party. Envision that after one year, injuries due to accidents in this community were down by 50 percent and deaths reduced by 75 percent.

While the process just described can occur and surely has occurred, it is an infrequent, almost random event. One could restate the scenario using a myriad of problems: cardiovascular disease, diarrhea, teen pregnancy, or AIDS. Irrespective of the problem, the scenario characterizes precisely the sort of action and outcome that PATCH seeks to establish as the norm. It is our hope that every community in the United States would have the *capacity*, not just the *will*, to carry out that process regardless of the health issue in question.

PATCH: SOME UNDERLYING ASSUMPTIONS

The PATCH program is grounded in several assumptions extrapolated both from the literature on community interventions and our own experiences.

1. Because volitional behavior is so critical to health promotion, citizen participation is essential. Citizen participation must be a first consideration in planning and setting priorities, and citizens' priorities need to be a constant point of reference throughout the process.

2. The network of State and local health agencies needs to be an integral part of health promotion in the United States. This network has been effective in mitigating infectious and environmental health problems. It can and is contributing significantly to the contemporary problems of chronic disease, unintended injuries, violence, and substance abuse. Failure to solicit the involvement and resources of public health offices is a rich opportunity missed.

3. Health promotion programs need a target and goal from which specific measurable objectives are established. Without some kind of concrete target, the chances of maintaining the productive energy of any group are limited.

4. The resources for local-level programs will invariably be scarce, and the expertise among the personnel needed to carry out those programs may be limited. Few communities have either the level of expertise or financial support found in the major community-based cardiovascular disease and cancer preventional trials. Therefore, efforts must be made to seek creative yet realistic means to apply the good lessons and insights learned from these important demonstrations, despite the existing limitations.

5. The conceptual framework, methods, and strategies applied in the PATCH program should by no means be viewed as innovative. PATCH is a combination of the principles and methods long used by community organizers, epidemiologists, behavioral scientists, and health educators. PATCH re-emphasizes and combines these critical elements.

WHAT IS PATCH?

PATCH provides a forum through which community health workers, health education professionals, and citizens plan, conduct, and evaluate health promotion programs at the community level. Working as a team, key representatives from the State health department, the local health agency, local community workers, citizens, and the CDC form an active partnership with the intent of putting into place health promotion programs designed to meet the priority health needs of the community. This program is based on the cooperative involvement of several key partners in health:

1. *The State Health Department.* Any State with a commitment to provide technical assistance and support to community-based health programs within its State is a candidate for the partnership.

2. *The Centers for Disease Control* (CDC). The CDC's Division of Health Education provides training and technical assistance to the State and community.

3. *The Community.* A PATCH community can be a city, county, district, region, or even a smaller unit such as a neighborhood. To be a candidate for the partnership, community members need to express their willingness and commitment to implement PATCH.

Like individuals, all communities are different. However, effective PATCH communities generally establish an organized framework that has a local coordinator, a core group, and a community group.

Local Coordinator. The local coordinator has primary responsibility for coordinating PATCH activities in the community, and is usually someone in a local or regional health agency who has responsibility for health education. The local coordinator makes the commitment to provide ongoing guidance to the process. This is an essential element for program maintenance.

Core Group. The core group consists of members of the community who make a long-term commitment to the PATCH effort. This group typically consists of 6 to 12 people who are interested in and concerned about addressing health issues and problems in their community. The core group's responsibilities include assisting with the program's administrative functions, helping to identify the resources necessary to accomplish the program's objectives, and assisting in implementing interventions.

Community Group. The community group consists of community volunteers who are willing to participate. Often the community group is comprised of private citizens, political office holders, and individuals from service organizations, health organizations, hospitals, neighborhood organizations, private companies, etc. The community group's role is one of active participation in establishing program objectives, serving on working committees, and assisting the implementation of interventions. PATCH strives to make their collective and individual views heard and acted upon.

HOW DOES PATCH WORK?

Many communities have active community groups firmly in place and they support well-conceived programs to promote health education. When that is the case, PATCH should become a part of their agenda. In communities where such groups are not yet established, however, the State health department will need to work with local-level leadership to alert community health education workers and other community members about the PATCH opportunity. Members who choose to be part of the core group will be responsible for identifying and recruiting the membership of a larger, representative community group. Before the PATCH process can begin, community members, represented by the local coordinator, must indicate their commitment to this process in a letter of interest to the State health department PATCH coordinator. The State must then document the level of commitment within the community and contact the CDC's Division of Health Education (DHE), expressing interest in becoming a PATCH partner. A State health department representative will then schedule an appropriate time for a representative from DHE to discuss the program with community members and to describe in detail the steps and phases of PATCH. At that time, the CDC provides a detailed description of the various roles to be played by participating agencies, a summary of the training component, and details about the program documentation requirements. Based on how relevant PATCH is to their mutual needs, the State and community health education workers will then make a joint decision on their commitment to the partnership. This bureaucratic series of commitments and confirmations is the most effective way the CDC can manage its PATCH technical assistance resources to the State. The long-range plan, of course, is to establish levels of competency in the States so they will be self-sufficient in replicating PATCH in other communities in their respective States.

After orientation, the partners plan the program's first session. There are five distinct yet interrelated phases to the PATCH process. Each phase consists of:
1. A period of preparation for the meeting that involves State and local health department staff, community members, and a representative(s) from CDC.
2. A one-half day training session that involves CDC staff, the State and local coordinators, and core group members as indicated.

3. A one-day meeting that involves all official agency PATCH staff and members of the community.

The five phases are described below. Each description begins with a highlight of activities in the preparation phase and is followed by highlights of the training session and the community meeting for that phase.

Phase I

Preparation begins with all partners committing themselves to participate. The local coordinator is responsible for assembling the core group. The core group develops a plan for recruitment of the community group (2). The CDC will provide all workshop materials and readings for participants in the training sessions.

In the one-half day training sessions, the skills necessary to conduct a nominal group process, personal and telephone interviewing, as well as record data are reviewed (3). During the community group session, participants will identify sources of data, generate names of potential opinion survey interviewees, prepare for personal interviews, and form working committees to manage the opinion survey, the behavioral risk factor survey, and other tasks as needed.

Phase II

Preparation begins after the collection of mortality data and opinion data is well underway. At this time the initial steps are taken for conducting the behavioral risk factor prevalence survey. This preparation includes identifying interviewers, selecting the sample size, identifying telephone prefixes/suffixes, and other logistical considerations.

The Phase II training session consists of preparing interviewers, monitors, editors, and supervisors to perform the behavioral risk factor survey. Following training, the State coordinator and the CDC staff member(s) remain through the first night of interviewing. The interviewing process generally takes approximately 2 weeks for 10 interviewers to complete a random sample of 800 interviews. The remainder of this session is used to meet with and receive updates from the committees formed in the first session.

Phase III

Preparation involves wrapping up any loose ends in data collection and then preparing the data for presentation and analysis. Recruitment of new members is again emphasized. At this time, participants will receive materials on the rela-

tionship of risk factors to health status and examples of objectives (4—6).

During the training, participants will discuss methods of presentation and terminology. They will also perform preliminary analysis and determine responsibility for each part of the presentation. In the community group meeting, all data are presented with appropriate comparisons made with national and State estimates. Depending on the group process used, citizens then identify priority health problems, set goals related to those problems,

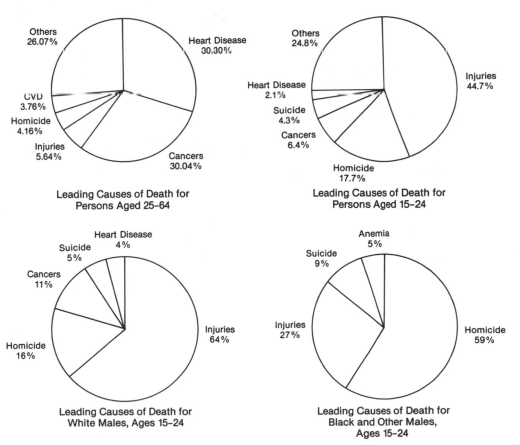

Figure 1. Data for Montgomery County, Ohio, 1980.

and write community-level objectives (7) that express the community's intention to resolve or reduce the problem.

Figure 1 illustrates the kind of mortality data communities typically use. Note the sizeable portion of homicide deaths for black males. This kind of information enlightens communities and often triggers important "why" questions that in turn lead to "what can we do" questions. Figure 2 gives an example of citizen opinion data collected in PATCH.

Next, group members generate ideas and develop an action plan that delineates roles for diffusing this information to the community at large in order to enhance community awareness.

Phase IV
Preparation focuses on completing the work initiated in the third session and getting participants ready to identify those behavioral and environmental factors that

are contributors to the health problems identified in the previous session. Information on risk-factor relationships and economic and social costs will be provided and discussed. The accomplishments of the third session and plans for the fourth session will be provided to new members and to those who were unable to attend the third session.

Figure 3 gives an example of how findings from the behavioral risk factor survey are presented. The Phase IV training session includes a review of the basic elements of the planning model utilized in the PATCH program (8).

The group session consists of three activities: analyzing and describing the major factors that are related to the communities' leading health problems; identifying health education strategies that may reduce these problems; and identifying persons with relevant competencies,

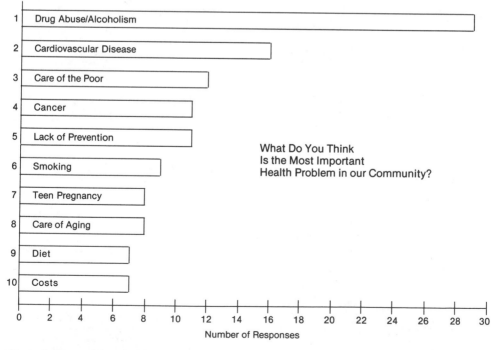

Figure 2. Responses to the Community Opinion Survey—Montgomery County, Ohio, 1984.

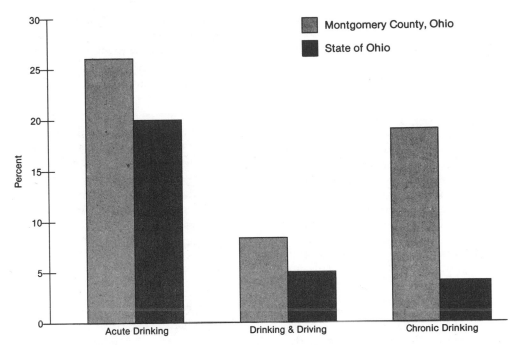

Figure 3. Reported Drinking Behaviors from the Behavioral Risk Factor Surveys—Montgomery County, Ohio (1984) and the State of Ohio (1983).

as well as services and resources currently in place in the community. At the conclusion of this session, committees are formed that will complete the brainstorming process for each of the problems identified. Previously formed committees will continue the process of informing the community at large about PATCH program accomplishments and recruiting or involving more members from the community.

Phase V

Preparations are made to finalize the inventory of community resources for each of the problems identified. Appropriate intervention and evaluation reference materials are assembled for distribution to training session participants.

In the training session, PATCH coordinators and core group members will, given the target problem(s), delineate existing skills, services, and resources that exist within the community in order to identify gaps; discuss intervention evaluation (9, 10); and discuss the design of intervention strategies for recommendation at the group session.

In the group session participants will review and discuss recommendations for an intervention plan of action. The action plan serves as a model that will change as the PATCH group modifies and refines its strategies. Rather than being the end of the PATCH process, Phase V marks a beginning. It nurtures a commitment to lasting change—change in which the "partners" become a normative part of the community's fabric.

WHAT SKILLS ARE NEEDED TO CARRY OUT PATCH?

Those of us who have a hand in PATCH view it as an ongoing source of continuing education. We are always learning;

and the structure of PATCH is sufficiently flexible to enable us to make modifications in the process as new insights are gained.

We have found that the PATCH process requires competence or skill in five general areas of health promotion work: community organization, data collection and analyses, problem specification and priority setting, intervention planning and implementation, and program evaluation.

As previously mentioned under the section on PATCH assumptions, the PATCH process and the skills required to conduct it are by no means new. The five areas of competence cited have long been basic staples for community health education workers. In PATCH, these skills are pressed into service at the outset. Moreover, without their application, progress is virtually impossible. Without culturally sensitive community organization, nothing happens. Without assistance in the collection of data that fairly represent a community's health status and citizens' viewpoints, problems cannot be meaningfully identified. Without problems identified as priority concerns by citizens, objectives and program targets may be of questionable importance and most assuredly will lack political support over time. Without precise program targets, health promotion programs, if they are generated at all, are likely to be blunderbuss efforts. And evaluation? In the PATCH philosophy, evaluation is not a tag-on activity: it is an integral part of the whole process. Good baseline data, precise objectives, and clear descriptions of interventions are the necessary ingredients of sound evaluation.

CONCLUSION

We believe that the PATCH process creates an opportunity for citizens and health workers to commit themselves to systematically improving the health of their community. The system enables them to document problems, activities, and progress. This documentation in turn serves them in the following ways:

1. It creates local, relevant news to enhance community awareness and interest.

2. It generates the kind of specificity and baseline information that makes applications for resources, become priorities for support, from either the public or private sectors.

3. It provides essential information to make program modifications, assess progress, and evaluate outcomes.

REFERENCES

1. Mahler, H. The meaning of health for all by the year 2000. Health 2000. *World Health Forum*, 1981; 2(1):5.

2. Tait, J.L.; Bokemeier, J.; and Bohlen, J.M. Identifying the community power actors: A guide for change agents. Ames, IA: North Central Region Cooperative Extension Service, 1980.

3. Gilmore, E.D. Needs assessment processes for community health education. *International Journal of Health*, 1977; 20:164.

4. U.S. Department of Health, Education, and Welfare. *Healthy People: The Surgeon's Report on Health Promotion and Disease Prevention*. Washington, DC: U.S. Government Printing Office, 1979, (DHEW [PHS] Publication No. 79-55071).

5. U.S. Department of Health, Education, and Welfare. *Model Standards for Community Preventive Health Services*. Washington, DC: U.S. Government Printing Office, 1979.

6. U.S. Department of Health and Human Services. *Promoting Health/ Preventing Disease: Objectives for the Nation*. Washington, DC: U.S. Government Printing Office, 1980.

7. Morrisey, G.L. *Management by Objectives and Results*. Reading, MA: Addison-Wesley, 1970.

8. Green, L.; Kreuter, M.W.; Deeds, S.; and Partridge, K. *Health Education Planning: A Diagnostic Approach*. Palo Alto, CA: Mayfield Publishing Company, 1980.

9. True, J.A. *Finding Out: Conducting and Evaluating Social Research*. Belmont, CA: Wadsworth Publishing Company, 1983.

10. Windsor, R.A. *Evaluation of Health Promotion and Education Programs*. Palo Alto, CA: Mayfield Publishing Company, 1984.

CHAPTER 48

Community Involvement in COPC

Craig Robinson

The ordinary layman lacks the knowledge to define his own medical needs and can rely only on the expert opinion of medical practitioners and public health authorities (1).

While participation in decision making by the individual patient is important for satisfactory care, it is perhaps even more so in community health care (2).

The goals of risk reduction and morbidity prevention in a defined community, with specific at-risk subgroups, requires that the community be understood and touched more intimately than is required by the mere offering of the health service. The goals of a COPC program necessarily involve attempts to change attitudes and practices both in the community at large and in particular individuals. COPC also involves the difficult task of drawing people into a program who may not be practice users, or convincing people to use services that are not a part of the traditional doctor-patient encounter.

The specific objectives of a COPC program will vary: to reduce cardiovascular risk, to improve perinatal outcome, to

limit disability from chronic lung disease, or to establish a COPC practice. In all cases, however, the program development problems are similar: How do we define the problem and the solution in this particular setting? How do we motivate people to understand and participate in the program? How do we gain the necessary support, in the community and on the outside, to carry the program forward? The practical solution to all three of these basic problems requires the involvement of the people who are at risk.

Community involvement should be seen as primarily an educational process that respects the knowledge and understanding people bring to it and takes advantage of the decisions and tasks required here and now. It is education based on purpose. Education is required to gain understanding, support, and participation as well as to contribute to personal and social development. Though many of us may think of ourselves as progressive in the health field, we carry around quite traditional and dysfunctional notions regarding education.

Certainly, both the methods and goals of education fostered by involvement are different from those of traditional education. John Dewey (3) characterized traditional education as:

. . . preparation for a more or less remote future as opposed to making the most of opportunity in present life and by static aims and materials as opposed to acquaintance with a changing world.

On the other hand, progressive education is based on the assumption that there is "an intimate and necessary relation between the processes of actual experience and education" (3). Community involvement is a powerful educational experience when it fulfills the two important criteria that Myles Horton, the founder of Highlander Folk School, judged necessary for successful adult education: that the purpose be important, clear, and shared, and that the process confer dignity upon the participants.

Since community involvement means different things in different contexts, it is important to clarify the meaning of the term in the context of COPC. The community, for COPC purposes, consists of those who will benefit from the program. It does not include representatives from all the agencies in the area, other providers or hospital administrators, the prominent and powerful citizens in a community, or others whose interests are opposed to the success of a program. These people may certainly be in the geographic area of the community and it may be that their help or cooperation would benefit the program. However, it would be dysfunctional to involve them in governance since their personal interests may conflict with those of the groups at risk. If people with influence or resources are needed, their help should be solicited by the community members who are served by the program. It is the community members who make the decisions, and those who are involved are selected because they represent the program's constituents. In some cases, there may be institutions, such as trade unions or tribal councils, that offer a functional means of elected representation in the program. Usually, however, the selection will be by those already in the program and follow such criteria as what constituency to have represented, leadership potential, and interest. Of course, who should be involved is determined by the particular problem being addressed. For example, women must be involved if the problem is maternity service improvement, workers if the issue is occupational health.

For many COPC programs, those who are most at-risk are those who are poor, powerless, overlooked, or otherwise vulnerable. The development of involvement and trust in the program by these people is important if they are to be reached. Paulo Freire's instruction to would-be revolutionists (4) holds some truth for the community-oriented health activist as well.

Many political and educational plans have failed because their authors designed them according to their personal views of reality, never once taking into account (except as mere objects of their action) the men-in-situation to whom their program was ostensibly directed . . . . They approach (the people) with projects which may correspond to their own view of the world, but not to that of the people.

Sensitivity to a community's attitudes, as well as to social and political networks, is facilitated when those being served are represented in the planning, implementation, and evaluation of a program. This requires flexibility on the part of the professionals involved, in problem identification and program design.

Another function is served by this involvement: the development of a solid base of support for the program in the community. Community involvement builds on the fact that those who are served by the program have the biggest stake in its continuation and growth. Those who have a stake in the program for themselves and for their neighbors are the most reliable allies of the COPC practice.

People develop a stake in a program for two basic reasons: because they believe it will improve their lot, and because they believe the program belongs to them. Both are required to develop the proprietary interest that stimulates support for the program. Myles Horton described the process that he witnessed many times in the communities where he worked:

If you get people involved, then creativity comes out of the people; it helps the 'leaders' to get things done. The power comes from the bottom instead of the top then people start educating each other . . . that is when you are going to get things moving (4).

Maintaining a COPC program is not just a matter of carrying out various program elements to address specific risks. It is also a matter of maintaining the basic structural requirements for COPC, that is, the survival of the practice itself and continued access to care for at-risk groups in the community. This must be done in the face of a health industry that, if not hostile, is at least indifferent to the basic precepts of COPC. For example, in our community, there has been an increase in unemployment and a corresponding increase in the number of people who are uninsured or covered by a public program. Hospitals and specialists have responded by developing even more draconian measures to keep out the poor to insure a favorable patient mix. A community that is organized around a primary care practice is much better prepared to respond to the continual and varied assaults on access to care.

A community cannot afford to rely on the medical marketplace to provide access to care nor to provide support to many worthy community health efforts. Hill-Burton, cost-based reimbursement, and the focus on specialist training have all conspired to give hospitals and specialists a disproportionate share of health resources. We are way out on the flat part of the cost-benefit curve, and resources are being diverted from primary care and community health. There are strong interests in every community who like it the way it is, or want to make it worse. It is important for us to take advantage of community involvement to develop our own coalition to support access to care for all our neighbors as well as special programs for at-risk groups. Good data are helpful, but politics must not be ignored. Community involvement offers the opportunity to affect the body politic.

The regional perinatal program of the Robert Wood Johnson Foundation represents a program whose continued viability really rested on changes in the body politic as much as on good statistics. The latter were attended to but not the former. In this program, easy access to the appropriate level of care was critical, especially for poor women, who were at higher risk. Even though the data appeared to support the program's effectiveness, program reviewers were pessimistic about the continuation of important elements of the program. They saw access to prenatal care threatened by trends in coverage offered by private and public insurance programs as well as by the lack of coverage by many at-risk women. Although hospitals and physicians were involved in the program design and implementation, where were the representatives of labor and business and women—people who had a stake in the program? The need to establish a coalition of support was apparently not addressed.

The second major clarification in the definition of community involvement concerns the meaning of involvement. For the purposes of COPC, involvement must mean ongoing participation in decision-making about the program. Kark notes that while practitioners have accepted the notion that it is important for patients to be involved in decisionmaking about their personal health care, there is less acceptance, although it may be even more important, for the community to be involved in decisions related to its health care (2). For Kark and the others who developed the program at the Polela Health Center, which served a Zulu community in South Africa, community involvement was important in completing specific public health tasks. However, they also recognized a more important result of community involvement:

> If health is about the quality of life, promoting community involvement is not only for the purpose of achieving specific goals such as building protected water supplies or changing diet. Community involvement is in itself a health activity, promotive of social well being and mental health (2).

The fact that community members do not have formal training in health care delivery, management, or planning is irrelevant to the need to involve them in important decisions about their community's health. Horton describes his problem with the traditional notion that one must not participate in decision-making without first having completed a formal education:

> What I think is wrong with the regular decision making processes is that they are so rarified and stratified. People are boxed in . . . . What seems to be crucial here is getting people used to making decisions . . . and setting up the processes in which this is possible (5).

For Horton, the process of involving the community in decisionmaking will serve to educate and empower. A transformation takes place when people who have felt powerless can participate in important decisions about the health of their community. Apathy and resignation are dispelled. It becomes possible to care about one's neighbors as people gain the confidence and ability to act in a public sense. Involvement in decisionmaking permits community members to convert what had been private personal problems into public problems. What was intractable as a private problem becomes manageable as a problem for the group. Creativity and learning are stimulated as solutions are explored. This is parallel to the process that takes place in a practice when it moves from the individual patient-by-patient shopkeeper approach to taking responsibility for the community. The intractable problems of a string of patients become manageable when those patients are perceived as members of a group with common risks. The practice is thereby empowered and creativity is stimulated.

Community involvement may also include the involvement of community members as staff in carrying out various program elements, particularly in the area of education and case-finding. People from the community are more effective at convincing their neighbors to participate in a program or change some behavior than are trained professionals. Class or cultural differences between teacher and student are strong barriers to reaching people.

Myles Horton believes that the literacy program developed by Highlander to serve black people living on the Sea Islands of South Carolina was effective because the classes were taught by local black people who had been in the program. Sidney Kark describes the successful use of community members trained as health outreach workers at the Polela Health Center. The early findings from the Vanderbilt University Maternal and Infant Health Outreach Worker (MIHOW) program indicate that pregnancy outcomes are better for high-risk women when the education is conducted by lay "natural helpers" rather than by professional health workers.

Community involvement is facilitated when the practice has a consumer governing board. The consumer board serves as a vehicle for the ongoing training not only of community members but also of the staff. The staff becomes accustomed to preparing and presenting policy and program options to the board and working out differences. In addition, the consumer board members, who have developed some pride in their program and knowledge of health issues, are ready to respond to threats both to the practice and to community health status in general.

However, community involvement need not stop with the board of directors. Particular COPC initiatives may require that members of particular groups be more involved than the board structure permits. These additional people may make up a committee of the board or they may form a separate association, which may or may not become incorporated. For example, if child day care were determined to be a community health need, the practice might organize a group of parents who would form a separate nonprofit organization or, alternatively, function as the day care committee of the existing community board.

The organizer's basic job is to help establish the decisionmaking process, help pose the problems that require decisions, introduce new ideas and people, provide encouragement, and facilitate education. Organizing a community's involvement should be a step-by-step process that exploits the tasks and decisions for the purpose of education. Tom Ludwig, an organizer who has worked with community people on health projects in Appalachia, the deep South, inner cities, and Native American communities, has outlined his organizing technique as follows:

• Help people set up a nonprofit tax-exempt corporation with a consumer-controlled board of directors.

• Help them believe that the solution they have chosen is correct, and brook no disagreement. Let disagreement be over such matters as location, whether to have a basement or not, or who to hire.

• Help them set up and conduct a banquet and invite only well-placed outside supporters to join them. (Aside from the education provided by the speakers, the banquet lends dignity to the cause and the people involved. It also develops a network of outsiders with influence who understand and sympathize with the project.)

• Help arrange a trip to a similar solution by a similar group in a similar location with a similar problem. Travel is not, in itself, important. It is the learning that is important.

• Help them get more information. Help them learn and help them teach (at a folk school, medical school, their own workshop— anything helps). Learning will take place unless the teacher impedes it.

• Help them get money from the system that oppresses them.[1]

Ludwig's rather curt directives to the organizer carry some important unstated principles. First, there is the linkage between decisionmaking and purpose and education. Second, decisionmaking involves having real power such as that held by a board of directors. Third, decisionmaking requires structure, including votes, officers, committees, and recording of minutes. Fourth, decisionmaking requires that some specific effort be put into organizing educational functions. Fifth, education is stimulated and advanced by bringing outside people to explain their experiences. Exposure to new people serves other purposes as well. It can help

---

[1] Thomas Ludwig, personal communication, January 17, 1986.

convey that the problem or the solution is not unique or strange in the world, although it may be locally. Involving outsiders develops support for the program beyond the community.

There must be clarity of purpose. As mentioned above, purpose motivates learning. It also provides the basis for group cohesion in the face of the inevitable differences and conflict as to the means of fulfilling the purpose of the program. Political scientist Carey McWilliams reflects on the role of purpose in group cohesion and the sense of community:

> Community demands purpose because in any case where men are vital to men they will get on one another's nerves and will need forgiveness from annoyance and conflict—and it is purpose which helps to provide the basis for forgiving (6).

CONCLUSION

Certainly, the COPC model is correct in taking advantage of the strategic position in a community of the accessible primary care practice. It is also correct to make use of the insights offered by epidemiology as applied to a practice and its community. However, sometimes underdeveloped, sometimes overlooked, and sometimes scorned is the opportunity for the primary care program to involve its community in addressing its own health problems. The AMA President of 1976 still speaks for many who are suspicious of the community's role. Regarding the consumer's role in health planning, he said, "passengers who insist on flying the airplane are called hijackers" (7). In fact, however, reducing morbidity and mortality rates in a particular community is more related to successfully involving the community in its health care than in skillfully applying medical technology. Those whom the medical shopkeepers fear as hijackers we in COPC welcome as copilots.

REFERENCES

1. Committee on the Cost of Medical Care, *Medical Care for the American People*. Chicago: University of Chicago Press, 1932.

2. Kark, S. *The Practice of Community Oriented Primary Care*. New York: Appleton-Century-Crofts, 1981.

3. Dewey, J. *Experience and Education*. New York: Collier Books, 1958.

4. Freire, P. *Pedagogy of the Oppressed*. New York: Herder and Herder, 1972.

5. Dropkin, R., and Tobier, A. *Roots of Open Education in America*. New York: The City College Workshop Center for Open Education, 1976.

6. McWilliams, C. *Political Arts and Political Sciences. Power and Community: Dissenting Essays in Political Science*. New York: Vintage Books, 1970.

7. Starr. *The Social Transformation of American Medicine*. New York: Basic Books, 1982.

CODA:

Patient and Community Involvement

Cecil G. Sheps, M.D., M.P.H.

The notion of including patient and community involvement in the design and delivery of health services, in diagnostic and treatment activities as well as disease prevention and health promotion has, in recent years, gained more popularity but not clarity of purpose, method or performance. There has been an unfortunate tendency, among some COPC enthusiasts, to take a purist stance calling for a full measure of community involvement, often times control, as the *sine qua non* of COPC and averring that anything less does not meet the requirements and is, hence, outside the pale. Involvement of individuals and groups in health activities are the means to an end. These ends are specific health achievement objectives. The target group varies greatly depending upon the sponsoring practice. To give a simple example, the target group for a hypertension screening program undertaken by the only physician in a community can readily focus initial attention on the entire community. This would clearly not be possible if the physician with this interest was one of several physicians practicing in the same community. Furthermore, the formal commitment of the practice to its patients influences its ability to

focus attention upon, and involve, its entire patient base. An HMO, for example, has a clearly designated population for whom it has formally undertaken responsibility whereas a free choice, fee for service practice cannot assume that all the patients it has seen, let alone their families, are prepared to welcome activities aimed at them, however well-meaning they may be.

Whether we are considering community, family or personal involvement in health care, there is much that can be said as well as much to learn. It is true of all of them and most especially about community involvement, that they are like motherhood, praised by all but interpreted differently in different places and by different people in terms of expectations, needs, rights and privileges. One thing is clear. The concept of the "provider" and the "consumer" developed in the past twenty years or so, must be discarded. This marketplace concept of a series of health care commodities or "products" that are offered, sold and bought is not only inconsistent with, but is obstructive to, the implementation of COPC. COPC calls for a continuous inter-action, a two-way street, a partnership which goes well

402

beyond the health professional ministering to patients. The latter, while often crucial, is however frequently not sufficient to complete the task nor, in some instances, even to start it. Thus, the concept of the consumer and the provider, so frequently used in many countries and especially in the U.S., is misleading and obstructive to the implementation of patient and community involvement.

The question can be raised as to whether community involvement is a means or an end: whether it is something like democracy, the practice of which has certain inherent values of itself, or whether it's something we need to put into operation because we know it will help us, in unique and essential ways, to do a better and more effective job in health care. This "means versus ends" question calls up interesting potential differences which, for the full achievement of COPC, are of little account. The single, compelling fact is that, without a certain measure of patient and community involvement, COPC is seriously deficient. The nature and depth of the involvement should be determined by the specific health achievement goals it is expected to assist the program or practice to reach.

Community participation is a process. The World Health Organization's definition is, "Community participation is the process by which individuals and families assume responsibility for their own health and welfare and for those of the community, and develop the capacity to contribute to their and the community's development" (1). Clearly, this bespeaks community involvement as a major strength and support for primary care which is crucial to its ability to maximize its effectiveness in much of what it undertakes to do, as well as broaden the scope of its services. Attention must be given to the difference between genuine and spurious community participation. The term has been used in various ways, some of them inappropriate, and therefore incorrect, so far as the basic operating principles of the COPC are concerned. It does *not* mean the paternalistic extension of centralized, professionally controlled health services to "penetrate" the "target" populations of poverty. However it *does* mean helping the poor organize at the family, neighborhood and greater community levels so as to understand their health problems, use health services more effectively, understand how other elements of their lives influence their health status and to join and work with others to promote and participate in measures and programs which will improve their capacity to live and function more fully. Though the gains to be made through this approach are presently greatest with the poor, there are significant gains to be made with virtually any type of population. It has application in all types of primary practices and programs.

The concept of a partnership is applicable here—one which involves the professional health personnel in a practice, its public (however this is defined) and politics. "Politics" is a nasty word in many contexts in the U.S. Nevertheless, if one thinks of it in terms of the process of change in community norms, expectations, institutions and services, it becomes clear that it is difficult, if not impossible, to develop and implement improved or new programs to achieve optimum health care for a population without taking political considerations, in this sense, into account.

It is useful to consider the ways and levels in which participation can take place. The simplest level, and easiest to achieve, is to provide the community with information. *Informing* the community is the first step. Producing the desired result— appropriate behavior and action based on adequate knowledge and desirable attitudes — is not a simple matter. The next level, even more complex and one with which most physicians and other health personnel have even less experience, is *consulting* the community. Here, too, the health professional continues to be in control but has decided that it would be desirable to obtain specific information about the perceptions, interests and probable reactions of certain types of populations to plans that are being developed so as to increase the probability of their success. This may, of course, also lead to recognition of the need to invite certain *population groups* to publicize their interest in certain health program developments and *to intercede* in the process so as help gain acceptance or political support where that is needed.

The most advanced form of involvement is that of active and formal participation of the community in the *policy making process*. The degree of community responsibility and authority may range from *voting* to *control*, with the latter being achieved by the community representatives forming the majority on the policy making body or having veto power over its decisions. It's helpful to be aware of this range of responsibility and the authority as, in the light of the objectives which have been identified at a point in time, type of community involvement which is needed is selected. Thus, there is a broad range of possibilities in what can be described as *community empowerment* in health which extends from providing information to giving the community full control over policy and even operations. Though U.S. physicians and other health personnel are generally unaccustomed to community control, there are a great many health care organizations in this country, large and small, which are organized and administered in this fashion, though not all in the same way. Some examples are many of the urban and rural health centers set up by federal and state agencies as well as some totally self supporting health care organizations. An outstanding example of the latter is the group health cooperative based in Seattle, Washington which has a membership of over 300,000 people and a medical staff of several hundred physicians.

J.C. Lukmonik, in her chapter, describes a very instructive series of examples of ways in which community involvement and responsibility have improved health care programs. They have done this through identifying and drawing attention to inadequately recognized health needs, participating in program design and implementation as well as evaluation and decision making for the future. Though most of her examples are from community health centers and other organized programs of care, some are advisory councils set up by solo practitioners, group practices or even larger health systems. Seifert's chapter gives a fascinating and stimulating account of what he has been able to accomplish with an advisory group in a solo, small town, primary care practice. Lukmonik concludes by making a most important point which highlights the fact that the principles of COPC, even if applied incompletely, can be productive in terms of the health of the community. "None of these practices are the full-blown model of COPC as outlined in the IOM study, *Community-Oriented Primary Care: A Practical Assessment.* Each has some elements of community medicine combined with a service delivery model that responds to problems beyond its own walls. Each is answering to the health needs of a known population and is a richer practice for involving the community. While none may have yet created the synthesis that is the conceptual model of COPC, each is somewhere on the way." To insist on the "all or nothing" view of COPC espoused by some dedicated protagonists is unnecessary, unrealistic and off-putting for the many individual programs and agencies to whom the goals and general principles of COPC appear interesting, appealing and relevant to their overall sense of purpose.

Freeman's chapter provides a useful framework for thinking about the very real ethical issues inherent in the assumptions made in the COPC approach to the community per se, as well as to erstwhile patients of a practice or the person who selects and comes to a particular practice only for certain specific services. In a heuristic and pertinent way, he discusses three "layers" of ethical principles which are pertinent to sorting out the ethical issues: the basic social contract of the community that applies to all persons in it, the social contract between society and the physician and contracts between individuals or groups of lay people and physicians that ". . . govern mutually-desired specifics of their relationship. . . ." This formulation is useful in finding one's way between professional control (and even arrogance?) and full, dignified interaction and cooperation.

Taylor describes a relatively unique set of responsibilities undertaken by the board of a cooperative dedicated to the conduct of a program of health promotion, health education and preventive care emphasizing feedback from the members regarding all aspects of the program. The evaulation of the effectiveness of the approach should prove useful.

The description, by C.F. Nelson et al. of the project of the Centers for Disease Control—a planned approach to community health—makes one impatient to await the findings. These should provide new guidance on community action and interaction with regard to behavioral health risks, thus contributing significantly to the effectiveness of health promotion activities, a subject which lies close to the heart of COPC.

In discussing various elements in, and approaches to, community involvement, Robinson's chapter provides a relevant and useful road map so that "the commu-

nity can be understood and touched more intimately than is required by the mere offering of the health service". In viewing community involvement, as he does, as an educational process, it's important to see it as mutual education, between the public and the health professionals as well as within the community itself. Robinson also makes the important point that community representatives, however selected, do not necessarily represent relevant sick or high risk populations unless this need is, where pertinent, recognized and attended to. His closing metaphor, that we should view the community as the co-pilot of the health service enterprise, is most felicitous.

Clearly, responsible involvement of patients, families and the community is fundamental to the goals and operation of COPC. Without some measure of it, COPC has no meaning. The achievement of COPC's overall purpose depends on the practice or program opening its doors outward — to become a place from which health activities emanate. Without some measure of involvement appropriate to the specific health objectives which have been identified, COPC cannot succeed. In such complex matters cooperation of all relevant parties is essential. This requires agreement, both as to the end to be desired and the methods of reaching it. As this author wrote some fifteen years ago, "At one time the provision of health care meant no more than the ministrations of select individuals, be they priests, herbalists or physicians. . . . Recognition is emerging that a new kind of partnership is needed in the development and operation of the nation's health services. This partnership would bring the needs and interests of consumers into the decision-making structure, not to deprecate the relevance of professional and technical elements, but rather to help focus the emphasis more sharply and increase the effectiveness of medical services in terms of community needs. . . . This situation calls for new adaptations on the part of the health professions. They must learn how to work within this new framework enthusiastically, confidently and well (2).

REFERENCES

1. World Health Organization. Alma-Ata 1978: Primary Health Care Report of the International Conference on Primary Care, Alma-Ata, USSR, 6-12 Sept. 1978. Geneva, 1978 (*Health for All Series*, No. 1), p. 50.

2. Sheps, Cecil G.: "The Influence of Consumer Sponsorship on Medical Services." *Milbank Memorial Fund Quarterly*, 50, No. 4, Part 2, pp. 41-69, October 1972.

Part VII.
Practice Management for COPC

Introduction

If not managed properly, the additional tasks of COPC may strain the energies and patience of the professional staff of a busy primary care practice, however committed to COPC they may be. In order to accomplish the COPC activities without deterioration in the central activities of direct patient care, particular attention is needed to develop efficient mechanisms to aid in practice management, particularly in smaller practices and programs. In particular, methods and tactics are needed to motivate and sustain the commitment of the professional staff, to delegate responsibility appropriately, and to monitor progress in implementing an emphasis program. Part VII offers suggestions on practice management strategies that enhance the COPC process.

COPC is not the prevailing mode of primary care in the United States and little is known about how to manage the COPC practice. By the nature of COPC, the practice itself will be required to make periodic adjustments in the way it provides services. While many adjustments may represent only refinements, they necessarily involve change and change is often difficult in any organization. In Chapter 49, Freeman reviews concepts of planned change from the organizational development literature, and illustrates them from his experience with a carefully developed and evaluated emphasis program. He suggests that while the change necessary for the emphasis program may be achieved initially, maintenance of the program over time may be problematic. He offers four approaches to help maintain a change in the practice pattern.

In Chapter 50, Reed proposes a simple estimation of the economic burden of creating a registry of the "practice community" as a target population for COPC.

He discusses the implications of investing in the process of defining the practice community in terms of the potential to generate additional practice revenues as a result of offering needed health services to individuals who currently are not active patients of the practice.

A major challenge to efficient practice management is the increased demand placed by the COPC activities on the storage and analysis of data. The last three chapters of this section deal with this important issue. Farley begins in Chapter 51 by addressing the structure and use of the basic medical record as the core of a COPC data system. He describes the several classes of information that can be retrieved to support direct patient care, practice management, and several of the functions of COPC.

Office automation is rapidly becoming commonplace and computer services are increasingly considered to be part of the cost of doing business.[1] Even those practices that have yet to invest in an automated data system often have one or more practitioners with a microcomputer and a growing knowledge of its capability. Many practices getting started in COPC have been aided by relatively simple microcomputer applications, developed by staff using commercially available software. In Chapter 52, Kamerow reviews the seven classes of software with potential application to COPC and briefly describes some of the important functions to which they can be put.

Most practices begin with a computer system that handles billing and other office management functions. While often visit-oriented rather than patient-oriented,

---

[1] A number of chapters describe specific computer applications to the processes and activities of COPC. The interested reader may wish to review the chapters by Trachtenberg et al. (Chapter 17), Schlager (Chapter 29), and Rosser (Chapter 32), in which computer applications are discussed in some detail.

these systems can nonetheless serve as important sources of data. In Chapter 53, Jacobs describes the use of billing systems to analyze data that describe the patient population, often going well beyond that which would be thought possible in a billing system. He also offers advice for the practice that is contemplating the installation of a billing system and would plan to use it for some of the basic COPC functions as well.

In the Coda, Culpepper further discusses ways in which office and practice management techniques can be used to expand the attention of the staff beyond the practice and into the community. He reinforces the need for the physician to delegate responsibility for monitoring the routine maintenance of the tasks of COPC.

CHAPTER 49

Implementing COPC:
Achieving Change in
a Small Organization

William L. Freeman, M.D., M.P.H.

A thoughtful and knowledgeable participant-observer of medical care, Dr. David Rogers, has noted that there are several barriers to implementing COPC, what he calls "non-health-related reasons for the failure of COPC systems to capture the hearts and minds of health professionals" (1).

Rogers listed five major barriers. Current reimbursement mechanisms reward "high tech" more than "community" medicine. Tertiary level specialists receive higher prestige than COPC specialists. Many physicians who think of themselves as "the captain of the ship" do not share well the cooperative responsibilities with others that COPC usually requires. Teaching lifestyle changes is unpopular with the potential teaching practitioners; being taught lifestyle changes is unpopular with patients. "Statistical compassion," i.e., translating statistics into the "cure and care" functions of health care, also is unpopular.

Dr. Rogers' points make sense to me. But there are additional important barriers to COPC. A way to see them is to look at obstacles to implement COPC in an organization that has few of the barriers on Dr. Rogers' list — the Indian Health Service (IHS).

IHS's system should foster COPC. Because IHS physicians are salaried it does not reward high tech care at the expense of community care. It emphasizes and gives prestige to primary, ambulatory care, not tertiary care. Most IHS physicians cooperate and share as members of multidisciplinary teams. IHS develops extensive epidemiological data, and bases clinical medicine on those data. IHS has many programs that emphasize prevention.

In my 8 years of experience in the Indian Health Service, however, I have seen that it also has problems implementing COPC. Many problems, such as inaccessible data, are topics covered in this book. I discuss here another problem: achieving and maintaining change in small organizations, such as a clinic or practice.

The Lummi IHS Clinic provides COPC to 5,000 American Indians who reside on or near the Lummi Reservation in Washington State. The multidisciplinary staff has special, COPC-based emphases including: maternal and child health; general diabetes and diabetic retinopathy; hypertension; immunizations; pap screening; fluoridation; infant car seats; sexually

410

transmitted disease; and prevention and control of tuberculosis.

The Clinic staff have implemented some COPC emphases only partially, and frequently after an extended struggle. The struggles concerned initial nonacceptance — not by the community but by the staff itself.

I have seen several reasons for non-acceptance by staff. Intra- and interdisciplinary turf problems limited the incorporation of some COPC programs into day-to-day clinical activities. Some staff disagreed with the importance of the specific COPC intervention. Some staff felt that the new activities were not in their "job description" or a legitimate part of medical care. Sometimes the Clinic did not have the extra organizational capacity to do the additional work of the COPC program — the "When you are up to your ears in alligators, it is difficult to remember that you came to drain the swamp" problem.

In my experience, then, COPC does not flower spontaneously, even when external conditions promote it. To implement COPC successfully requires thoughtful management. Two kinds of studies are relevant to the problem. Studies of organizational management have focused on behavior, motivation, and change in usually large organizations. Studies of quality assurance have focused on changing providers' behavior at the time of the encounter.

A recent article reviews the organizational development studies about planned change (2). A useful book by active consultants in organizational change summarizes lessons learned and practical approaches used, based on case studies (3). I will summarize the major points of the article and book, modifying some elements to be more relevant to implementing COPC in small organizations.[1]

There are three primary stages of change. In the first stage of "unfreezing,"

individuals and the group perceive and accept the need for change. In "moving," the second stage, staff replace old values and behaviors with new ones. The group, in the third stage of "maintenance" ("refreezing"), lock the new values and behaviors in place by supporting mechanisms.[2]

These stages are conceptual divisions of a process that is more fluid and mixed than linear in time. At any given moment, part of the change process may still require unfreezing, part may be in the maintenance stage, and part may be in the moving stage. Within that understanding, these conceptual stages imply that there are different problems and solutions specific to each stage. In small organizations, two entities must go through these stages successfully for the change to be implemented and maintained: the individual members of the organization and the organization itself as a group.[3]

Thus there are two dimensions to institutional change in a small organization: the stages of the process (unfreezing, moving, and maintenance), and the participants (individuals and groups). Tables

---

[1] I am indebted to Borje Saxberg, Ph.D., Robert Wood Johnson Clinical Scholars Program and Department of Management and Organization, University of Washington, Seattle, who gave me both the article and the book.

[2] The article calls this stage "refreezing," following the phrasing in the original work by K. Lewin (*Field Theory in Social Science*, New York: Harper and Row, 1951). But COPC does not seem frozen in place once established. Rather, it requires constant attention, else the organization often returns to pre-COPC behavior. "Maintenance" more accurately describes the COPC situation.

[3] Buller, Saxberg, and Smith (2) give four levels of participants: the individual, group, organization, and environment. Almost all organizational development studies are about large bureaucratic organizations. COPC practices have the size and characteristics of the "group" in these studies. Findings about the "organization" level have less relevance to COPC; I have not included them. David Rogers' article, quoted earlier, well describes the impact of the "environment" on COPC.

TABLE 1. Factors Affecting Implementation of Change

	INDIVIDUAL LEVEL	GROUP LEVEL
UNFREEZING	— Self-ability to change — Ambiguity of change — Linkage of behavior to rewards — Perceived value of rewards — Individual's trust of sponsor — Congruence with personal values — Pressures to change	— Others in the group are seen to be adopting the behavior — Belief that change is appropriate — Receptivity to sanctions — Congruence with group's process & structure — Intra- & inter-professional role conflicts
MOVING	— Congruence of initial values & expectations with actual outcomes	— Congruence of initial values & perceptions with actual outcomes
MAINTENANCE	— Congruence of people, processes, & structures — Transmission to individual's replacement — Congruence of individual's changes and adaptations with implemented change	— Congruence of people, processes, & structures — Transmission to next generation of staff — Congruence of other, routine, organizational adaptations and changes with implemented change

1 and 2 give in a two-by-three format, first, factors that affect implementation of change, and second, approaches to modify those factors.

Resistance to "unfreeze" by an individual is often due to the potential threats, fears, and insecurities that change precipitates. If the change is unclear, people may be excessively unsure of their ability to meet it. Perceived potential loss of job security, self-esteem, rewards, status, control and power, or competence increase people's resistance to change. If the perceived sponsor of change is not trusted by the individual, or if the expected new behaviors are incongruent with one's established norms, resistance likely will increase.

Resistance to "unfreeze" in small organizations is often due both to the resistances of the individuals (above), and also to the threats, fears, and insecurities felt

by the *group* itself. For instance, change in one part of the group may affect other, apparently unrelated, parts, by requiring these other parts to accept new responsibilities. The change may be incongruent with group norms, e.g., with what medical practices "are supposed to do" (as defined by the staffs of most practices in the community), or with the *actual* decisionmaking process and structure of the organization. If most staff see that only a small minority in the organization has adopted the change, that staff may be reluctant to change because it would be going against the majority of the group. A problem specific to organizations in health care is turf — inter- and intraprofessional disagreement about roles and responsibilities.

Change may not reach implementation after the "unfreezing" stage if the change is not supported in the "moving" phase.

TABLE 2. Approaches to Implement Change

Stage:	INDIVIDUAL LEVEL	GROUP LEVEL
UNFREEZING	— Reduce concerns about ability by providing *training & education* early in change process — Reduce perceived ambiguity by having all staff *participate* in planning the changes, & keeping all staff *informed* — Adopt new reward system *clearly linked* to desired behavior — Make changes *attractive* to staff — Make changes in *small steps*, to maintain close congruence between existing & new values & behaviors — Sponsor of change should be seen as *trustworthy & credible* — Communicate *need to change*	— *Maintain communication within group*, for staff to see that others in group see need to change & are adopting changes — Obtain cooperation & agreement of the *informal leaders* of the group — *Reward group*'s behavior [not just individual's] — Make change's structure & process *congruent with group's style of decisionmaking, structure, & processes*

MOVING	— Repeatedly address *confusion* about roles, processes, & structures
	— *Continued feedback & information:*
	  — periodic work-team meetings
	  — organizational "sensing" meetings
	  — renewal conferences
	  — performance reviews & evaluations
		— *[Same as for "Individual level"]*

MAINTENANCE	— *Change performance appraisal, personnel, & reward* systems to reinforce the new behaviors — *Select & train new staff* to reinforce the new behaviors — *Enhance the competence* of current staff	— *[Same as for "Individual level"]* — *Avoid overload* of implementing too many changes [COPC plus all others] at once — *Maintain support* for the change in the organization by outside validation, public rewards, etc.

For instance, if the staff see that the rewards they expected to receive for adopting the change (e.g., increased self-esteem, more satisfying job, personal and personnel rewards) do not come forth, or, worse, that nonadoption is rewarded or adopters receive more hassles, staff will likely stop adopting the change.

The change may be adopted temporarily but falter in the "maintenance" stage. If the reward system (e.g., performance appraisal) and the selection and training process have not been changed to include the desired behavior, maintaining COPC will be more difficult. Routine changes or adaptations that individuals or the group make, even if not directly involving COPC, may inadvertently reverse the implementation of COPC or make its maintenance more difficult.

Having a small organization adopt COPC usually requires the sponsor to diagnose accurately the specific problems in the change process, and to manage each problem. Table 2 gives approaches that are likely to convert resistance to change into opportunities that support adoption of COPC. Two characteristics are not explicit in Table 2. First, implementing and maintaining COPC is not a one-time effort. Resistances change over time. Changes in the organization (e.g., new staff) or the environment (e.g., budget cutbacks, requirements to put more personnel time into billing) may mean new pressure to neglect COPC. Second, "congruence" is of major importance. For example, not all staff want more challenging jobs; employees who want a less challenging position will resist adopting COPC behavior if it represents more challenge to them. Thus taking the "human potential" approach of giving more challenge to a person is most appropriate for those staff whose values are congruent with it.

Tables 1 and 2 may appear to imply that implementation of COPC is a formidable procedure. In fact, most small organizations experience only a few of the many difficulties; the Tables list most of the possible problems and their solutions.

A problem not discussed in the Tables is information overload. Often a major element of COPC is prevention. Many

COPC practices ultimately deliver that service to the individual recipient in the provider-patient encounter; high compliance rates by providers are critical to the success of those programs. These COPC practices encounter a major problem: "the non-perfectability of man ... due to man's limitations as a data processor rather than to correctable human deficiencies" (4). When in the clinical encounter with the patient, practitioners often are noncompliant with their own standards of care; frequently compliance changes little in spite of education or exhortation.

Clem McDonald's studies (5) show that providers change most when presented brief, appropriate information at the time of the encounter. Even when providers *want* to provide a service, such as doing periodic pap smears, they do it much less frequently if they themselves have to work through the chart during the encounter to assess if *this* patient needs a pap at *this* visit. If providers see highly visible reminders during the encounter that "this patient needs a pap now," the rate of compliance with their own standards increases significantly (Figure 1).

An example of how these principles apply in practice is the Pap Emphasis Program of the Indian Health Service Clinic mentioned above.

Age-specific cervical cancer death rates for American Indians are two to three times those of the U.S. population. In January 1978, the IHS Clinic started a Pap Emphasis Program with three major elements: assign one nurse to be responsible for it; put a highly visible reminder on the charts for patients due for a pap; and use a system ("tickler file") to track when patients were due for a pap.

A nurse accepted the challenge of having responsibility for increasing the pap rate. She developed the system; she also got the credit for the success of the program. Because she felt responsible for the program and "owned" it, she cajoled the

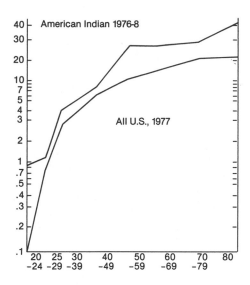

Figure 1. Cervical Cancer Death Rates Age-Specific, per 100,000.

physicians and other nurses to comply with her reminders. She also taught the other nurses, increasing their interest and compliance to encourage "overdue" patients to have a pap done during their visit. She used McDonald's approach without using a computer. She kept a tickler file of dates the next pap was due. The date of next pap was made obvious on every chart, and updated by her. When the next pap was in fact due, she attached a highly visible color sticker to the Problem List.

The evaluation of the outcome was impressive. A crossover quasi-experiment had occurred naturally. A nearby private

	Total N	P.E.P.	Screened	X^2	p
7-74 to 6-76:					
CLINIC	76	without	45%	6.22	<.02
COMPARISON	72	with	64%		
7-78 to 6-80:					
CLINIC	100	with	73%	10.2	<.01
COMPARISON	80	without	49%		

Figure 2. Screening Rates: Comparison Between Practices.

practice, serving members of an Indian Reservation about 50 miles away, had an almost identical pap recall program in the early 1970s, but the program had lapsed by 1978. The rates of screening paps were markedly higher in each setting when their programs were in place than when they were not.

Comparing the rates between the two sites during the same two time periods, when one site had and the other did not have a special program in place, again showed the marked positive effect of the programs. The naturally occurring crossover quasi-experiment excluded "maturation" and "historical change" as possible explanations for the improvement noted by the evaluation (6).

The Clinic's Pap Emphasis Program has been evaluated twice more. It continues to function well, but it stopped twice for brief periods. Both times the nurse in

	Total N	P.E.P.	Screened	X^2	p
CLINIC:					
7-74 to 6-76	76	without	45%	14.7	<.001
7-78 to 6-80	100	with	73%		
COMPARISON:					
7-74 to 6-76	72	with	64%	3.53	.05<p<.1
7-78 to 6-80	80	without	49%		

Figure 3. Screening Rates: Change Within Each Setting.

charge of the program had changes imposed on her responsibilities, workload, and time available. She solved those conflicts by putting the Pap Emphasis Program on "hold." Both times, once the Clinical Director found out about the conflicts, he adjusted the situation to permit continuation of the program.

A similar sequence occurred in the comparison private practice clinic in the mid 1970s. Two additional physicians entered the practice; its pap recall program was disrupted because the nurse doing the program had more responsibilities, more work, and less time. The nurse did not tell the physician in the practice who had established the pap recall program. In this case, the program did not operate for several years, until the senior physician found it was not working.

DISCUSSION

The experiences of both the Indian Health Service Clinic and the nearby practice illustrate a few of the points mentioned above. Both groups "unfroze" and "moved" the staff to adopt a COPC-linked program. Both buttressed physicians' processing of encounter data with external (noncomputerized!) reminders. Both had problems "maintaining" the program, because the sponsors of the change did not continue to pay attention to it.

The major problems occurred in the "maintenance" phase; some methods might have "refrozen" the COPC program more effectively. Some approaches include: asking for summary statistics every quarter or half-year; publicly and periodically reporting the statistics to the entire staff; periodically reminding the staff of the need for the program; and adding "maintenance of the pap program" to the job descriptions of the people responsible.

SUMMARY

Barriers external to primary care practices are only part of the difficulty in implementing and maintaining COPC. Practices experience resistances to implementation and maintenance similar to general resistances that occur in many small organizations; organizational management studies help identify potential problems and their solutions. The information overload of the primary care chart in the setting of insufficient time during the provider-patient encounter also is a problem; informational and memory aids (computers, manual tickler files, or checklists) that are integrated in the system of care help improve that problem.

REFERENCES

1. Rogers, D. Community-oriented primary care. *Journal of the American Medical Association* 1982; 248:1622.

2. Buller, P.F.; Saxberg, B.O.; and Smith, H.L. Institutionalization of planned organizational change: A model and review of the literature. *The 1985 Annual: Developing Human Resources.* San Diego: University Associates, 1985.

3. Lippitt, G.L.; Langseth, P.; and Mossop, J. *Implementing Organization Change.* San Francisco: Jossey-Bass, 1985.

4. McDonald, C.J. Protocol-based computer reminders, the quality of care and the non-perfectability of man. *New England Journal of Medicine* 1976; 295:1351.

5. McDonald, C.J., et al. Reminders to physicians from an introspective computer medical record: A two-year randomized trial. *Annals of Internal Medicine* 1984; 100:130.

6. Cook, T.D., and Campbell, D.T. *Quasi-Experimentation: Design and Analysis Issues for Field Settings.* Boston: Houghton Mifflin, 1978.

CHAPTER 50

Estimating the Economic Impact of COPC Activities on Primary Care Practice

Frank M. Reed, M.D.

In the last 5 years there has been considerable interest in the United States in developing the concept and identifying the function of community-oriented primary care. In a medical environment of increasing complexity, with more requirements attached to practice, any new activity, including COPC, must be seen as an opportunity with incentives rather than just another burden to the practice. In the Institute of Medicine study (1), it was noted that most of the existing models of COPC in the United States are found in the public sector of medicine. It is also true, however, that the line between public and private medicine is narrowing with the advent of other than fee-for-service schemes in the private sector.

Increasingly, the name of the game is enlarging the size of the population served by each practice, in order to survive in an environment where fewer dollars are available for each life at risk. It would seem that COPC might be viewed as marketing strategy, provided the direct and indirect cost of this marketing could be shown to be reasonable and even recapturable by increasing the practice's share of a particular community. Whereas in private medicine, the ultimate capture of additional

revenue would be the payoff, one could hypothesize that in the public sector rewards and success could be gained by reaching an ever-increasing percentage of the targeted populations with programmatic goals.

Regardless of the economic model of health care delivery, adequate expense analysis must be undertaken before embarking on major projects of COPC. A primary focus of COPC is, of course, to target health problems of persons not currently defined as active patients. Using a registration document that identifies the age, position in family, and sex of all family members of active patients is one way to generate such an at-risk practice community. If such a system is tied with an automated medical information system (not a necessity but certainly a very useful tool), one can then design a method for assessing the direct cost of defining the practice community. Such a formula might look like this:

$$C_{COPC} = (C_{pt} + C_{de}) \times (N_{rp} - N_{ap})$$

C_{COPC} is the cost of a practice COPC registry; C_{pt} is the cost of personnel time to register family members other than active patients; C_{de} is the cost per active patient of entering and maintaining registered patient data; N_{rp} is the number of registered patients; and N_{ap} is the number of active patients.

For example, assume the following:

Personnel cost: (@ $8/hour or $0.13/minute) $0.04/person (reg)

Data cost: Cost of storing data — $1.00/person/year

Registered patients: 4,000

Active patients: 2,000

The annual cost of the registry would be $2,080. With an offset of an average $36/visit, the practice would need 58 registered patients to become active (i.e., new) patients per year as result of COPC effort (true growth).

The total cost of COPC using a "practice community" is the registry cost above and the direct cost of the activity itself.

If one then has the ability to monitor practice growth before COPC is instituted, and also control for other economic seasonal and growth factors in the practice while measuring the active visitation rate following institution of COPC (non-trivial but achievable measures), one can get a sense of the economic impact of COPC. For example, if the cost of registering a patient is $.05, the receptionist's time is $.15, the annual cost of storing that information is $1.00, and there are 3,000 registered patients in a practice that had 4,000 visits from 2,000 patients, then the total would be $4,200 per year. If one could show a practice growth rate of 100 new patients per year at an average of $42 per visit, one could break even on COPC registry costs for that year and anticipate long-term gains from the acquisition of additional patients from the registered families.

Furthermore, one can develop a series of rates by which to understand the character of the practice, because the proportion of family members visiting can be analyzed from year to year. This can be particularly useful when attempting to target, for example, a pediatric population. One can have a sense of the potential number of pediatric patients through the family registration and can study penetration trends into that subgroup of patients.

From a marketing standpoint, especially in rural areas, community members are viewed as potential patients. However, COPC can just as effectively be aimed at health problems of community groups without the need to take them on as patients, if the fundamental economic analysis above is favorable. In other words, knowing what the cost burden is on the practice allows one to undertake additional projects without the need to capture revenue. In a sense, these volunteer efforts will always have costs associated with them, but these costs can be justified if patient recruitment is sufficient from other activities. Thus, there are two possible types of COPC activities from a fiscal point of view: those that may result in potential revenue production and those in which revenue production will occur only rarely or coincidentally, if at all. The particular balance of these activities in a practice may, in large part, determine fiscal viability of various undertakings. Some examples may help serve to illustrate these points.

The use of family-oriented charting systems in registration of entire families during individual visits is an example of increasing health care access to community segments while optimally increasing practice growth and yielding revenue. An additional example would be enrolling subsets of registered patients in special programs, such as influenza immunizations for inactive patients, again in the hope of ultimately gaining many of these community members as active patients. A third example, with little if any economic return for a practice, would be the targeting of special groups such as smokers for public information seminars. Theoretically, success in attaining smoking cessation should decrease revenue to the practice because of the consequent reduction of health problems in ex-smokers. Nevertheless, most would agree that comprehensive primary health care certainly requires the promotion of smoking cessation, at least among patients, and ideally throughout the community in which the practice is established. Another way to address the practice community is by gaining access to previously defined community segments. Organizations with a health focus such as geriatric groups often have fairly comprehensive lists obtained from the Postal Service, voting registration lists, etc., which can inexpensively be obtained for targeting health problems within these groups.

CONCLUSION

Addressing the practice community beyond the active patients presents a challenge that can be viewed either as a burden or an opportunity. A simple model for expense analysis of COPC activities can provide a yardstick for choosing activities that are feasible and affordable.

REFERENCES

1. *Community Oriented Primary Care: A Practical Assessment*, Vol. 1. Institute of Medicine. Washington, DC: National Academy Press, 1984.

CHAPTER 51

Data Organization:
The Practice as a
Laboratory for COPC

Eugene S. Farley, M.D., M.P.H.

"I look at the earth, sea and sky and all contained therein and am filled with wonder. . . . I observe, but do not 'see,' I 'see' but do not understand."

THE PHYSICIAN AS PARTICIPATING OBSERVER AND NATURALIST

The word physician is derived from the Latin *physicus* and the Greek *physikos*, meaning scientist. This association of nature and science is basic to the modern concept of physician. The dictionary definition of the word includes the legal, "A person licensed to practice medicine," and the inclusive, "Anyone who heals or exerts a healing influence." In his attempts to heal and to explain healing, the physician has not always used science but has acquired some of the trappings of magic, superstition, ritual, and religion. Thus today the term *physician* has connotations of healing, knowledge, science (biological, psychological, and sociological), and faith. The role of healer requires the physician to juggle these seemingly contradictory concepts of science, magic, and faith and integrate them into a usable whole to help those he serves.

The continuous expansion of knowledge and the development of new tools and methods for disease prevention and healing allow the physician to better serve his patients as a "scientist" who deals with "nature." But as a healer the physician often acts on the edge of science. To better understand the edge of science he must try to understand the healing process in its full breadth. To develop this understanding he must use scientific concepts. These concepts are a basic part of the education and training of both naturalists and physicians. They include careful observation and recording of what is happening, organization of the data collected from the observation, and analysis or explanation of the data in the light of current knowledge or developing theories. The physician is asked to observe (look at, listen to, examine, study) the patient and his environment in order to identify his problems (diagnose) and participate (treat, help) in their resolution. The physician assumes these responsibilities for observation and participation when he accepts the care of an individual as a patient. A community-oriented primary care (COPC) physician assumes these responsibilities for observation and participation for care of the patient and uses this access to the patient as an entry point into the community. He extends this responsibility to work with the community as well. The COPC physician accepts the opportunity to look at and care for the individual patient in the context of his environment, both family and community. He has access to the patient and community at many different entry points, and therefore has opportunities to follow through and study the natural history of individuals and communities.

The primary care physician's access to people and problems in their "natural" state causes him to ask questions and seek answers that may be different than those asked by other physicians. To formulate the appropriate questions and develop the answers requires the improvement and use of skills that are basic to all physicians. These include observation and participation. Being a physician or naturalist requires collection of appropriate data, organization of the data to facilitate analysis, analysis of the data, and decisionmaking based on that analysis.

OBSERVATION

Observation includes data collection and data organization. Data collection includes taking histories and conducting physical and laboratory examinations and special studies. Data on individual patients are organized and entered into the chart. Aggregate data obtained from many patients are analyzed to identify such factors as family (or household), area of residence, age and sex, diseases, and problems of the population served and to learn about the community.

PARTICIPATION

Participation involves making decisions on the basis of problem definition based on data analysis (diagnosis for the individual, family, and community). Decisionmaking involves the formulation of a plan

(treatment, intervention, or nonintervention) for the individual, family, and community.

COPC physicians must observe, collect, organize, and interpret data at a broader level than other practitioners. By definition they are community based and therefore must be able to reach out to define, understand, and serve a community. To do this they need data systems that help them to care for the patient and to understand the family, community, and society of which that patient is a part. This chapter describes simple, manual organizational systems for practice-acquired data that meet some of the needs of COPC.

ORGANIZATION OF THE DATA SYSTEM

The Medical Chart. Traditionally, practice-acquired data are organized in the medical chart to support the care of the individual patient. The medical charts, therefore, form the basis of the data system. Other data, which in themselves may originate from the medical chart, can be found in the accounting system for collecting payments and paying bills and taxes. COPC practices require organization of the practice-acquired data for better definition of the problems of the population and community served, better understanding of needs, and provision of appropriate care to their communities.

The "System." Practice data systems have been developed to function effectively with or without computers to meet many of the needs of COPC practices for teaching, service, and research. The systems have been proven functional and practical in the daily practice of medicine. They are not restricted to the exigencies of the pure practice model, the pure research model, or to the incompletely thought-out, "good idea" model. They provide easy entry (recording) and retrieval of information to facilitate patient care, practice management, chart review, provider education, and research.

The data organization systems appropriate for COPC practices allow the practices to serve as "laboratories" from which old knowledge is studied and new knowledge is developed. This is achieved in part by improving the ability to record, retrieve, and analyze the variety of data collected routinely in caring for a patient. Appropriate data handling methods facilitate the provision of comprehensive and continuous care and allow identification of what has not been done in care of the patient. They allow study of the individual patient and the population of patients served and identification of population related problems. They facilitate patient care, practice management, appropriate use of resources, outreach, application of new knowledge, continuing medical education, audit, identification of new knowledge and problems, and evaluation of old knowledge and problems.

The basis of a system of data organization for COPC is the patient's health record. The chart should contain a structured and defined database, flow sheets, problem-oriented notes, and other components as needed and discussed below. A good data system also identifies the family (or household) by the household folder (charts of all members of the family or household can be filed in the same folder) and by family number, which identifies the family and the patient's relative position in the family.

The practice population is characterized by the age and sex register and by the morbidity, diagnostic, or problem index. This index contains and enumerates the problems identified in the patient population and allows retrieval of all individuals in the practice with those problems. It allows study of groups of patients with the problem or disease, and facilitates review, outreach, audit, and application of new knowledge to patients with the identified

problems. Its use requires coding of problems, preferably using the "international classification of health problems in primary care" (ICHPPC), which was developed by an international group of primary care physicians for use in active office practice.

The data that characterize the community are organized by the method of filing the medical record. Geographic filing, or filing by census tracts, allows household folders or charts of all of those who live in a defined area or census tract to be filed together. This is simplified by color coding the family or household folder by area of residence. It allows easy relation of Census Bureau sociodemographic information of specific census tracts to the population served from that census tract. It allows problems seen in the practice to be related to geographic areas or population groups.

The following components are recommended for a data system that facilitates service and research in COPC practices. Each will be discussed in detail.

1. Encounter form.

2. Age/sex registry.

3. Individual patient charts.

4. Family or household folders.

5. Geographic filing of household folders to facilitate outreach, community identification, and epidemiologic studies.

6. Morbidity or problem index.

The individual components of any data organization system are interdependent and therefore must be developed as part of an integrated system. There must be a clear understanding of the purpose of each component. In a COPC practice each component must be developed in a way that facilitates patient care, provider education, audit, outreach, practice management, and research. The ease of recording and retrieval are an important aspect of any system, and the system must work for episodic as well as comprehensive visits so the patients are able to receive comprehensive care even through episodic visits. It is instructive to examine the potential for each of the components of the practice data system that supports COPC, as listed above.

1. Encounter Form

The encounter document should serve as a billing, routing, and scheduling slip, a problem and medication list, a prescription pad, and computer entry document. The ideal encounter has yet to be developed for practices that use computers as part of their data system. A different type of encounter form that contains some of the same attributes, but does not contain an updated problem or medication list is needed for practices without computers. Problems of maintaining an up-to-date medication list have been resolved in part by a modified prescription pad that makes a carbon copy to place on the medication list. An excellent one has been developed by the family practice program at the University of Arizona.

2. Age/Sex Registry

An age/sex registry is of basic importance to any practice in which there is to be effective outreach, review of charts by age cohorts, management decisions based on the population served, and research.

There are many ways to develop an age/sex registry. The simplest and cheapest consists of having a three-by-five card, blue for male, pink for female, for each patient in the practice. On the card is written the patient's name, address, and date of birth. The card is then filed alphabetically with others of the same sex under year of birth. This is done only once for each patient no matter how many times he or she visits the practice. This gives a running count of the patients in the practice by age and sex.

For a new practice this should be done from the first day patients are seen. For an established practice the cheapest and simplest approach is to pick a starting date and fill out a card the first time any patient, old or new, is seen in the practice after that date. For an already established practice to develop a complete age/sex registry that includes all patients presently in the practice it is necessary to go through all of the active charts and fill out an age/sex card for each patient. This can be done, but is more costly than just picking a date and starting because it requires time and effort to catch up, and all charts in the file may not be active.

To keep an age/sex register updated it is essential that the cards of individuals who have not been seen within the previous 2 years be pulled once a year, preferably as near January 1 as possible.[1] Updating of the age/sex registry can be done most effectively by identifying on the visible edge of the folder containing the chart the last year anyone in that folder was seen. This can be done by writing or identifying the actual year with a piece of colored tape representing the year in which someone in that folder was seen. On January 1 of each year those folders with no markings indicating a chart in them was active within the last 2 years are pulled. The age/sex cards of the individuals whose charts are in that folder can then be pulled and either placed in the folder before the latter is filed with inactive charts or filed in an age/sex registry of inactive patients. If and when an individual from one of the households represented by the folder returns to the practice, the inactive folder and age/sex card are pulled and filed with the active folders and age/sex cards.

---

[1] International convention in family practice defines an active patient as anyone in a family or household that has had at least one member seen in the practice during the past 2 years.

3. Individual Patient Charts

The data in patient charts define and characterize the individual. The database in the chart must be organized to allow rapid recording and retrieval of the data so they will be collected and used. The patient chart should include several important components.

Front Sheet. Perhaps the most important component is the front sheet or personal identification section that contains data on the individual and family. It serves as a quick reference and reminder for the provider and has some of the functions of an index with greater details inside. Specific elements suggested for the front sheet include data identifying the individual (name, date of birth, place of birth); race; ethnicity; religion; education; date first seen in practice; identification number, i.e., family and position in family; occupation and dates; list of selected past illnesses of individual and family members; list of previous hospitalizations, surgery, injuries, and serious illnesses; immunizations (past, present, and future); allergies; skin tests with dates and results; habits (drugs, alcohol, tobacco, marijuana, stimulants, sedatives, other); lifestyle (exercise, nutrition, sleep); housing description (when indicated); overseas or foreign travel; military service or equivalent; other health care providers (name, specialty, and address); contraception education; and health education.

The chart must allow these data to be collected over a period of several more episodic visits as well as during more extensive in-depth visits. There must be a clear way to determine whether the questions have been asked so they will not have to be repeated on each visit. The chart must facilitate use of data aggregated over time as well as data collected during any individual visit.

Relationships and Support Systems. This section should include information on the family, community, social, institutional, organizational, and household systems available whether used or unused; genogram, including parents and grandparents at least and children and grandchildren; list of specific family members with names and birth dates and state of health with particular emphasis on selected specific diseases. The genogram can be set up to do all or part of this to avoid redundancy. This section should also include information to describe functional family and community relationships and support systems. These should reflect not only genetic relationships, but functional supportive, destructive, or nonsupportive relationships as well.

Development and Health Maintenance. This section contains developmental guidelines, screening, health maintenance and promotion, and prevention information, that are age-related and designed with specific disease processes in mind. The section must be developed with the concept of dealing with these issues in an individual from conception to the grave. Its basis is the individual and family life cycle with recognition of developmental stages and tasks. It should contain, according to age: growth and development charts; education and advice guidelines; screening recommendations and dates done; Denver developmental forms; obstetrical forms; adult developmental and screening recommendations with emphasis on developmental stages and tasks such as used in pediatric age groups. This will encourage development of the ability to recognize and respond to problems of adult development, and to recognize and respond to problems associated with known or suspected risk factors.

Progress Notes and Flow Sheets. Progress notes are structured to allow rapid recording and retrieval of data entered and to allow rapid comparison of findings in a semi-flow sheet manner. This minimizes the writing time of the provider and the typing time of the transcriptionist. They are structured to allow aggregation and comparison of data gathered during episodic as well as health maintenance visits. They reduce the need for repeating parts of the examination done on previous visits and allow a complete database to be developed on the health status of the individual, whether that person is seeking episodic or continuous care. The progress notes facilitate the doctor's role in defining the health problems of the patient and responding to them appropriately. The notes must facilitate the physician's ability to be an advocate for the health maintenance of the patient seeking care.

Progress notes should be structured in a semi-flow sheet format to allow rapid recording and retrieval of information; easy transcription; indexing of laboratory data, special studies data, and referrals; and accumulation of data needed for comprehensive care even during episodic visits. The progress note flow sheet also should contain an index checklist which identifies any lab or special studies ordered during the last visit. This assures that results are sought on the followup visit.

Laboratory and Special Studies Reports. The in-office laboratory forms can be designed to be shingled and form a flow sheet without the need for transcribing. Out-of-office laboratory reports may need to be transcribed into a flow sheet format, or they may be inserted into the chart in sequence without transcription. Special study reports should be inserted by category and may or may not have a specific index tab.

Correspondence, Consultations, Referral Notes. These can be entered into the chart in the order in which they occur. They are indexed on the progress note flow sheet on the day of the visit.

Summaries: Hospital Discharges, Records from Other Physicians. These can be entered into the section in dated order.

Review of Systems. Periodic system review (ROS) and history updating is necessary in the care of any patient. The progress note structure must allow such an updating to fit into the time sequence of the notes and still be identified as an updating. To facilitate this the ROS can be developed on a color-coded sheet that can fit into the sequence with the progress notes or be glued onto the progress note of that date. This allows quick identification and review of the ROS by anyone caring for that patient.

Special Studies. Special studies can be identified as having been ordered or done on a part of the progress note set aside for such indexing. When done they are then inserted on specific forms or sheets in the special studies section of the chart.

Family and Social History. Family and social history updating can be done on another color-coded form to be placed in sequence in the chart, glued into the progress notes in the appropriate sequence, or recorded directly onto a color-coded family history form as part of the genogram and family section.

Past History. Past history updating requires use of the "front sheet," which serves as the cumulative summary and index for individual's past illness and family history of illness.

4. Family or Household Folder

Within each folder of a family or household there can be a family chart. This family chart contains data important to all of the family and are not unique to the individual. Information in this chart will unavoidably overlap with some of the family-related information in the individual chart. Some feel this is the proper place for the genogram, but with so many reconstituted families, or families with adopted children, it becomes difficult to have one genogram serve all of these members effectively.

The family chart contains information needed to identify the family life cycle, the stage it is in at the time of the entry into the chart, and the developmental tasks associated with that stage. COPC practices need to develop the tools that create a functional awareness of the importance of the family and its developmental stages.

If the practice provides family-oriented care, families or households need a recognized provider who cares for all the members of that family, unless members prefer to be cared for by someone else in the practice. This way of providing care is important for care of the individual and for knowledge of exposures, risk factors, and support systems. Filing the charts of all members of a household together in a common household folder facilitates this care. Family or household members who leave the household to set up a new one for marriage, work, or other reasons need to have their charts removed to the folder of their new household.

Filing individual medical records together in a family folder ensures that all providers caring for individual members will have access to the charts of all members on each visit. It will encourage them to think in terms of living groups, allow them to encourage members to get the care needed, and make it possible to know the members of the household.

5. Geographic Filing of Household Folders

Filing charts by area in which the individual patient lives facilitates recognition of community concepts and factors in the lives and care of the patients seen. It allows environmental, physical, cultural, and social factors to be more clearly related to the community. It facilitates chart identification and retrieval, outreach to the patients, and practice management.

To gain the maximum benefit of such a filing system, census tracts are used to define the geographic unit. This allows identification of predetermined boundaries with an accurate counting of the individu-

als living in that area. It allows regional data to be shared. It lets those doing studies identify whether the population in the practice represents a significant part of the population in the area or geographic unit studied.

Geographic filing of folders requires changing the system of identifying charts, assigning the correct census tract number to each household in the practice, assigning a color-code to each census tract, color-coding household folders to match the color code assigned each census tract number, and filing household charts alphabetically within the census tract.

6. Morbidity Index

A morbidity index is a record of the problems identified among the patients cared for in the practice. It allows patients with previously identified problems to be grouped together, studied, reviewed, reached out to, and served. It requires coding the problems identified with a standard code, such as the International Classification of Health Problems in Primary Care (ICHPPC) or the International Classification of Disease (ICD).

A morbidity index can be developed with simple cards, over-leafed ring binders, or a computer. The over-leaf or card system requires each card or page to be numbered. The number of each page is the code number for the problem. For ease of analysis these sheets have places for the names of 10 male patients on one side and 10 female patients on the other side. The number of patients with the identified problems is easily determined by simple counting of the cards.

Whether the morbidity index is developed with a computer or by use of hard copy, an entry document is needed. The encounter form can serve as this entry document since it contains the information needed to make entries into the data system. The encounter form or data entry document can also serve as the billing document, routing slip, and appointment slip. If the practice is computerized, the encounter form or data entry document can also contain the problem list, prescription pad, and medication list.

SOME PRACTICAL MATTERS

As the charts are developed and put together, bulk and costs can be kept down by not providing each chart with its own heavy manila folder cover. The front sheet should serve as the front cover and the last patient visit progress sheet as the back cover. Both sides of the paper should be used, and most forms and dividers should be on standard weight paper. Greater ease of use is likely if the data can be read from front to back like a book.

Various types of fasteners may be used. If progress notes are not of the shingled type and dividers are not made of too heavy stock, one of the quickest, cheapest, and least bulky fasteners is the staple. Though they hold well, they can be removed quickly and new sheets can be inserted readily. They do poke more holes in the paper, but this can be handled by reinforcing the edge of the front sheet and the progress note sheet. If transcription of the progress notes is done, the last progress sheet page can be inserted loose in the chart, to be fastened in when it is full.

The most effective and cheapest transcription can be done when each individual provider uses a small portable dictating unit. The charts are stacked in the sequence in which they are dictated. The dictated cassette is placed on top of the completed charts and taken to be transcribed in sequence. Transcription is done on the loose progress note sheet, which contains notations of the providers from that visit. A specific system of transcription allows the charts to be completed and refiled quickly. The encounter form is handed to the patient to take to the receptionist or billing clerk upon comple-

tion of the visit. The billing clerk gives the patient one sheet as a receipt if paid, or as a bill if unpaid. It also serves as an appointment slip or reminder for the next visit with the name of the provider for that visit, the time of the appointment, and the purpose and length of the appointment. One sheet is kept for the billing office and one can be retained as a control document or as a data entry document if that entry is done separately from the billing entry.

CONCLUSION

The concepts presented in this chapter can serve as a framework for the development of a data organization system for practices interested in being involved in service and research appropriate for COPC. There is enough flexibility in the concepts to allow individual input and development of appropriate alternative forms that achieve these goals.

The systems described here do not make a physician a naturalist. However, they should provide the physician an ability to serve the population and community more effectively than is possible in traditional practices. It allows the physician to truly develop his practice as a "laboratory," to become a better observer of and participant in the care of his patient and community, to evaluate old knowledge better, and to develop new knowledge based on experience gained in practice. All of these concepts are important to the future development of COPC. As a part of COPC, appropriate data organization can and will change the whole concept of how primary care is practiced.

427

CHAPTER 52

COPC Applications
for the
Microcomputer

Douglas B. Kamerow, M.D., M.P.H.

The collection and analysis of data is central to the practice of community-oriented primary care. Every aspect of the COPC process involves the manipulation of information (1). Data are required to define a community; to identify the community's health problems; to institute a program to address priority needs; and, finally, to evaluate the effectiveness of the interventions selected. Currently available microcomputers and inexpensive software can aid in each step of this process. After reviewing the basic types of software available, this chapter will suggest some applications for the microcomputer in each of the steps listed above.

TYPES OF APPLICATIONS SOFTWARE

For each type of software, two representative commercial products are given, one for each of two of most popular microcomputers, the IBM Personal Computer and the Apple MacIntosh. Similar commercial software is available for almost every type of microcomputer. These examples do not, of course, imply endorsement of the particular products, as there are many others that perform equally well. In addition, there are also extremely low-cost

public domain software products that will perform many of these functions. They are usually available through local computer user groups.

Word Processing (WordPerfect, Microsoft Word)

The most commonly used microcomputer application is word processing, allowing text to be entered, changed, and printed in many formats. Many programs also have "mail merge" capabilities, allowing the rapid creation of many similar letters or documents with the name or certain lines personalized for each addressee.

Database Management (DBase III, Overview)

This type of software can be thought of as a giant card file. Information can be entered onto individual cards (usually called "records"), which can then be sorted by any of the components in the record (Figure 1). For example, suppose each record is a patient and the data stored for each patient include demographic and clinical material. One could then list those with a certain diagnosis, calculate the average age of those patients, or determine if a certain diagnosis was more common among one ethnic group.

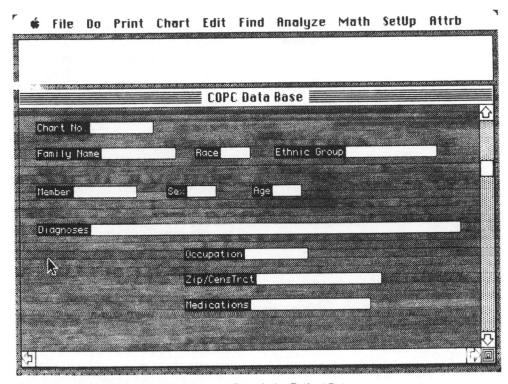

Figure 1. Computer Screen Set Up to Accept Descriptive Patient Data.

Spreadsheets (Lotus 1-2-3, Excel)

First popularized for financial accounting and forecasting, spreadsheets now have much wider application. They are useful whenever columns or rows of numbers need to be manipulated and displayed. For example, in figuring the costs of a screening intervention, the information on unit cost for each of the components (materials, labor, overhead) need only be entered once. Then any aspect of the calculation can be changed at will; all totals will be instantaneously recalculated. Thus one can quickly predict what it would cost to add a nurse, to screen twice as many persons, or to use a new supplier of materials.

Graphics Programs (Graphwriter, Microsoft Chart)

Data are best understood when displayed graphically. These programs enable one to easily create bar, pie, and line graphs either by entering the data manually or by using data directly from a spreadsheet program. Some spreadsheet programs have the ability to do simple graphs themselves. Graphics software can also be used in exploratory data analysis, as outlined by Breckenridge and Like in their chapter in Part 2.

Statistical Software (Statpro, StatWorks)

Mainframe computer systems are no longer necessary to do most simple (and some complex) statistical analyses. These programs can do chi square and t-tests as well as many descriptive and inferential procedures. Data may be entered into the program or imported from a spreadsheet.

Telecommunications (Smartcom II, MacTerminal)

Using an inexpensive device called a modem connected to the microcomputer and a telephone, this software allows the transmission of data to any similarly equipped machine. Thus material may be shared between microcomputers, with mainframes, or with a group of other users via a "bulletin board" set up for that purpose. In a community-wide or regional system, data may be gathered in several remote locations and telecommunicated to a central analysis point.

Integrated Programs (Symphony, Jazz)
These programs combine some or all of the above capabilities into one integrated package. Although each individual component, such as the spreadsheet, might not be as powerful or fully functioned as a stand alone product, most general functions are available. Thus the operator only has to learn one system of commands, and data are easily shared among all of the program's parts. For convenience and economy, these products deserve close examination.

MICROCOMPUTER APPLICATIONS IN COPC

The microcomputer can help organize patient information to better understand what community is being served or, perhaps more importantly, what community is *not* being served. A database program can be used to answer questions about the population currently served: How old are they? For whom do they work? Where do they live? Which members visit most frequently? Which are never seen? The answers to these questions can then be tabulated to describe the active patient practice, the first step to expanding into the community. Community or regional data can be obtained to compare with data from the practice to learn what parts of the community are not being served. Telecommunications can make the transfer of such data much easier, and graphics programs are useful in displaying any differences found.

A comparison of the diagnoses most common in the defined practice with those available from community or other sources can be used to determine the major unaddressed problems in the community. For example, if community data indicate a high black population but practice data show few hypertensives, then community outreach around this issue is probably needed. Or if a search of diagnoses turns up a few cases of lead poisoning among patients with the same zip code or in the same census tract, then all children in that area (and perhaps others living in that area as well) should be screened for lead.

The use of a database system to categorize all patient demographic, occupational, and diagnostic data allows extrapolations to be made from a few members of the population to all members who share the same characteristics. If three Indochinese immigrants reactivate tuberculosis, for instance, then others at risk can be screened. More ambitiously, database and spreadsheet software could be used to record results of a community survey, with graphic and statistical manipulation of the results. Such a survey could be used to guide COPC activities, much as was done in the Tarboro-Edgecombe Health Services System (2).

Word processing and mail merge programs facilitate contacting members of the community for screening programs. Files of those contacted and their responses and outcomes can be put on a database system. The whole process, if large and complicated, can be tracked with project management software to ensure that persons and materials are available at the right places and times. Educational materials may be produced easily using the right software.

Finally, to evaluate the effectiveness of interventions, followup letters and questionnaires can be composed with word processing and mail merge software. Database managers are easy to set up as an automated "tickler" file, to track high-risk persons for certain milestones or procedures. Any kind of record keeping is easier with the help of microcomputers.

Computers are no more nor less than a way of systematically storing and retrieving data. They can be very useful during every step of the COPC process. The investment of a modest amount of time and money can result in the simplification of many laborious tasks, as well as give individual practices the ability to perform powerful displays and analyses of their data.

REFERENCES

1. Nutting, P.A.; Wood, M.; and Conner, E.M. Community-oriented primary care: A status report. *Journal of the American Medical Association* 1985; 253:1763-1766.

2. Institute of Medicine. *Community-Oriented Primary Care: A Practical Assessment*, Vol. 2. Washington, DC: National Academy Press, pp. 163-186.

CHAPTER 53

Creative Uses of
a Practice Billing System
to Support COPC

Joseph Jacobs, M.D., M.B.A.

Computerized billing systems have become increasingly important in medical practice. The independent primary care practitioner has become more dependent on his billing system to help ensure economic survival in a competitive health care marketplace. The introduction of automation to the practitioner's office usually first involves financial billing as a high priority over other functions because of the imperative to maintain cash flow. Patient scheduling and reminders are usually next in priority, then automation of clinical monitoring activities because of the added expense of software and additional hardware to support such activities.

This chapter offers the clinical practitioner an optimal way to use a relatively simple automated billing system to address one of the three components of a COPC model. In my discussion I assume that readers may be able to access some elements of their billing systems and either have some programming skills or some programming support available.

COPC is defined as having three components: a practice actively engaged in the delivery of primary care, a defined community whose health care needs are being addressed by the practice, and a

process by which a community's health care needs are addressed. The COPC process consists of four steps: 1) defining and characterizing the community, 2) identifying the community's health problems, 3) modifying the health care program to address priority health care needs, and 4) monitoring the effectiveness of program modifications. The focus of my discussion is on the first three steps. My discussion is based on my experiences while I was a house officer in the Department of Maternal and Child Health of the Dartmouth-Hitchcock Medical Center in Hanover, New Hampshire.

Most billing systems for the health care industry are able to provide sufficient information for the American Medical Association's Standard Billing Form. This form requires the use of patient insurance numbers, date of encounter, location of encounter, physician codes, diagnostic codes, and procedures codes. Much of these data, if properly manipulated by a computer, may provide primary care practitioners information about their practice without having to engage in expensive and complicated surveys. It is possible to use the computerized billing system to define subsets of the community being served, by looking for patients with certain chronic conditions with further breakdown by age and sex. Patients with diabetes, hypertension, etc., may be readily identified through the typical billing system.

EXAMPLE

The Department of Maternal and Child Health of the Dartmouth-Hitchcock Medical Center, Hanover, NH, serves the people of the Connecticut River Valley. The Clinic is a multispecialty group practice whose staff also serve as the attending physicians of the Dartmouth-Hitchcock Medical Center and provide clinical instruction at the Dartmouth Medical School. The Department of Maternal and Child Health is composed of a section of obstetrics and gynecology as well as a pediatrics section.

The staff of the pediatrics outpatient section felt the need to consider the health care issues of the adolescent population within the community being served by the Hitchcock Clinic. Having recognized this need, the decision was made to determine the extent to which adolescents use the services of the outpatient department. Attendant upon examining the care provided to the adolescent population, several additional questions were raised:

1. How many clinical encounters are generated by patients in the adolescent age group, 13 to 17 years?

2. What is the socioeconomic status of these patients?

3. Where do these patients live?

4. What are the most frequent diagnoses being made?

5. Where are the patients being seen in the Medical Center? Are they being seen in the pediatrics, internal medicine, family medicine clinics, or the emergency room?

6. Is there justification for hiring a pediatrician who would concentrate on adolescents?

Questions 1 to 3 fall into Step 1 of the COPC construct, defining and characterizing the community. Question 4 addresses Step 2, identifying the community health problems. Questions 5 and 6 indirectly address Step 3, modifying the health program to address priority health care needs.

It became apparent that access to a data system that contained the necessary variables to help in answering these questions was imperative. The Hitchcock Clinic required that an "encounter form" be filled out by house staff and attending physicians after each outpatient encounter. Data extracted from this form would then be entered into the Clinic's financial billing system to generate charges for outpatient visits. Standard billing systems commonly use ICD diagnoses codes as required by many insurance companies. The Hitchcock Clinic encounter form captured some additional information. For example, all house staff and attending physicians were assigned unique identifying codes. Again, procedure required putting one's code on the form after each encounter. The clerical staff provided additional information on the form such as clinic codes and checked off the approximate time of day the patient was being seen.

Followup discussions with the data processing personnel revealed that most of the data elements seen on the encounter form were indeed computerized for billing records. With the permission of the administration of the Hitchcock Clinic, it was decided to create a database on magnetic tape with certain data elements extracted from the billing system. Each data record corresponded to an outpatient encounter. The hospital numbers were "hash coded" to preserve patient confidentiality, but it could be determined if an individual patient made multiple visits

Fields 1–6					
1	2	3	4	5	6
Hospital No.	Encounter date	Date of birth	Age at encounter	Department code	Clinic code

Fields 7–11				
7	8	9	10	11
Physician code	ICD-9 code	Method of payment	Zip code	Sex

Figure 1. Data Elements Extracted from the Patient Billing System.

to the clinic. The extracted data elements are shown in Figure 1.

Data extracted from the billing system were on patients 0-18 years of age who were seen as outpatients from July 1, 1977 to June 30, 1978. Approximately 37,000 encounters were identified within these age groups.

Method of Analysis

Analysis of the data was done with a series of computer programs written in the BASIC programming language rather than using a statistical package (at that time, it was easier for me to write short programs in BASIC than learn how to use an unfamiliar statistical program). Each program was modified to access the individual fields of the database. Encounters were sorted by the month of encounter (field 2) and then by age (field 4). Sorting in this manner made it possible to obtain a frequency distribution for each age group (<1, 1-2, 2-3, etc.). Frequency distributions were done for each month, thereby revealing the gross number of encounters within the pediatric age groups. The frequency distributions made it possible to address question 1 (above) by determining the number of clinical encounters generated by patients in the 13-17-year age groups.

The next issue to be addressed was the socioeconomic status of these patients. A general idea of socioeconomic status was obtained by looking at field 9, method of payment. To avoid skewing the analysis, the database was sorted by patient hospi-

tal number (field 1), keeping all identical hospital numbers together and then obtaining the method of payment from field 9. If, for example, a patient was seen five times over the course of the year, chances were the payment status would have remained the same. This facilitated getting the total number of patients in the database as well as a frequency distribution of insurance type. The number of patients on public assistance, private insurance, and self-payment could then be determined.

This same technique was then applied to question 3, where do these patients live? Again, after aggregating the database by hospital number, a frequency distribution was done on field 10, zip code. This became useful in determining referral patterns by community. Zip codes were particularly useful because virtually every town in New England has its own. This also was useful in identifying areas of high need, especially if there were no physicians practicing in that community. This part of the data analysis enabled support of Step 1 of the third COPC component, defining and characterizing the community.

Step 2 of the third COPC component, identifying the community health problems, was done in the following way. Field 8, ICD-9 diagnosis code, enabled question 4 to be addressed, what are the most frequent diagnoses seen? This issue was addressed in two ways. First, the database was sorted by month of encounter, then a frequency distribution of ICD-9 codes was obtained. A monthly profile of the clinic was then obtained, which grossly revealed some of the health needs of the community.

Modification of the health care program to address priority health care needs of the adolescent community could only be done after first determining how the adolescent community used the outpatient facilities. The type of clinic used by adolescents was determined by doing frequency distributions of the clinic types on a monthly basis. The number of patients seen in the pediatrics, internal medicine, and family medicine clinic as well as in the emergency room was determined. Analysis of workload among house staff was also done as a monitoring tool by looking at field 7, physician code, and doing simple counts of encounters by month.

DISCUSSION

The microcomputer industry is slowly evolving toward some degree of unanimity among the various software and hardware products. IBM and Apple Computer have made office automation in the small practice eminently possible. Medical billing software has become readily available for computers made by these companies and others that produce compatible systems.

If it is possible to extract encounters from the billing system as described, two questions immediately come to mind. The first relates to the practitioner's anxiety about embarking on a venture that may well spell disaster: how does one keep from ruining this crucial database? Implementation of the automated financial billing system should have included an archiving system for routine backup of files. This would be imperative even if one were not planning to do the described data extraction. Extracting the data elements involves reading data from the billing database, not writing data to it. If the main database is on a hard disk, then the extracted elements should be copied onto a floppy disk or magnetic tape for safe processing. Analysis will be slower, but at least the main database will not be affected if something goes wrong.

Once the data elements are extracted and transferred to another medium, processing the data to address questions about the practice population becomes an issue.

There are software packages that enable some very sophisticated statistical manipulation of data elements, equal to what one may find on mainframe computers. If a practitioner has an IBM PC or a compatible system at the office and one at home, then processing could be done at home (busy practitioners may find that home is the only place where they have the time).

A frequent concern often arises over the "myth of IBM compatibility" when, for example, the practitioner has an IBM PC compatible computer in the office and an Apple computer at home. If both the office computer and the home computer have telecommunications capability through a modem, there usually is no problem in transferring data, although the transmission process may be slow or subject to poor telephone transmission, especially in rural areas. Poor transmission can often be eliminated by physically bringing both machines together in the same room and using two telephone extensions if the practice has multiple lines (obviously, this would have to be done after hours). If the billing system's data can be extracted and saved in a "text" format, it would be possible for a local computer store or club to convert the data from IBM format to Apple format.

What if the practice is not currently automated? This obviously presents an opportunity for some degree of planning. The most crucial step is determining what one wants out of a billing system. Six types of functions are usually found in an automated billing system:

1. *Accounts receivable or the ability to generate a bill for each encounter.* Computerization tends to be more accurate than "hand tallies." The "shoe-box method" of billing is unreliable.

2. *Patient scheduling.* The system allows appointment schedules to be set up.

This can be essential in a busy, growing practice.

3. *Automatic recall of patients.* Notices may be sent to patients 2 weeks before a scheduled visit as a reminder. One should be able to do an analysis of which patients are "chronic cancelers." Office hours may not be convenient for certain clients in a practice.

4. *Automated clinical data.* History, clinical examination, and laboratory data may be computerized to varying degrees. Keep in mind that the more data that are computerized, the greater the expense.

5. *Drug prescription information.* Medications prescribed with allergies listed may also be computerized. Some systems may even include the ability to warn of possible drug interactions. This may be a useful alternative to computerizing the whole medical record as a balance between cost and effective patient monitoring. Practitioners may decide to look at their own prescribing patterns as a quality assurance tool.

6. *Ad hoc reporting.* This refers to the ability to go to the computer and request certain kinds of reports that are predetermined. The situation described in the case presentation is an example of ad hoc reporting whereby information is generated through comparison of some data elements. A typical question posed to the system through ad hoc reporting might be: "List all patients with the diagnosis of diabetes who have not been seen in the last 3 months." Some systems may not allow entry in such a free form, but more expensive systems do have this capability.

A system that would enable this kind of analysis would be ideal. It must be kept in mind, however, that increased capacity and flexibility in the system generally increases costs. When a practitioner does invest in a financial billing system, ideally a system should be chosen that would allow some degree of access to some of the data elements. This access makes it possible to get answers to questions by using other types of software, such as statistical programs and programs that generate graphs.

It is important to keep in mind that the price of computer hardware is constantly falling relative to the degree of sophistication. The price may be the same, but the number of features may increase, as in the case of color TV sets over the last 15 years. Specific recommendations regarding hardware and software tend to become obsolete soon after they are published, so none are made here. However, the uses of the data and the information these systems provide to the primary care practitioner do not become obsolete.

CONCLUSION

The experience presented here represents a simple approach to using a financial billing system to support COPC in a large outpatient setting. Billing systems in smaller practices may enable practitioners to engage in a similar exercise by providing a gross description of the communities they serve. A wealth of information may also be obtained about the health care needs of a community and possible areas of intervention, as well as a mechanism of monitoring intervention strategies.

CODA:

Practice Management for COPC

Larry Culpepper, M.D.

The chapters of Part VII address many of the day-to-day issues encountered in developing and running a practice aspiring to community-oriented primary care. COPC activities are frequently motivated by one or two practitioners and are sustained with limited resources and the good will of other staff members. For such beginnings to result in effective redirection of practice goals, the initial activities must be successful. They must be seen as productive of improved patient health, not too taxing on support staff, and personally rewarding to the practitioners. Previous sections have discussed various approaches to initiating COPC activities, identifying useful initial targets of concern, and working with others in the community. However, all COPC efforts eventually require, as crucial to their success, the development of information about the practice itself. Development of much of this information can be integrated with practice management routines.

Need for data about activities in the practice can be defined for each of the four COPC steps. To paraphrase them, data regarding practice clinical activities are needed for each of the four COPC steps including:

1. Defining and characterizing the *practice's involvement* with the community;
2. Identifying the portion of community morbidity *seen within the practice*;
3. Identifying appropriate targets and methods of *modifying practice health care programs* as part of overall COPC program development to address priority health care needs;
4. Monitoring the effectiveness of *practice clinical activities* in support of such program modifications.

Much has been written about development of practice information systems. However, most such efforts have a goal of developing information regarding practice activities without relating them to community needs outside the practice. The efforts discussed in the chapters in this section stand out as having this latter undertaking as a primary intent. In the discussion that follows, each chapter is commented upon briefly, and ways in which the efforts presented could be augmented to address overall community issues, rather than focusing solely on practice patients, are examined.

Farley's chapter includes an excellent discussion of a model medical records system. This is an elegant system, eminently operational and, potentially, totally manual. Critical steps in identifying the desired database for a practice and planning the conversion of practice systems have been discussed previously (1). Likewise, the components of a complete practice record system such as Farley proposes have been presented in detail (2-16). These references are highly recommended to the reader considering adopting this approach.

The most critical concept of Farley's chapter is that a practice medical records system should be designed with its purposes and goals clearly in mind. To be successful, a practitioner or group developing information about practice activities and their impact in the community must undertake a planning effort which goes beyond that necessary for the simple processing of patient charts and bills on a day-to-day basis. Once the practice's information needs are clearly defined, Farley presents practical tools for collecting and maintaining the required data.

While the proposed system is practical *in toto* for a new practice, the simultaneous conversion of all recordkeeping to such a system by an ongoing practice would be overwhelming. Fortunately, individual components can be adopted sequentially with modest staff effort. A good way to start is to simply adopt the encounter form, age/sex register, and year of visit tagging of patient charts.

The encounter form serves as a very efficient tool, facilitating patient flow and communication among staff (9). In most States the encounter form can be constructed as a superbill. This eliminates the need to complete insurance forms, or to produce separate bills or receipts for patients paying at the time of visit. Such a form can be used to have the patient check the accuracy of demographic and insur-

ance information, to record Workers' Compensation or other special insurance information, to collect information on activity to be billed from the visit, and by the practitioner to indicate orders for procedures (lab, x-ray, immunizations, etc.) as well as desired future appointment information. If a practice has prepackaged patient information packets, the practitioner can signal the secretary to provide the patient with those appropriate by using the encounter form. In addition, a box on the encounter form can be used as a standing order to the practice nurse to audit and complete routine health maintenance activities.

The initiation of the age/sex registry (3) along with the flagging of patient charts with the year of last visit may be done with very little effort on the part of support staff. A number of medical record product companies distribute an adhesive tape with the current year (e.g., "87") printed repetitively. If, as Farley proposes, the outside of a patient chart is marked with such tape at the first visit each year, over several years this provides a very convenient way for staff to deactivate old records. This approach results in time and space savings.

The final startup effort recommended is the acquisition of a very large map of the practice area to be posted prominently on a wall close to patient examining rooms where practitioners and staff will constantly see it (not in the waiting room). Such maps can be obtained from commercial vendors. Alternatively, large census tract maps are frequently available from city or county planning departments, often at no charge. Once posted, these become a daily reminder of the outside community. Patients can identify where they live or work to the physicians. They also are useful in planning home visits or for reference in discussing community trends. If Farley's recommendation that charts be filed by geographic region is followed, such regions can be marked on the map for easy reference.

The revision of record formats and changing of office files usually require a more ambitious effort. An alternative to filing all patient charts in a single household or family folder is to create a separate household file with only a family chart in it. These can be filed separate from patient charts and maintained only for those household units for which the practitioner feels particularly motivated to keep such information. This may be a useful way to test the concepts represented by such information gathering and as an interim step on the way to converting all records to the Farley system.

COPC activities, including conceptualizing and implementing a practice COPC information system, are very susceptible to failure based on human factors. Freeman provides us with an excellent review and a vivid example of such factors in action. Instituting new practice routines usually requires at least 3 to 6 months of reinforcing the change before new norms of behavior are accepted. Freeman has done an excellent job of emphasizing the fluid nature of such changes and the need to manage their impact at both individual and organizational levels.

Visible reminders of the COPC related activities involved in such change may be very helpful in promoting new COPC norms of practice activity. The addition of a wall map in a practice's "inner sanctum" is one such reminder. A second is the production of comparative data using components of the practice's data system. Depending on the size of the practice, a comparison can be drawn between a solo practitioner's present and previous activities, between a group's physicians, or between practice teams. In networks of health centers, inter-center comparisons can be drawn.

I have found the mere presentation of comparative data to be a very powerful motivator of physician behavior change. In research, this is known as the "John Henry Effect." If physicians know that their patients belong to a study control group, the relevant outcome of the control group shows significant improvement over a previous baseline without any intervention other than study involvement (the physician-level equivalent of the placebo effect). In promoting practice behavior changes, feedback of comparative data seems to have a marked effect which lasts for 2 to 3 months. Frequent modification of the style and content of feedback helps keep it interesting and effective.

A further consideration in planning COPC changes involves a practical application of Freeman's advice to carefully consider staff and plan appropriately. As many physicians will admit, there are few professionals worse than physicians at carrying out routine activities on a reliable basis. Physicians have emphasized throughout their training the need for unique responses to each patient. Consequently, periodic health maintenance, surveillance, and similar activity requiring regular attention are not supported well if left solely in the physician's hands. Such efforts are improved by the delegation of these duties to other staff, many of whom have had training emphasizing the need for reliability in such repetitive activities. This requires overcoming a frequent physician perception that "it's not done right if I don't do it." A compromise may be to generate (using a microcomputer) a physician tickler notice. This may be added to the comments section of an encounter form (e.g., "remember flu vaccine," or "get occupational hx").

Jacob's presentation is an eloquent reminder that highly organized medical centers do not have a good understanding of the health issues and needs of their surrounding communities. The potential for a small group of COPC-aware physicians in such organizations having a major impact also is apparent from Jacob's presentation. The development of an organized set of information which begins to address the four steps of COPC activities by one group in a medical center may foster similar activities by other tertiary care health professionals. Once again, this chapter reinforces the need for a carefully thought-out information system.

While Freeman primarily addresses the human dilemmas of mounting COPC efforts in a practice, Jacob's example begins to illustrate some of the additional complexities of such effort in a tertiary care setting. In such a setting, not only may motivations be suspect, but issues related to the need to maintain integrity of databases and ensure confidentiality of information may become major concerns to be addressed in pursuing COPC efforts.

Kamerow's chapter on the potential of the microcomputer for assisting COPC practices provides an introduction to a potentially valuable practice tool. The microcomputer was highly experimental until the early 1980s, but in the past 5 years there has been a tremendous expansion of their memory capacity, computing power, and reliability. This has led to the creation of microcomputers, particularly the Apple Macintosh family, that a health worker with no prior computer exposure can be quite comfortable using after half a day's effort.

Spreadsheet and database programs, in particular, are tools that can allow the busy practice to intelligently target and mount COPC community efforts that heretofore would have been impossible. Such systems can be extremely useful for the surveillance, practice outreach, and reminder functions alluded to by Kamerow. As he notes, the integrated software packages (such as Excel for the MacIntosh) are particularly recommended.

Database programs generally are not included in integrated software packages. A number of database software develop-

ers have produced families of increasingly complex database packages. These usually begin with a glorified filing system program, have as an intermediate step a complete "flat" database program (one large file), and have at the upper end a complex relational database program (several linked files). The dramatic increase in power and versatility of these increasingly complex software packages is matched by increasing difficulty in initial programming, but generally not by greater difficulty in actually using databases once they are set up. Such families of databases allow one to start with a simple, easy to learn and use program that is somewhat limited in capacity. As the practice's computer sophistication increases, upgrading to a more complex database program in the same family is possible. Fortunately, files created using the simple database software are generally easily converted for use by the more complex programs in the same family. Thus, data initially accumulated does not have to be reentered.

As discussed in these four chapters, development of information about practice activities is critical to community-oriented primary care. Development of such information, as well as the overall development of COPC activities, must be done in a manner sensitive to individual and group personnel issues. In complex organizations, attention must also be paid to ways in which the COPC activity may be viewed by others in the organization and how it will affect them. Use of microcomputers may facilitate development of COPC activities. To become truly community oriented, a practice's efforts must reach beyond the established patient population to address the needs of others in the defined community population. The following discussion reconsiders the chapters of this section with particular emphasis on examples of how this last challenge can be met.

One method of expanding a practice's

information base to include a group of nonpatients is to "register" all household members at the enrollment of the first visiting patient from that household. This is particularly feasible using a microcomputer database. The simple entry of other household members' names, dates of birth, and sex, along with the date of entry and identification of the index patient, provides an excellent expanded database. Using such information, the practice can track its success in attracting other household members to enroll as patients. Such nonenrolled household members may be included in patient education or outreach activities such as childhood immunization or elderly flu vaccine efforts. To update and maintain such a system for all households in a practice will involve considerable effort due to the frequent moves made by a subset of the population. For instance, households that are composed of four or five college roommates can be expected to have high turnover. Such households might be excluded from this effort depending upon the intended COPC focus of the practice.

A second method of encouraging community orientation using an information system is the establishment of an employer roster. This can be developed either as a manual or computer application. For this, patients are asked to identify their employer and provide limited additional information about the work setting (such as type of products, exposure to toxic environments, or information about the employer's health program). Over time, the practice will develop an information base about its area's employers, as well as a roster of its patients working for each employer. Such information may be of particular use in surveillance of work-related conditions, or in aiding development relationships with community employers. If the location of major employers is added to the practice's large map, community and environmental influences

of work sites may also become more readily identifiable. An analogous effort might be used to develop information about other community groups, such as those defined by residence in a high-rise or housing project.

A further addition to a COPC practice's record system may be problem-oriented community records. Such records are analogous to the individual patient's chart or the household chart. However, the "patient" for this chart is the particular target population. In any practice, there may be numerous target populations depending on the energy of the practitioners. The formal recordkeeping of the community diagnostic activities and interventions performed may be very useful in defining future directions and assessing progress.

Analysis of practice information available in most conventional billing systems may provide information of great value to COPC efforts. Issues related to barriers to access for community residents seeking care at the practice may be investigated. For instance, an analysis of diagnoses made on the first visit by various patient groups may be illuminating. Such patient groups may be defined by insurance status (welfare vs. Blue Cross/Blue Shield vs. no insurance), by location of residence (low income vs. high income area, or close vs. distant from the practice), by employer group, or by age group. The analysis of first-visit diagnoses for such groups may find that some groups seek care early for preventive measures, while others wait until a serious acute or chronic illness forces a visit. Such data may help a practice target community education or outreach efforts. Similarly, analysis of return visit rates for such groups may identify continuity and compliance issues that should be addressed at the community level.

A second example of the use of practice diagnostic information is to use it to identify community "sentinel events."

Such events may alert the practice to morbidity of concern at the community level. A major group of sentinel events includes those that should never happen. Even one such event in a practice is a signal for community concern. The diagnoses of rubella, whooping cough, or toxic exposures are examples. The geographic localization of drug-abusing patients, or teens using alcohol, may alert a practice to a major concern within a school; other sentinel events may identify problems at a particular work site.

Such expanded uses of practice data are very much in keeping with the system proposed in Farley's chapter. In addition, the practitioner may expand the usefulness of his practice data by linking it to data on the community collected by others. To illustrate this, Freeman's presentation of the Indian Health Service Pap Emphasis Program will be reconsidered.

Freeman presents the ups-and-downs of a nurse-supported Pap surveillance system. This effort was undertaken prior to the development of microcomputers as potential practice tools. As noted, the major limitation recurring in this specific effort involved time constraints and work pressure on the nure. Clearly, the aid of a microcomputer would make this task much easier. In addition, it would allow several additional analyses of the resulting data from a community perspective. Such analyzed data might easily identify patient subgroups at high risk of never receiving or not returning as recommended for Pap smears. If one neighborhood or employer group, or other community subpopulation, stood out as being in special need of followup, this would allow efficient targeting of practice community education or outreach efforts. Beyond this, the practice could take a major step to expand the value of its data by linking it to other information as indicated above.

Considerable information usually is available about the health status of communities from State, county, or city health departments. This may include information about morbidity or causes of mortality. In a city or rural area for instance, most practitioners can learn the number of cervical cancer deaths (or other analogous information) for their communities by census tract. Such information can help a practice identify its participation in caring for the total community burden of the particular health problem (total community morbidity − practice morbidity = residual community morbidity). Using some of the techniques already discussed, an audit could be performed to assess practice barriers to access, inadequate continuity or compliance, or similar issues for patients with the problem. Such analyses usually suggest potential changes in practice routines or community education and outreach targets.

Comparison of practice information to community data also may allow the practice to identify ways in which its enrolled population is concurrent with, or differs from, general community trends. For example, an analysis of data on the obstetric population seeking prenatal care at the Brown Univerity Department of Family Practice model unit has recently been completed. As a first step, data published by the Rhode Island Department of Health was reviewed to define "social high risk" census tracts in the surrounding neighborhood. All census tracts meeting at least two of the following three criteria were identified: greater than 40 percent of residents below the 200 percent poverty line; more than 20 percent of residents who speak English with difficulty; more than 20 percent of pregnant residents delaying enrollment for prenatal care until after their first trimester. Next, the prevalence of three conditions in patients attending the practice for prenatal care were identified for each census tract. This information was then superimposed on the initial "social high risk" census tract map.

HIGH RISK CENSUS TRACTS
BASED ON 1983 STATE VITAL STATISTICS

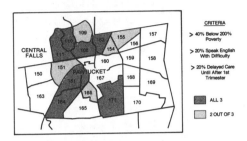

HIGH RISK CENSUS TRACTS
**MORE THAN 7 PATIENTS ≤ 17 YEARS OLD
BASED ON 1982–85 PRACTICE DATA**

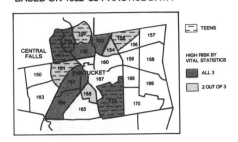

HIGH RISK CENSUS TRACTS
**>10% ILLICIT DRUG USE
BASED ON 1982–85 PRACTICE DATA**

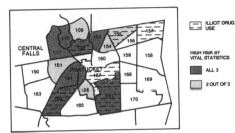

HIGH RISK CENSUS TRACTS
**> 30% THIRD TRIMESTER ENROLLMENT
BASED ON 1982–85 PRACTICE DATA**

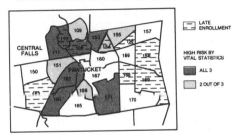

Figure 1. Social High Risk Areas.

As can be seen in Figure 1, three distinct patterns of overlap emerged. For the practice's teen population there is no census tract with more than seven patients 17 years of age or younger that is not also a social high-risk census tract (complete overlap). There was partial overlap between social high-risk census tracts and location of practice prenatal patients using illicit drugs. Finally, there was considerable lack of overlap between social high-risk census tracts and those for which more than 30 percent of patients waited until their third trimester to seek prenatal care. The identification of such practice patterns provides information which now is being used for community education and outreach to specifically address the identified concerns for each census tract.

CONCLUSION

This discussion has attempted to synthesize and expand upon the chapter of this section on practice management for COPC. As Farley's introduction eloquently points out, we may observe but not see, or see but not understand. It is hoped that the tools discussed in this section may help COPC physicians to observe *and* see health issues that affect practice patients and other community residents. They also may help practitioners begin to see factors in the community environment that affect health. With support of these tools, the creativity and ingenuity of COPC oriented practitioners will lead to an increase in the understanding of health issues in communities. This will begin to fulfill Farley's vision of the physician as participating observer and naturalist.

REFERENCES

1. Culpepper, L. Guidelines for the revision of practice data sets. *Journal of Family Practice* 1980; 11:437.

2. Farley, E.S. Jr.; Treat, D.F.; Froom, J.; Henck, SH.H.: Culpepper, L., et al: An integrated medical record and data system for primary care: Introduction. *Journal of Family Practice* 1977; 4:949.

3. Froom, J. An integrated medical record and data system for primary care: Part 1: The age-sex register: Definition of the patient population. *Journal of Family Practice* 1977; 4:951.

4. Froom, J. An integrated medical record and data system for primary care: Part 2: Classification of health problems for use by family physicians. *Journal of Family Practice* 1977; 4:1149.

5. Froom, J.; Culpepper, L.; and Boisseau, V. An integrated medical record and data system for primary care: Part 3: The diagnostic index: Manual and computer methods and applications. *Journal of Family Practice* 1977; 5:113.

6. Froom, J.; Culpepper, L.; Kirkwood, C.R., et al: An integrated medical record and data system for primary care: Part 4: Family information. *Journal of Family Practice* 1977; 5:265.

7. Farley, E.S. Jr.; Boisseau, V.; and Froom, J. An integrated medical record and data system for primary care: Part 5: Implications of filing family folders by area of residence. *Journal of Family Practice* 1977; 5:427.

8. Froom, J. An integrated medical record and data system for primary care: Part 6: A decade of problem oriented medical records: A reassessment. *Journal of Family Practice* 1977; 5:627.

9. Froom, J.; Kirkwood, C.R.; Culpepper, L., et al. An integrated medical record and data system for primary care: Part 7: The encounter form: Problems and prospects for a universal type. *Journal of Family Practice* 1977; 5:845.

10. Treat, D.F., and Boisseau, V. An integrated medical record and data system for primary care: Part 8: The individual patient's medical record. *Journal of Family Practice* 1977; 5:1007.

11. Newell, J.P.; Bass, M.J.; and Dickie, G.L. An information system for family practice: Part 1: Defining the practice population. *Journal of Family Practice* 1976; 3:517.

12 Bass, M.J.; Newell, J.P.; and Dickie, G.L. An information system for family practice: Part 2: The value of defining a practice population. *Journal of Family Practice* 1976; 3:525.

13. Newell, J.P.; Dickie, G.L.; and Bass, M.J. An information system for family practice: Part 3: Gathering encounter data. *Journal of Family Practice* 1976; 3:633.

14. Dickie, G.L.; Newell, J.P.; and Bass, M.J.: An information system for family practice: Part 4: Encounter data and their uses. *Journal of Family Practice* 1976; 3:639.

15. Fry, J. Information for patient care in office based practices. *Medical Care* 1964; 2(Suppl. 2):35.

16. Levinson D: Information management in clinical practice. *Journal of Family Practice* 1978; 7:799.

Part VIII.
Getting Started:
Resources, Allies, and a Critical Mass

Introduction

In any new undertaking, the first steps are often the most difficult. Too frequently we make an initial foray into uncharted terrain alone and largely unprepared, only to find we have taken our first steps in the wrong direction. COPC is still an innovation in the primary care system of the United States, and a number of unexpected obstacles lurk in our path. COPC is not a short-term effort, and evidence of substantial progress may come slowly at first. However, careful preparation for the initial activities is essential; and it is definitely worthwhile to spend some time initially to develop allies and a resource base.

In some settings colleagues in the same or neighboring practices may be interested in COPC and forces can be combined. Joining fellow travelers through the unmapped territory of COPC can be important for enriching the experience, developing a wider range of strategies, developing a broader base of support, and sharing the workload.

In some settings, patients and members of the community may be important allies to include in the initial phases. Strategies for patient and community involvement in the COPC process are described in Part VI, where the chapter by Seifert describes a stepwise approach for incorporating the patients as partners in the COPC program.

The chapters of Part VIII offer a wide range of possibilities for developing a critical mass for COPC. Some are most useful in specific settings, while others are more broadly applicable. The first two chapters explore the potential support roles of two important institutions available to most primary care practices and programs. COPC has been characterized as the reunion of the traditions of primary care and public health (1). In Chapter 54,

Kozoll, Stewart, and Rhyne describe the local health department as an important ally in developing a COPC program. They review some of the potential support roles and discuss an exciting new approach by the Health and Environment Department of the state of New Mexico. An important new ally for COPC may be the product of the current economic environment. Financial pressures on many community hospitals provide new incentives for reaching out into the community and cooperating with primary care practices, particularly those who are addressing a defined population. In Chapter 55, DeVito, Carmichael, and Zubkoff review the incentives and the potential role that the community hospital may play as collaborator in COPC activities. Two examples from different hospitals in the Miami area are described.

Part VIII continues with five chapters that offer valuable suggestions for developing a critical mass for a COPC practice or program. First, Massad describes, in Chapter 56, the development of a coalition of community health centers in an urban area and outlines considerations for practitioners wishing to form formal alliances among health programs in a variety of settings. Hartye and Andrews are independent rural private practitioners who have collaborated in COPC activities. In Chapter 57, they offer suggestions for developing a COPC practice in rural settings, dealing with issues in manpower, program development, and financing. In Chapter 58, Schlager writes from his experience in an urban private practice and describes approaches for starting COPC in settings that do not appear conducive to COPC. In Chapter 59, Gold reviews information resources and sources of potential program support in rural areas. She stresses the importance of seeking information sources and developing allies early in the development of a COPC program. She reviews many of the important sources of support that deserve the early attention of the COPC practitioner. Finally in Chapter 60, Furey describes a federal program to develop health consortia in remote rural areas and discusses their application to COPC.

The next two chapters offer suggestions for generating different types of resources for use in supporting the COPC activities. In Chapter 61, Taylor describes an innovative prepaid membership approach that both generates an important margin of revenue for COPC activities, as well as encourages involvement of members in the COPC activities of the practice. In Chapter 62, Shonubi describes the use of students as a critical resource in many of the community-based activities involved in characterizing and defining the community and identifying the important health problems.

Finally, in Chapter 63, Newman examines the diversity of community-based programs that may exist within the community. They represent important sources of information and program support and may be relevant to practitioners in a variety of settings.

REFERENCE

1. Mullan, F. Community-oriented primary care: An agenda for the '80s. *New England Journal of Medicine* 1982; 307: 1076.

CHAPTER 54

COPC Support Roles
of State and Local
Health Departments

Richard Kozoll, M.D., M.P.H.
Brian Stewart, P.A., M.P.H.
Robert L. Rhyne, M.D.

Community-oriented primary care offers an important opportunity for collaboration between the local health department and the primary care practices and programs that serve the community. In order to foster collaboration, the New Mexico Health and Environment Department's Health Services Division has adopted a policy of coordinating and integrating its activities with those of primary medical care providers. Among our efforts has been the establishment of an Office of Primary Care Epidemiology capable of assisting sites attempting to implement community-oriented primary care. This chapter reviews both external and internal forces capable of moving other State and local health departments to assume this role. It also suggests specific support functions of particular value to COPC practices.

HISTORICAL CONTEXT OF STATE AND LOCAL HEALTH DEPARTMENT ACTIVITIES

The rise of State and local health authorities in this country during the mid-nineteenth century may be related to industrial development, the growth of cities, and the need for sanitary control of sewerage and water supplies. Challenges to new health authorities were confined for the most part to prevention of communicable diseases such as tuberculosis, enteric infections, and diphtheria. Health department activities became environmental inspection, immunization, and infectious disease casefinding and treatment, and the tools to carry them out became the new disciplines of vital statistics, disease surveillance, and epidemiologic analysis. Maternal and child health activities, including services for individual women and children, were added through a wave of liberal Federal legislation in the second decade of this century. This, along with the advent of venereal disease control in the mid-1930s, set the precedent for health department operation of clinic-based personal health services. Accompanying this development was a decrease in the total physician/population ratio brought about by the Flexner report on medical education in 1910. The rationale for health department-run "preventive clinics" would not be challenged until the 1950s and 1960s.

In the mid-twentieth century, State and local health departments began adapting to sweeping changes in health care. Concern shifted from communicable disease

448

control to prevention and control of heart disease, cancer, dental caries, and other chronic problems significantly related to personal lifestyles. Physician numbers began increasing, and the family practice movement changed its orientation to caring for the "total patient and family," including clinical preventive services. By the mid-1960s Federal resources were primarily diverted into financing medical and hospital care, leaving health department roles less clear and often relegated to "plugging up the gaps" in personal health services. "Turf" issues between State and local health authorities and medical care providers became both more widespread and more serious.

Developments over the last two decades are causing State and local health authorities, rapidly increasing numbers of private medical care providers, and public and private third-party payers to face serious resource limits. Federal grants and State and local appropriations to health departments are shrinking and will increasingly require avoidance of duplication of effort and the setting of priorities.

This historical description is presented to set the stage onto which COPC has arrived. COPC, as a discipline, has great potential for connecting health authorities to medical care providers and "firming up" the health department role.

COPC APPEAL TO HEALTH DEPARTMENTS

Health departments have traditional strengths in the disciplines of health problem surveillance, epidemiologic and statistical analysis, health promotion and education methodology, and health planning. These skills are often missing in the medical practice setting and are required to implement COPC. Reliance of COPC practices on State and local health departments for technical assistance in these areas would improve communication between the organizations, orient practice activities towards State health priorities, and help consolidate a role for the department unrelated to operation of personal health services.

Another point of appeal of COPC relates to uninsured or other populations without complete primary care service. Many in these populations, an important target for COPC practitioners, frequently receive categorical services at health department clinics. Promotion and support of COPC practices by a health department would increase the volume and enhance the quality of medical care received by this group.

A third point relates to networks of federally subsidized nonprofit clinics that have arisen in most States. Many health departments are already involved with supporting, coordinating, or funding nonprofit primary care. This activity is often loosely related to the overall mission and goals of the department and may be a source of tension within the agency. COPC technical assistance should be seen by these health agencies as a bridge between public health and medical care and a vehicle for better integrating primary care services into their mission and activities.

A fourth attraction is the potentially rich morbidity database offered by primary care practices. Aggregation of such data collected by individual COPC practitioners offers the health department new and badly needed information for setting priorities.

A final point relates to increasing competition and corporatization of primary medical care. Categorical personal health services such as family planning, well-child care, immunization, and venereal disease treatment, the "bread and butter" of local health department activity, are now items in the marketplace. Health departments are already or will soon find themselves competing for these patients with increasing numbers of primary care physicians and clinics, prepaid plans, urgent care centers, hospital outpatient departments, and work site clinics. It is questionable how long the Federal or State legislatures will see fit to fuel this competition with separate subsidies to all of them. COPC support has potential for restoring programmatic substance to health departments that become devitalized by loss of funding for personal health services.

RESOURCE NEEDS OF COPC PRACTICES

Health department COPC leadership or support should also have appeal to primary care practices. Expertise or manpower absent in the practice staff can often be found in the local or State health department. One particular area of appeal would be centralized clinical data processing by the department. Separate systems of clinical data gathering, storage, analysis, and dissemination by each COPC practice is expensive in both time and money and may in fact pose a major barrier to COPC implementation. Ability of a health department to centralize these functions for primary care data collected by each practice, as well as public health data collected by the health agency itself, may be the answer to this problem.

Another need relates to lack of familiarity by many primary care practitioners with the literature and experience base for successful characterization of and intervention against common health problems. As a consequence, many COPC practices may repeatedly "reinvent the wheel" and lose time and energy in the process. Health department staff, particularly at the State level, often have this knowledge or experience or can quickly access those who do. As there are a finite number of common health problems, health departments providing this assistance should soon find themselves with regional resource networks that can be "tapped" by COPC practitioners.

Another resource constraint experienced by many COPC sites will be lack of practice manpower to carry out health problem characterization or interventions. Local health departments offer public health nurses and other staff who may have marginal time to devote to such projects.

Finally, COPC requires a level of epidemiologic and statistical expertise uncommon among primary care providers. While training may alleviate this problem in the long run, health department consultation at critical points during a COPC effort may offer a more realistic short-term approach. In addition to facilitating the COPC study at hand, repeated consultation to a practice will assist with development of epidemiologic and statistical skills at the site.

NEED FOR COPC RESEARCH

It is unlikely that COPC will be widely embraced by either medical practices or medical school training programs until its efficacy, at least for certain primary care problems, can be demonstrated to be both feasible and inexpensive. Field research on COPC is badly needed and will require central design and administration. Many health departments have the capability of leading or supporting such research. Important by-products of research of this kind would be standard methodologic "kits" and problem-specific "databases" that could be adapted by COPC practices for their local situations. Until COPC has a secure base of United States research experience, it is likely to remain little more than a "buzzword" for many enlightened practices.

NEW MEXICO'S PLAN — ONE STATEWIDE MODEL

The New Mexico Health and Environment Department is one of several State health authorities that operate State and local programs and offices under a single administrative structure. Since 1980 and the passage of the New Mexico Rural Primary Care Act, the Department has had a statutory mandate to:

. . . provide for a program to recruit and retain health care personnel in health care underserved areas; develop plans for and coordinate the efforts of other public and private entities assisting in the provision of primary health care services through eligible programs; provide for technical assistance to eligible programs in the areas of administrative and financial management, clinical services, outreach and planning; and provide for distribution of financial assistance to eligible programs . . . .

Since July 1985, the Health Services Division of the Department has operated an Office of Primary Care Epidemiology for the purpose of providing technical assistance to primary care sites interested in implementing COPC activities. Augmenting the Office is the part-time contract service of a physician epidemiologist on the faculty of the University of New Mexico School of Medicine. His consultation ties in the resources of the Medical School with those of the Department. Central to our model is linking the resources of local health departments to COPC practices.

The Office has realized success with a number of COPC technical assistance activities. Specifically, the Office has:

- Created a resource center with written materials, census data, population projections, maps and epidemiologic "tools" for use by COPC sites;

- Created a network of Medical School and Department resource persons knowledgeable about COPC and willing to donate time to COPC sites;

- Created microcomputer applications for abstracting local census and vital statistics data for use by primary care practices and local health offices;

- Inventoried and developed experience with accessing a variety of sources of health data for use by COPC sites;

- Supported four demonstrations of systematic COPC activity through community characterization, problem identification and problem characterization stages of the COPC process;

- Assisted with the development of a research design to test the efficacy of COPC in the Southwest in conjunction with the University of Arizona, University of New Mexico, and University of California at Los Angeles Schools of Medicine and the Arizona Department of Health;

- Provided elective rotations for health science students and residents of the University of New Mexico.

Plans over the next 3 years are to systematically extend technical assistance to other primary care providers and sites, assist with the performance of the research project, support the four demonstration sites through the program modification and evaluation stages of COPC, and continue to develop or assemble materials and resource persons of statewide value to COPC practitioners.

SUMMARY

A rationale for a role for State and local health departments in supporting COPC is presented. One model for assuming this role is being developed in New Mexico. Important elements include a statewide focus, a medical school coalition, centralization of data and consultants needed by COPC sites, involvement of local health departments with COPC practices, and the setting of priorities for primary care by the State health authority. Other State and local health departments may wish to consider similar involvement on this important interface between public health and medical care.

CHAPTER 55

Toward Community-Oriented Care: The Role of the Community Hospital

Carolee A. DeVito, Ph.D., M.P.H.
Lynn P. Carmichael, M.D.
William Zubkoff, Ph.D., M.P.H.

"Management has no choice but to anticipate the future, to attempt to mold it and to balance short-range and long-range goals . . . Lacking divine guidance, management must make sure that these different responsibilities are not overlooked or neglected, but taken care of as well as humanly possible (1)."

Though some, like Drucker (1), might even argue that the community hospital should anticipate obvious changes towards a COPC orientation to health care delivery, most would probably agree that today's community hospitals are at least struggling for survival and are therefore receptive to innovation. For many reasons, including prospective payment mechanisms, community hospitals are seeking aggressive plans to increase numbers of admissions and shorten length of stay.

Therefore, it is reasonable to depict today's community hospital as an organization seeking to both find new markets and to expand outreach program activities. The community hospital is interested in developing defined constituencies, both physicians and patients, and must con-cern itself with the wants and needs of these constituencies. Most certainly, the community hospital would like to cultivate satisfaction among its constituencies — a sense of community identity and loyalty.

Whether the community is represented by geographic boundaries or not, it is likely that the community hospital will be interested in defining this constituency/community. Those interested in primary care or COPC can look to their experiences and their patients' experiences in community hospitals as opportunities to promote COPC; that is, the current needs of the community hospital can be exploited as at least an important, if not dominant, piece of the system-wide community-oriented approach to patient care.

In addition to the predisposition to support defining and characterizing the community, community hospitals want patients, their family members, and their friends to return to them when they are in need of acute care. Their relationship to the patient at discharge is thus a rather difficult one these days: they want the patient to be discharged in a timely fashion; they want all care that is associated with the hospital, including post-hospital placement, to be viewed favorably; they do not want premature rehospitalizations; they want to know what happens to the patients between acute care hospital stays; and they want to be selected as the site of care if rehospitalization is ever needed.

Those interested can work with administrators to help move the community hospital toward COPC, specifically because this move is consistent with achieving a defined "constituency."

Hospitals should be likely targets/ receptive targets of COPC program activities for several reasons: they collect a lot of information about individuals; they deal with patients and family members at critical times; they see large numbers of patients for whom community-oriented approaches to care may be very important; they have contact with family members; and they must coordinate with community agencies and multiple physicians and other providers caring for an individual.

STRATEGY: WHAT CAN AND CANNOT BE DONE EASILY?

Defining the Community

Cooperative efforts through the community hospital will easily identify users of the hospital site. Just a little more effort through information gathering or record abstraction can produce information about family members and significant others as well. As with other provider records, usual information gathering in the community hospital rarely produces information to characterize the population or subpopulations of a specific geographic area, and unless restricted by their payer, both patients and physicians often frequent more than one hospital site. Insight concerning the specific utilization patterns in the community can help define the limits of denominator data which can be retrieved through the community hospital vehicle.

Defining Needs

Currently, hospital records are a rich source of at least two kinds of information: information needed to care for the patient during the stay, and information needed to place the patient in the appropriate level of care after the stay. This information is found in the emergency room and admissions departments, the medical record itself, old medical records for the same individuals or their family members, nursing assessments done at admission and throughout the stay, and social service and discharge planning records.

Serious problems associated with information gathering from the community hospital are numerous. They include the ability to measure health and health status, the ability to translate measures of health status into service needs, and all of the methodological problems associated with gathering information in a standardized, valid, and reliable manner. Depending on the specific goals of an individual investigator, the resources available for development, and the leadership at a specific community hospital site, information retrieval can range from one-shot abstraction of data already collected, and perhaps online, to forms modification, to training of personnel, to record information, and even to system-wide mechanisms to share information as a usual part of the institution's responsibilities.

At the very least, both the departments of nursing and administration, as well as the medical records committee, can be helpful in defining the significance of information that is routinely gathered.

Matching Needs With Community Resources

In some way, the community hospital shares information with community providers, including agencies to whom they refer patients, institutions at which they place patients, and physicians who will care for those patients. Again, the first step toward understanding the usefulness of information routinely gathered, the appropriateness of the match between needs and services provided, the information flow to community providers, and the potential for program enhancement is a careful review of the existing process at any community hospital site of interest.

Monitoring the Match Between Needs and Services Rendered

This part of the COPC model is unlikely to be in place but is likely to be of interest to many at the community hospital, including those with planning department responsibilities. However, certain groups of patients (e.g., some frail, elderly individuals) may be followed by community agencies with service coordination or case management responsibilities. These agencies are potentially rich resources of information to the community hospital for the identification of gaps in the need-utilization process for care.

WHAT HAS BEEN DONE? TWO EXAMPLES FROM SOUTH FLORIDA

Continuity of Care for the Public Patient

In many metropolitan areas, medically indigent persons receive primary medical services at community clinics and secondary and tertiary care at a public hospital. Continuity of patient care between the clinics and hospital is universally endorsed but rarely occurs. Typically, the patient seen in a community clinic who is referred to the public hospital may encounter several circumstances incongruous with continuity of care.

There may be admission problems, for example. The patient cannot be directly admitted and is sent to the emergency room with a note or a phone call; the note is collected on arrival by a clerk; the professional who received the call is off duty; the patient is triaged on the basis of the apparent circumstances, and vital

information from the referring provider is not obtained; if the patient is sent home, the clinic is not advised nor is the patient referred back to the clinic; if the patient is admitted, the clinic is not informed of the admission diagnosis or patient's location.

There may also be problems during the course of hospitalization. The attending physician may not seek information about the patient from the referring provider; the clinic may not be kept informed of the patient's progress, complications, or even death; clinic physicians may not have medical staff appointments at the hospital and thus may not have professional visits with the patient.

The time of discharge can present a new set of problems. For example, the discharge plan is not sent to the clinic; the patient is not given an appointment at the clinic; the prescribed therapeutic regimen does not take the patient's circumstances into account; the patient is given return appointments to specialty clinics at the hospital; a copy of the discharge summary is not sent to the clinic without a signed release by the patient; the patient may feel deserted and unwanted by the clinic and not actively seek future care from the clinic. As a consequence, the patient frequently leaves the hospital with a management plan that is difficult to follow, if not impossible, and without professional monitoring to care. The initial illness recurs and the patient returns to the hospital: the "revolving door syndrome." Proposed solutions to such problems require active participation by hospital and clinic, including administration, medical staff, and nursing staff with ongoing trade-offs and benefits. The focus must include maximizing use of available information concerning the patient's needs.

Example of Specific Strategy

Jackson Memorial Hospital (JMH) is a 1,350-bed general hospital operated by a nonprofit corporation, the Public Health Trust, for the Metropolitan Dade County government. It serves as the tertiary medical center and is the major teaching hospital of the University of Miami School of Medicine. Along with a network of community-based health centers, it provides virtually all of the medical services to medically indigent persons in the entire county. The University of Miami/Jackson Memorial Health Center houses an extensive variety of medical care, professional, educational, and research programs.

The Family Practice Service (FPS) at JMH has responsibility for various ambulatory care programs, a 41-bed general medical inpatient service, and an approved family practice residency with 36 positions. The purpose of the inpatient service is to provide direct access to patients referred from one of the 11 primary care programs scattered across the county.

In a typical teaching hospital mode, the Family Practice Inpatient Unit is staffed by seven family practice residents and two attending physicians. But the relationship between the inpatient unit and the community health centers provides the opportunity for continuity of care, indeed rather atypical of indigent care.

Specific strategies were employed to foster a COPC approach from the perspective of the Department's inpatient responsibilities. Inpatient units were established, staffed by the Family Practice Service, to which the patient may be directly admitted. Clinic physicians were given medical staff privileges on the Family Practice Service. Necessary administrative and recordkeeping mechanisms were provided: the referring clinic physicians contact the medical director of the unit when admissions are considered; patients are admitted directly to the hospital in the names of the attending and referring physicians; discharge planning begins as a usual part of inpatient care through coordination by a case manager and review at regular continuing care meetings; attending physicians maintain contact with the referring physicians, and include them in the care planning process; appointments are made at the clinic for the continuing care of patients, including available specialty services located at the clinic; continuing care plan outlines are completed by attending physician just prior to the discharge with copies mailed to the patients and referring physicians; and copies of the discharge summaries are sent routinely to the referring clinic physicians.

The Role of a Community Hospital in the Evolution of COPC for Older Persons

A description of "good" health care for the aged (2) includes an emphasis on restoring functional ability, support systems, a broadened approach to health assessment, and continuity of care. This patient-centered view calls for an emphasis on long-term care needs in relation to usual activities rather than limiting professional responsibility to acute episodes or specific diagnoses. The extent to which our contemporary health care system, which reflects society's technological imperative, meets the challenge of long-term "caring" appears limited.

For example, Medicare does not pay for prescription drugs outside the hospital, eyeglasses, hearing aids, or a variety of outpatient and in-home services, "even though such services may be effective in delaying institutionalization" (3). However, the need to address long-term care issues is obvious.

Older persons are likely to have relatively longer lengths of stay than others and they are at risk for rehospitalization since a large proportion of their hospitalizations are associated with acute exacerbations of chronic conditions. Thus the community hospital may provide a unique opportunity to initiate responsive long-term care programs because of its dominance in the health care industry as well as the high utilization rate among the elderly (4).

South Shore Hospital and Medical Center is a private, nonprofit, fully licensed and accredited 178-bed general hospital serving the southernmost tip of the City of Miami Beach (Florida) Island and is located about 5 miles from the University of Miami Medical Center Campus. South Shore Hospital and Medical Center is the only hospital and primary health center for this 3.5 mile-catchment known as South Beach. South Beach has approximately 46,000 permanent residents, 60 percent of whom are over the age of 65 (source: 1980 U.S. Census and interim estimates). The characteristics of this elderly, ethnically diverse community are reflected in the hospital utilization data, which show the highest percent elderly of any acute care hospital in the Nation, over 90 percent, with a median patient age of 80 + years on an inpatient basis.

South Beach has gained the attention of the University of Miami School of Medicine as a "natural geriatric laboratory" for developing and testing innovative approaches to the care of older persons. The hospital also recognized the opportunity to evolve as a model geriatric care center and in recent years has been the hub of cooperative efforts among many organizations, including the University of Miami School of Medicine, Dartmouth Institute for Better Health, the Miami Veterans' Administration Medical Center, and the Geriatric Community Resources Steering Committee.

Under the leadership of the Department of Family Medicine, an affiliation between the School of Medicine and South Shore Hospital and Medical Center was formalized. The Department of Family Medicine has responsibility for planning, evaluation, and research at the South Shore site. Through this responsibility, a close working relationship has developed between the Department, South Shore Hospital and Medical Center, the Veterans' Administration Medical Center, and community service providers. A wide variety of collaborative programs and projects has been instituted in the past several years.

A model discharge planning program was developed including functional health status assessment mechanisms and a meaningful data system, as one of three national sites in a Kellogg Foundation-supported program to develop assessment technology in acute care hospitals serving the elderly. The first clinical geriatric fellowship was developed, along with one of only two geriatric medical psychiatric units in South Florida. Programs were instituted for specialized nursing inservice and education staff development. Education programs were developed, including community-oriented continuing medical education and the "Topics in the Care of Older Persons" inservice education series. An Administration on Aging grant subcontract was instituted with the Dartmouth Institute for Better Health, Self-Care for Seniors Program Evaluation; an Arthur Vining Davis Foundation grant was obtained to disseminate the program throughout community sites; and the Caregiver Training Program was developed. A National Center for Health Services Research generic drug evaluation contract was also implemented. Planning and implementation were undertaken for the Veterans' Administration Medical Center Adult Day Health Center Program and Lifeline Program. The Geriatric Assessment and Planning (GAP) Program was developed and implemented, focusing on continuity of care, as one of 24 national sites (the only site in Florida) in the Robert Wood Johnson Foundation Program for Hospital Initiatives in Long-Term Care. Finally, Geriatric Assessment and Planning (GAP) Program components were disseminated to other Department of Family Medicine sites.

The primary focus on COPC goals demanded tailoring services to needs rather than to reimbursement, as a fully integrated, case-managed, health and personal care service system with an enrolled population, central care provider, and realistic financing. The overriding tasks have been to use specific information about functional ability to link patients with services and to monitor service needs, thereby promoting the least restrictive level of care and, as often as possible, living at home. The mission includes mainstreaming the essential components into the usual activities of each provider while defining mechanisms to foster continuity among providers, credibly passing the baton from the acute care setting to community-based providers. The systematic identification of acute and long-term health care problems, the cost-effective matching of unmet needs with resources and services available on site or in the community, and the development of new programs where service or reimbursement "gaps" exist has become the primary organizational goal. The goal has been approached through an incremental process with strong organizational commitment and community leadership.

Brief Program Overview

In its present form, the Geriatric Assessment and Planning (GAP) Program is a service provided to all South Shore Hospital and Medical Center inpatients 65 years and older, and, after discharge, to those who are discharged with community-based service recommendations. An interdisciplinary team assesses pre-hospital status and status on admission; on about day three of the stay, assessment rounds (at the bedside and including family, if possible) are conducted. Functional status is translated into need-equivalents, and service recommendations are made. Patients are linked[1] to community-based services at discharge and followup assessments are conducted. "Fast followups" are used for specified high-risk individuals (e.g., service recommendations refused by patient/family/physician, patients who are confused and live alone). Routine followups (assessment and relinkage) are conducted 3 months after discharge, then at subsequent targeted dates or every 6 months until community-based services are no longer recommended. Though a wide range of cooperating agencies participates by notifying the program office of patient enrollment[2], services provided, patient discharge, and referral to other services, all information management and staffing is housed at the Medical Center. Additionally, certain outpatients are referred for GAP team evaluation as a consultative service to community physicians and agencies.

The Consortium represents sophisticated medical components targeted at the key event of hospitalization of the frail elderly person. The goals throughout the program's development included actually changing the care process by mainstreaming the technology of functional assessment and monitoring, as part of the hospital responsibility, and creating mechanisms to credibly "pass the baton" of care among community-based providers. The role of the hospital post-discharge varies depending on the agency and physicians responsible for care. The assumption guiding the program development was that the ability of the frail older persons to live independently will be enhanced by carefully and continually matching needs to services. Our service coordination model

---

[1] Patients and agencies also are contacted at specific time and day that services were scheduled to verify receipt of care. Any problems are resolved.

[2] In calendar year 1985, 1,672 linkages were confirmed to a total of 47 agencies in 14 different services categories.

is offered to all discharged patients in need regardless of ability to pay, while services are provided largely by the multitude of community-based agencies available and in coordination with primary care as well as specialist providers.

Each step of the Geriatric Assessment and Planning (GAP) Program development was supported ideologically and financially by the Medical Center-Consortium as well as developmental grants. The charge at each step was to produce a meaningful program of services, monitoring and financial arrangements which would persist under usual circumstances (i.e., not grant- or waiver-dependent). Each component had to be self-supporting at the close of each grant period. We now have the capability to determine service needs likely to maintain individuals (who were at high risk for institutionalization and expensive service utilization) living at home. Additionally, quantifying needs, service recommendations, and utilization have formed the basis for sound program development in the future. The extent to which individual primary care physicians are involved in the hospital-based program varies considerably, but the coordination of hospital efforts (planning and resources) has been enhanced in relationship to all primary care physicians whose patients are hospitalized at least once at South Shore Hospital and Medical Center.

WHAT DO YOU REALLY NEED IN PLACE?

Organizational Interest

The important actors at any community hospital site who can promote the COPC process have to be identified and, somehow, their interest has to be cultivated into informal or formal commitments.

Meaningful Data

Mechanisms have to be set in place, or existing ones have to be identified, so standardized information is available for the site, for communication among sites throughout the community, and optimally, for comparison to other activities represented in published or unpublished works. In addition to requirements for standardization (reliability and validity), the information that is gathered must be important. For example, it is likely that measures of problems, functional ability, and social situation will be critical to the COPC program in addition to traditionally recorded medical diagnostic information.

The Ability to Use Information

First, mechanisms have to exist or be devised to assemble the gathered information (information syntheses). Though this task may be facilitated ultimately by computers, the design of minimal and routine data handling activities is the more fundamental effort. While lots of free time and outside resources may be necessary to develop a sophisticated product, this step can really begin with a careful look at how information currently is used at the community hospital. For example: Who assigns a patient identifier or pay status? Who classifies patients to meet JCAH staffing requirements, to justify referrals? What forms are used routinely for intra-hospital transfers and referrals or for inter-agency discharges, transfers, or referrals? Who else within the institution could use new information or synthesis of existing information important to those interested in COPC?

Second, mechanisms have to exist to pass the information along in a timely and useful form to community providers. Again, this task could be as sophisticated as an online, real-time, common database, but could begin as a careful understanding of information routinely passed along, e.g., transfer forms.

Third, mechanisms have to be devised to sum up the information for the population of interest. This task could take the form of elaborate data analyses, but clearly could begin with targeted case reviews by interested individuals or groups of individuals.

Community Interest and the Ability to Make Changes

There is likely to be a great deal of variability in the ease of implementing changes systemwide or filling gaps in the need-service match. These activities may be much easier for certain settings, certain population segments (e.g., certain age groups of patients), or already organized groups such as members of a specific health maintenance organization. Though the goal of communitywide interest and collaboration may be difficult to approach, it may be quite feasible to organize meetings of groups of providers (such groups undoubtedly exist in most communities) as forums for the discussion of needed changes and as "think tanks" for implementation plans.

The Ability to Target Efforts

It is unlikely that even a well-funded effort will be able to address a wide range of COPC-related problems and solutions at any given time. Thus some of the most significant and yet tiresome efforts have to be directed at establishing priorities among desired goals and targeting efforts. Though the promoters of COPC really do have to be politically sensitive, systemwide progress is most likely when priority-setting and targeting result from standardized information collection and information use.

REFERENCES

1. Drucker, P. F. *Management: Tasks, Responsibilities and Practices.* New York: Harper and Row, 1974, p. 121.
2. Kennie, D.C.: Good health care for the aged. *Journal of the American Medical Association* 1983; 249(6):770.
3. Johnson, E., and Williamson, J. *Growing Old.* New York: Holt, Rinehart, and Winston, 1980, p. 118.
4. DeVito, C.A., and Zubkoff, W. Role of acute care hospital in long-term care — a model program on South Miami Beach. *Journal of the Florida Medical Association* 1985; 72:258.

CHAPTER 56

Building a Coalition
for COPC

Robert J. Massad, M.D.

A health worker or a health facility with waxing enthusiasm for COPC will encounter early obstacles to its implementation. Among these impediments will be some for which the response should be the formation of a coalition or consortium with other providers. This paper describes some of the problems for which coalition-building may be a solution and the steps required to build a coalition. It also shares some observations gleaned from experience in the development of a coalition of inner city health centers.

RATIONALE: THE NEED FOR A CRITICAL MASS

The science of physics has contributed to everyday parlance the concept of "critical mass," by which is meant the existence of sufficient size to sustain a chain reaction. The common meaning of the term critical mass is relevant in the development of COPC projects.

A single provider or small health center will have difficulty sustaining the vision and the energy required for the successful development of COPC. The crush of daily responsibilities and recurring crises can be distracting from longer term plans. In the words of a popular wall poster from a few years ago, "When you're up to your 'ears' in alligators, it's hard to remember that your original intent was to drain the swamp." On such occasions it is helpful to work with others who share this vision of a drained swamp, to whom commitments for a dry swamp have been made, and who, moreover, can help shoot a few alligators.

Another reason for trying to develop an enhanced mass is that a single provider may be too small to have a measurable impact on a community. Also, a wealth of data may describe the health status of a community but it may be reported in geographic or political units that exceed the service area of a single provider. In that instance, banding together with the other providers offering services in the area may be necessary if consequences of an intervention are going to be measurable or capable of being evaluated.

Finally, in addition to finding colleagues who can sustain your energy and enthusiasm, add to your ability to impact on the community, and assist in conforming your service area to those for which statistics are gathered, the resources and staff available in a single office or center may be insufficient to undertake a COPC project. Combining resources may be the only solution to the problem.

STEPS IN BUILDING A COALITION

Consideration of the structure and membership of the desired coalition is a critical preliminary step. In most contexts the fully participating members will probably be other primary health care providers, but additional constituencies in the community may be valuable in enabling or supportive roles. Examples of some of these constituencies are public agencies, community organizations, political bureaucracies, and educational institutions; their potential role is described below.

In an environment with multiple primary care providers and a complex panoply of regulatory agencies, public health facilities, and other resource-rich organizations, coalition membership should probably be limited to the primary health care providers. In that case, the other relevant actors can be recruited for a steering committee or advisory group to which the coalition has a reporting relationship. This structure will encourage support from the wider community while limiting coalition membership to those with similar problems and interests, i.e., other primary care providers. In a small community with few primary care providers, the coalition membership can be expanded to create the critical mass required for success. Each structure will have distinct advantages and disadvantages, but the difference will affect the goals and the methods of coalition function.

The next step in the formation of a coalition is to survey the resources of the community for potential colleagues. One must discover who is out there, what their mission is, and what resources they may possess that will further COPC activities. It is important to cast a wide net and search beyond the line of health providers.

Is there a college with statistical or epidemiologic resources? Does the Health Systems Agency (HSA) gather valuable data and is it possible to excite someone there about the challenge of improving the health of the community? How about the Department of Health, a hospital, or a medical school?

An important first step in coalition formation is the development of a constituency for COPC from the community. Depending on local conditions it may be necessary to organize and educate such a community group, but there may already exist grassroots organizations of tenants, block associations, etc. Members of boards of directors of provider organizations may be helpful in this effort as may members of community planning boards of other political advisory groups.

Community members will usually need neither extensive education nor convincing about the basic tenets of COPC; they are likely to see it intuitively as correct and self-evident. The reasons for early community involvement are several. The community can help articulate its health care issues and concerns. It can be an important force to help motivate others to participate in or to support COPC — especially other providers or political leaders. More importantly, community collaboration can help the providers maintain their focus on the COPC goals and force progress by requesting periodic accountability. Finally, community participation can provide the personnel for the work of COPC — from door-to-door surveys to community outreach.

STIMULATING COLLABORATION

In order to get the providers together for collaboration it may be necessary to identify several common, nonthreatening problems that would benefit from cooperation. Early collaboration may not be directed at COPC but at problems that involve the self-interest of those with whom collaboration is sought. Important survival issues facilitate energetic participation but can be scheduled for your convenience and may provoke feelings of competitiveness that do not contribute to generosity and trust. Cooperation might better be fostered around items like joint purchasing or the performance of a community-wide needs assessment. In these early stages it is necessary that the initiator be prepared to sacrifice some priorities for the sake of the group process and in order to establish an atmosphere of trust and compromise for the sake of consensus-building.

Providers who do not have a tradition of group collaboration will need a framework that protects individual prerogatives and interests. Operating rules should be established early for managing issues that threaten conflict between an individual's self-interest and that of the group. It is always better to have the rule established before the issues arise that require their invocation. One example of such a rule is that decision-making will be democratic with assurance of protection for the minority, e.g., all decisions must be reached by consensus.

If the coalition is able to develop an independent staff capacity, the staff must demonstrate impeccable integrity. Even the appearance of favoritism or coalition with individual members will destroy the environment needed for successful cooperation. Until an atmosphere of trust has been established, participants will refuse to let down their defense of self-interest or to share their problems openly with others.

Several goals of the coalition must be incorporated into the formative stages. One of these is the establishment of credibility with other providers, regulators, and funding agencies. If, for example, the coalition develops as an entity that speaks with a single voice and where individual interests are merged, those who are inter-ested in operating in the community will learn that their interests will be served by seeking out the coalition early. If, in contrast, unified interests are not maintained, those whose interests are served by "divide and conquer" strategy will see no need or advantage in acknowledging the coalition.

Balanced against the need for democratic decision-making and consensus building is the need for agility and flexibility in exploiting opportunities. Rules of operation must ultimately entrust some workable number of people with the ability to pounce on opportunities for the group to pursue grants or negotiate projects; in short, to speak for the group. The tension between these conflicting needs can be great and will change with the maturation of the coalition.

OBSERVATIONS

Although the initiator of coalition formation must be prepared for the long haul and not be discouraged by the inevitable frustrations and difficulties, there is some help in the environment. The current climate of funding agencies — Federal and philanthropic foundations — favors coalition support. "Networking" has become a catchword of the helping professions in the 1980s and this can be exploited.

Finally, it is vital that success for the group not be defined in such an expansive manner that it cannot be experienced early. Nothing succeeds like success. Set goals in terms of the process of coalition development, such as improving the degree of collaboration or the relationship with the community. In this way, success can be achieved and appreciated and will encourage greater efforts.

Coalition-building demands thoughtfulness, planning, hard work, and good humor. Its rewards are greater effectiveness and the fun that comes from collegial relationships.

Acknowledgment

The author is grateful to Christel Brellochs of the Community Service Society of New York and to his colleagues on the Bronx Committee for the Community's Health for their contributions to this paper and for the experience from which it originated.

CHAPTER 57

Starting COPC
in a Rural Setting

Jim Hartye, M.D.
Mark Andrews, M.D.

Community-oriented primary care is desirable, but can it work in a rural private practice? How can one get community outreach projects started in the isolation of a rural private practice? A busy medical practice doesn't leave much time or energy for such niceties of community practice, and practicing in a rural area isolates one from the powers that run Federal, State, and institutional programs that affect local communities.

As two practitioners in this situation, we have found that COPC can be accomplished in a rural practice. There are three important elements in developing a community orientation in a rural practice: manpower, appropriate programming, and financing. These issues are common to any setting, but have unique dimensions in the rural private community clinic settings in which we practice.

MANPOWER

One of the first decisions affecting manpower is whether or not to maintain a community board of directors for the office. Community boards can be an integral link with the strengths and resources of the community and a potentially vital force in community outreach efforts.

There can be problems in the use of community boards. Some boards back away from serious involvement, leaving everything in the provider's hands. Other boards take total control and lead the office in very politicized directions. The attitude of the provider can make a difference. Boards will be as active as they are encouraged to be and will attract new members based on the roles they expect to play, i.e., a complacent board will attract complacent new members. Over time, the potentials can be brought out if the appropriate energy can be maintained.

The board should be made up of individuals from each of the surrounding communities. They can serve to publicize activities and give feedback on issues the community feels are important. Secondly, the board experience becomes an important tool for health education in the practice and community. By using rotating 3-year terms, a number of community members are educated in the issues affecting the community's health. The provider must consistently instill a sense of involvement and enthusiasm for dealing with health care issues beyond the confines of the medical office itself. Over time the board will begin to take responsibility and even initiate ideas and activities. Empowering others in the community without losing control of the medical aspects of the practice is a fine line to walk.

A second critical manpower issue is how to staff the office. This is probably the most overlooked aspect of planning. However, in a small rural practice it is the most important factor in long-term stability of any program one initiates. Several things are worth keeping in mind:

■ Hire people who are self-motivators. The physician cannot afford to spend a lot of time making sure that everything is getting done.

■ Try to choose individuals who reside in various regions of the community. This helps exposure and outreach.

■ Try to select people that others in the community would normally go to for advice. Office employees in a rural community practice are often on call 24 hours a day, 7 days a week.

■ Look for and maintain role flexibility across work positions in the office. Besides being smart business practice, it also allows each member of the office team to be freed up for involvement in outreach programs.

■ Plan to gradually train each employee in basic aspects of first-aid, common illness, and communication skills. In rural areas they are going to be used as paramedics whether they are prepared or not.

A third critical manpower issue involves community outreach. In most cases this means community health workers. Several different models have been proposed for the role of outreach workers. It is beyond the scope of this discussion to review them in detail.

As we see it, there are several roles that community health workers can play:

Advisor — giving health information and advice to community members on things they normally would not bother to ask a professional.

Sentinel — recognizing problems and needs that are not being taken care of by the health care system and helping identify effective ways to approach filling those needs.

Caseworker/Advocate — helping community members plug into the complex health care system in order to get their needs met and to remind providers of the primacy of the patient's needs over the expediency of routine or mediocre care.

Organizer — helping shape appropriate outreach programs and involving their community in making them work.

Community health workers, through their training process and work in the field, represent a significant education tool and force for behavioral change in the community and the health care system. It is this potential for long-term impact on attitude and lifestyle that is most promising. The health workers can improve patterns of professional health care utilization, both in the doctor-patient relationship and the system-patient relationship. They can also identify which needs the community is most open to working on at a given time.

Once it is decided to utilize community health workers in some fashion, the next step is to identify the appropriate people to train. The ideal type of individual is one that others already tend to go to for advice, not those who are always offering advice. These tend to be very different groups. In general, one looks for individuals with greater visibility and more frequent contact with other community members. In a rural setting there are certain places to start looking — the corner stores, the barber shops, the beauty salons, and the churches. Rural physicians and their office staffs readily come to know who these natural advisors are. The physician can also do an informal or formal survey of patients to see who they go to for advice on medical or personal problems besides their doctor.

Having chosen potential outreach workers, one needs initially to establish goals and structure a training program. A number of well-developed and organized "health awareness" programs are available that may serve as a source of didactic knowledge for a training program. This simplifies organizational efforts and avoids "reinventing the wheel." With a little tailoring and individualization, meaningful programs can be created with a minimum of time and energy. Additional efforts often need to be focused on listening and communication skills and local resource awareness to round out program structure.

The "Community Health Awareness Training" program that we have run locally spans approximately 10 weeks and includes about 22 hours of instruction. Classes are taught by a variety of health care and social work professionals including physicians, dentists, pharmacists, and nurse practitioners. Following the basic training phase of the program, participants remain active as "Community Health Promoters" by attending six annual continuing education sessions. Involvement of local area "helping" professionals in training serves to develop and strengthen interagency linkages and introduces those professionals to the concept of the program.

Another question is whether to coordinate all of the training oneself or hire someone else to do all or part of it. Coordinating this takes a lot of time and energy that most practitioners do not have, so we recommend getting someone to handle the practical details, but at the same incorporating aspects of the training that are important to the physician.[1]

It would be a common mistake to think that the individual training of the community health advisors is the most important goal. Equally important aspects of any such program are:

- Monitoring the effectiveness of training. We use pre- and posttesting to evaluate the basic transfer of didactic knowledge base.
- Monitoring advice given by the trainees. We have a simple reporting system for the advisors to use in order to monitor the quality and quantity of their functioning over time. A staff member can go over the short forms monthly with the advisors to obtain more extensive data.
- Continuing education sessions for the advisors. We currently provide bimonthly sessions on topics chosen by the advisors or based on the questions they are frequently asked.
- Getting important feedback on which issues seem most important to the community. We use monthly data collection from the advisors.
- Monitoring behavior changes in the trainees. We do Serial Health Risk Assessment Surveys.

The manpower to run the long-term coordination of the community health advisors/promoters can be done by volunteers from the program, but may best be maintained by a part-time staff member from among the trainees. We chose the latter in order to allow for longevity and for expansion of the program as the advisors/promoters come across recurrent problems in the community worth organizing around.

A final manpower issue is that of the critical mass it takes to overcome the huge inertia of an isolated and busy medical practice. Even though our offices are about 2 minutes apart, our linkage has been crucial to getting started. In our case, it was a natural alliance of outlying practition-

---

[1] A full discussion of the details of health advisor training is well beyond the scope of this chapter, but we would be glad to share details of our program with those who inquire.

ers in a nearby area. For others the linkage may not be as easy. Perhaps learning to share tough cases and clinical strengths with local colleagues is the first step to such a relationship. As rural practitioners we need to have supportive questioning of our thought processes on a regular basis to keep from becoming stale and outdated.

By linking up, the group can attract publicity, interest and funding. Another advantage to linkage is that a number of the start-up costs can be shared.

PROGRAM DEVELOPMENT

Appropriate program development begins with identifying issues important to the particular practice. One can use practice profile data and local statistics to identify important disease categories and problem areas in the population being served that need special attention. One can survey and evaluate available human services in the area to identify gaps that need to be filled. Examples in our area include substance abuse services, respite care and transportation from outlying areas to available services. As discussed previously, one can use community board members and community health workers as sentinels for problems of particular importance in the community. One can also use community forums as a means of identifying health concerns and mobilizing community interest.

The next step in program development is to locate or develop resources to deal with the identified issues. Academic medical centers provide a variety of expertise if the proper contacts are made. Research methodology, epidemiology, and program design are areas where academics can often be of assistance. In our experience, this type of assistance has been welcome in exploring methods of measuring outcome and methods for doing surveys and questionnaires. One problem we have found, however, is finding academicians who are willing to help us with our programs rather

than having us become raw data sources for research topics of interest to them. The longer we have worked in this area, the more we find local people with the expertise and energy to help and support our efforts. It has always been helpful to have technical support that is cognizant of local nuances.

Another important aspect of appropriate planning is to start out with small projects. It is important to start with projects that one can handle with a minimum of time and effort. It is always better to start with a small success than some huge project that never gets off the drawing board.

A final aspect of program development is the proper use of existing local human resources services. The hardest part is often finding out what services are available and by whom. It has taken us a few years and we are still finding people in the area involved with providing community services whom we do not know. Awareness of local human resources is an important part of training office staff and outreach workers. To facilitate this, a human resources directory for the area is an important early tool to develop. In our area we collaborated with the local United Way to compile and publish such a directory. It has served as a teaching aid but has also identified gaps in services that should be available in our area.

FINANCING

How can we finance community-oriented primary care programs in a private practice setting? Federal programs are attractive but they are also precarious and can gain or lose funding unpredictably. What good is a program that raises hopes or brings to light an important issue if it does not have the longevity to carry through? Many beautiful ideas and plans have withered in rural areas due to lack of long-term funding. Our approach to COPC has been tempered by this pessimistic realism.

Financial stability is possible only if one "stays lean" and funds programs on the margin.

Every office has times in the week that are slower than others. Take advantage of this. Use slower time to free staff members to do COPC work on a rotating basis. In this way it is possible to finance early projects on the margins of the present budget. One of our first programs was a home visit health education project. Each person chose an identified chronic disease or high-risk group. One person would go out on Wednesday and Thursday afternoons of most weeks, since these tended to be our slower office days. Staff members rotated to free up each other. There was little expense (just travel) and no charge for the visit. The only other hidden cost was some consulting time on what questionnaire to use in evaluating the project. There are some weeks when it's too busy in the office, but not enough to lose continuity. It wasn't an earth shattering project, but it was a good place to start.

There are structural ways to put aside money from the practice if one can afford to do so. We have a part-time community worker in the budget, and we give the community board 25 percent of our surplus to fund other programs.

The development of local funding is becoming more important year by year. Sources of financial support can be found in related city or county agencies depending on the focus of the project. The local United Way has been very helpful and supportive. They seem interested in new programs and reaching new people that they may not reach with their other programs. The United Way is also a good source of information on what local and regional industries may be included to support homegrown community-oriented programs. Local industry may also be helpful by providing services or even lending personnel for programs from which they may derive some direct benefit.

Industry is increasingly interested in the areas of employee wellness, health promotion, and disease prevention, partly because it can reduce their ever-rising health insurance premiums. Because these types of programs may be demonstrated to decrease costs and inappropriate health care utilization, they could be increasingly supported by industry in the future. In organizing community outreach efforts one can easily combine the interest of industry with the needs of the family and community and thereby gain an important ally in program development. And finally local churches, Ruritans, and home extension groups, are excellent sources of in-kind services, especially in rural areas.

We do use some outside funding but we are cautious when we do, since Federal, State, and foundation money tends to be given in clumps of 1 to 3 years. We feel that it should be used for larger one-time start-up costs or training. We try to avoid creating a dependency by using such funding for a part of the program that will need continued funding when the grant runs out or administrations change. In our case the State Office of Rural Health Services has been a wonderful supporter financially and technically. Many States have such agencies, which foster not only access to care but also quality of care.

CONCLUSION

It *is* possible to do community-oriented primary care in a rural private practice. Being in a rural area may make it easier to identify the resources that are available. Being in private practice actually increases flexibility to do creative programming. After all, well done community-oriented primary care is just part of a thorough approach to the practice of good medicine.

CHAPTER 58

Starting a COPC Practice
in an Unfriendly Atmosphere

Charles E. Schlager, M.D.

The majority of primary care providers work within a milieu that is not supportive of activities that go beyond the provision of direct services to patients as they present one-by-one to the practice. Most practices are organized to financially support the members of the medical care team that provide service in the facility. Local physicians, in general, do not freely exchange data for a variety of reasons, one of which is a protectionist attitude toward the presumed active patient population. Exchange of information is primarily on an individual patient basis, and little attempt is made at appraisals of the aggregate problem or the aggregate solution. Hospitals are also reluctant to exchange aggregate information or projections primarily out of fear of loss of the competitive edge. These forces, along with the perceived financial burden of clinical research at the primary care level, obstruct the development of community-based and community-specific evaluations.

In some areas, there are intra-disciplinary conflicts and inter-professional problems that cause the flow of data to be very difficult. Some examples of these obstructions can be seen in the secondary and primary care provider turf battles, and the allopathic/osteopathic medicine conflicts. If these or other similar impediments exist, community-oriented primary care will make slow progress. Lack of fluoridation of many municipal water supplies speaks to this lack of appreciation of community-oriented applications of medical services.

A physician, in the position of practicing in a community with no defined support for characterizing itself from a medical standpoint, must use other strategies to introduce this philosophy into the planning system. My experience with community-oriented primary care began in 1970. The event that highlighted the sense of community was the onset of open rioting in the city streets. With the sounds of tanks and gunfire, everyone said, "I think there is a community problem." This episode alone was worth more than anything else in beginning community-oriented medical planning. Within a few months, there was a combined effort — by the hospital, the medical society, a group of private practitioners, the government, the volunteer agencies, and the private citizens — to establish a system of medical care that would be responsive to the people's needs. You might label this strategy as use of civil unrest. This is not recommended, but if it occurs it can be effective in producing a change.

Another strategy that can be used is to develop a group of physicians within the community who share a strong interest in COPC. A group of four or five dedicated physicians, working together, will influence the community much more than five individuals working outside an organized system. It is important to have the official name of your group state your purpose, for example, Family and Community Health Associates. Within this group, each individual can develop interests and spheres of influence, such as professional education, continuing medical education, public health, women's health, care of the handicapped, etc. Within the scope of these interests, each physician should join actively in community groups. By employing this strategy, the physicians and the group will gain the respect of the community and be identified as community physicians.

Within the practice, it is wise to start with simple organizational techniques. Structure your medical records so that a current profile of your practice is at your fingertips. With information such as this, attendance at community meetings becomes a definite sharing experience. Members of the community will respect your projections if they are based on accurately obtained data and observations. The age and sex distribution of your practice is an excellent starting point.

Another simple strategy is to characterize your practice geographically. This characterization can follow census tracts, townships, counties, zip codes, or whatever subdivisions are most practical in your area. This intimate knowledge of your practice is essential to develop credibility as a data source within your community. Armed with these data, a physician will become an opinion leader in development and planning groups. Many communities have

not assessed medical practice needs and have little or no experience in medical manpower planning. In this milieu, a COPC physician can use his organized data base to begin the evaluation process. With simple techniques and the use of national norms, a plan for the development of practice modalities can be accomplished by the COPC physician. Local census data, extrapolation of growth trends, real estate development, sewer and municipal water supplies, provide the data upon which to make these projections. The actual work for the project can be done by well-motivated college students as study projects or during vacation employment. The physician group serves as the monitor or project manager. This strategy frequently produces income for the group while the characterization of the community is being carried out.

In many communities, there is a lack of definition regarding primary care problems that present in the office of practicing physicians. There are many questions as to the distribution of these problems and the referral patterns to secondary and tertiary centers. This information is especially helpful to local and area hospitals when planning services. Following the characterization of your practice and the development of some projections for your community, this information becomes very important as resource data to local area hospitals for these purposes. Again, this activity can produce income that will allow for the continued activities in practice characterization and COPC to develop.

At the present time, there are many third-party payers who are trying to collect data for feasibility studies with regard to the development of local HMO's, PPO's, and other alternative care delivery systems. Again, a well-characterized practice can serve as a data source for these types of surveys. Frequently, the third-party payers are in a position to reimburse the practice for these data. Since the characterization data are used in several areas, and once collected and collated require very little modification, the fees for collection of these data are multiple and profitable to the parent organization.

Another strategy is the need in many areas for the local residency training programs to document disease profiles in the residents. In these two areas, a COPC physician, who is accustomed to classifying a practice, can make a proposal to these programs and serve as the resource for the development of such a program in a residency. Again, these services are well compensated.

These examples are listed not to exhaust the possibilities, but to stir the imagination. To be ready for these opportunities, however, you must begin now to characterize your practice. This can be done, first, by developing a good age and sex profile. This can be accomplished totally by your office staff and needs no input from you. The next step would be to create a profile of diagnoses that present in your office setting. Again, this can be accomplished by manual methods and the use of presently available coding systems such as ICHPPC-2. The next area of characterization should be a survey of your practice geographic distribution. This can be done by plotting the addresses of your patient population on an area map. All of these parameters can be compared to reported national norms and community census data.

After your interest is stirred by this characterization exercise, it will soon become evident that this type of activity would be easily developed into computer applications. With the introduction of a computer system into the COPC, the horizons are much broadened. There are several systems available to physicians at the present time at reasonable cost, and the investigation of these modalities surely deserves your attention. My advice for any physician who is beginning his or her trek into community-oriented primary care is to start in a very controlled and small way, but start immediately.

CHAPTER 59

Finding Additional Resources for Special Problems Outside the Mainstream

Marthe Gold, M.D.

The multiple tasks associated with implementing a COPC model require access to and facility with many types of skills. This chapter is intended for health care providers with an interest in COPC who find themselves in practice where there is no infrastructure upon which to build. By this, I mean practices that lack specific academic or government affiliation and need to gather momentum and support from without. Typically, these will be rural practices. The apparent problems of isolation and lack of resources that such practices face are not only circumventable, but can be sources of strength for project development. Rural communities, with their attendant isolation, often lend themselves to readier definition by reason of their discreet geographic boundaries, cultural homogeneity, and finite number of health care services. The dearth of immediate institutional support will provide actions that should serve to more firmly establish a program in the community because of the broad base of other contacts necessarily formed. In settings where large institutions do not prevail, there is often less entrenchment of systems to contend with and easier access to other community groups and leaders with whom to

work. Approaches to garnering information and further resources outside of the mainstream are discussed in this chapter.

An early step in COPC, the first attempt at demographic and epidemiologic definition of a community (well discussed by others in this volume), will help delineate the most prominent health care problems of your area. Whether or not you are newly arrived in your community, the compilation and review of information relating to distributions of age, income, employment, occupation, and race in the region will help in the generation of hypotheses about the community's health care needs.

Demographic information is present in census data and is readily available locally from county planning offices. Large area maps with dwellings enumerated corresponding to census tracts are also obtained here and will often provide a logical, geographically defined denominator with which to work. The local office of the Department of Social Services can provide information about numbers of persons receiving Medicaid benefits. Using census information of numbers of residents living at 125 percent or less of poverty income levels as a denominator and Medicaid recipients as a numerator will give a reasonable indication of the proportion of indigent persons with significant financial barriers to care. Compilation of local morbidity and mortality rates and comparison with State and U.S. rates for unfavorable health indicators is an important step that may begin to channel project efforts in a specific direction. Crude death rates for major categories, broken down by geographic area, are available from such sources as State health departments, local health systems agencies, and county health departments. Maternal and child health indicators, potential markets for preventive services including infant mortality rates, percent of women receiving early prenatal care, and percent of low birthweight infants (all collected from birth certificates) can be obtained from these agencies. Information regarding immunization status of children on entry to school is available through county health departments and area schools.

The collection of these data serves the COPC process in two ways. The presence or absence of a set of discordant values between a given health-related characteristic of your population and other populations can help the next round of information gathering and project planning. Priorities are likely to be different for a community composed disproportionately of elderly indigent persons with an excess burden of stroke deaths than those identified for a population with a high birth rate and poor perinatal outcomes. High rates of accident deaths suggest different community problems and intervention strategies than do high rates of cancer deaths.

Sometimes, however, data exploration merely points to an "average" community with "average" indicators, providing no enlightenment as to what path to take. The second benefit of the information gathering work will help here: the process of obtaining objective data is accompa-nied by invaluable subjective and anecdotal material about the area, coupled with the less quantifiable resources of allies and contacts (to whom homage is paid in the remainder of this section).

During the initial foraging efforts you may hear from persons furnishing the data that in their view a given rate or statistic over- or underrepresents a problem. Their concerns, joined with the epidemiologic data that you have gathered, should set off a second round of agency contacting. I use "agency" in a generic sense to note any type of organization/individual of any size with any information or resources of possible relevance to health priorities for your community. Included are local offices of State and Federal Government programs, local government agencies, voluntary organizations, community leaders, educational institutions with health care programs, regional health systems agencies, the State health department, local hospitals, and local health care practitioners.

Local offices of State and Federal Government programs (e.g., WIC, Headstart, Office of the Aging, Mental Health) can be sources of more descriptive information about the populations that the particular programs serve. They may have health professionals on staff (nutritionists, educators, psychologists, social workers) with complementary areas of expertise.

In most cases, local offices of voluntary organizations (e.g., American Heart Association, Planned Parenthood, American Cancer Society, American Lung Association) will have developed educational programs and materials that may be appropriate to the focus of your work. Underused medical equipment may be available for screening programs, and volunteers who work for these organizations may be available to help do the screening. An innovative project addressing areas of major interest to such organizations may attract financial support from the local or national office.

Among local government agencies, the public health nursing service and the county health department keep accounts of reportable diseases, run screening and immunization clinics, and have personnel with public health perspectives. Information about area health indicators is often available through these agencies filtered through the eyes of people who have a great deal of interface with the community. Also, county planning departments are familiar with transportation networks, water supplies, and waste disposal, and any attendant problems.

Local officials and community leaders (church, government, school, union, industry) are usually very familiar with the concerns and problems of various sectors of the population.

Health care professional training programs can be a source of personnel. Their students may be available to participate in large screening and surveying efforts. A medical school within traveling distance, particularly one with a community medicine perspective or department, is a valuable source of statistical and academic support for a program.

Because of their planning function, regional health systems agencies are repositories of much of the health status indicators for their domain; these are divided into small geographic units. In addition to supplying morbidity and mortality rates, these organizations know about health care resources in the region, including outpatient programs and services. Early knowledge about the priorities of your health systems agency may provide valuable political support in the future.

As the major collector of health statistics, a vast resource for health professionals and epidemiologic expertise, and a funder of programs, the State health department can be of great help in program development implementation. Contacts with various sections specific to areas

of your interest (e.g. maternal and child health, cancer, infectious disease, chronic disease) can give you access to comparative health indicators throughout the State and Nation. Departments with programs in place on a community basis in areas similar to your own can facilitate useful information exchanges. In cases where the State health department has identified specific health problems on an aggregate basis in your community that are congruent with your own interests, they may become a source of funding.

The hospital that serves your community should be cultivated as a natural ally for a COPC. Most rural hospitals are voluntary, with a community board committed to delivery of good health care to the area. Many rural hospitals are small and particularly vulnerable to problems of low occupancy, and it is important for their survival that they are seen by the residents of their service area as a credible source of primary hospital care. Linking the hospital to a project by use of its clinical services, data sets, or specialized health care personnel can extend the potential of a program to undertake more comprehensive services, at the same time bringing good feelings and more patients to the hospital from the community. Programs undertaken with institutions, and grants written in conjunction with established health care facilities, are generally in a stronger position than individual practitioners, both in the eyes of the community as well as with outside funding sources.

Other practitioners in the community can often provide important perspectives about local health care problems. They are potential co-workers in clinical and educational initiatives that are undertaken, and if involved early in evaluation of community needs, they may provide considerable help.

In addition to confirming or refuting of the importance of the health care problems you have already identified, contacts in the above agencies will serve other purposes. Certainly you may find a need to shift your focus to an area that appears more pressing by virtue of the strength and/or breadth of information you receive from these sources. But more importantly, you have begun building alliances for further help. The future resources that these agencies may provide are significant. The political support engendered by interesting other community and outside organizations and individuals in your work is vital. Conversely, friends are readily lost when agencies with a stake in health care are disenfranchised or discredited.

Public and private agencies with programs in place addressing health problems that your project also addresses may feel implicitly criticized and may therefore be competitive rather than cooperative. Designing complementary approaches to shared problems creates coalitions rather than adversaries. Other health care providers may see in your descriptions of "denominators" an attrition of their fee-for-service patients; any program defining denominators outside of its own clinical practice must be sensitive to the perceived financial or professional implications for other practitioners. Administrators and boards of hospitals with borderline occupancy rates may see in your preventive emphasis the specter of still more empty beds.

Support is more likely in such circumstances when increased use of outpatient facilities, market expansion, or other sweeteners can be seen as possible consequences.

New programs, no matter how carefully planned, will tread on toes. The building of coalitions for support is important for the long-range success of a program, particularly where cold winds blow. Associations with other organizations and individuals become valued intellectual and emotional resources. Especially when one

individual is the primary source of energy for a project, there will be inevitable bouts of floundering and inertia. These can be tempered by the interest and encouragement of others. This help is vital to the well-being of the COPC practitioner working outside the realm of formal institutional support, and hence to the programs shaped.

POSTSCRIPT

The preceding directions and advisories are culled from the mistakes and successes associated with our use of a COPC methodology to develop a cardiovascular risk reduction program in a financially depressed agricultural area of upstate New York. As salaried physicians in a local hospital, working in a newly started fee-for-service practice, part of our time was devoted to assessing the primary health care needs of the service area. From statistical data gathering conducted over the first 6 months, it was evident that the cardiovascular and stroke crude death rate for the area was significantly higher than State and national averages. This was chosen as a focus after discussions with a variety of agencies and individuals. Two years later, a project is in place in two contiguous and demographically similar towns in the service area of our hospital (total population approximately 2,500). The project screens free of charge on a house-to-house basis all persons 16 and older for hypertension and elevated blood glucose. Other components of the project include: collection of standard demographic information; collection of information about use of health care services, usual sources of care, and perceived barriers to care; assessment of community perception of health services needed; assessment of knowledge about cardiovascular risk factors, with individual education provided by community health workers at time of survey and screening; referral for rescreening (without charge) for any individual from one town with abnormalities identified, who has no usual source of care or has financial barriers to care to our hospital's cardiovascular risk reduction clinic; treatment of any of the above group as needed by our clinic on a sliding scale basis; followup with other community physicians to assess control status of persons they provide care for; and community educational programs. Community-wide re-screening is planned 2 years after initial screening for control status.

Financial support for this program has come from a local foundation and the State Health Department's Heart and Hypertension Institute. Medical students served as community health workers for the first two summers of the project, with funding from their school. Grants currently pay for part-time community health workers. A part-time nurse coordinator (who has trained the community health workers, provides followup for persons with screening abnormalities, and works on educational program development) and a family physician (10 percent time) are currently paid out of grant funds. Our hospital provides clerical and laboratory support. Computer time and statistical support is provided through the University of Rochester Department of Preventive and Family Rehabilitation Medicine. Educational materials and programs have come from the local chapter of the American Heart Association and the State Health Department.

CHAPTER 60

Achieving a Critical Mass in Rural Areas: The Role of the Primary Care Consortium

Kathleen E. Furey Martin, Ph.D.

This chapter discusses a practical approach to developing a critical mass for COPC in rural areas. Practices located in rural areas often face difficulties in systematically providing high-quality health care, due in part to the sparseness of the population, the magnitude of area between population pockets, and a general scarcity of providers. The latter is due in part to the quality of life of the few practitioners. The low population base will often support only one provider, who is on call virtually 7 days a week with little opportunity for continuing medical education, vacations, and time spent with family. Following patients through hospitalization is difficult, because it means time spent away from their primary functions that can be ill afforded.

The frequent result is an overworked physician who feels inadequately trained and badly needs some free time. Many choose to leave their rural practice for additional training or enter a system with adequate backup and support. The practitioners who remain have little time to study, implement, or monitor a COPC model.

As part of a 1984 initiative by the U.S. Public Health Service, several rural consortia were funded. The primary purpose of this initiative was to ensure that well-trained primary care physicians entered rural practices and remained there. This included having board-eligible obstetrician-gynecologists, internists, pediatricians, and family physicians available to rural communities. A secondary result in many of the pilot areas was the beginning of a COPC system.

The Public Health Service, through the Bureau of Health Care Delivery and Assistance (BHCDA), traditionally targets its rural resources toward areas defined as medically underserved, funding nonprofit organizations that agree to serve all persons regardless of ability to pay. The Public Health Service grant makes up the operating deficit of such organizations that results from provision of free or reduced fee services. The BHCDA is also responsible for determining which areas most in need of critical health manpower will be available for service by National Health Service Corps scholarship recipients. The goal of rural consortia was to ensure a critical mass of well-qualified practitioners to serve a rational medical trade area. It was highly desirable that these practitioners admit and follow their patients through hospitalization.

Operationally, the process involved identifying areas with less than three practitioners or lacking needed specialty care; locating the rational medical trade area (e.g., a reasonable distance from which patients could be drawn which included a hospital); identifying available health care programs in the area; identifying priority health needs of the population involved; developing a network in which the available programs participated without duplicating effort; and recruiting practitioners to meet the unmet health needs identified.

TWO EXAMPLES

The process may best be described by briefly examining two areas that attempted to develop a consortium. One western area covered a large county in which a private practitioner, a small hospital, a federally sponsored practitioner, and the county health department all provided services. The total county population was 12,253, and the residents of the area range along the economic scale and are comprised of several religious and ethnic groups. Because of the size of the area, its remoteness from urban centers, and the diversity of the programs offered, however, the services overlapped and the providers operated without backup. The general practitioners who settled in the area generally left after 2 years for further training and did not return. The State health department had identified pre- and postnatal care, pediatrics, and emergency services as the most critical needs of the area but had not been able to address those needs. The population was not adequate to support an obstetrician-gynecologist or a pediatrician at any of the freestanding sites.

By combining the services offered into a countywide network, it was possible to bring an obstetrician-gynecologist, a family physician, and a pediatrician into the system. The obstetrician-gynecologist and the pediatrician operated at varying sites on a rotating basis. While it is too early to assess the impact of this cooperative program, the communities involved have reacted enthusiastically to the idea and the various organizations involved have created an independent governing board that oversees policy for the network. Continuing medical education is provided by the State, which agreed to fly specialists into the area to conduct classes and to continue their investigation of the special health needs of the area. High-risk pregnancies must still be handled out of the area, but the OB-GYN and family practitioners are able to follow routine deliveries.

Several elements were critical to the early success of this effort. The county had a population base large enough to support specialty care; a health care system did exist, although it was fragmented and weak; and knowledge existed regarding the health needs of the area.

Three additional elements were important in establishing the initial network. First, the network organization that was founded applied for and received a BHCDA grant to offset losses due to the provision of free or reduced-rate care. This enabled the consortium to offer care to the entire community without significant financial risk. The grant also enabled them to perform some minor remodeling and renovation work. Funding provided an incentive for beginning the network, ensured financial stability, and carried reporting requirements with it. The required reports include a yearly needs/demand survey and semiannual clinical and administrative performance reports. This last point is important as the reporting provides a way to monitor the effectiveness of the program over time. These reports, in conjunction with monitoring by the State health department, will provide valuable information necessary for fine tuning the programs offered.

Second, the network had access to the recruitment pool of NHSC scholars, which was also critical to the implementation of the network. The State as well as the county had been unsuccessful in their efforts to interest private physicians in the area, especially specialists. They were successful, however, in attracting the obligated scholars who knew they would be practicing in a group-like setting. Whether they will elect to remain in the area after their obligations are fulfilled is not yet known. Recruitment of replacements into the network should, however, be possible if they elect to leave.

Third, representatives of the national, State, and local organizations were willing to devote an enormous amount of time and energy to developing the consortia. Development of the network was not easy, nor was it a quick process. Initial services were begun within 6 months of the beginning of the consortia initiative, full services took approximately 18 months to fully implement.

A second example focuses on a parallel effort begun in the same State in the more sparsely populated east-central region. The sole practitioner in the targeted area was a physician's assistant whose preceptor was located 84 miles to the north. The area is surrounded by mountains and national parks. It was hoped that a network could be developed in which at least one additional provider could be supported. This provider would serve the predominantly adult population and provide support for both the PA and his preceptor. This effort was not successful for a variety of reasons.

First, the population base served by the PA was very small and spread over great distances. This made financial support of an additional provider questionable. Next, the commute between the two sites involved was too great, especially in bad weather. Third, the communities involved were very individual oriented, not organized, and not particularly interested in cooperative ventures. The area is a frontier area which will require some other solution to meet its needs.

Experience shows that cooperative efforts like rural consortia are beginning across the country, especially between small hospitals and practitioners. In fact, many of the areas and organizations that applied for BHCDA consortium funding but did not receive it have reported that they joined together anyway. Reasons given included: they were previously unaware of other health programs in their area; the process of developing a grant proposal resulted in exciting ideas that were inexpensive to implement; and cooperation and treating the community as a whole was an appealing idea worth trying.

CONCLUSION

Consortia provide a practical way to ensure critical mass, backup, and provision of specialty care. The federally sponsored consortia ensure the additional benefit of being able to monitor progress toward goals through the required reporting mechanisms. However, even in the absence of Federal funding, consortia or network ventures in general may be an important step toward a practical approach to COPC.

CHAPTER 61

The Membership Concept:
Achieving Critical Mass
for COPC

Henry Taylor, M.D.

This chapter describes an innovative approach to starting a COPC practice or program. It is based on a membership concept that offers a package of health promotion and disease prevention benefits to a prepaid group. Not only does this approach generate a small pool of unrestricted capital for COPC initiatives, it also encourages the involvement of a group of community members in various aspects of the overall program.

The general approach is based on four assumptions. These are:

1. That a COPC practice can offer a package of benefits to a membership.
2. That these benefits can be designed to support the goals of health promotion and disease prevention.
3. That the practice can finance these services with a nominal, prepaid, annual membership fee, and
4. That those in the community who are interested in relating to the practice can, and will, choose to do so, while others will come for just their acute medical care.

The concept of having members join a practice to receive benefits for a nominal

annual fee impacts on all four functions of the COPC process. This unique relationship with a segment of the population identifies individuals in the community and reaches out to encourage their involvement. The membership dues provide a basis for further fund raising as well as a limited source of unrestricted capital for new initiatives in COPC. The advantages are similar to a cooperative, but they are combined with the tax advantages of a nonprofit corporation.

PENDLETON COMMUNITY CARE: AN EXAMPLE

Pendleton Community Care is incorporated as a not-for-profit corporation with a majority of its board of directors elected by the membership. Membership is open to anyone, with benefits provided for a minimal annual membership fee. Acute care is financed separately, allowing annual membership fees to remain constant at $10 per person or $25 per family since 1982.

The membership benefits cover a variety of preventive care, self-care, and health education services. For 1986 they include: a voice in the organization, non-emergency house calls for homebound patients, a free blood pressure check, a quarterly newsletter, health education classes, telephone consultations (which may involve prescribing over the phone), an annual physical screen (half-price to members — $17), a reading room, and free prescription refills.

In the first year, 10 percent of the county joined to receive benefits and support the fledgling institution. There was a drop after the practice actually opened, but we have maintained a core of support without any major membership recruitment efforts. Recent changes in the practice appear to be increasing membership this year. These trends are diagrammed in Figure 1 which also shows the revenues earned from membership fees.

The membership fees cover the costs of providing membership benefits. In addition, they subsidize money-losing community services such as home visits, Medicare assignment, and Medicaid patients. There is enough left over to facilitate

experimenting with new programs without having to go through the lengthy (and overly restrictive) process of requesting outside funding.

DEFINING AND CHARACTERIZING THE COMMUNITY AND ITS HEALTH PROBLEMS

Offering benefits to a self-defined membership is a tool that allows the COPC practice to move beyond its "numerator" population to a target population interested in health. This is fundamentally different from a target population defined by the practice as being at risk for a particular disease.

Members can represent a defined constituency for the practice. This may range from an informal group that works with the practice in specific COPC activities to a formalized governing body, as for Pendleton Community Care. By progressively working with subgroups in the population, the entire community will gradually be represented in the practice "denominator."

Too often, health care providers feel an epidemiologic analysis identifies and establishes priorities for all the health problems in a community. Community members, however, may have a radically different perspective. The membership concept offers an opportunity to integrate epidemiologically defined health needs with the needs and demands felt by the community.

MODIFYING THE HEALTH PROGRAM AND MONITORING ITS IMPACT

Working with members in the community facilitates the process of defining and intervening in community health problems. Membership benefits can provide an environment that encourages lifestyle change to improve health. For example, some members of Pendleton Community Care want to explore private funding to

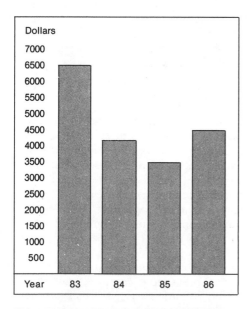

Figure 1. Income from Pendleton Community Care Membership Fees.

build a swimming pool or wellness center in the basement of our proposed new building. In addition, a health risk appraisal is included in the annual physical screen for members.

The members themselves can represent an important first step in introducing lifestyle change to the community. They presumably will be the most interested in new programs and ideas relating to health. In addition, through their informal social networks, the concepts will spread naturally through the community.

A TOOL FOR DEVELOPING A UNIQUE RELATIONSHIP WITH THE COMMUNITY

The membership concept affirms an individual's right to choose a particular style of health care. Just as patients select their doctor, members join to receive benefits. For example, approximately one-fifth of our patients are members and almost two-thirds of our members are patients. People choose which of our services they wish to receive. They may get their acute medical care at another physician's office, while they participate in membership classes, receive the newsletter, or use telephone consultations to decide if they need to see their regular physician.

Fundamental to the membership concept is the fact that the members have the right to choose to join or not. However, they reflect any biases the practice introduced through the particular composition of the membership benefit package. Therefore, benefits directed at prevention, health promotion, and health education should extend the COPC practice beyond a disease orientation so the membership will have a bias toward wellness.

By having the members pay an annual fee, the relationship is extended over time. It is hoped that they will do more than just go to one question-and-answer session on AIDS or a class on death and grieving. Because classes are free to mem-

bers, they may come to classes such as one on Alzheimer's disease to gain an insight into the care of an elderly relative. In addition, the providers gain a new awareness of the community by interacting in a different way with members outside the office. We feel it is the antithesis of the one-stop "Doc-In-The Box" style of medical practice.

Because anyone can choose to be a member, Pendleton Community Care cuts across social lines. The telephone consultations ranged from requests for treating influenza with tetracycline, to home remedies for colds or dehydration, to one request for blood tests for chronic mononucleosis (after a member read about the condition in the *Harvard Medical School Health Letter!*).

Offering membership services in the areas of wellness, prevention, and health education integrates a COPC practice into the current consumer health and wellness movement in the United States. It provides visible evidence of how the practice is different from "just a doctor's office." For example, a pregnant weaver asked if the naphthalene in the wool she was using would pose a risk to her baby. To more effectively research these questions with our microcomputer, we currently subscribe to the Combined Health Information Database.

From the perspective of the COPC practice, membership services form a bridge from providing good primary care to true community participation. Pendleton Community Care and the services it offers is an example. A practice can take the first steps towards COPC by offering services to a membership, listening to their needs, reactions and ideas, and then developing a dialogue about how to solve priority health problems.

MARKETING AND FINANCING

The membership concept can be part of an overall marketing plan for the practice.

However, do not overlook the fine ethical line between advertising that sells an unnecessary "product" and that which informs the public about services to meet their needs. One of the postulates of COPC is that having a truly community-responsive practice is not only good business, but also good medicine.

The membership dues provide a small, but significant, source of unrestricted capital for new program development. In addition, the members themselves are a key to grassroots fundraising efforts. They form a pool of people willing to help with local bake sales, moving to a new office, or holding quilt raffles. Their involvement in various activities can indirectly stabilize the practice and expand the patient base.

Community attitudes should be a major factor in deciding whether to undertake a new venture. For example, there was considerable local controversy over whether Pendleton Community Care should seek Federal funding for a new building. The local mountaineer sentiment is to be as independent as possible; some sincerely want to do their part to limit the national debt. To help the board decide, we polled the community membership in one of the quarterly newsletters. While they were not totally opposed, they encouraged the board to explore private funding sources thoroughly, an option that proved fruitful.

DISCUSSION

While Pendleton Community Care has demonstrated that the membership approach works well in a rural, nonprofit setting, it could apply to other situations also. For example, a private practitioner in a nearby county rents a pool in the basement of his office to patients who want to lose weight. If they prepaid him on an annual basis, this would be the start of a membership relationship. Alternatively, a community health center that already offered comprehensive services

might not have enough capital to offer evening health education classes to its community. Establishing a prepaid program of classes or workshops would not only provide some unrestricted funds, but could engage interested community members in active collaboration with the practice. From this focused beginning the practice could begin working with the health promoters in its community.

Interagency cooperation is a challenging aspect of community participation. Potential conflict arises when membership benefits duplicate other services in the community, such as a wellness center, local birthing classes, school health programs, or a health department PAP smear clinic. It is easy to underestimate the resources required for effective liaison with other agencies.

A potential liability of the membership concept is the time and energy needed for membership development. Paperwork, managerial time, and accounting are all increased. Given the goals of COPC, however, this appears to be a worthwhile investment. Pendleton Community Care's modest membership program definitely pays for itself and enhances the practice with few liabilities. Nevertheless, each practice needs to examine its own goals and the extent of community demand for particular services.

Finally, development and growth of such a program can be slow. While Pendleton Community Care has some very committed members, we have not fully implemented all aspects of the concept in 3 years. The main lesson is that COPC is a dynamic process of growth, not a single static model. The membership concept is a structural tool to facilitate that process within the community.

CHAPTER 62

Students as a
COPC Resource

Pat Shonubi, B.S.N., M.S.

The resources to develop a COPC practice are often difficult to obtain. For practices involved in health manpower training, the students themselves may be an important resource for COPC. Using students as a resource and simultaneously providing them with a first-rate educational experience, however, is not always simple. This chapter describes the use of students and residents in early and continuing attempts to achieve full development of COPC within the Residency Program in Social Medicine (RPSM) at Montefiore Medical Center in the Bronx. The mission of the RPSM is to train primary care physicians for underserved inner city communities. Since its founding in 1970, it has trained 72 internists, 52 pediatricians, and 61 family physicians and has offered dozens of medical students brief preceptorships in community health centers (1, 2). To do this adequately, we believe it is necessary to introduce trainees to the knowledge, skills, and attitudes necessary for COPC. Also, to affect the health of the community in which we train and practice, we must use the strategies inherent to COPC.

MEDICAL RESIDENTS AS A COPC RESOURCE

The first vehicle for involving residents in COPC projects is the orientation month which begins in the fourth month of the internship. The orientation begins with a series of didactic and interactive seminars on health beliefs and health practices, and a community tour to see the Bronx and meet with local community leaders and organizations. Later, residents are asked to develop collectively a community-based project which they design, plan, and implement with faculty support. Guidelines for the project are that it must be in the community, that data collection and analysis are essential, and that evaluation must be performed.

The resident projects provide important information for the overall COPC approach. For example, in carrying out a community hypertension screening program, residents, with faculty help, developed an instrument for data collection and devised a patient education and followup system for those found to have high blood pressure. Before the instrument could be used, faculty worked with residents in deciding how many families to interview, how to gain access to homes, how to choose apartment houses, how to work as a team, and how to integrate their findings into the ongoing health center work. Similar screening programs and community assessment were started with pairs of medical students and were continued by separate groups of residents and students. Other efforts have yielded information about community perceptions on a variety of health issues.

Another training vehicle consists of core courses in COPC. Residents can elect 1-month courses in Understanding the Health System and Health Teams, and Community Assessment, Epidemiology, and Research. During the course of their 3-year training, residents are expected to develop an additional individual or collaborative social medicine project that addresses the broader context of projects, for example, lead screening, programs to provide health care for the homeless, and school health education projects, as well as literature reviews on the health status of various ethnic groups in the practice population. While some projects make only a small contribution to the overall COPC program, some have laid the foundation for obtaining grant funds that the health center uses to address community health problems.

MEDICAL STUDENTS AS A COPC RESOURCE

Our work with preclinical and clinical level medical students has been both highly and loosely structured. In the early 1980s we received funds from the Robert Wood Johnson Foundation to develop a training program in COPC for medical students interested in primary care. We designed an 8-week program of structured lectures, clinical preceptorship, and community work that has been detailed in a recent book (2).

The 8-week program places students in a community health center for 2 days of clinical precepting with a primary care practitioner, offers them 1-1/2 days of seminars a week, and reserves 2-1/2 days for the performance of a community project. In the first 2 weeks students are taught how to gather data in the community, how to set goals with their preceptors, and how to orient themselves to primary care delivery at the sites. In weeks 3 and 4 they learn interviewing skills, how to use community and center resources, and the importance of cultural issues in the delivery of care. They also use this time to share information on their projects. Weeks 5 and 6 cover the health delivery system and its components. Weeks 7 and 8 provide the students opportunity to share their personal reflections on the system, their career goals, and the outcomes of the projects they undertake.

Unlike the residents who design their own projects, student projects are often partially designed by the preceptor or other center staff before the students' arrival. Students are expected to gather literature and community data, perform surveys, design programs for the project, and meet frequently with project preceptors to discuss progress and get guidance.

For example, Valentine Lane Family Practice, a four-practitioner practice, has always encouraged student placement. Early groups of students summarized the location of the practice population on large maps and took pictures of several areas to give practitioners information on where their patients lived. Later, new students went to local health departments and gathered health and population data to describe the health problems in the community. These preliminary data were used to solicit State grants for prenatal care and funds for the medically indigent programs. Currently, students are involved in characterizing the practice population to allow practitioners to compare the practice with community data. Students are also surveying areas in the community that are not covered by the practice. These data will be used to develop marketing strategies for the practice.

RESOURCE REQUIREMENTS

The successful use of students in projects requires some previous planning by site staffs and those responsible for the students' education. We have been in both positions. The preplanning work is manageable even for busy practices. Our experience of having both residents and students from schools in our area and other parts of the country seeking placement with us leads us to believe that many trainees are available in various levels of training with 1-2 months available elective time to participate in project development. Often they seek both a clinical and community experience. When they request only a clinical experience, we have been able to persuade students to accept a combination program of half-time clinical and half-time project work. We continue to market our program and the opportunities for site placement by announcements in local school publications that list electives for students. We have used simple application forms to help us select students or have conducted phone conversations in which we try to determine students' past experience in working independently and with the kinds of populations we serve. While we have not done any studies on these as measures of student success, we feel these are strong indicators for a successful placement with us.

Another requirement for using students is the preceptor or project coordinator who may act as both faculty and project manager to ensure continuity of the COPC projects. In our early beginnings, students and faculty learned side by side how to assess health problems in the community. We started our early COPC efforts with the help of faculty from the Sophie Davis

Biomedical program in New York City, which had skilled community faculty. Sidney and Emily Kark also led seminars in COPC for our faculty and trainees for a year.

CONSIDERATIONS FOR USE OF TRAINEES IN A COPC PROGRAM

1. Structuring the Training Experience

Arriving trainees require a variety of experiences to meet their training program's goals and their personal goals. It is wise to solicit these before placement and to negotiate which ones the student will be able to meet during the placement. The expectations of the site should also be made clear. We have used written evaluation forms before the start of the experience, which ask the students to list their goals for the placement. In evaluations at the end of the experience, we ask the students to rate on a scale of 1 to 5 how well their goals were met.

Students have listed goals that range from learning about the culture of the inner cities to enhancing their outpatient experience. Others have wanted to learn epidemiology. Others have come for the experience of working in inner-city environments. Similarly, when we offered formal didactic programs we asked students to rate how the goals for each seminar were met. We also feel that early in the placement, oral feedback should be solicited from both student, preceptor, and site about the placement success.

2. The Role of Preceptor, Faculty, and Project Manager

When the roles of preceptor, faculty, and project manager are carried out by different individuals it is important that all concerned understand clearly what they can expect to get or must give to each during the experience. We have encouraged physicians in our practice to involve themselves not only in the students' education but in the management of COPC projects.

This provides a role model for the students and keeps the COPC and clinical practice together.

3. Student and Practitioner Knowledge of COPC

Some assessment of both students and preceptors must be made concerning the attitudes, knowledge, and skills that foster COPC. We have designed independent reading programs for students and preceptors to enhance their knowledge of COPC. Much work still needs to be done in this area. We have been very fortunate in having students from the Sophie Davis program, which has a formal educational program in community assessment, and we have used their students to conduct surveys in several areas of our communities.

4. Tension Between Service and Training

As the practice tries to integrate the academic needs of students with its own need to provide service, the realities of time in a busy practice must be planned for and dealt with. Specific time should be set aside to deal with student concerns regarding their experiences and the project. Frequent lunch meetings with the students have been the most common vehicle for such interaction. Also, students' activities can be seen as disruptive by other staff in the practice who are not directly involved with the student or preceptor. Much friction can be decreased by arranging early in the student experience some time for the student to talk with other staff and find out about the jobs of others working in the facility. This interaction often gives other staff permission to interact with the student and keep informed about activities in the project.

5. Ownership of the Project

It has been our experience that projects that come purely from student interest rather than community, practice, or pre-

ceptor interest have short life spans. Students are often willing to compromise on individual wishes in the interest of furthering COPC at the site.

6. Sense of Completion

Often students are unable to see their efforts as being part of a larger effort to accomplish COPC. Some discussion about the nature of COPC and the length of time it takes for a practice to make small advances in COPC is necessary to give students, if not a sense of completion, at least a sense of continuity in their efforts.

SUMMARY

Our use of trainees as an important resource for COPC projects has evolved over time. We are still experimenting with ways best to encourage the development of projects and to integrate student-initiated projects into the day-to-day operation of the practice. It is clear, however, that integration is critical to balancing the requirements of both an educational experience for the trainees and the long-term pursuit of a COPC approach in our program.

REFERENCES

1. Boufford, J. I. Primary care residency training: The first five years. *Annals of Internal Medicine* 1977; 87:359.
2. Massad, R. Training for inner city family practice: Experience of the Montefiore Medical Center. In: *Urban Family Medicine*, Birrer, (ed.). New York: Springer-Verlag (in press).
3. Boufford, J. I., and Shonubi, P. A. *Community Oriented Primary Care Training for Urban Practice.* New York: Praeger, 1986.

CHAPTER 63

Community Resources
for COPC

Jeffrey Newman, M.D.

Each stage of the COPC process requires expertise and resources not normally available to the primary care practitioner. Thus as the traditional individual care oriented practice becomes more and more community oriented, the need for collaboration with other health care providers and community agencies becomes evident. The health care team, rather than the individual practitioner, becomes central to the practice. The individual clinician's potential for leadership and initiative may be critical for the development of the team, but collaborative relationships will be essential for success.

For example, an initiative to prevent low birthweight in a clinic population may lead to an awareness that in the community at large, most mothers of low birthweight babies do not have access to good primary care. Working together with community agencies and other primary care providers, along with community groups such as Healthy Mothers/Healthy Babies, outreach programs can be developed to reach these underserved mothers.

Potential collaborators with the COPC practitioner include public health agencies, health care facilities and schools, business groups, voluntary agencies,

media, professional societies and foundations, as well as local, State, or Federal government programs. This chapter will briefly outline the ways in which these resources can be used in COPC practice.

SOURCES OF HELP

Public Health Agencies

Some have viewed COPC as a concept combining clinical and public health practice; at the very least public health agencies can provide epidemiologic, clinical, and educational support to the COPC practitioner. They may also afford links to other resources described below.

State public health programs concentrate on preventive services, such as family planning or immunization clinics, but may provide the full range of primary care services for certain populations; State public health departments generally provide home health care as well.

At the Federal level, several agencies of the U.S. Public Health Service have actively supported COPC. This includes the Community Health Centers Program, the National Health Service Corps, and the Indian Health Service. The Centers for Disease Control (CDC) will provide epidemiologic support in certain circumstances. Resources of the National Institutes for Mental Health, the Office of Disease Prevention and Health Promotion, and the Office on Smoking and Health can provide support for COPC programs in these areas.

An example of effective State and Federal collaboration with local resources and practitioners is the diabetes project sponsored jointly by the Colorado Department of Health and the CDC. Epidemiologists from the University of Colorado School of Medicine used the database of a federally funded community health center to identify gaps in primary care for diabetics in the Denver area. A program to provide the needed care has been established through collaboration among primary care clinicians, the Department of Health, and the School of Medicine.

Health Care Facilities

Primary care services provided by hospitals, HMO's, and private sector practices can be used as resources in COPC. Public relations considerations, or residual humanitarian instincts, will sometimes include these institutions to provide help for programs focusing on providing care for high risk populations, such as the elderly, or the examples of prenatal care and diabetic care mentioned above.

Professional Schools

Collaboration between COPC practitioners and health profession students and faculty can be productive. COPC projects may merge educational and community health objectives. Student projects may include community surveys, resource directories, and planning, implementation, or evaluation of COPC activities. Besides health profession schools like medicine, nursing, or dentistry, other university programs can be approached; for instance, epidemiologists may be helpful in survey work or software development.

Voluntary Agencies

The enthusiasm and expertise of voluntary agencies such as those for specific diseases like heart, cancer, diabetes, arthritis, mental retardation, etc., or more prevention-oriented groups such as Mothers Against Drunk Driving, Healthy Mothers/Healthy Babies, and others can provide consultation, materials, and manpower to aid COPC efforts in their areas of emphasis.

Professional Societies and Foundations

Professional societies, such as State medical societies or other State professional societies, can provide important contacts to facilitate COPC programs. Foundations can provide needed financial support. While the large national foundations are usually best known, most areas have smaller foundations with a local focus. The practitioner should make an effort to contact local foundations to determine their specific areas of interest.

Media

Television and radio stations, as well as newspapers and other printed media, are sources of needed information and can be used for publicity once COPC programs are underway.

Government

Many local, State, or Federal agencies outside the public health realm can provide resources to COPC practice. The Bureau of the Census can provide detailed, block by block information of epidemiologic importance. Support from city councils can be very supportive to local COPC efforts.

Business

While some business support can be garnered as a public relations or community service function of the business, the best approach to businesses is to point out cost savings from preventive programs directed at employees. Some businesses will have occupational health expertise that can be of help.

CONCLUSION

The COPC practitioner frequently needs to take a leadership role in initiating and maintaining COPC practices. However, formulation of a successful team effort involves collaboration between numerous groups, including other health programs, government agencies, educational institutions, and businesses.

COPC and Medical Shopkeeping

H. Jack Geiger, M.D.

The driving forces and directions of any health care system change over time, and those changes may profoundly affect attempts at innovation. New formulations and concepts, in turn, may be seriously influenced by the prevailing health care climate—even to the point of blurring their original purpose. Although only a few of the papers in the preceding section discuss the issue explicitly, I believe their cumulative message is the difficulty of developing community-oriented primary care in a system that is currently focused on other concerns, and the danger that the real meaning and purpose of COPC may be lost in some attempts at implementation.

Two decades ago, the driving force in U.S. health care was *improvement of access* and, in particular, the initiation and improvement of primary care services for the poorest, sickest and highest-risk segments of the Nation's population. The explicit goals were improvement of health status and reduction of the gap between the healthiest and the sickest populations. Underlying this thrust and its specific manifestations—Medicaid, Medicare, the development of community health centers and the entire panoply of related programs—was a belief that health care *planning*, by both governmental and private sources, based on specific information about populations and communities, was essential to improvements in health status. The need for more funding, both public and private, was also recognized.

Today, in a dramatic and pervasive change, the driving force is *cost containment*, both public and private, the operative method is *competition*, and the primary goal for health care providers is *survival in the marketplace*. Access to health care, and improvement in health status, are rarely addressed directly as goals, as answers to the question: what is a health care system *for?* Rational and centralized planning, particularly for the underserved, is rejected. The underlying belief is that competition in a health-care "marketplace" will produce the most efficient, the most appropriate and the most effective medical care and thus—while reducing the dollars devoted to medical care—will produce the biggest improvements in health status.

In short, Adam Smith has replaced John Grant. In this world view, unless there is a compelling financial or competitive reward, there is no reason for primary care practitioners or other providers to be community-oriented. Instead, the pressure is to become (in Julian Tudor-Hart's striking phrase) "medical shopkeepers," motivated primarily to increase their trade and unconcerned with the health status of those who do not come through their doors seeking services. Indeed, under many competitive fixed-payment or capitation schemes, the poorest and the sickest are likely to be seen not as an unmet medical care challenge but as a financial risk to be avoided.

Few providers are in fact so narrowly motivated, but the overall change in direction is undeniable. It intensifies the difficulties of developing community-oriented primary care. Worse, it raises the risk that activities described or promoted as community-oriented may really be, in whole or in part, entrepreneurial efforts aimed at increasing patient flow, cash income, or competitive advantage.

Numerous instances of resistance to community and population-based orientations are, in fact, cited by the authors of these papers. It is noted, for example, that "local physicans will protect their practices and their incomes, may exchange individual patient data but not aggregate information." Or again, "practitioners may see 'denominators' as threatening attrition of their fee-for-service patients; administrators of hospitals with borderline occupancy rates may see in your preventive emphasis the specter of yet more empty beds." It is, at the least, arguable that a physician who rents out his basement swimming pool to community clients in the name of "weight reduction" is less community-oriented than entrepreneurial.

And it is certainly unclear that the marketplace sale of a "benefit package" including a half-price screening examination, a "free" blood-pressure check, a health education newsletter and other unspecified preventive services constitutes an exercise in community-oriented primary care,

particularly when 40 per cent of the buyers obtain their curative primary care services elsewhere and 80 per cent of the index practice's acute-care patients do not choose, or lack the means for, the additional benefit. It is noteworthy that this activity is graphically described in terms of the dollars generated, and not by any demographic, diagnostic or geographic definition of the recipient group.

Other papers describe activities which are clearly desirable in their own right but which are not necessarily a part of a coherent plan meeting the basic criteria of COPC. A hospital's attempts to improve the continuity of care and the quality and appropriateness of geriatric services are admirable, but without a defined population denominator or aggregating arrangements designed to approximate the community as denominator, they may lack the epidemiological dimension that is central to COPC.

These are hardly new problems in the development of COPC. With the exception of the direct provision of services by the public sector our health care system, after all, has always been entrepreneurial to a substantial degree. Nor are some of the problems unique to marketplace incentives and goals; Tudor-Hart's criticism, it must be remembered, was made of physicians working in a national health service. The new and important risk is that all sorts of health care activities and programs that reach out to recipients or involve community in some way—even when "community" really means an undifferentiated marketplace—may be accepted as part of COPC. If that happens, the concept will lose its meaning—and its future.

There are other, more positive lessons that emerge from these papers. First among them is the likelihood that, in the near future, it will be much easier to begin COPC programs in rural than in urban areas. In larger and underserved rural areas, at least, competition is likely to be less marked; when both manpower and resources are in short supply, cooperation is likelier and the integration of separate components is easier. The definition of rural denominators may be easier, and population turnover is probably lower. These assets, in turn, reflect an aspect of community that is important in COPC: "community" is more than a denominator; it implies a degree of social cohesion and a willingness to see problems as shared and solutions as requiring cooperation rather than competition.

In urban areas, progress in COPC is likeliest, in the immediate future, to begin through the cooperative efforts of programs for the poor and underserved, particularly community health centers joining in formal coalitions. There are two immediate goals, both relating to the idea of "critical mass": to achieve a critical mass of manpower to plan, deliver and evaluate additional services or improve existing ones, and to achieve a combined target population large enough to permit defined numerators and denominators for the characterization of populations in need, the rational planning of interventions, and the evaluation of results.

A third area of early promise for COPC is in public-private partnerships involving primary care practitioners and public health departments or other public health agencies, sometimes in cooperation with nonprofit voluntary health agencies. In a fiercely competitive, cost-containing and increasingly privatized environment, health departments (and many private practitioners) may feel themselves to be marginal. In COPC, new roles may be found and new, pooled strengths identified. Again, rural communities, counties or States may lead the way, but a number of metropolitan governments are now beginning "medical homesteading" plans to establish primary care practitioners in underserved areas—and to support them with the strengths of public-agency data

sources, computer resources, and planning and evaluation skills.

Almost every initiative described in the preceding pages recognizes the community itself as a resource, and as a partner in coalitions for COPC. In a competitive and entrepreneurial environment, difficult questions emerge: are community workers to be volunteers, or paid? If the latter, who pays them? To whom does their loyalty belong—to the sponsoring providers or to the community? The last question may have great influence on their perception by the community as they go about their roles as advisers, sentinels, advocates and organizers, for it will be crucial to make clear that such workers are not, in effect, marketing agents for particular providers and are, rather, resources for the public health.

Finally, these papers suggest a slow but steady growth in the development of practice profiles. Primary care providers' participation in this first step may prove to be the critical process in the intellectual re-orientation away from case-by-case interests to a truly population-based community orientation, easing the way for further COPC developments. The rapid proliferation of office-practice microcomputers, and the growing availability of software to make practice profile construction easy, may prove to be the common denominator of all attempts to initiate practitioner participation in COPC.

Since shifts in the fundamental directions of health care systems are cyclical, there is reason to hope for a change to more COPC-supportive health care environments in the not-too-distant future. The goal, during the interim, should be to keep the concept and the definition of community-oriented primary care intact, to concentrate on the easiest and likeliest sites, and to achieve modest but steady growth.

Part IX.
Information Resources for COPC

Introduction

There is a considerable body of information of interest to the COPC practitioner that is available but often difficult to access, because it does not bear a COPC label. In Part IX, three authors have assembled information in three specific areas of interest. In Chapter 64, Berman offers a brief tour through the national data sets that are available to describe the health status and practices of national population samples. In many cases, these data are available and may be of use as a first approximation of the health problems of the community. In Chapter 65, Mickalide focuses on those information resources useful in the health promotion and disease prevention activities that should be a central component of many COPC practices. Finally in Chapter 66, Voorhees has selected and annotated a collection of the most useful literature describing the theory and practice of COPC. Each should serve as a rich source of information in these three important areas.

CHAPTER 64

Data Sources for COPC: National Health Surveys

Leatrice H. Berman, M.A.

National surveys are rich data sources for COPC. The purpose of this chapter is to list several important surveys, describe their content and suggest their utility to COPC practitioners. Chapter 19 has already discussed the ways in which questionnaire items and methods in these surveys can be useful to COPC practitioners as models for the development of their own tools when collecting original data. However, this chapter will bring into focus how one can access these findings.

Generally, the results of these surveys can be useful in two ways. First, if the practitioner needs descriptive health data for a specific community population or target group beyond that which is available in patient data bases of primary care practices or local secondary data sources (e.g., public health departments, hospitals, health systems agencies or special surveys), one can look to the overall findings and subgroup analyses (e.g., white females with family incomes of $10,000-$20,000) of these national surveys to get suggestive data on problem prevalence, health status, etc.

Second, if one has a local data set, it is useful to see the extent to which comparable findings exist in similar population sub-

sets of national surveys. For example, in assessing the utilization patterns, unmet health needs or prevalence of specific problems in Puerto Rican children in Chicago, it might be quite useful to compare one's findings with those found in the New York Puerto Rican population as part of the Hispanic Health and Nutrition Examination Survey. This comparison can help to evaluate the significance of local findings or can raise useful hypotheses about why such patterns might be different. These hypotheses either lead to a greater understanding of problems particular to Chicago's Puerto Rican children, methodology problems related to the local survey or methodology problems related to comparing national and local data sets (see below). Nevertheless, these comparisons can be rich in moving COPC methods and program strategies forward.

One word of caution is in order. Sole reliance on national data to characterize local health needs or problem prevalence can be risky due to population differences. For example, there are regional differences among Mexican-Americans, health problem differences that correspond to lifestyle and exposure and sampling differences for which statistically it is very difficult to account. Margins of error can be quite high in extrapolating national data, which yield information on typical patterns across the country, to small geographic areas that have their unique features.[1] On the other hand, the estimation of local health problem prevalence based on findings of comparable substratum of national data sets—called synthetic estimation—can be very useful if the variance on the variable of interest is not so great that the estimation would be so far off. Furthermore, estimation can be valid if the geographic or population comparisons make sense, such as using urban substratum data to estimate prevalence for comparable urban populations.

Frerichs[2] believes that stratum-specific prevalence rates on conditions that show less variability among respondents from studies such as the National Health Interview, National Health and Nutrition Examination Surveys, or national blood pressure data, can be very good estimates for local populations. These synthetic estimates will get one closer to the truth than an expert, are less accurate than a primary data collection effort but are also far less expensive. There is a tradeoff between cost and accuracy.

Second, for practice program-related decisionmaking, what is the threshold of accuracy required? Does it make a difference in mounting a program whether estimates are 20-30 percent higher or lower than actual? Based on these tradeoffs and specific program area of interest, a COPC team can make a decision on whether synthetic estimates from national surveys will be useful to its purpose.

_____

[1] Personal communication with N. Hearst, University of California, San Francisco, and School of Public Health, University of California, Berkeley.

[2] Personal communication with R. Frerichs, Professor of Epidemiology, UCLA, School of Public Health.

Several national surveys from which data can be obtained are reviewed in the following charts:

1. National Health Interview Survey (NHIS).
2. National Health and Nutrition Examination Survey (NHANES).
3. Hispanic Health and Nutrition Examination Survey (Hispanic HANES).
4. National Survey of Personal Health Practices and Consequences.
5. National Medical Care Expenditure Survey (NMCES).
6. National Medical Care Utilization and Expenditure Survey (NMCUES).
7. National Ambulatory Care Survey (NAMCS).
8. National Institutes of Mental Health, Epidemiologic Catchment Area Study (NIMH, ECA).
9. Rand's Health Insurance Experiment (HIE).

A few introductory comments can assist in understanding the data that are potentially available from these surveys. Most of them with the exception of the National Ambulatory Care Survey provide data directly from a population household sample. The Health and Nutrition Examination Surveys and Rand Survey additionally provide data from medical examinations and laboratory analyses. The Medical Care Expenditure/Utilization Surveys and the Rand Study also review health insurance claims or provider data (including Medicare and Medicaid and employer health insurance data in the former).

The National Ambulatory Medical Care Survey collects provider data from physicians' office visits and does not report population data—just data with respect to problems among patients seen.

CHART 1

SURVEY	*POPULATION BASE*	*DATA TYPE*
National Health Interview Survey (1981)	Civilian, non-institutionalized, multi-stage probability sample continuous (weekly) additive 41,000 households (107,000 persons) 3% non-interview rate	Self-report data: yields prevalence data and distribution of measurements

CONTENT CATEGORIES
Acute Illnesses[1] and Injuries[2]
Selected Chronic Conditions
Disability Days[3]
Limitation of Activity due to Chronic Conditions[4]

Measures of Health Care Utilization
    Hospital Discharges
    Hospital Episodes
    Hospital Days/year and/episode
    Dental visits
    Physician visits

Child Health Supplement (1981)
    Child Care and Relationships and Residential Mobility; Breastfeeding; Motor and Social Development; Birth; Prenatal Care; Hospitalizations and Surgery; Supplemental Conditions; Weight; Vision; Dental; Medicine Use; School Behavior; Behavior Problems Index; Social Effects of Ill Health; Sleep; and Seat Belts.

Health Promotion and Disease Prevention Supplement (1985)
    Individual health behaviors and knowledge of health practices: general health, nutrition, injury control and child health, high blood pressure, smoking, stress, exercise, alcohol use, dental care, occupational safety and health.

Reference: U.S. Vital and Health Statistics *Current Estimates from the National Health Interview Survey: U.S. 1981.* Series 10, Number 141 (DHHS Pub. No. (PHS) 82-1569.) Hyattsville, Maryland: NCHS, October, 1982, 82 pp.

---

[1] Defined as those episodes which last less than 3 months and involve medical attention or at least 1 day or more of restricted activity.

[2] Injuries by class of accident: 1) motor vehicle; 2) at work; 3) home; 4) other.

[3] Temporary and long term: restricted activity, bed-disability, work-loss, school-loss (in relationship to specific conditions).

[4] 1) Persons unable to carry on usual activity; 2) persons limited in amount/kind of usual activity; 3) persons limited but not in their usual activity; 4) persons not limited.

CHART 2

SURVEY	POPULATION BASE	DATA TYPE
National Health and Nutrition Examination Survey (1976-1980)	27,803 sample persons, yielding 20,235 examined persons Civilian, non-institutionalized stratified, multi-stage, probability cluster household sample (4 years) (oversample poor, elderly, pre-school children)	a) Standardized, direct medical examination[1] including tests and procedures used in clinical practice b) Self-report data: yields prevalence data and distribution of health related measurements

CONTENT CATEGORIES

Medical History (6 months-11 yrs)
   birth weight, prematurity, developmental-congenital conditions, medication/vitamin usage, neurological conditions, lead poisoning, accidents, hospital care, disability, diarrhea, pica, vision, other chronic conditions, URI, allergies, kidney and bladder disease, anemia, speech and hearing, lung and chest conditions, participation in food programs, outstanding/untreated health problems, school attendance.

Medical History (12-74 yrs)
   TB, medications, hospital care, nutrition, acute and chronic disease, tobacco, tea, coffee usage, physical activity, smoking, weight, height, vision disability, exposure to pesticides, gastrointestinal problems, menstrual-pregnancy history, current untreated health problems, anemia, diabetes, respiratory conditions, hearing, speech, liver, gallbladder conditions, kidney and bladder disease, allergies, hypertension, cardiovascular conditions, stroke, arthritis, (back and neck problems stressed), participation in food programs

Dietary
   Dietary Recall (24 hrs)
   measures of calories, cholesterol, fat, unsaturated fats, protein, carbohydrates, specific vitamins and minerals; food frequency yields - daily/weekly consumption of food groups including salt, vitamins, minerals
   7 Day Recall
   Special Diets (12-74 yrs)
   HX, prior medications, barriers to purchase groceries or eating foods

Behavior (25-74 yrs)
   behavior associated with coronary heart disease

Household
   relationships, age, sex, race, occupation; household income; veteran status; housing information; participation in food programs

---

[1] Special attention given to nutrition, hearing, thyroid gland, cardiovascular, respiratory, muscular-skeletal/neurological systems.

CHART 2

CONTENT CATEGORIES

Clinical Procedures
 Spirometry (6-24 yrs) (e.g., FVC, FEV1, peak flow)
 Electrocardiogram (25-74 yrs)
 Body measurements (e.g., height, weight, skinfolds)
 Puretone audiometry (4-19 yrs)
 Speech recording (4-6 yrs)
 Allergy tests (6-74 yrs)
 X-ray cervical - lumbar
   spine (osteoarthritis, degenerative disc)
 X-ray chest
 N-multistix urine test (6-74 yrs)
 Urinary Sediments (20-74 yrs)
 Gonorrhea (12-40 yrs)
 Analyses for pesticides (12-74 yrs)
 Glucose tolerance (diabetes in adults)
 Liver function tests
 Anemia - related lab
 Biochemical nutrition (e.g., vitamin A, C, albumin)
 Serum LIPIDS
 Biochemical Tests - toxics (e.g., leads, pesticides, metabolites, carboxyhemoglobin)
 Hematology
 Kidney function
 Syphilis

Reference: Vital and Health Statistics: *Plan and Operation of the Second National Health and Nutrition Examination Survey 1976-1980.* Programs and Collections Procedures. Series 1, No. 15 (DHHS Pub. No. (PHS) 81-317) Hyattsville, Maryland, Office of Health Research Statistics and Technology, July, 1981, 144 pp.

As one will note from the following charts, some surveys sponsored by the Federal Government are continuous or recurrent; others are special one-time surveys. Some surveys sample across the country and others—particularly the Hispanic HANES, NIMH Epidemiologic Catchment Area Study and the Medicaid data from NMCUES—deal with particular geographic areas; therefore, generalizing from them is more difficult.

Most of these studies are fielded by the U.S. Government, but the Rand Survey, although federally funded, was carried out by the Rand Corporation in Santa Monica, California. All the charts provide references to basic descriptive material, which provide further details. Many of these materials either embody or refer one to the basic instruments and protocols of the survey. Most of these surveys have published findings either as part of the National Center for Health Statistics' *Vital and Health Statistics Series* (as indicated from the reference) or in the form of special reports.

This chapter does not inventory the extensive findings from these surveys, but library work with good reference librarians or a call to respective study offices is always a direct and quick way to access necessary material. Most studies have pub-

CHART 3

SURVEY	POPULATION BASE	DATA TYPE
Hispanic HANES (1982-1984)	Mexican Americans (Southwest and California) 7,462 out of 9,894 (75%); Cuban Americans (Dade County, Florida) 1,364 out of 2,244 (60%) Puerto Rican Americans (New York) 2,846 out of 3,793 (75%)	Same as HANES. More attention paid to interview portion.

CONTENT CATEGORIES

Same as HANES:

Expanded components listed only:
  Diabetes[1]
  Hypertension[2]
  Dental care/caries
  Immunization
  Tuberculosis
  Alcohol consumption
  Drug Abuse
  Depression
  Nutrition
  Functional Impairment
  Gallbladder ultrasonography
  Gallstones
  Impedance audiometry
  Toxics: lead/pesticides; reproductive hazards
  Detailed questions on health services utilization and health needs assessment[3]
  Measures of acculturation[4]
  School attendance and language use (6 months - 11 yrs)

Reference: U.S. Vital and Health Statistics. *Plan and Operation of the Hispanic Health and Nutrition Examination Survey 1982-1984*. Programs and Collection Procedures. Series 1, No. 19, DHHS Pub. No. (PHS) 85-1321. Hyattsville, Maryland: NCHS, September, 1985.

---

[1] In relationship to obesity and dietary intake; sequalae, including kidney, cardiovascular, retinal changes, and limitation of activity.

[2] Expanded control status categories, screening, diagnosis, treatment modalities, compliance with RX, health care visits, related conditions, risk factors, and sequalae.

[3] Usual source of care, waiting time, travel time, satisfaction with care received, and barriers encountered in receiving care.

[4] Cuellar, Harris, Jasso, 1981 (shortened version).

CHART 4

SURVEY	POPULATION BASE	DATA TYPE
National Survey of Personal Health Practices and Consequences (1979-1980) Wave I and Wave II	Civilian non-institution-alized population ages 20-64. Probability, three stage, stratified, cluster sampling 3,025 Wave I Interviews (81% response rate) 2,436 Wave II Interviews (81% response rate)	Telephone interviews (interview-reinterview year later); descriptive statistics, distribution of measures, and prevalence data.

CONTENT CATEGORIES

Personal Health Practices
   general habits[1]
   dental
   high blood pressure
   breast exam
   smoking
   pap smear
   alcohol use
   exercise

Self-perceived health
status/limitations and health problems (prevalence of health conditions and limitations);

Health care utilization
Compliance with medical advice
Social support
Psychological well being
Occupation-related health factors
Life events
Selected socio-demographics

Reference: U.S. Vital and Health Statistics. *Highlights From Wave I of the National Survey of Personal Health Practices and Consequences: U.S. 1979.* Hyattsville, Maryland: NCHS. Series 15, No. 1 (DHHS Pub. No. (PHS) 81-1162) June, 1981.

Eisenstadt, R.K., and Schoenborn, C.A. *Basic Data from Wave II of the National Survey of Personal Health Practices and Consequences: U.S. 1980.* Warberg Paper. Number 13. NCHS. Office of Analyses and Epidemiology, October, 1982.

---

[1] E.g., eating, drug taking, sleep patterns.

---

lic use tapes for purchase that enable local users to analyze the data further according to their specific needs and to formulate specific correlations and subgroup analysis of the national data set. However, several of these tapes are costly. Often, local academic health survey policy centers or State health planning departments

CHART 5

SURVEY	POPULATION BASE	DATA TYPE
National Medical Care Expenditures Study April 1977-1978	14,000 Civilian non-institutionalized probability sample	Household survey; six interviews/ household (3 month recall); survey of physicians and facilities used by sample of interviewees; survey of employers and insurance companies covering interviewees.

CONTENT CATEGORIES

Household Survey:

Ethnicity and household composition.

Use of medical services (medical, hospital, dental)
   reason for visit, site of care, office waiting times.

Charges for services
   ancillary services (e.g., x-rays, lab); prescription medicine and other expenses (e.g., eyeglasses, contact lenses, hearing aids, wheelchairs); long term care expenses for persons currently institutionalized for health reasons and not living at home.

Sources of payment.

Access to health care and barriers to care
   condition for which care is being sought, sick leave, health concern or worry.

Conditions and accidents
   seriousness and time frames related to seeking professional help.

Disability days (number, type), limitations of activity

Health insurance coverage
   premiums, deductibles, benefits and Medicaid program coverage and income eligibility.

Status of income tax filing
   amount of itemized medical deductions.

Employment status
   hours worked, occupation, barriers to employment, welfare status.

Income and assets.

Medical Provider Survey:
(for sub-sample of household survey participants)

   Patient visits
   Diagnoses
   Charges
   Sources of payment
   Physician characteristics and practice settings (sub-sample of providers)

CHART 5

Employee-Union Survey (combination mail-telephone):
(for sample of household survey participants)

Health insurance coverage
Number of employees covered
Distribution of employees by wage levels
Total amount of employer payments for health insurance
Amount of premium paid by employees

Health Insurance Claims Survey:

Claims paid for persons insured by four Blue Cross/Blue Shield insurance plans.

OVERALL ANALYTIC OBJECTIVES

1. Financial burden of illness (illness-use-expense correlations, diagnosis specific) including impact on out of pocket expenses, loss of wages, loss of productivity and cost of medical care to the public.

2. Factors that affect demand for health services among different population groups, especially the relationship between health insurance coverage and use/costs of medical care.

3. Changes in participation and eligibility in Medicaid including impact on pattern of service use, expenditures, out-of-pocket payments (for groups at different socio-economic levels and for select chronic and acute health problems).

4. Changes in patterns of access to care with particular reference to beneficiaries of federally supported programs and to the relationship between health care costs and access.

5. Corporate and personal income tax provisions and their effect on patterns of use for specific population groups and tax revenues overall.

6. Patterns of use for type, breadth and depth of health insurance coverage including patterns of coverage for different population groups and the extent and nature of coverage for catastrophic illness, dread diseases and extra cash benefits.

Reference: Bonham, G.S., and Corder, L.S. *NMCES Household Interview Instruments.* Instruments and procedures 1. Hyattsville, Maryland: NCHSR. April, 1981. [Publications and Information Branch, Rm. 7-44, 3700 East-West Highway, Hyattsville, Maryland 20782]

---

have these tapes. The availability of public use tapes is either indicated in the references listed or can be checked by calling the National Center for Health Statistics (NCHS: Hyattsville, Maryland), the National Center for Health Services Research (NCHSR, Rockville, Maryland), the Health Care Financing Administration (HCFA, Baltimore, Maryland), or the National Institute of Mental Health (NIMH, Rockville, Maryland), depending on which agency sponsors the survey.

CHART 6

SURVEY	POPULATION BASE	DATA TYPE
National Medical Care Utilization and Expenditure Survey (NMCUES) 1980-1981	Civilian non-institionalized, multi-stage probability sample; 6,000 households yielding data on 17,900 individuals. Four state Medicaid household stratified[1] probability samples, civilian, non-institutionalized: California, Texas, Michigan, New York; 4,000 households yielding data on 13,700 individuals.	Panel survey[2] entailing five household rounds of in-person and telephone interviews[3], 3 months apart yielding self-report data; interview included the use of a computer generated cumulative summary of responses to be used in: updating health care charges, sources of payments; reducing double reporting, missing data; and improving validity. Analysis of Medicare and Medicaid administrative records corresponding to eligible interviewees. Payment records of the Medicaid recipients in the national sample were not obtained. Instruments used in national household and State Medicaid household components were identical.

CONTENT CATEGORIES

Household Survey:

Sociodemographics: geographic identification, family size, composition, marital status, age, sex, race/ethnicity, veteran status, education, employment, income.

---

[1] Stratified by four Medicaid eligibility groups a) aid to blind/disabled; b) aid to the elderly (those receiving SSI); c) AFDC; d) state-aid only.

[2] Panel survey involves multiple, longitudinal data collection in contrast to a cross sectional survey which represents a set of prevalence data at a specific, single point in time.

[3] In Round 3, 83 and 58% of the interviews were conducted by telephone in the national and state surveys respectively; in Round 4, similarly 88 and 65% of the interviews were done via telephone.

CHART 6

Health Status:
  conditions (morbidity), disability (bed days, loss of work and reduction of usual activities), activity limitations, functional limitations[4] (subsample of persons 17 years and older).
Access to Health Services:
  Barriers to care, unmet needs, usual source of care.
Utilization of Health Services (Medical, Hospital and Dental):
  By provider[5] per illness episode, visits and procedures; site of care with special emphasis on use of hospital emergency rooms and outpatient departments[6] and reasons for selecting these sites.
Use of Health Care Supplies:
  Prescribed medicine, non-prescribed, other medical (i.e., eyeglasses, orthopedic equipment, hearing aids, diabetic items, ambulance services).
Health Care Charges:
  Total charge per episode or flat fee per series[7].
Sources of Payment:
  Amount of payment by source, out of pocket expenditures.
Health Insurance Coverage:
  Extent, premium costs, Medicaid eligibility and beneficiary characteristics with an emphasis on whether individual was subject to Medicaid "spend down" rules; reasons for no coverage when relevant.

Administrative Survey

Medicaid:
  Periods of eligibility and aid category (national and state sample), claims data and provider data (state sample only) including type of claim, recipient characteristics, services received, total charge, amount Medicaid paid and amount paid by other sources.
Medicare:
  Services, charges, amount paid per episode of illness and per year (national and state Medicaid samples).

---

[4] Based on Stewart et. al. *Conceptualization and Measurement of Health Habits for Adults in the Health Insurance Study.* Vol. 11, Physical Health in Terms of Functioning. (Contract No. R - 1987/2 - HEW.) Santa Monica, California: The Rand Corporation, 1978.

[5] Chiropractors, speech therapists, faith healers, psychologists, nurses, medical and osteopathic doctors.

[6] All visits to separate clinics were recorded as separate visits even if made on same day at same institution.

[7] Flat fees were prorated among services rendered.

References:

National Center for Health Statistics, Bonham, G.S. *Procedures and Questionnaires of the National Medical Care Utilization and Expenditure Survey.* Series A, Methodological Report No. 1. (DHHS Pub. No. 83-20001) Washington, D.C.: U.S. GPO, March, 1983.

Dobson, A., Scharff, J., and Corder, L. Six Months of Medicaid Data: A Summary from the National Medical Care Utilization and Expenditure Survey. *Health Care Financing Review.* 4: 3: 115-121, March, 1983.

CHART 7

SURVEY	POPULATION BASE	DATA TYPE
National Ambulatory Medical Care Survey (NAMCS)	Annual, multi-stage national probability sample of office based physician practices[1] and a randomly assigned seven (7) day period of visits from which a systematic random sample of visits is selected[2]. Combined 1980-1981 samples included 5,805 physicians of which 1,124 were ineligible when screened; of the 4,681 eligible physicians, 3,676 or 78.5% responded.	Encounter data (filled out on a standardized patient record form) per visit. Statistics are presented on provision and use of services and trend data 1975—most recent survey is presented; physician specialty profile records (e.g., pediatrics, internal medicine, general surgery); reports describing selected diagnoses and specific age-sex groups are available as part of Series 13, Vital and Health Statistics (e.g., drug utilization in practice).
National Ambulatory Medical Care Complement Survey (1980)	Multi-stage, stratified probability sample of non "office-based" physician practices sampled by professional grouping (e.g., federally employed, teaching, pathology). Eligibility based on providing any direct patient care in the following locations: private offices; non-hospital based free standing clinics; groups or partnerships, Kaiser, Mayo Clinics, neighborhood health centers, and non-family planning privately operated clinics. Locations out of scope included ERs, hospital outpatient departments, college or university infirmaries, industrial outpatient facilities, family planning clinics, government operated clinics.	Encounter data (same as NAMCS) used to measure volume and characteristics of ambulatory patient office visits made to physicians who see patients not as their principal professional activity and in the settings listed (as a percentage of total estimated ambulatory volume to U.S. physicians). Data was inflated to provide national estimates.

SURVEY   POPULATION BASE   DATA TYPE

5,000 physicians were screened
by telephone in random sets of
500 to yield eligible physicians;
2,008 physicians were contacted
and on the basis of screening
procedures, 1,118 physicians
were ineligible leaving a final
sample of 328 physicians out of
which 245 completed forms according to NAMCS visit sampling procedures.

[1] Included in the sample are visits to physicians classified as being engaged in "office-based, patient care" by the American Medical or American Osteopathic Associations. Excluded are visits to physicians principally engaged in teaching, research or administration as well as telephone contacts and visits made outside the physician's office. Excluded from the physician universe are also those practicing in Alaska, Hawaii and those specializing in anesthesiology, pathology or radiology.

[2] A range of 20% sample for large practices to 100% sample of seven (7) days for small practices.

CHART 7

CONTENT CATEGORIES

Patient Characteristics:
  Age, sex, race, ethnicity (Hispanic, non-Hispanic).

Physician Characteristics:
  Professional identity (medicine, osteopathy); type of practice (solo/other).

Visit Characteristics:
  Major reason for visit:
    Acute problem, chronic problem, routine; flare-up; post-surgery/post-injury; non-illness care.

Patient Complaints (in own words)

Specific Reason for Visit:
  Since 1980, the Reason for Visit Classification for Ambulatory Care has been used which provides an extensive listing by reason and symptom.

Accidental Injury or Product Related Illness:
  Agents of injury or illness and location by home/work other.

Principal Diagnosis:
  16 categories from (ICD-9-CM)

Diagnostic Services:
  Limited exam and HX; general exam and HX; clinical lab test; x-ray; blood pressure check, pap test; ECG, vision test, endoscopy; mental status exam.

Therapeutic Services:
  Drugs (prescription/non-prescription); injection; immunization/desensitization; diet counseling; family planning; medical counseling; psychotherapy or therapeutic listening; physiotherapy; office survey.

Duration of Visit.

Prior Visit Status:
  New patient; old patient, new problem; old patient, old problem.

Referral Status:
  Referred by another physician/not referred by another physician.

Description of Visit:
  No follow-up planned; return at specified time; return as needed; telephone follow-up planned; referred by another physician; returned to referring physician; admit to hospital.

References:
U.S. Vital and Health Statistics. *The National Ambulatory Medical Care Survey, U.S., 1979 Summary.* Series 13, No. 66 (DHHS Pub. No. (PHS) 82-1727) Hyattsville, Maryland: Public Health Service, National Center for Health Statistics, September, 1982.

U.S. Vital and Health Statistics. *Patterns of Ambulatory Care in Obstetrics and Gynecology: The National Ambulatory Medical Care Survey.* January, 1980—December, 1981. Series 13. No. 76. Hyattsville, Maryland: Public Health Service, NCHS (DHHS Pub. No. (PHS) 84-1737). February, 1984.

U.S. Vital and Health Statistics. *The National Ambulatory Medical Care Complement Survey, U.S. 1980.* Series 13. No. 77. Hyattsville, Maryland: Public Health Service, NCHS. (DHHS Pub. No. (PHS) 84-1738). May, 1984.

CHART 8

SURVEY	POPULATION BASE	DATA TYPE
NIMH Epidemiologic Catchment Area Program (ECA) 1980-1982	Five Site Study: New Haven, Connecticut; Baltimore, Maryland; St. Louis, Missouri; Durham, North Carolina; Los Angeles, California.	In person interviews and year after re-interviews (Wave 1 and and II) to yield prevalence and annual incidence and health service use data.
	3,000 individuals each from unique households[1] selected from multi-stage probability sampling involving a mixture of random, systematic and/or cluster sampling (differed slightly per site). Completion rates[2] range from 75-80% eligible respondents;	Same instruments and standardized procedures used across sites including: use of highly trained, non-clinician interviewers; re-interview of a subsample by clinicians to measure validity and error; and computerized-algorithmic scoring of symptoms to arrive at DSM-III diagnoses. Structured interview was adapted from the Renard Diagnostic Interview[4].
	500 institutionalized individuals residing in long term hospitals, prisons and nursing homes; institutions both within and outside of immediate catchment area were sampled.	For the small number of individuals unable to complete interviews, a proxy informant interview was conducted to obtain maximum amount of comparable diagnostic and service use data.
	Total sample approximates 20,000 individuals; 60% female[3]. Oversampling occurred for special populations of interest: elderly, Black, Hispanic; oversampling methodology was different by site.	

[1] Household Surveys include currently resident household members *and* those temporarily in "non-institutionalized group quarters," i.e., acute care hospitals, dormitories, hotels, barracks, half-way houses and jails.

[2] Completion rates are computed by dividing the number of completed interviews by the entire number of eligible respondents after eliminating vacant households and non-household addresses.

[3] The higher female rate of response was due to women's increased longevity and the fact that men are more difficult to locate for interviews.

[4] Helzer, J.E., Robins L.N., Croughan J.L., Welner, A. Renard Diagnostic Interview: Its reliability and procedural validity with physicians and lay interviewers. *Arch. General Psychiatry*, 38: 393-398, 1981.

CHART 8
SURVEY   *POPULATION BASE*   *DATA TYPE*

Statistical adjustments corrected
for low completion rates in some
subgroups[5].

CONTENT CATEGORIES

Sociodemographic Characteristics.

Administration of the NIMH Diagnostic Interview Schedule (DSM-III):

Presence, duration and severity of individual symptoms (i.e., has the symptom ever occurred and what has been/is the degree to which it limits activity; whether a physician or other professional has been consulted; whether medication has been taken to treat it; and whether every recurrence was explained by medical illness, alcohol or other drug intake.)

Use of health, specialty mental health and other human services over the lifetime and over the year prior to interview.

OVERALL ANALYTIC OBJECTIVES

1. To acquire prevalence rates of specific mental disorders as defined (more uniformly) by DSM-III;

2. To establish combined community resident and institutionalized population rates to represent the total population;

3. Identification of the treated and untreated prevalence rates of both the severe mental disorders, found in higher concentrations in institutions, as well as the less severe disorders found more frequently in the community;

4. To establish longitudinal data on the course of specific mental disorders in terms of new case onset (incidence), recurrence or remission rates;

5. Data on the use, by persons with specific mental disorders, not only of specialty mental health services, but also of the entire range of general medical and other human services that compose the U.S. de facto mental health services system including analysis of factors influencing use of services;

6. The utility of DSM-III diagnostic categories as currently defined, to discriminate useful subgroups in both untreated and treated populations—a test of the DSM-III hypothesis that its operational criteria are useful discriminators;

7. Production of epidemiologically derived data on the correlation of disorders (i.e., factors influencing development and continuance of disorders);

8. Demonstration that replicable results can be obtained from multiple psychiatric epidemiology surveys when methods are standardized.

---

[5] Post stratification weights were computed to inflate the influence of age-race-sex groups with low response rates so that the sample percentages in a given age-sex-race group were equivalent to the 1980 Census for the catchment area.

CHART 9
SURVEY
Rand Health
Insurance Experi-
ment

POPULATION BASE

2,750 families[1] (8,000 individuals) from six sites: Dayton, Ohio; Seattle, Washington; Fitchburg, Massachusetts; Franklin County, Massachusetts; Charleston, South Carolina; Georgetown County, South Carolina.

70% participating for three years, 30% participating for five years; low income families were over-sampled.

Unbiased allocation—assignment model was used for 16 different experimental health insurance plans.[2]

DATA TYPE

Self administered medical history questionnaires (used at enrollment and exit).

Medical screening examination—clinical/lab findings (60% of enrollees at enrollment, 100% at exit).

Biweekly health use reports (not described below).

Provider claims data (not described below).

Tracer disease reports presenting measurement methods and prevalence findings.

CONTENT CATEGORIES

Demographic and Socioeconomic Variables (baseline interview).

Medical History Questionnaire

Children 0-4, 5-13 (separate forms-items distinct for.0-4 vs. 5-13 are indicated below)
 Form A: General Functioning and Health Habits:

> Height and weight
>
> Developmental milestones and satisfaction with general habits—eating, sleeping, bowel and advice from physicians concerning these
>
> General health status
>
> Health concern
>
> Functional limitations including activity limitations
>
> Health perceptions
>
> Fluorides
>
> Diet with limited food frequencies and 24 hour recall

---

[1] Ineligibles: persons mainly heads of households 61 years of age and older at time of enrollment; military; institutionalized; Medicare eligibles.

[2] Overall analytic objectives of this study primarily relate to the effect of differing health insurance coverage, experimentally contrived, on health status, use and costs of health services. In the context of this inquiry, which will not be described herein, much data are available on health conditions, health status, use of and attitudes about medical care and valuable instruments are available for adaptation.

Form A (0-4, 5-13 continued)

   Immunizations
   Safety
   Symptoms list
   Medicine taken
   Learning (5-13)
   Getting along (5-13)
   General well being (5-13)
   Behavior problems (5-13)

Form B (Disease-Specific):

   Colds (0-4)
   Ear Infections
   Eczema
   Allergic skin rash
   Anemia
   Lead poisoning
   Cancer
   Fever convulsions
   Epilepsy
   Convulsions
   Tonsils
   Adenoids
   Missing limbs
   Drug allergy
   Other
   Medical appliances
   Anticipated future health expenses
   Transportation to health
   Fluoride treatment
   Teeth and gums (5-13)
   Eyesight and hearing (5-13)
   Asthma, hay fever, other plant allergies (5-13)
   Kidney, bladder, urine infection (5-13)
   Bedwetting (5-13)

Adults 14 + :

Form A:

   Height and weight
   General health
   Health worry
   Functional and activity limitations

   Eating habits, diet including limited food frequency and 24 hour recall

   Weight problems
   Sleep and exercise
   Safety
   Smoking
   Drinking

General well being (mental health)
Social activities
Life events
Symptoms
Health perceptions
Medical opinions (attitudes)
Satisfaction with medical care
Opinions about effects of health care
Dental care
Medicine taken

Form B:

Eyesight
Glaucoma
Hearing
Hay fever or other plant allergies
Teeth and gums
Pimples or acne
Goiter or thyroid trouble
Joint problems
Cardiovascular symptoms and conditions
Chronic lung or bronchial conditions
TB
Stomach pain and problems
Kidney, bladder, urine infections
Kidney disease
Cholesterol
Anemia
Diabetes symptoms, conditions
Cancer
Hemorrhoids, piles
Hernia
Varicose veins
Condition related physical and activity limitations
Missing limbs
Drug use (sleeping pills, tranquilizers, sedatives)
Surgery

Reproductive health and female use of preventive screening procedures
Other illnesses
Medical care attitudes and advice received
Medical appliances
Future health expenses
Transportation to medical care
Fluoride treatment

Medical Screening Exam:

Disease Condition	Screening Test	Population
Acne	Facial skin graph	≥ 14 with relevant condition
Alcoholism and Liver Disease	Blood alcohol level Total Bilirubin SGOT	≥ 14 + (all)
		≥ 6 months of age (all)
Anemia	HCT Hemoglobin Mean Corpuscular Volume	
Cardiovascular	ECG	≥ 25 yr. except pregnant women ≥ 14 with related complaint
	Chest x-ray	Men ≥ 30; Women ≥ 35 ≥ 14 with relevant complaint
	Serum cholesterol	≥ 14 (all)
Abnormal Child Growth/Development	Head circumference	0-2 yrs.
	Length/height	0-2 yrs.
	Weight	3 mos.–5 yrs.
	Denver developmentals	3 mos.–5 yrs.
Dental Disorders	Decayed-missing-filled index	≥ 3 (all)
	Gross decay index	≥ 3 (all)
	Simplified oral hygiene index	≥ 3 (all)
	Periodontal index	≥ 14 (all)
Diabetes	2 hr. Post-load Glucose	≥ 14 except diabetics
Drug Usage	Urine screen	≥ 14 (all)
Glaucoma	Tonometry	≥ 40 (all)
Hearing Disorders	Pure tone threshold Audiometry	≥ 4 (all)
	Tympanometry	≥ 4 except those with recent ear surgery
Hypertension	Sitting blood pressure	≥ 14 (all)
	Standing blood pressure	For those on anti-hypertensive medication
Joint Problems	50 foot walk; grip strength; joint size; rheumatoid factor hand x-ray	≥ 14 with relevant complaint
Gout	Uric acid	≥ 14 (all)
Kidney Disease	BUN/Creatinine	≥ 14 (all)
	Dipstick blood and protein	Women 6 Men 14
	Microscopic UA	Men 14
	Urine culture	Women 6

Lead Poisoning	Blood lead level	1 yr.–5 yrs.
Obesity	Height, weight, body mass index	≥ 2 (all)
Respiratory Problems	Spirometry	≥ 14 (all)
	Chest x-ray	≥ 25 except pregnant women
		≥ 14 with relevant history
TB	"	"
Thyroid Disease	T4	≥ 14 (all)
	T3 uptake	Pregnant women,
	T7	women on birth control pills or taking thyroid medication
Tonsil Disease	Tonsil exam	0–19 yrs.
Ulcer, Stomach Pain	Serum pepsinogen	≥ 14 (all)
	Blood type	
	Saliva for secretor status	
	Urine pepsinogen	
Varicose Veins	Exam	Women ≥ 20 and Men ≥ 14 with relevant condition
Visual Disorder	Near, Far vision	≥ 3 (all)
	Pinhole acuity correction	
	Motility	
	TNO Stereocopic Test	3 yrs.–14 yrs.
Immunization Status	Serum antibody	1 yr.–10 yrs.

517

Tracer Reports:

Acne
Anemia
Angina Pectoris/selected ECG abnormalities
Asthma
Chronic airway obstruction and shortness of breath
Congestive heart failure
Convulsions
Dental conditions
Diabetes mellitus
Eczema
Hay fever
Hearing disorders
Hemorrhoids
Hernia
Hypercholesterolemia
Hypertension
Hyperthyroidism and Hypothyroidism
Joint disorders
Otitis Media
Stomach pain and peptic ulcer
Urinary tract infection
Varicose veins
Vision disabilities

References:

Personal communication, Caren Kumberg and Dr. Robert H. Brook, Rand Corporation, April, 1985.

Smith L.S., et al. *The Health Insurance Study Screening Examination Procedures Manual* (R-2101-HEW) Santa Monica, California: The Rand Corporation, September, 1978.

Medical History Questionnaire Forms.

Berman D.M., et al. Conceptualization and Measurement of Physiologic Health for Adults, Vol. 4. *Angina Pectoris* (R 2262-4-HHS) Santa Monica, California: The Rand Corporation, June, 1981.

CHAPTER 65

Health Promotion and Disease Prevention Resources for COPC Providers

Angela D. Mickalide, Ph.D.

Locating sources of accurate and timely patient education materials can be a challenging task. To simplify this search, a resource guide for practitioners interested in becoming involved in health promotion and disease prevention activities has been compiled. The following listing of clearinghouses, professional organizations, projects, and references is intended to be of assistance to community-oriented primary care providers.

CLEARINGHOUSES

The Federal Government operates various clearinghouses and information centers for consumers and health professionals. Provision of publications, referrals, and responses to inquiries are encompassed within services offered. Descriptions of selected health information clearinghouses and information centers excerpted from the National Health Information clearinghouse *Healthfinder* are presented below.

The *National Clearinghouse for Alcohol Information*, P.O. Box 2345, Rockville, Maryland 20852; (301) 468-2600, gathers and disseminates current information on alcohol-related subjects, responds to

requests from the public as well as from health professionals, and prepares and distributes bibliographies on topics relating to alcohol.

The *Cancer Information Clearinghouse*, National Cancer Institute, Office of Cancer Communications, Building 31, Room 10A-18, 9000 Rockville Pike, Bethesda, Maryland 20892; (301) 496-4070, collects information on public and patient education materials and disseminates it to organizations and health care professionals.

The *Office of Cancer Communications*, National Cancer Institute, Cancer Information Service, Building 31, Room 10A-18, 9000 Rockville Pike, Bethesda, Maryland 20892; (301) 496-5583, answers requests for cancer information from patients and the general public. A toll-free telephone number (800 4 CANCER) is available.

The *Consumer Information Center*, Pueblo, Colorado 81009; (202) 566-1794, distributes consumer publications on topics such as children, food and nutrition, health, exercise and weight control. The Consumer Information Catalog is available free from the Center and must be used to identify publications being requested.

The *National Health Information Clearinghouse*, P. O. Box 1133, Washington, D.C. 20013; (703) 522-2590 (in Virginia); (800) 336-4707, is a service of the Office of Disease Prevention and Health Promotion. The NHIC helps the public locate health information through identification of health information resources and an inquiry and referral system. Health questions are referred to appropriate health resources that in turn respond directly to inquirers. In addition, NHIC prepares a series of resource lists and fact sheets *(Healthfinders)* on a variety of health topics. Current available titles are listed in Table 1.

Three other relevant resources available through the NHIC are:

■ *Office of Disease Prevention and Health Promotion Publications List*

■ Locating Funds for Health Promotion

■ DHHS Nutrition Publications for Consumers: A Selected Annotated Bibliography.

The *High Blood Pressure Information Center*, 120/80 National Institutes of Health, Bethesda, Maryland 20892; (301) 496-1809, provides information on the detection, diagnosis, and management of high blood pressure to consumers and health professionals.

The *National Highway Traffic Safety Administration*, NES-11 HL, U.S. Department of Transportation, 400 7th Street, S.W., Washington, D.C. 20590; (202) 426-0123, works to reduce highway traffic deaths and injuries. The agency publishes a variety of safety information brochures, conducts public education programs to promote the use of safety belts and child safety seats, and informs the public of the hazards of drunk driving. A toll-free hotline (800-424-9393) is available for consumer complaints on auto safety and for requests for information on manufacturing flaws and recalls.

TABLE 1. Recent *Healthfinders* available from the National Health Information Clearinghouse (NHIC)

Selected Federal Health Information Clearinghouses and Information Centers (December 1985)

Electronic Bulletin Boards for Health Information (October 1985)

Financing Personal Health Care (May 1985)

Health Fairs (September 1984)

Health Promotion Software (October 1984)

Health Risk Appraisals (May 1985)

Health Statistics (January 1985)

Herpes Information Resources (September 1984)

Home Health Care (December 1985)

Indochinese Health Information Resources (November 1984)

Locating Audiovisual Materials (July 1984)

Medications: Sources of Information (January 1985)

National Health Observances 1986 (December 1985)

Posters for Health Promotion (November 1985)

Spanish Language Health Information Materials (June 1985)

Stress Information Resources (August 1984)

Toll-Free Telephone Numbers (May 1985)

Vitamins (February 1985)

Weight Control (November 1985)

The *National Injury Information Clearinghouse*, 5401 Westbard Avenue, Room 625, Washington, D.C. 20207; (301) 492-6424, collects and disseminates injury data and information relating to the causes and prevention of death, injury, and illness associated with consumer products. Requests for general safety information are referred to the Consumer Product Safety Commission.

The *Project for Patient Education in Family Practice*, S.S.M. Family Medicine Center, 2900 Baltimore, Suite 400, Kansas City, Mo. 64108; (800) 821-6671. maintains a Patient Education Library of approximately 50,000 books, pamphlets, and leaflets addressing the most common complaints encountered by primary care physicians. Materials are available for three levels of patient education: basic, intermediate, and advanced. A comprehensive resource library on health and nutrition fraud is also available for patients and health professionals.

The *Prevention Education Resource Center*, Association of Teachers of Preventive Medicine, 1030 15th Street, N.W. Suite 1020, Washington, D.C. 20005; (202) 682-1698, is an outgrowth of the ATPM/CEDH Curriculum Development Project, funded by the W. K. Kellogg Foundation. Currently in early stages of development, the Center will provide information on materials, resources, and program activities to improve and expand the teaching of preventive medicine in undergraduate, graduate, and continuing medical and nursing education.

The *President's Council on Physical Fitness and Sports*, 450 5th Street N.W., Suite 7103, Washington, D.C.; (202) 272-3430, conducts a public service advertising program and cooperates with governmental and private groups to promote the development of physical fitness leadership, facilities, and programs. It also produces informational materials on exercise, school physical education programs, sports, and physical fitness for youth, adults, and the elderly.

The *National Clearinghouse for Primary Care Information*, 8201 Greensboro Drive, Suite 600, McLean, Va. 22102; (703) 821-8955, provides information services to support the planning, development, and delivery of ambulatory health care to urban and rural areas where there are shortages of medical personnel and services. Although the Clearinghouse will respond to public inquiries, its primary audience is health care providers who work in community health centers.

The *Office on Smoking and Health*, Technical Information Center, Park Building, Room 1-10, 5600 Fishers Lane, Rockville, Md. 20857; (301) 443-1690, offers bibliographic and reference services to researchers and others, and publishes and distributes a number of publications in the field of smoking.

PROFESSIONAL ORGANIZATIONS

COPC providers may augment their health promotion/disease prevention knowledge and skills through membership in various professional organizations. Associations whose publications, conferences, and outreach efforts focus on preventive medicine are listed in the Appendix to this chapter. However, the listing is intended to be selective rather than exhaustive. Local chapters of several national associations should be contacted in addition to local and State health departments.

PROJECTS

Two national initiatives, one Federal and one academic, deserve special citation for their potential contribution to patient education in health promotion and disease prevention.

The U.S. Preventive Services Task Force

In 1984 the Department of Health and Human Services convened the U.S. Preventive Services Task Force composed of prominent researchers, clinicians and scholars to review the scientific basis of over 100 clinical preventive interventions and to develop a set of age- and sex-specific recommendations for the use of preventive services in clinical settings.

The U.S. Preventive Service Force consists of 21 senior level individuals from the research and health communities. They were selected for their contribution to knowledge in preventive services, not as representatives of particular organizations, associations, or institutions. The members, most of whom are physicians, represent a variety of disciplines including epidemiology, health economics, behavioral science, medical sociology, health education, nursing, osteopathic medicine, and allopathic medicine.

The U.S. Preventive Services Task Force is collaborating with the Task Force on the Periodic Health Examination to develop recommendations concerning history and physical assessment, laboratory and screening investigations, immunizations, and physician counseling of patients regarding behavioral risk factors (e.g., nutrition, exercise, smoking, substance abuse, stress management, injury control, contraception). The Task Force's final report will contain all of its recommendation together with an implementation guide discussing the behavioral and structural issues that influence the integration of preventive services into clinical settings.

Selected topics to be addressed in the implementation guide include: the impact of setting (solo practice versus group practice versus health maintenance organizations); the use of computerized medical records, flow sheets, and other curing systems; the role of nonphysician health care personnel in providing preventive services; physicians' skills in delivering health education and counseling; and reimbursement for preventive services. For further information, contact Angela D. Mickalide, Ph.D., Staff Coordinator, U.S. Preventive Services Task Force, Office of Disease Prevention and Health Promotion, 330 C Street, S.W., Washington, D. C. 20201, (202) 472-5370.

The Association of Teachers of Preventive Medicine (ATPM)/Center for Educational Development in Health (CEDH) Curriculum Development Project

An instructional system for teaching clinical health maintenance has been established through collaboration between ATPM and CEDH at Boston University, with support from the W. K. Kellogg Foundation. The instructional system was designed to facilitate attainment of specific competencies essential to the practice of clinical prevention. The objectives were identified in a study of physician performance conducted with the cooperation of the American College of Physicians, the American Academy of Family Physicians, the American Academy of Pediatrics, and the American College of Obstetricians and Gynecologists.

Key competencies include those needed to plan a practice-specific program for health maintenance, adapt the program to the needs of individual patients, carry out procedures for health and risk assessment, and implement selected modalities of intervention for risk reduction.

Portions of the instructional system have been extensively field tested in nursing and medical schools across the United States. The educational materials have been revised in the light of field test results and are now ready for wider dissemination. The 18-volume ($210.00) instructional system consists of three modules: The Epidemiologic Basic of Clinical Prevention, Management for Preventive Services, and Clinical Health Maintenance. The third module encompasses such preventive medicine issues as smoking, hypertension, nutritional aspects of cardiovascular disease, occupational health, breast cancer, and immunizations. The instructional system may be used as part of a comprehensive program for preclinical, clerkship, and residency training; in a less extensive but systematic approach involving multiple phases of the curriculum; or in a more limited way to enrich a small segment of the curriculum.

For further information, contact Hannelore Vanderschmidt, Ph.D., Director, ATPMF/CEDH Curriculum Development Project, Boston University, 67 Bay State Road, Boston, MA 02215, (617) 353-4528.

Selected List of Professional Organizations Offering Preventive Medicine Information Relevant to COPC

Alcoholics Anonymous World Services, P.O. Box 459, Grand Central Station, New York, NY 10163

Ambulatory Pediatrics Association, 1311A Dolley Madison Boulevard, Suite 3A, McLean, VA 22101

American Academy of Family Physicians, 1740 West 92nd Street, Kansas City, MO 64114

American Academy of Ophthalmology, P.O. Box 7424, 1833 Fillmore Street, San Francisco, CA 95819

American Academy of Pediatrics, 141 Northwest Point Road, P.O. Box 927, Elk Grove Village, IL 60007

American Alliance for Health, Physical Education, Recreation, and Dance, 1900 Association Drive, Reston, VA 22091

American Association of Public Health Dentistry, 10619 Jousting Lane, Richmond, VA 23235

American Association of Retired Persons, 1909 K Street, N.W., Washington, DC 20049

American Cancer Society, 90 Park Avenue, New York, NY 10016

American College of Cardiology, 9111 Old Georgetown Road, Bethesda, MD 20814

American College of Obstetricians and Gynecologists, 600 Maryland Avenue, S.W., Suite 300 East, Washington, DC 20024

American College of Physicians, 4200 Pine Street, Philadelphia, PA 19104

American College of Preventive Medicine, 1015 15th Street, N.W., Suite 403, Washington, DC 20005

American College of Public Health Physicians, Nassau County Health Department, 240 Old Country Road, Mineola, Long Island, NY 11501

American Council on Life Insurance/Health, Insurance Association of America, 1850 K Street, N.W., Washington, DC 20006

American Dental Association, 211 E. Chicago Avenue, Chicago, IL 60611

American Diabetes Association, 2 Park Avenue, New York, NY 10016

American Dietetic Association, 430 North Michigan Avenue, Chicago, IL 60611

American Health Foundation, 320 E. 43rd Street, New York, NY 10017

American Heart Association, National Center, 7320 Greenville Avenue, Dallas, TX 75231

American Hospital Association, Center for Health Promotion, 840 North Lakeshore Drive, Chicago, IL 60611

American Kidney Fund, 7315 Wisconsin Avenue, Suite 203-E, Bethesda, MD 20814

American Lung Association, 1740 Broadway, New York, NY 10019

American Medical Association, 535 North Dearborn Street, Chicago, IL 60610

American Nurses' Association, 2420 Pershing Road, Kansas City, MO 64108

American Optometric Association, 243 N. Lindberg Boulevard, St. Louis, MO 63141

American Osteopathic Association, 212 E. Ohio Street, Chicago, IL 60611

American Pharmaceutical Association, 2215 Constitution Avenue, N.W., Washington, DC 20037

American Podiatry Association, 20 Chevy Chase Circle, N.W., Washington, DC 20015

American Psychiatric Association, 1400 K Street, N.W., Washington, DC 20009

American Public Health Association, 1015 15th Street, N.W., Washington, DC 20005

American Red Cross, National Headquarters, Health Services, 17th and D Streets, N.W., Washington, DC 20006

American School Health Association, P.O. Box 708, Kent, OH 44240

American Society of Allied Health Professionals, 1101 Connecticut Avenue, N.W., Suite 700, Washington, DC 20036

American Society of Internal Medicine, 1101 Vermont Avenue, N.W., Suite 500, Washington, DC 20005

Arthritis Foundation, 1314 Spring Street, N.W., Atlanta, GA 30309

Association for the Advancement of Health Education, 1900 Association Drive, Reston, VA 22091

Association of State and Territorial Health Officials, 1311A Dolley Madison Boulevard, Suite 3A, McLean, VA 22101

Association of Teachers of Preventive Medicine, 1030 15th Street, N.W., Suite, 1020, Washington, DC 20005

Asthma and Allergy Foundation of America, 1835 K Street, N.W., Suite P900, Washington, DC 20006

Center for Health Education, Inc., Coggins Building, 1204 Maryland Avenue, Baltimore, MD 21201

Coalition of Hispanic Mental Health and Human Services Organizations, 1030 15th St., N.W., Suite 1053, Washington, DC 20005

Doctors Ought to Care, HH-101, Medical College of Georgia, Augusta, GA 30912

National Center for Health Education, 30 East 29th Street, New York, NY 10016

National Council on Patient Information and Education, 1625 I Street, N.W., Suite 1010, Washington, DC 20006

National Medical Association, 1012 10th Street, N.W., Washington, DC 20001

Society of Behavioral Medicine, P.O. Box 8530, University Station, Knoxville, TN 37996

Society of Prospective Medicine, 1101 Connecticut Avenue, N.W., Suite 700, Washington, DC 20036

Society for Public Health Education, 703 Market Street, Suite 535, San Francisco, CA 94103

Society for Research and Education in Primary Care Internal Medicine, 4200 Pine Street, Philadelphia, PA 19104

Society of Teachers of Family Medicine, 1740 West 92nd Street, Kansas City, MO 64114

CHAPTER 66

Community-Oriented
Primary Care:
An Annotated Bibliography

Ronald E. Voorhees, M.D.

Community-oriented primary care (COPC) encompasses the fields of epidemiology, primary care, and community medicine, as well as drawing on the understanding of communities and health services that has been gained through study and experience in the social sciences and education. It is a wide-ranging field, and the literature of COPC is correspondingly wide-ranging. While it is necessary and desirable for COPC practitioners to coordinate efforts with experts in these areas, it is also beneficial for health care providers at all levels to gain an understanding of these fields as well. It is in this spirit that this annotated bibliography is offered.

Since this volume is produced with the primary care practitioner in mind, this brief guide to the literature of and about COPC is designed to serve three primary objectives. First, writings are given that provide a conceptual base for planning and implementing COPC in an existing or planned practice setting. Articles and books are presented that illustrate the historical development of the COPC concept, as well as those describing the current state of development and those pointing out possible directions for the future. Second, the chapter attempts to provide

an access point to the tools and resources needed to carry out COPC projects. Resources available to assist the practitioner in an ongoing process of community participation, planning interventions, and evaluating those interventions are presented.

Third, a selection of examples of projects illustrating elements of COPC is included to provide an idea of the scope of ongoing developments.

Due to the broad scope of literature that is relevant to COPC, this is by no means an exhaustive bibliography. An attempt has been made to provide a sense of the foundations of COPC and to open new doors for inquiries into expanding its practice. References in this chapter provide a broad introduction to the field; references for more specific areas of interest are found in the other chapters of the book.

FUNDAMENTAL WRITINGS ON COMMUNITY-ORIENTED PRIMARY CARE

The works listed here are important in developing the concepts that encompass the current theoretical framework and practice of COPC.

Connor, E., and Mullan, F. **Community-Oriented Primary Care—New Directions for Health Services Delivery**, National Academy Press, 1983. This collection contains the papers presented at the first major conference on COPC in the United States, convened by the Institute of Medicine in 1982. The proceedings bring together currents in medical practice, community health, and medical education to present a coherent vision of a new format for the practice of primary medical care. Both theoretical issues and practical applications are presented. Together with the 1984 IOM study, the book provides a cogent view of recent developments toward implementing COPC in the United States.

Community Oriented Primary Care - A Practical Assessment (vol. 1); and Case Studies (vol. 2), Institute of Medicine Report, National Academy of Science Press, April 1984. This two-volume work sets out an operational model for COPC from an observational study of seven existing practices that incorporate elements of COPC. (All of the sites are described in detail in volume two.) The study attempts to synthesize what is known regarding the operations, costs and health impacts of COPC as currently practiced. The study concludes that a fully operational model does not yet exist in the United States, but that one is needed in order to study COPC's potential impact and costs. The need for practical information for practitioners who wish to move toward COPC is expressed. The case studies are a very useful exposition of the variety of projects and practices that have been developed.

Kark, S.L., **The Practice of Community Oriented Primary Health Care**, Appleton-Century-Crofts, 1981. This is a major work in the develop-

ment of COPC as a discipline. The book discusses the nature of community health care, including curative and preventive services, and relates them to the functions of the health care team. A chapter on community diagnosis and health surveillance addresses the determinants of health and quantitative methods for setting priorities for programs. The roles of a wide range of health workers are considered, and examples of COPC practice are given for projects carried out in urban and rural areas in maternal and child health and cardiovascular risk factor reduction. Major contributions have been special issues of the **Israel Journal of Medical Sciences** and **Public Health Reports**, which lay a firm theoretical and practical groundwork for what is there termed community-oriented primary health care (COPHC). Some of the individual articles are included separately in the bibliography, but articles that were left out may also be of value; browsing these issues is a useful endeavor.

Kark, S., and Abramson, J. H. (eds.). Community Focused Health Care, **Israel Journal of Medical Sciences, 17(2-3)**, February-March, 1981. Establishes a model for COPC, developing relationships of epidemiology and primary care; articles provide specific approaches that were developed in Israel to meet community-defined needs.

Abramson, J.H. et al. (eds.). Trends in primary health care: A joint South-African-Israel symposium, **Israel Journal of Medical Sciences,** 19(8), August, 1983. A variety of articles further define current and future trends in primary health care services, including the integration of primary and community health services, uses of epidemiology in primary care, and other important aspects of community-oriented care. Includes a number of examples of project design and evaluation.

Second Binational Symposium: United States-Israel—Papers on the role of epidemiology in assessment of need, program development, and resource allocation. **Public Health Reports,** 99(5); 1984. A very strong collection covering a variety of practical and policy-related issues in the development of community-oriented care.

THE HISTORICAL AND CONCEPTUAL BASIS OF COMMUNITY-ORIENTED PRIMARY CARE

Since the concepts of community-oriented care arose in response to specific historical situations, it is artificial to separate these two topics. They are presented here as a continuum of thought that has led to the current conceptualization of COPC.

Pickles, William N., **Epidemiology in Country Practice**, John Wright, 1939. The classic writings of an English country physician who realized that his community general practice was an ideal setting for epidemiologic investigation that would benefit his practice as well as contributing to medical knowledge.

Kark, Sidney L., **A Practice of Social Medicine**. E. & S. Livingstone, 1962. Describes the health care studies and experiments of the Karks in South Africa, including descriptions of a variety of community health services and epidemiological studies of malnutrition among schoolchildren.

Seipp, Conrad, ed., **Health Care for the Community: The Collected Papers of Dr. John B. Grant**, Johns Hopkins Press, 1963. From the preface by Cecil Sheps, "The student will find a logical, rational, holistic discussion of the major elements . . . of health services . . . the veteran of program development and administration will find a systematic reorder-

ing of many of the problems and pitfalls . . . bringing them into focus . . . [and] leading directly to corrective action." The book is a collection of Dr. Grant's writings on the nature of health services in the United States and China.

Geiger, H.J., The Neighborhood Health Center. **Archives of Environmental Health** 14:912, 1967. Discusses the relationship of the community health center to the health system as a whole in terms of both professional and community orientations, affirming the CHC as the "hub" of the system from the community viewpoint. Explores the constraints and opportunities of neighborhood health clinics in improving the health of marginal populations.

The Margaret S. Brogden Memorial Symposium, **The Johns Hopkins University Medical Journal** 124(5):239 (1969). This symposium provided a forum for raising issues related to the interaction of the health system, particularly the university health center, and the community. Papers covered a wide range of issues concerning the roles of faculties, students, and hospitals in community health, and on future directions in medical care.

Deuschle, K.W., Community Oriented Primary Care—Lessons learned in three decades, in Connor and Mullan, eds., *op. cit.*, p. 6. Four diverse settings are described that illustrate elements of COPC, and the common features are discussed, namely community participation, the bridging of cultural differences, the epidemiologic assessment of health status, and the use of local community health workers.

Preventive and Community Medicine in Primary Care, Fogarty International Center, NIH, Series on the

Teaching of Preventive Medicine, Vol. 5 (USDHEW, PHS, NIH, DHEW Publ. (NIH) 76-879, USGPO #017-053-000051-5). Proceedings of a conference in cooperation with the Association of Teachers of Preventive Medicine on developing skills and knowledge of community and preventive medicine for family physicians. Papers discuss developing competency-based objectives in preventive medicine for family physicians and residents, and preventive strategies in primary care.

Lipkin, Mack, Jr., and William A. Lybrand, eds., **Population-Based Medicine**. Praeger, 1982. Papers presented at a Rockefeller Institute/Institute of Medicine conference in Italy in 1980. Discusses the need and presents strategies for regaining a population-based perspective in medicine.

Haggerty, Robert J., Klaus J. Roghmann, and Ivan B. Pless, **Child Health and the Community**. John Wiley & Sons, 1975. A community orientation for guided research and program development for working toward a greater orientation to health for all children. Discusses the identification of unmet health needs and the organization of services to meet them. Contains sections on integrating individual health behaviors and family and community functioning with the utilization of health services. Describes the impact of specific Federal and State legislation on health services in the functioning of a neighborhood health center. A very thorough and well-organized approach.

Kark, S.L., and J.H. Abramson, Community Oriented Primary Care— Meaning and Scope. In: Connor and Mullan, *op. cit.*, p. 21 (1983). A

distillation of the broad experience of these two authors. This paper expands on and points the way to a new form of medical practice: "In our view what is needed is a change in orientation of responsibility for care of all the people." They lay out the essential features of COPC·that have been expanded upon in this book, pointing out the features that set COPC apart and beyond primary care.

Geiger, H.J., The Meaning of Community Oriented Primary Care in the American Context. In: Connor and Mullan, *op. cit.*, p. 60, (1983). Dr. Geiger addresses six common fallacies widely held about what COPC really involves, and stresses the need for actions to be taken that involve the community and the health team. He raises the question of whether the wide-ranging health impact of community health centers might have been due to their elements of COPC, and discusses some of the constraints facing COPC in the present political situation.

Kark, S.L., and E. Kark, An Alternative Strategy in Community Health Care: Community Oriented Primary Health Care, **Israel Journal of Medical Science**, 19(8):707, 1983. This paper points out the lack of cooperation between public health and medical care and the need to close this gap at the primary care level, involving those groups that have "intimate face-to-face association and cooperation," and argues that the main functional unit of the health system should be primary care, not hospital-based care. Discusses epidemiologically-initiated community projects in childhood growth and development and the Community Syndrome of Hypertension,

Atherosclerotic diseases, and Diabetes (CHAD).

Deuschle, K.W., and S.J. Bosch, The Community Medicine-Primary Care Connection. **Israel Journal of Medical Science**, 17(2-3):86, 1981. In describing the East Harlem (NYC) Neighborhood Health Center, the article provides a conceptual base for the interaction of population-based community medicine and individually-based primary care.

Several articles have appeared in the medical literature describing the development of COPC in the United States and advocating its further implementation:

Mullan, F., Community-oriented primary care: An agenda for the 80's. **New England Journal of Medicine**, 30:1076 (Oct. 21, 1982). Urges the cooperation of the community and primary care movements to form a system of care that is in "constant awareness . . . of the overall problems of the community."

Madison, D.L., The case for community-oriented primary care, **Journal of the American Medical Association** 249(10:1279, (3/11/83).

Nutting, P., Community-oriented primary care: A promising innovation in primary care. **Public Health Reports** 100(1):3, 1985.

Nutting, P., Community-oriented primary care—a status report. **Journal of the American Medical Association**, 253: 1763, 1985.

Rogers, David E., Community-Oriented Primary Care. **Journal of the American Medical Association**, 248: 1622, 1982. A frank discussion of the barriers presented by the current policies and priorities within the health system and other obstacles that must be overcome in order to realize the full potential of COPC.

Nutting, P.A., Community-oriented primary care: An integrated model for practice, research and education. **American Journal of Preventive Medicine**, 2(2) 1986 (in press). Presents an operational definition and criteria for quantifying the implementation of COPC methodologies within a primary care practice. Discusses the need for data to evaluate the costs associated with (and perhaps saved by) COPC.

Nutting, P.A., Community-oriented primary care: an examination of the United States experience. **American Journal of Public Health**, 76:279, 1986.

EPIDEMIOLOGY IN PRIMARY CARE

The application of epidemiology in guiding and evaluating interventions at the primary care level presents a different set of problems than when applied in experimental studies. A sampling of books and articles is presented here that directly approach these problems.

Kark, S.L., **Epidemiology and Community Medicine**, Appleton-Century-Crofts, 1974. A thorough text on the conceptual and operational basis of community health, its appraisals and intervention. Section 5 establishes the common ground of community medicine and primary health care, and gives a case history of the development of the health practice in Jerusalem that was developed using community-oriented planning. Specific approaches are given in applying COPC principles to problems of infectious diseases, homebound patients, perinatal care, and the CHAD project.

Dever, G.E.A., **Community Health Analysis—A Holistic Approach**, Aspen Systems Corp., 1980 (400 pp.). A courageous effort to integrate a wide spectrum of influences into an operational framework for the consideration of community medicine. Begins by considering models of health beliefs and disease causation, then joins this with planning and evaluation techniques, basic statistical and epidemiologic methods, and health status indicators. It is conceptual rather than methodological and is thus good as an entry level book, but also contains a moderate level of useful detail. Chapter 8 develops methods for determining health service areas and performing accessibility analysis. The book attempts to minimize the effects of the author's statement that "health must be lived, and can only in small part be delivered."

Bauman, K.E., **Research Methods for Community Health and Welfare—An Introduction**. Oxford University Press, 1980. Written for "non-researchers," this book is designed to provide the knowledge base to evaluate studies that have been carried out, increase communication between "users and doers" of research, and increase the use of research in decisionmaking. It provides an introduction to causal thinking and covers study designs for interventional and noninterventional trials.

Mullan, F., Community-oriented primary care: Epidemiology's role in the future of primary care, **Public Health Reports**, 99(5):442, 1984. Describes the potential of COPC for improving the effectiveness and efficiency of medical practice, and points out the need for the application of clinical epidemiologic approaches to primary care in order to close the feedback loop from the community diagnosis to the functioning of the practice.

Abramson, J.H., Application of epidemiology in community oriented primary care, **Public Health Reports**, 99(5):437, 1984. Describes the special focus of epidemiology in COPC;

it is customized, practical information that is needed to address common problems in order to benefit a specific community through the practice of clinical medicine. The article notes that this type of epidemiology is not currently taught and stresses the need for its development as well as that of sites where it can be practiced and taught.

Palti, H., Use of control groups in evaluating the effectiveness of community health programs in primary care. **Israel Journal of Medical Science**, 19(8):756, 1983. Discusses the problems of control groups in studies of primary care practices (small population size, randomization difficulties, "contamination" by communication among subjects). Describes designs that may be useful in COPC projects, including examples of experimental, quasi-experimental and matching studies, and designs using external comparison groups.

Doron, H., Planning community-oriented primary care in Israel. **Public Health Reports**, 99(5):450, 1984.

COMMUNITY PARTICIPATION

Perhaps what seems to be the most difficult component of COPC for health providers to grasp is that of community participation in the design and delivery of health services. The writings presented here will hopefully illustrate the range of benefits that derive from active community participation, as well as provide some practical insight into its development.

Salber, Eva J., **Caring and Curing:. Community Participation in Health Services**. Prodist, 1975. A clear, insightful book that approaches community participation from the side of those who participate. The book is a collection of interviews of people who participated in various aspects of a community health center, and allows the participants to share their own unique insights concerning their personal involvement in the health system and insight into their own lives and the lives of the people of the community.

Salber, E.J., Where does primary care begin? The health facilitator as a central figure in primary care. **Israel Journal of Medical Science**, 17(2-3):100, 1981. Proposes that all professionals, even primary care providers, are second-contact persons, and describes the use of lay providers in North Carolina to identify problems and facilitate services, in order to meet the unmet health needs that do not reach the health system. Also discusses the long-term hazards of short-term projects that do not provide for project continuation after the funding period.

Geiger, H.J., Community control—or community conflict? In **Neighborhood Health Centers**, Hollister, R.M., B.M. Kramer and S.S. Bellin, eds., p. 133. D.C. Heath, 1974. Addresses the conflict between professional and community goals and values in controlling and setting goals for health systems, using examples from the Columbia Point (Boston) and Tufts-Delta (Mississippi) Health Centers. Lessons: Priorities come from people in communities, not providers; changes are necessary in organizations to give people greater control over the provision of health services; conflict is usually inevitable in the change process and must be dealt with appropriately.

Hatch, J.W., and E. Eng, Community participation and control: or control of community participation. In **Reforming Medicine**, Victor W. and Ruth Sidel, eds., p. 223. Pantheon Books, 1984. A challenging essay in a challenging book that addresses the fundamental questions of community par-

ticipation: "For what reason?", "In what way?", and, "By whom?" Discusses the reasons for the successes and failures of projects developed under the Office of Economic Opportunity and Community Health Planning initiatives and points the way toward a broader definition of health that allows communities to solve the underlying causes of ill health.

Freire, P., **Pedagogy of the Oppressed**, Pelican Books, 1972. An important work on education for community development. The book explores the developing of "critical consciousness" for change through a process of education that empowers community members to act.

Pritchard, P.M.M., Community participation in primary health care. **British Medical Journal**, 3:585 (Sept. 6, 1975). Describes the formation of a community participation group in coordination with a group medical practice in the United Kingdom, and the meaningful input it was able to make in the operation and scope of services offered by the practice.

Appleton, Sherwood, **Challenge for Tomorrow:. Towards community care and caring. Total health and well being and enrichment of the quality of life; a proposal for a community mental health-initiated model "Human Support" project in the province of Prince Edward Island**. 1976. As evident in the title, this report describes an ambitious, holistic proposal for a community need-based health system with multiple in-puts from the community at multiple stages of its development and implementation.

Ragland, Sherman, and Harlan K. Zinn, eds., **Citizen Participation in Community Health Centers: An annotated bibliography and theoretical models**. National Institute of

Mental Health, DHEW Publication No. (ADM)79-737, 1979. "The purpose . . . is to provide CMHC board members, CMHC administrators and staff, public officials and interested citizens [e.g., providers] with a selected list of references that might help them to understand, develop, and modify the governing or advisory boards of CMHC's." Contains sections of the characterization of catchment areas, community development, coordination of service and community groups, the effects of citizen participation, and evaluation of participation efforts.

Sheerin, Ian, and Laurence Malcolm, **The Parklands/Queenspark Health Survey: An exercise in community participation**. Health Planning and Research Unit, Christchurch, New Zealand, 1978. Describes a community health needs assessment that used community participation in the development of the assessment and in the planning of services for a new regional health plan. Uncovered the need for prolonged, active participation rather than one-time, passive administration of a questionnaire.

MacCormack, C.P., Community participation in primary health care. **Tropical Doctor**, 13(2):51, 1983. Describes advantages of community participation in health in terms of cost-effectiveness, community self-action, increased commitment to use of community-planned services, and increased effectiveness of health education. Discusses the need for a commitment to the community on the part of the medical staff.

Seifert, M.H., The Patient Advisory Council concept, in Connor and Mullan, *op. cit.* 1983. Discusses the formation and functioning of a patient advisory council involved in a cooperative decisionmaking process for a pri-

vate, primary care medical practice as it relates to each of the aspects and phases of COPC development. Dr. Seifert's practice has been featured on national media and is a useful model of this approach.

Prins, Agma, Community participation in health action through structured problem solving - Lessons learned in the socio health program of the Togo Rural Water Project, **Public Health Reviews** 12, (3-4):322, 1984. Describes a "Socio-Health Program" that illustrates the concept of integrated community participation and health education as "a continuous learning process during which a community clarifies, acquires, and actively applies knowledge, skills, and organizational capacities to the resolution of its own problems."

Hopp, C. and H. Pridan, Community participation in a Community and Family based Primary Health Care program, **Public Health Reviews** 12(3-4):348, 1984. Discusses the problems of engendering community participation in communities that do not perceive themselves as disadvantaged, and describes self-motivation and initiation as needing to be fostered in such if community participation is to be successful.

UNDERSTANDING THE COMMUNITY, ITS CULTURE, AND ITS ORGANIZATION AND DEVELOPMENT

Adair, John, and Kurt Deuschle, **The People's Health: Anthropology and Medicine in a Navajo Community**. The engaging story of the interaction of Western medicine and traditional Navajo culture, coming together to form an effective health care delivery system through the collaboration of anthropology and medicine. Contrasts Navajo and physicians' views of health and disease, and how both can learn from each other. The essential nature of cultural understanding and community involvement is evident throughout. A delight to read in addition to its educational value.

Clark, Margaret, **Health in the Mexican American Culture** (Second edition). University of California Press, 1970. Through the barrio population of Sal Si Puedes in 1955, this book explores patterns of community family and religious life and the ways in which they affect access to and appropriateness of health services. Gives recommendations for improving the effectiveness of services and the quality of interaction between the community and health care providers.

Pearsall, Marion, **Medical Behavioral Science: A Selected Bibliography of Cultural Anthropology, Social Psychology, and Sociology in Medicine**. University of Kentucky Press, 1963.

Kleiman, Arthur, **Patients and Healers in Context of Culture**. Emphasizes the need and process of understanding the cultural context in which medical care is delivered.

Hatch, J. and E. Eng, Health worker roles in community oriented primary care. In: Connor and Mullan, *op. cit.*, p. 138, 1983. Points out the disparity between community priorities and values and those of providers, and that the usual community diagnostic tools may not be sufficient to "understand how a community operates and feels." Examples are given of the nature of beneficial, cooperative efforts in and with communities. They find the challenge of COPC is to translate between and link communities and professionals and to enable communities to take full advantage of the opportunities for change.

TRAINING AND EDUCATION FOR COPC

To realize the full potential of COPC, it is necessary to train health workers who have the necessary skills and attitudes to put the principles into practice. A variety of approaches have been or are being developed toward this purpose, centering around early and extended contact between students and communities. Examples are presented here.

Shonubi, Patricia A., and Jo Ivey Boufford, **Community Oriented Primary Care—Training for Urban Practice**. Praeger, 1986. (161 pp.) This new book presents a curriculum for an intensive 8-week summer program in COPC, developed for preclinical medical students in a practical format that greatly increases its adaptability for training programs elsewhere. The goals of the course were to expose students to health care issues in a participatory manner and to assist in their clarifying of career choices. Seminars are presented with tips on presentation, and suggested readings are given. The book also serves well as an introduction to COPC for practicing physicians who were so fortunate as to attend such a program.

Abramson, J.H., Training for community oriented primary care. **Israel Journal of Medical Science**, 19(8): 764, 1981. Stresses the inadequacy of current programs for training COPC practitioners, the need for more functioning COPC sites as training facilities, and the need for integrated training in health needs appraisal, organization of care, and evaluation.

Boufford, Jo Ivey, Medical education

and training for community-oriented primary care. In Connor and Mullan, *op. cit.*, p. 167, 1984.

Novick, L.F., C. Greene, and R.F. Vogt, Teaching medical students epidemiology: Utilizing a state health department. **Public Health Reports**, 100(4):401, 1985. A description of a course in epidemiology for medical students taught in conjunction with the Vermont Health Department, allowing exposure of students to a population perspective of health care.

Prywes, Moshe, The Beersheva Experience: Integration of medical care and medical education. **Israel Journal of Medical Science**, 19(8):775, 1983. A very interesting description of a comprehensive organized medical and health system that is organizationally integrated with the health training institutions, allowing a high level of focused primary care and appropriate training of health workers.

Kaufman, Arthur, ed., **Problem-Based Education: Lessons from Successful Interventions**. Springer, 1985. Analogous to a community problem-solving approach inherent in COPC, this book presents a discussion of a problem-based educational approach, using as examples a variety of programs both within the United States and internationally.

Kark, S.L., et al., Community medicine and primary health care: a field workshop on the use of epidemiology in practice. **International Journal of Epidemiology**, 2(4):419, 1973. A detailed description of a field study course for Master's degree candidates in public health that attempted to provide students with a working knowledge and skills for the epidemiologic evaluation of communities and health services in a variety of project activities.

Shah, U., Epidemiology training: a necessity for primary health care. **Jour-nal of Epidemiology and Community Health**, 39:194, 1985. Argues for all members of a health team to be trained in community epidemiology and for communities to provide locally determined input into district planning in India.

Kurtzman, C., and D. Block, Preparation of nurses for community orientation in primary health care in Israel, **Israel Journal of Medical Science**, 19(8): 768, 1983. Presents an experimental course for nurses in community assessment and planning of nursing interventions. Argues that community orientation should not be reserved for Master's level specialization but should be offered at all levels of nursing education.

The following is a list of examples of ongoing attempts to broaden the community orientation of medical education, selected from the proceedings of the Institute of Medicine's 1982 conference on COPC. (Connor and Mullan, eds., **COPC—New Directions for Health Services Delivery**.) Each is briefly discussed in the book.

Greep, J., Training for COPC in the Netherlands and around the world, p. 250.

Hansen, K.F., Can Area Health Education Centers promote COPC? The Colorado experience, p. 258.

Mettee, T.M., and J.H. Medalie, Departments of Family Practice as vehicles for promoting COPC, p. 264.

Obenshain, S.S., New Mexico's Primary Care Curriculum, p. 269.

Segall, A., C. Margolis, and M. Pryes, The Beersheva Experience, p. 276.

SELECTED EXAMPLES OF COPC PROJECTS

This section contains only a very limited sampling of the scope of projects that have been carried out. Other projects may be found in this volume and the two reports from the Institute of Medicine.

The following two articles deal with the development and evaluation aspects of a major COPC project. The project, the Community Hypertension, Atherosclerosis, and Diabetes Project (CHAD), carried out in Israel, was able to show a significant reduction in the prevalence of risk factors for cardiovascular diseases.

Hoop, C., A Community Program in Primary Care for Control of Cardiovascular Risk Factors: Steps in Program Development, **Israel Journal of Medical Science**, 19(8):748, 1983.

Abramson, J.H., et al., Evaluation of a Community Program for the Control of Cardiovascular Risk Factors, the CHAD Program in Jerusalem, **Israel Journal of Medical Science**, 17(2-3): 201, 1981.

Davies, A.M. and R. Fleishman, Health Status and use of Health Services as reported by older residents of Baka Neighborhood, Jerusalem, **Israel Journal of Medical Science**, 17(2-3):138, 1981. This study reports an interview of residents over 60 years of age, documenting a high degree of unmet needs that were only partially soluble by existing or possible health system services. Argues for improved community support.

Strasser, T., The uses of hypertension registers, in **Hypertension and Stroke in the Community**. WHO, Geneva, 1976.

Shorr, G.I., and P.A. Nutting, A population-based assessment of the continuity of ambulatory care. **Medical Care**, 15(6):455, 1977. Describes a method of measuring the continuity of patient care from community screening procedures through initial and followup examinations.

Smith, D., and P. Schnall, Hypertension surveillance system: An outcome approach, in **Assuring Quality Ambulatory Health Care: The Dr. Martin Luther King, Jr. Health Center**. Boulder, Westview Press, 1978.

Barnett, O., et al., A computer-based monitoring system for follow-up of elevated blood pressure. **Medical Care**, 21:400, 1983.

Morrell, D.C. and W.W. Holland, Epidemiology and Primary Health Care, **Israel Journal of Medical Science**, 17(2-3):92, 1981. Describes the fruitful cooperation between epidemiologists and primary care physicians at the St. Thomas Hospital Medical School, London. Reports on studies and subsequent interventions initiated by both groups, covering clinical and community projects.

The two publications of the Institute of Medicine also describe practices that have incorporated elements of COPC into their operation. Volume 2 of **Community Oriented Primary Care: A Practical Assessment** (1984) consists of detailed descriptions of seven sites that were studied to assess their use of the COPC model. The earlier conference proceedings, edited by Connor and Mullan (1983) also contain examples of functioning in a variety of settings, though in less detail.

EDUCATIONAL TOOLS—A SAMPLING

A broad range of sensitivities, attitudes, skills and knowledge are needed to realize the full potential of COPC. As the former are learned by effort and experience, this section deals only with the latter categories, and presents a brief sampling of the broad literature on epidemiology and community medicine that are very practical in their orientation and presentation.

Morris, J.N., **Uses of Epidemiology**, Churchill Livingstone, 1975 (3rd edition). A very excellent starting point for studying epidemiology "from the inside out." As described by the author, it is a "personal account" and thus contains much more than a review of techniques; it vividly presents a way of thinking. Sections on community diagnosis, health and services, risks to individuals and populations, and clinical epidemiology lead to the heart of the book—"In search of causes." In no sense presents epidemiology as the dry subject many were once taught that it was.

Kessler, I.J., and M.L. Levin, eds., **The Community as an Epidemiologic Laboratory: A Casebook of Community Studies**. Johns Hopkins Press, 1970. A selection of programs that illustrate the uses of epidemiology in defining community health needs in five categories: comprehensive studies of disease in total populations, epidemiologic surveys of specific diseases, social surveys, psychiatric surveys, and national health surveys. The primary focus of the book is epidemiologic methodology, and should be helpful to those designing or evaluating health surveys.

Rosner, E., **An Introduction to Biostatistics**, Duxbury Press, 1982. A basic text in biostatistics, clearly written, with examples from the medical literature and problems (with solutions) for self-teaching and evaluation.

Fowler, F.J., Jr., **Survey Research Methods**, Sage Publications, 1984. " . . . intended to provide perspective and understanding to those who would be designers or users of survey research, at the same time providing a sound first step for those who actually may go about collecting data." A well-organized text covering sampling, question-naire design, coping with nonresponse, and interviewing skills.

Abramson, J.H., **Survey Methods in Community Medicine**, Churchill Livingstone, 1979. (219 pp.) "The purpose of this book is to provide a simple and systematic guide to the planning and performance of investigations concerned with health and disease and with health care . . . an ABC to the design and conduct of studies." This is a thorough, step-by-step guide to carrying out a survey, from planning through sampling, data collection, and interpretation. Fairly methodological; may not be a "first book."

The following books are concise works on epidemiology and contain sections on community health appraisal, information systems, and prevention strategies:

Barker, D.J.P. and G. Rose, **Epidemiology in Medical Practice,** Churchill Livingstone, 1984.

Farmer, R.D.T., D.L. Miller, **Lecture Notes on Epidemiology and Community Medicine**, Blackwell, 1984.

Dever, G.E.A., **Epidemiology in Health Services Management**, Aspen Systems Corp., 1980. Chapters 10 and 11 deal with using epidemiologic assessment as a means for focusing on health problems using the planned interventions as a marketing tool.

CONCLUSION

Community-Oriented
Primary Care:
The Challenge

Paul A. Nutting, M.D.

Community-oriented primary care offers
an exciting variation for the delivery of
primary care services. It has the potential
to improve the quality of care and the
health status of a defined population. For
the practitioner so inclined, COPC offers
the rewards of expanding one's health care
activities beyond the confines of the examining room.

Two important features of COPC remain as unanswered questions. First, the
costs of transforming a primary care practice or program into a fully developed
COPC program are unknown. The practice of COPC involves activities not generally considered a requirement for the
practice of other forms of primary care.
These marginal costs are probably relatively modest, but their magnitude is
unknown. Clearly, the costs will vary
greatly as a function of the setting, the
number of problems addressed concurrently, and the rigor with which the activities are performed. In some settings, the
practice of COPC will increase the number of primary care services provided, thus
generating revenue in a fee-for-service
practice, but incurring additional costs in
prepaid programs.

Second, there are virtually no good data

on the marginal impact of COPC activities. The process of identifying and mounting an emphasis program to deal with a
community health problem is assumed to
have an impact on the health status of
the particular population that is greater
than that achieved by a traditional model
of primary care. The magnitude of that
margin of impact, however, is unknown.

The practitioner interested in moving
toward the COPC model can be heart-
ened by the knowledge that the move
need not be all-or-none. The COPC
model can be approached in simple and
reversible steps from which retreat is possible if the costs in time and effort are too
severe. For practitioners interested in
incorporating some of the principles of
COPC into their practice, the following
stepwise considerations are offered.

First, take an inventory of the resources
that can enhance the likelihood of success.
This can be done by seriously reflecting
on five questions:

How committed am I to trying COPC?
One's own personal commitment is critical
and should be judged objectively and without bias. Initiating a COPC practice
requires a great deal of time and personal
commitment and can be a lonely under-

taking. It probably is not appropriate to undertake the challenges of COPC during times of personal or professional stress. Similarly, those experiencing transition in their personal lives might do well to retain an interest in the principles of COPC, but temporarily postpone efforts to implement them.

Do I have professional colleagues equally committed? The commitment of the other professional staff is important. At least one other fellow traveler committed to the principles of COPC can make the journey through largely uncharted terrain less hazardous and less lonely. Importantly, the division of labor that allies within the practice or in other community programs will allow more time for family and personal growth.

Is the practice or program on reasonably stable ground, in terms of both financial and professional growth? The costs of initiating COPC activities are largely unknown, and cannot be assumed to generate additional income. The practice that is struggling financially or that is in a period of rapid transition in terms of personnel, physical facilities, or definition of goals may have a full agenda without taking on the challenges of COPC. On the other hand, practitioners who have established their practice and are looking for more excitement in their professional life may find that moving toward a COPC model is less expensive (and professionally more rewarding) than seeking new challenges in an expensive hobby.

Is there sufficient interest and commitment among the community or target population that I would address? Important allies in the COPC process, often not relied upon heavily enough in the early and difficult initial phases of COPC, are the patients and community participants. What constitutes the community and who the key participants are must be defined early in the process, and will vary greatly from one setting to the next. However the com-

munity to be addressed with the COPC process may be defined, the commitment of that community and its major participants can be an extremely important resource to recognize and incorporate at the time of the initial decision to implement COPC.

Do I have access to a reasonable amount of data on the community? Depending on how the target community is defined, there may or may not be a great deal of data available, a difference that can be critical in the early stages of defining and characterizing the community, and identifying its major health problems. For practices that plan to start with the active patient population, it is helpful (but certainly not necessary) to have an operational data system within the practice. For those planning to address a geographic community, a few hours spent with the epidemiologist at the local health department, will provide an important reconnaissance of the available data and a reasonable assessment of the effort required in the early COPC activities.

If the initial inventory of resources continues to engender interest in moving toward the COPC model, the following may prove to be useful suggestions.

First, define your community in a manageable way. Starting with the active patients of your practice or with the households of your active patients may be a more than adequate initial challenge. An expansion of the definition of the community will be relatively easy downstream.

Develop allies for the COPC effort, within your practice or program, within the community you plan to address, and wherever possible among other practices and/or community programs. Developing allies means gaining partners, and part of the price may involve modification in the initial goals and timetables that you have set for yourself. Remember, however, the practice of COPC is a long journey over rough and largely uncharted territory. Fellow travelers are important and well worth the inconvenience of altering the initial travel plan.

Don't rush—maintain modest and achievable expectations. Although difficult to appreciate at the beginning, many of the early successes will appear small, but will be viewed later as the most critical in the history of your efforts. Plan them carefully and accomplish them well. Subsequent progress (and success) will build on initial efforts and the stability of that foundation is critical.

Plan for initial success. Nothing reinforces commitment and generates new allies like an initial success. Taking on the most critical (and often the most vexing) health problem of the community at the outset is extremely risky. A good strategy is to direct initial efforts at a visible problem for which there is considerable enthusiasm, but particularly one for which success is achievable and will be apparent when achieved. Attempting to reduce cardiac mortality, for example, through a community-based blood pressure control program is a frequently selected COPC emphasis program. It also may be exactly the wrong problem for the *initial* effort. Success, even if achieved, will occur too far in the future and may be modest relative to the community's total cardiac mortality. Long before the data show that the initial efforts had an important impact, your allies will have moved on to other areas of their personal interest.

Finally, maintain a healthy perspective. You are among the first to discover and explore the territory of COPC. Those few that have gone before you are the pioneers—and you are one of the early settlers. There is not a great deal known of how to accomplish COPC in your setting. You will very rapidly become one of the experts. Document your experiences, for you are helping to develop the field. On your experience we will develop the future editions of this book. Let us hear from you.